Yasser El Miedany
Editor

Pediatric Musculoskeletal Ultrasonography

Springer

Editor
Yasser El Miedany
Medway Foundation Trust
King's College London
London
UK

ISBN 978-3-030-17823-9 ISBN 978-3-030-17824-6 (eBook)
https://doi.org/10.1007/978-3-030-17824-6

This Springer imprint is published by the registered company Springer Nature Switzerland AG
The registered company address is: Gewerbestrasse 11, 6330 Cham, Switzerland

Wherever the art of medicine is loved, there is also a love of humanity.

Hippocrates

Everyone has a soulmate who supports, encourages, and motivates them to achieve their ambitions in life. This book is dedicated to mine as well as all the special people in everyone's life.

Preface

The use of musculoskeletal ultrasonography in rheumatology clinical practice has expanded swiftly over the past decade as an outcome of the technological developments and implementation of the window of opportunity concept in most of the inflammatory musculoskeletal conditions. Ultrasound booked its place as the "rheumatologist's stethoscope" as it enabled the treating health-care professional to diagnose, prognosticate, and monitor disease activity as well as response to management. In contrast to other imaging modalities such as X-ray and magnetic resonance, ultrasound has clear advantages, namely, good tolerability, no radioactivity, ability to scan both joints and soft tissue at one sitting, and its dynamic facility, which enables direct correlation between clinical and imaging outcomes. In spite of some concerns regarding standardization, the use of ultrasound in rheumatology is expected to grow further as prices of the machine fall and the opportunity to practice improves.

In contrast with musculoskeletal ultrasonography in adults which has been thoroughly studied and become a well-established tool for patients' assessment both in research and clinical practice, musculoskeletal ultrasonography use in pediatrics is still limited. This is surprising, given the great potential and advantages of this technology for the assessment of the musculoskeletal system in children. Ultrasound is well-tolerated by children; therefore, it can be considered a typical first-line modality for a wide array of pediatric musculoskeletal imaging indications. Being readily accessible in both emergency and outpatient settings, ultrasound allows the health-care physician/sonographer to perform a dynamic assessment of the musculoskeletal system without using ionizing radiation or sedation. Unlike MRI, which requires the clinician to select a focal area of concern, ultrasound enables the evaluation of multiple joints or lesions in a single session and permits the operating person to rapidly compare abnormal structures to the contralateral side. Panoramic images also allow an expanded view and can be useful when assessing larger lesions. In addition, musculoskeletal ultrasonography started to book its place in patients' monitoring as it facilitates the ability to detect subclinical synovitis in children with JIA.

There are significant differences between joints of adults and children due to the age-related peculiarities of bone and joints in the immature skeleton, such as the presence of non-ossified cartilage and of a physiologically enhanced Doppler flow attributed to nutrient vessels. Therefore, this book was formatted to cover a whole range of musculoskeletal ultrasonography in pediatrics. In the first section, the fundamentals of pediatric musculoskeletal ultrasonography are discussed. Two chapters have been dedicated to sonoanatomy and differences between adults and children. Each approach to the relevant pediatric sonoanatomy is accompanied by clinical pearls to aid readers acquire as well as interpret ultrasound images of the area of interest with ease, provide guidance for successful intervention, and avoid pitfalls. This is followed by the second section which covers a whole range of anatomical sites, shoulder and arm, elbow and forearm, wrists and hands, hip and thigh, knee and leg, as well as ankle and feet. Scans for normal sonoanatomy as well as possible pathology are included. The third section discusses the use of ultrasonography in juvenile inflammatory arthritic conditions such as inflammatory arthritis and spondyloarthritis. In response to several of our colleagues' requests, we dedicated a specific section for musculoskeletal ultrasonography in standard practice, reporting US scans and US-guided interventional procedures in pediatrics. Section 5 discusses the use of US in children with sports injuries, whereas the last section summarizes advances in pediatric musculoskeletal ultrasonography.

The main theme of this book was to deliver a very practical and reader-friendly guide. On one hand, it describes a "how-to-do-it" approach, while, in the meantime, it delivers the evidence and advanced knowledge base of the relevant pathological sonographic appearances of the various musculoskeletal tissues. The illustrations and figures were meticulously selected to give the reader a clear guide toward implementation in real-life practice. Focusing on the major values of ultrasound in pediatric musculoskeletal conditions, this book with its 20 chapters is expected to fill an important void in the current literature. It represents what can be considered to be the best current thinking on the role of ultrasonography in the assessment of pathology, diagnosis, and treatment of different musculoskeletal pediatric diseases. Therefore, this work can serve as both excellent introductory and a very good reference resource for future reading.

This book has been the outcome of cooperative effort of a large international group of leaders in musculoskeletal ultrasonography. They have done a superb job in producing authoritative chapters including vast amounts of scientific and clinical data to create state-of-the-art descriptions of sonographic changes encompassed by different rheumatic diseases. Special thanks to Professor Angelo Ravelli who wrote the book's foreword and to everyone who helped me bring this book to light.

Personally, I feel privileged to have compiled this work and am enthusiastic about all that it offers to our readers. I hope you too will find this edition a uniquely valuable educational resource.

London, UK Yasser El Miedany

Foreword: A Beautiful and Well-Deserved Textbook of Pediatric Musculoskeletal Ultrasonography

In the past two decades, there has been important progress in the management of juvenile idiopathic arthritis, which includes the shift toward early aggressive interventions, the availability of newer and potent therapeutic agents, and the development of innovative treatment strategies. These advances have increased considerably the potential to achieve disease remission or, at least, minimal levels of disease activity and have consequently moved the therapeutic aims increasingly toward the attainment of an inactive disease status. In addition, they have made it important to identify patients with a high likelihood of developing erosive joint damage precociously, so as to institute appropriately aggressive therapy at an early stage of the disease. These issues have raised the need for sensitive methods that enable a precise definition and monitoring of the synovial inflammation process. Of the diagnostic tools currently available, ultrasonography is best suited for these purposes.

Ultrasonography has several advantages over other imaging modalities, including noninvasiveness, rapidity of performance, relatively low cost, ability to scan multiple joints in the same session, comparison between symptomatic and asymptomatic sites, dynamic study, repeatability, and high acceptability among children and parents. In addition, it does not involve exposure to ionizing radiations, does not require sedation, and is the only imaging technique that can be coupled with the conventional approach to patient assessment in the clinic. Recent studies in children with juvenile idiopathic arthritis have shown that ultrasonography may be more accurate than clinical evaluation for demonstrating joint inflammation and enthesitis, has the ability to detect subclinical synovitis, may improve patient categorization into the current classification schemes, and could alter the selection of patients who are candidates to receive synthetic or biologic disease-modifying antirheumatic drugs. Moreover, it was found to possess the potential to measure the integrity of articular cartilage and to capture early bone erosions. Owing to its capacity to precisely locate inflamed areas, ultrasonography can provide a guidance to corticosteroid injections into the joints, tendon sheaths, or other periarticular structures.

There are, however, several challenges with the use of ultrasonography. It is the most operator-dependent imaging technique, its validity is highly related to the properties of the machine used, and it has a limited value for the assessment of some musculoskeletal areas, such as the axial skeleton. Furthermore, it requires continuous practice after appropriate training. Specific problems encountered with its application in children are related to the unique features of the growing skeleton, which include age-related variations in the thickness of the articular cartilage and incomplete ossification. A thorough knowledge of the sonoanatomy changes at the different growth ages is, therefore, essential to distinguish physiological appearance from pathological findings. To overcome this shortcoming, the availability of normative data regarding the influence of different ages, stages of growth, and puberty is critical. In younger children with chronic arthritis, the difficulties are compounded by the development of distinctive abnormalities, such as disturbance of bone growth and maturation. It has also been argued that to consider any Doppler signal as a sign of synovitis might be problematic owing to physiologically enhanced blood flow. A number of initiatives aimed at improving the reliability and standardization of ultrasonography assessment in the pediatric age group are ongoing under the umbrella of the EULAR and the OMERACT.

In recent years, the clinical and research interest in musculoskeletal ultrasonography in children has grown sharply. There is, therefore, an urgent need of educational initiatives and teaching materials that help the practitioners who wish to apply this imaging modality to gain the necessary background and skills. This textbook edited by Yasser El Miedany meets fully these requirements and represents a major achievement in the field. It includes a series of chapters written by the leading international experts in pediatric musculoskeletal ultrasonography, which address all aspects related to the use of this technique in children and adolescents and provide the readers with all theoretical and practical information necessary to perform an appropriate assessment of their patients. The first section illustrates the fundamentals of musculoskeletal ultrasonography, from the most detailed technical aspects to the comparison of sonoanatomy between children and adults, to the spectrum of tissue pathology and clinical application. In the second section, the authors present a thorough description of the ultrasonographic findings in individual anatomic sites, including joints, vertebral spine of infants and neonates, and nerves. The features seen in inflamed joints and periarticular structures in patients with juvenile idiopathic arthritis and spondyloarthropathies are described in the third section. The last three sections are dedicated to the application of ultrasonography in standard clinical practice and in sport medicine and to an update on the recent advances in this area of imaging. All chapters are enriched with a vast and accurate iconography, which make more enjoyable the readings and offer valuable examples and references for comparison with ultrasonographic assessments actually performed in the clinics. In conclusion, I wish to congratulate Yasser El Miedany for accomplishing such an important, timely, and prestigious editorial engagement. I'm sure that this textbook will encounter a great success and will become a fundamental manual for all physicians and other health professionals who are interested in pediatric musculoskeletal ultrasonography and wish to embrace this imaging procedure in their clinical and research activities.

Angelo Ravelli
Università degli Studi di Genova
Genoa, Italy

Division of Rheumatology
IRCCS Istituto Giannina Gaslini
Genoa, Italy

EULAR Center of Excellence in Rheumatology 2018–2013
Zürich, Switzerland

Contents

Contributors

Domenico Barbuti Radiology Department, IRCCS Bambino Gesù Children's Hospital, Rome, Italy

Alessandra Bruns, MD, M.Sc Division of Rheumatology, Sherbrooke University, Sherbrooke, QC, Canada

MSK Ultrasound Courses, Sherbrooke University, Sherbrooke, QC, Canada

Pediatric Rheumatology & Musculoskeletal Ultrasound, McGill University, Montreal, QC, Canada

EULAR Working Group Anatomy for the Image, Zürich, Switzerland

OMERACT Ultrasound Pediatric Group, Zürich, Switzerland

Michael S. Cartwright, MD, MS Department of Neurology, Wake Forest School of Medicine, Winston-Salem, NC, USA

Anna Ciechomska University Hospital Wishaw, Wishaw, UK

Paz Collado Department of Rheumatology, Transitional Care Clinic, Hospital Universitario Severo Ochoa, Madrid, Spain

Jeimylo C. de Castro, MD, FPARM, RMSK, DABRM Physical Medicine and Rehabilitation Department, The Medical City-South Luzon, Santa Rosa, Laguna, Philippines

SMARTMD Center for Non-Surgical Pain Interventions, Makati City, Philippines

Yasser El Miedany Darent Valley Hospital, King's College London, Dartford, Kent, UK

Rheumatology and Rehabilitation, Ain Shams University, Cairo, Egypt

Mohamed Adel Eltomey, MD, EdiR Radiology & Imaging Department – Faculty of Medicine, Tanta University, Tanta, Egypt

C. Hernández-Díaz Musculoskeletal ultrasound Laboratory, Instituto Nacional de Rehabilitación "luis Guillermo Ibarra Ibarra", Mexico city, Mexico

Waleed A. Hassan Benha University, Banha, Egypt

Alka Karnik Nanavati Super Speciality Hospital, Mumbai, India

Adham Aboul Fotouh Khalil Egyptian School for Musculoskeletal Ultrasonography, Cairo, Egypt

Stefano Lanni, MD, PhD Reumatologia Pediatrica, Clinica de Marchi, IRCCS Ca' Granda Ospedale Maggiore Policlinico, Milan, Italy

Goumy Laurence Pediatric Department, CHU, Angers, France

Alice Leahy Paediatric Rheumatology, University Hospital Southampton, Southampton, UK

Tomasz Madej Children's University Hospital, Lublin, Poland

Silvia Magni-Manzoni Pediatric Rheumatology, IRCCS Bambino Gesù Children's Hospital, Rome, Italy

Clara Malattia, MD, PhD Clinica Pediatrica e Reumatologia, Istituto Giannina Gaslini, Genoa, Italy

Dipartimento di Neuroscienze, Riabilitazione, Oftalmologia, Genetica e Scienze Materno-Infantili, Università degli studi di Genova, Genoa, Italy

Carlo Martinoli Division of Radiology Ospedale Policlinico San Martino, Genoa, Italy

Department of Health Science, University of Genova, Genoa, Italy

Maribel Miguel-Pérez, MD, PhD Unit of Human Anatomy and Embryology, Department of Experimental Pathology and Therapeutic, Faculty of Medicine and Health Sciences (C.Bellvitge), University of Barcelona, Barcelona, Spain

Ingrid Möller, MD, PhD Unit of Human Anatomy and Embryology, Department of Experimental Pathology and Therapeutic, Faculty of Medicine and Health Sciences (C.Bellvitge), University of Barcelona, Barcelona, Spain

Instituto Poal de Reumatologia, Barcelona, Spain

Mohammed A. Mortada Zagazig University, Zagazig, Egypt

Esperanza Naredo Department of Rheumatology, Bone and Joint Research Unit, Hospital Universitario Fundación Jiménez Díaz, IIS-FJD, UAM, Madrid, Spain

Johannes Roth, MD, PhD, FRCPC, RhMSUS University of Ottawa, Ottawa, ON, Canada

Division of Pediatric Dermatology and Rheumatology, Children's Hospital of Eastern Ontario, Ottawa, ON, Canada

Jousse-Joulin Sandrine Rheumatology Department, Cavale Blanche Hospital and Brest Occidentale University, Brest, France

Eman A. Tawfik, MD Department of Physical Medicine and Rehabilitation, Faculty of Medicine, Ain-Shams University, Cairo, Egypt

Francis O. Walker, MD Department of Neurology, Wake Forest School of Medicine, Winston-Salem, NC, USA

Daniel Windschall, MD, PhD Pediatric Clinic, Asklepios Hospital Weissenfels, Weissenfels, Germany

University of Halle-Wittenberg, Halle, Germany

Federico Zaottini Division of Radiology Ospedale Policlinico San Martino, Genoa, Italy

Department of Health Science, University of Genova, Genoa, Italy

Part I

Fundamentals of Pediatric Musculoskeletal US

1 Musculoskeletal US in Pediatrics: Physics and Techniques

Silvia Magni-Manzoni and Domenico Barbuti

Introduction

Musculoskeletal ultrasound (MSUS) represents an imaging tool particularly suited in pediatrics due to several advantages over other imaging modalities [1]. In the past decades, the developments in transducer technology and advances in the quality and presentation of MSUS images particularly favored knowledge and new insights in the appearance of joints at different developmental ages [2-6]. The awareness on the underlying physics and the use of appropriate technique specific for the musculoskeletal assessment in children and adolescents are fundamental for the correct acquisition and interpretation on MSUS findings [7, 8]. The present chapter will present the basic physical concepts, techniques, and main pitfalls in the use of MSUS.

S. Magni-Manzoni (✉)
Pediatric Rheumatology, IRCCS Bambino Gesù Children's Hospital, Rome, Italy
e-mail: silvia.magnimanzoni@opbg.net

D. Barbuti
Radiology Department, IRCCS Bambino Gesù Children's Hospital, Rome, Italy
e-mail: domenico.barbuti@opbg.net

Ultrasound Waves and Their Properties

Ultrasound (US) imaging is based on mechanical (sound) waves with frequencies ranging from 1 to 20 MHz. The waves are created by an electric current applied to piezoelectric crystals located on the footprint of a transducer, which is used for emitting sound waves and for receiving reflected echoes.

As all mechanical waves, sound waves are characterized by a frequency (the number of a complete wave cycle per second, expressed in Hertz, Hz), a length (the distance, in meters, between two close peaks of compression or rarefaction), and an intensity (amplitude of the peaks, usually measured as watt/cm^2, Pascal or deciBel). The higher the frequency, the shorter the wave length.

The velocity of the sound waves depends on the density of the material they encounter along their pathway: the higher the density, the higher the sound waves velocity.

US waves in tissues are handled differently between different tissue layers. They can be partially absorbed, partially transmitted, and reflected on border of different tissues, depending on their density and, therefore, their acoustic impedance: tissue with high density need less energy to start undulating than tissue with little density. An impedance change arises when US waves cross borders between tissues of different acoustic impedance, creating different grades of reflection, absorption and deflection of the waves. This is the base for the generation of echoes (Fig. 1.1).

Y. El Miedany (ed.), *Pediatric Musculoskeletal Ultrasonography*,
https://doi.org/10.1007/978-3-030-17824-6_1

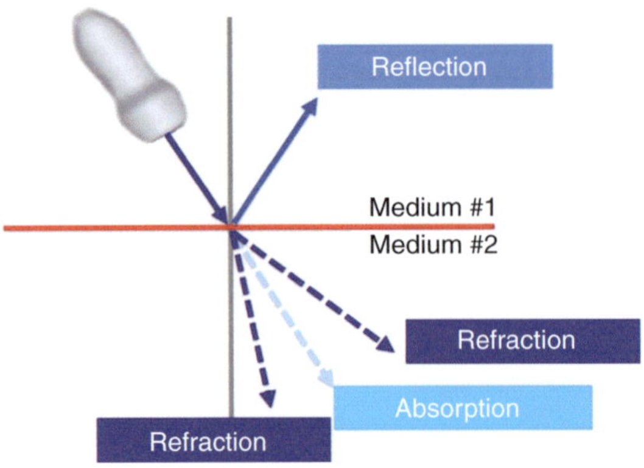

Fig. 1.1 Physical mechanisms which occur when an US wave crosses the border between medium with acoustic impedance #1 and medium with acoustic impedance #2

The US waves are gradually weakened when crossing media (absorption). The loss depends on tissue density and content and is proportional to the US frequency: the higher the frequency, the greater the loss and the lesser the penetration of the US wave.

Reflection is observed when the US waves meet the layer between tissues of different impedance; the degree of reflection depends on the surface structure (smooth versus rough, straight or bent) and on the angle between the US beam and the tissue surface. Finally, scattering of the US beam provokes deflection of the US waves, which can be responsible of artifacts [9].

Focus

In transducers, multiple crystals create multiple individual waves that run in a bundle which converges proportionally to the dimensions of the crystals in the proximal part (Fresnel's zone) and diverge in the distal part (Fraunhofer's zone); the focus represents the point of transition between the proximal and the distal zone and acts as a lens (Fig. 1.2).

In modern transducers, multiple lens, or focuses, can be used and need to be constantly optimized during the US assessment to create detailed images of the area/areas of interest, located at different depth from the surface (or the transducers' footprint) [10–12].

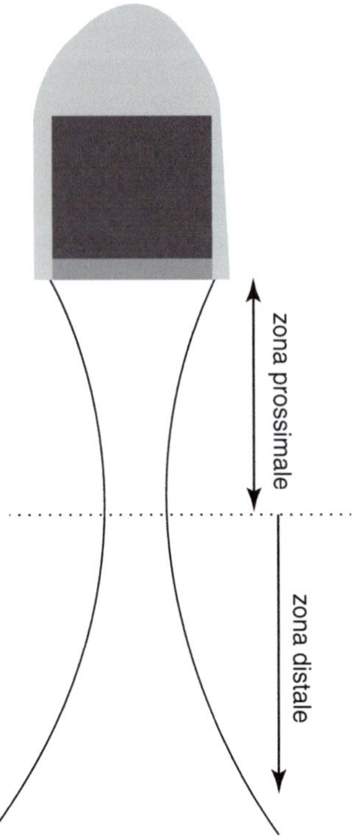

Fig. 1.2 Shape of the bundle of US waves, which converges in the proximal part and diverges in the distal part. The focus is the area of transition between the two parts, where the highest resolution is reached

Resolution

Resolution defines the minimal distance between two neighboring structures that can still be perceived separated. The lateral resolution represents the discrimination of objects side by side at same depth, and is mostly dependent on the beam width; the longitudinal and axial resolution is the discrimination of objects in direction of the US beam and are mostly dependent on the frequency. The higher the frequency, the smaller the depth and the better the resolution (Fig. 1.3).

US Equipment and Properties

US devices usually consist of transducers, which emit and receive US waves; cables to connect transducers to the system, made of hardware and

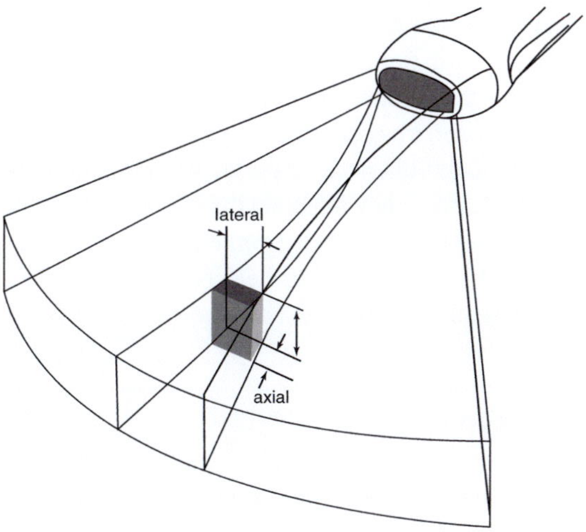

Fig. 1.3 Spatial resolution of the ultrasound beam

software, for the processing of the US signals; a display monitor; a keyboard; a storage system; and documentation facilities.

The transducers crystals are responsible of the US beam emission and represent the "sensitive" part of the transducers. A good contact of the transducer to the skin with enough US gel (or surrogate) to eliminate air is mandatory for optimal transmission of US waves into the tissue and acquisition of correct images. The waves are then partially absorbed; some US waves, particularly at the border of different tissues, are partially reflected. At this point, the crystals act as US wave receivers: reflected US waves create an electric signal within the crystals, with an amount of energy dependent on the energy of the reflected waves and amplified accordingly. More reflected waves will impact the crystals with more energy and will be represented as a brighter signal (more echogenic); moderate reflection will show poor echo; no reflection will not be detected and will appear as "echo-free" or anechoic.

The spatial location of the reflecting structure is defined by the time interval between the emission and the reception of the US waves: the deeper the structure, the longer the US beam needs to travel to it and back form it; the longer the US beam takes to travel, the deeper the position of the corresponding structure. The US image is composed by the representation on the display of the processing of US signals, which depends on their energy and time interval to and from the different structures encountered.

US Parameters

The *gain* defines the overall amplification of the incoming US signals (echoes) and depends on the output gain, the size of the subject, and the area under investigation.

Since reflected echoes from deeper structures have to pass through much more tissue than those from the superficial structures, they undergo much more absorption. To compensate the signal loss due to this effect, the signal can be proportionally amplified through the *time gain compensation* (TGC), which therefore should be constantly optimized during the US assessment. Of note, recent equipments may include automatic TGC.

The speed of the image update defines the *persistence*, or *frame rate*. Higher frame rates, with fast series of individual images, reduce the susceptibility to motion artifacts, but are usually coupled with a reduced resolution. More persistent image update allows the creation of a final displayed image through series of individual images, with increasing tissue density information and resolution, but at the cost of a slower displayed image.

The US signal can undergo a pre-processing, during the US assessment, with modulation of the signal quality and the sensitivity of crystals. Depending on the characteristics of the US manufacturer, there might be a post-processing, after the acquisition of the image, by modulating contrast, gray gain, etc., on frozen images.

Color and Power Doppler

A relevant aspect of MSUS examination is the possibility to detect synovial, tendinous, or muscular inflammatory hyperemia, which can be detected through color and/or power Doppler examination. It is worth to note that specific knowledge and experience are required when examining children by US, for not confusing physiological vascularization, within and around musculoskeletal structures, with pathological hyperemia.

The Doppler effect is a physical phenomenon in which the frequency of a wave that hits a moving body undergoes a variation that is directly related to the speed of the body itself. The Doppler technique compares the two frequencies and measures the difference between them. The obtained information can be represented as dot-by-dot color spots on the image elaborated in B-mode in an area defined in a box. Depending on the manufacturer, the size of the color/power Doppler box is predefined or can be decided by the operator. The box should always include the area of interest up to the skin surface. Since the main interest in rheumatologic diseases is in detecting low flows eventually present in synovial hypertrophy, Doppler parameters should be adjusted to assess low flows with low speed, applying low wall filters (WF) and pulse repetition frequency (PRF) between 700 Hz and 1 MHz. The gain should be progressively increased until random Doppler signal (also called "noise") appears in the color/power box, and then progressively decreased to reach a value just under the noise threshold. The flow inside the vessels appears as color spots that can be visualized in different scales, according to manufacturer features and the operator preferences. While the power Doppler scales generally show only the presence of blood flow, the color scales display also the direction from and toward the transducer [13, 14].

Transducers

Transducers' features [15] are of most importance for the investigation of small and relatively superficial sites, such as the musculoskeletal structures in pediatrics.

Modern transducers usually use a range of frequencies (multifrequency probes) and, therefore, allow the study of both superficial and deep structures in children at the same time, combining good penetration and resolution. The most recent generation of ultrasound equipment, with frequencies up to 20 MHz, allows highly detailed depiction of submillimetric structures located just a few millimeters from the probe footprint. For investigating deeper musculoskeletal structures, a good option is the use of a multifrequency probe at about 6–13 MHz.

Currently, linear-array transducers at variable sizes are available for musculoskeletal examinations, including large (>40 mm), medium-sized (<40 mm), and small-field-of-view (hockey-stick-shaped) probes. The selection of the most appropriate transducer primarily relies on the frequency to be used for the examination of a specific musculoskeletal area or structure. In case of small superficial structure with possibility of little contact to the skin, hockey-stick probes are particularly suited; on the contrary, for imaging deeper structures, high-frequency large-diameter transducers have the best potential, since they maintain the US beam shape to greater depths with less divergence, whereas they tend to have a large near-field beam width and a poor lateral resolution at shallow depths.

Handling

During evaluation of the musculoskeletal system, the probe should be handled with maximum stability over the region of interest, avoiding compression as much as possible. The stability of the transducer can be obtained by placing the long, ring, and little fingers of the examining hand directly on the patient's skin or on a stable surface while holding the probe with the thumb and the index finger. With this grip, the examiners can easily translate the probe along its short axis at a given angle minimizing rotational changes [16].

Probe Positioning

The patient must be positioned in a proper way to make the examination comfortable both for the patient and the operator, regardless of the examined anatomical region [17, 18]. The angle of the ultrasound beam must be perfectly perpendicular to the examined structure, for avoiding artifacts and granting the acquisition of a correct image. It is recommended to perform longitudinal and transverse scans, and sometimes also oblique and unconventional scans, for a detailed assessment of the musculoskeletal structures. Recommended standard probe positioning for specific musculoskeletal sites are presented in the corresponding chapters.

US Software

In the recent years, different softwares improved the visualization of US images. They have different characteristics depending on the manufacturer, and their potential values still need to be extensively explored in children.

In compounding mode, the digital beam former steers the US beam at several steering angles during real-time acquisition rates [10], therefore reducing image artifacts (e.g., speckle, clutter, noise, angle-generated artifacts) and showing a sharper delineation of tissue interfaces and better discrimination of lesions over the background, especially in structures composed of specular echoes, such as tendons and muscles [9]. The beam *steering function* has been applied to B-mode imaging to obtain a parallelogram format with lateral sides parallel but oblique instead of a rectangular field of view. Oblique lines-of-sight run along the depth axis and can better display anisotropic structures, such as tendons or ligaments, in their oblique course from surface to depth.

Even when examining the relatively small musculoskeletal structures in children, it may be useful the widening of the field of view, which is often limited to 4 cm or less, due to the size of the best-suited transducers. The *extended field-of-view technology* uses specific image registration analysis to track probe motion and reconstruct a large composite image during real-time scanning over long distances and curved body surfaces. For instance, it allows to show large fluid collections and overview of the examined area.

In the recent years, the *3D technology* has been applied to US [10, 19, 20]. Dedicated 3D-volume transducers sweep the US beam throughout the tissue volume by tilting the scanhead with a mechanized drive along the z-axis; after volume scan acquisition, the monitor displays reconstructed slices according to longitudinal, transverse, and coronal planes, which can be oriented within the volume block for detailed analysis by shifting around any of the spatial axes. This technology might be useful in a better understanding of physiological findings and vascularization in children's joint; however, 3D probes are usually larger and more difficult to handle than standard probes, and experiences in this regard in children's joints are scarce.

An additional innovative technique is the *elastosonography*, first used by Krouskop et al. in 1987, which allows to obtain information on the hardness and elasticity of soft tissues, particularly useful in the case of nodules or muscular lesions. It represents a sort of electronic palpation and is based on a simple principle: the compression of the tissue examined with the ultrasound probe produces a distortion, less in hard tissues and greater in soft tissues, which can be detected and quantified through a reprocessing of data obtained by US. The software displays an elastographic image in which the framed lesion is colored depending on its hardness, according to a chromatic scale usually ranging from red/green, in structures with greater deformability (i.e., soft nodules), to blue, in those with minimal or no distortion (i.e., hard and inelastic nodules). This technique, initially mainly used in diffuse hepatic changes and in thyroid nodules, proved to be very useful in the study of suspected tendons', muscles', and synovium alterations and of soft tissues in general [21].

Artifacts

Ultrasonographers should be aware of several artifacts that can occur and may be useful in the interpretation of findings, or, on the contrary, contribute to misinterpretation. Artifacts can be due to physical phenomena or to faulty scanning technique.

In fact, while some artifacts reduce the diagnostic power of the scan (reverberation, mirror effect, partial volume, doubling, empty tendon artifact), some others can be extremely helpful in the differential diagnosis (posterior acoustic enhancement, acoustic shadowing, comet tail, ring down and rain artifacts) [14, 22, 23]. Some artifacts can be avoided if the scan is performed in a proper way and the US equipment is properly set; others are caused by physical characteristics that cannot be changed. Nonetheless, they must be understood in order to avoid diagnostic mistakes.

Here is presented a list of US artifacts with their main features.

Posterior acoustic enhancement: an increase in echo intensity in tissues posterior to a fluid collection. It may not be detected when the fluid collection is small or spread over a large area (Fig. 1.4).

Acoustic shadowing: a weakening or absence of echoes posterior to a gas collection (high absorption of the beam), a bone surface (high reduction of the beam) or calcification. Lateral acoustic shadowing: it occurs when the ultrasound beam is tangential to tissues with different acoustic impedance. The wider the impedance

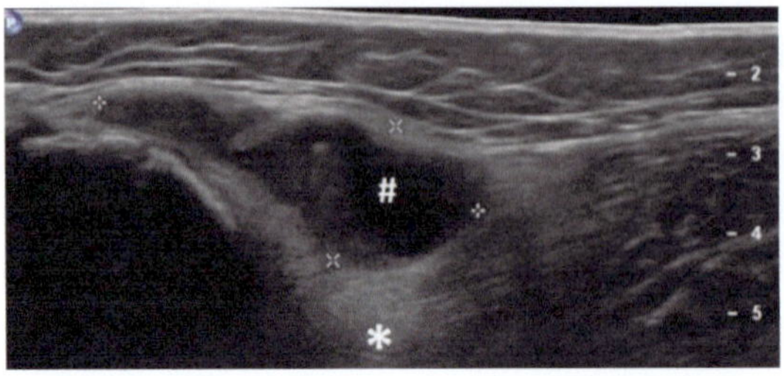

Fig. 1.4 Posterior acoustic enhancement is marked by *, deep to the fluid collection, marked by #, in a proliferative and essudative bursitis in a 10-year-old girl with juvenile idiopathic arthritis

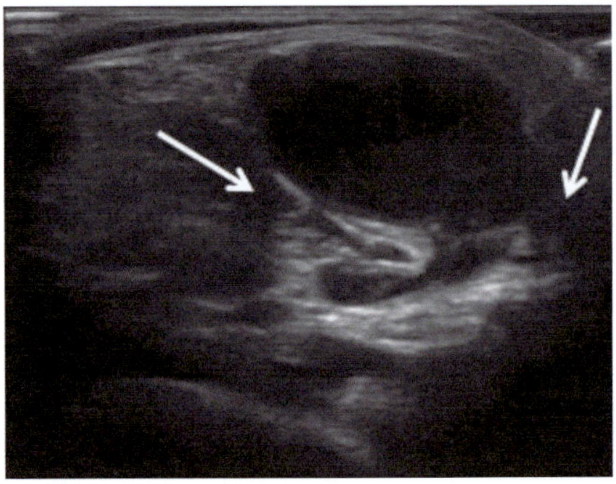

Fig. 1.5 Lateral acoustic shadowing aside a Baker's cyst (arrows) in a 5-year-old boy

difference, the more visible is the artifact (Fig. 1.5).

Rain effect: a reverberation artifact due to the gain curve. This is an important sign because it occurs when soft tissue overlies a fluid collection. It appears as a band of low-to-medium echoes lying parallel to the transducer and apparently arising from the soft tissue and moving down through the fluid.

Reverberation artifact: due to its appearance, this artifact is also referred to as "ring-down artifact" and "comet tail artifact." It is caused by the reflection of the ultrasound beam several times back and forth between two nearby interfaces. The multiple echoes thus created reach the transducer before the next pulse transmission and produce multiple copies of the anatomy.

Reverberation artifacts are commonly seen at soft tissue-to-gas/bone/metal interfaces.

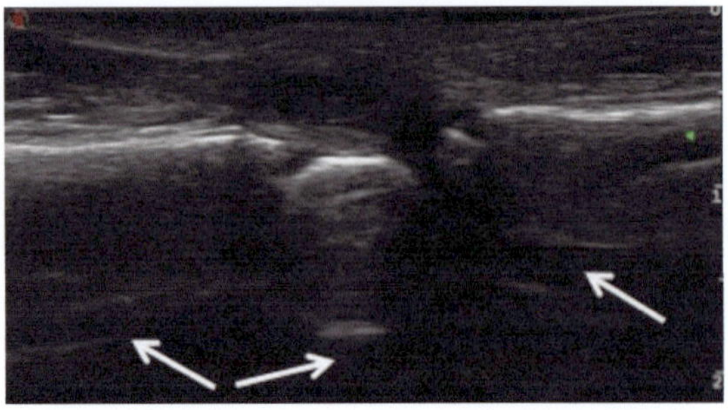

Fig. 1.6 Mirror artifact with specular reverberation of the metacarpal head, the distal diaphysis of the metacarpal and of the proximal part of the proximal phalanx of the III digit in a 9-year-old boy

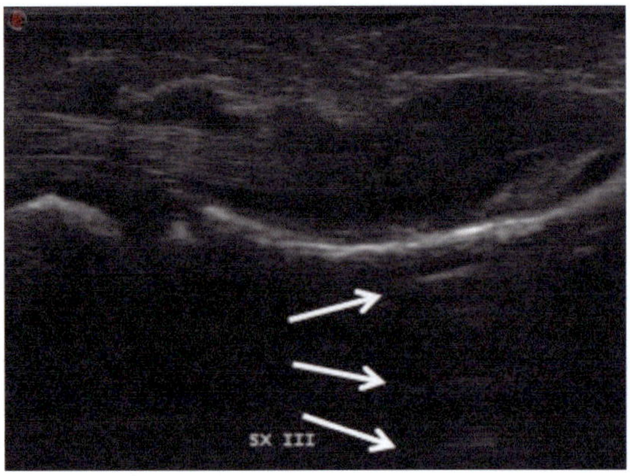

Fig. 1.7 Duplication and triplication (arrows) of the bone profile of the III right proximal phalanx in a 9-year-old boy with tenosynovitis of the flexor digiti propri tendon

Mirror artifact: a duplication of the image occurring when the beam meets a highly reflective interface causing reflection and reverberation phenomena (Fig. 1.6).

Partial volume artifact: a noise that occurs when the US beam is wider than the scanned structure or the structure itself is just partially sectioned so that it is surrounded by tissues with different acoustic impedance. For example, if the beam sections a fluid collection that is narrower than the beam itself, a partial volume artifact will occur.

Duplication and triplication: occurs when the US beam crosses two tissues with different acoustic impedance. It appears as a duplication or a triplication of the image when the structure measures less than one centimeter and as a deformation, enlargement, or interruption when the object is larger (Fig. 1.7).

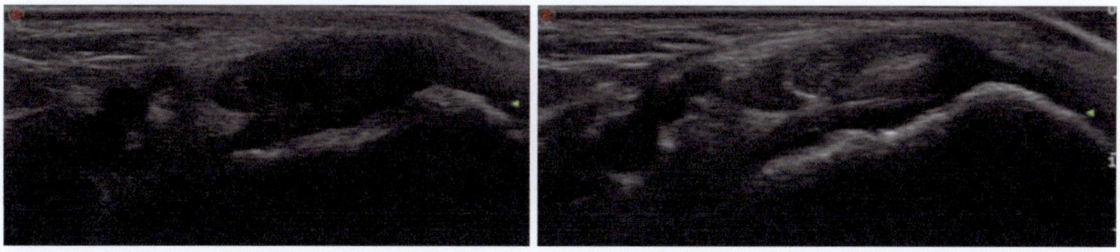

Fig. 1.8 Empty tendon artifact

Empty tendon artifact: occurs when the ultrasound beam is not perpendicular to the tendon, on both longitudinal and axial scans. The tendon appears, homogeneously or in some parts, hypoechoic without the normal fibrillar echotexture or totally anechoic (anisotropy), because of the relative obliqueness of the US beam to the fibrillar texture. The peculiar fibrillar pattern can be easily documented by slightly tilting the US beam perpendicular to the tendon course (Fig. 1.8).

References

1. Magni-Manzoni S. Ultrasound in juvenile idiopathic arthritis. Pediatr Rheumatol Online J. 2016;14:33.
2. Barbuti D, Bergami G, Vecchioli Scaldazza A. Role of ultrasonography of the knee in the follow-up of juvenile rheumatoid arthritis. Radiol Med. 1997;93:27–32.
3. Spannow AH, Pfeiffer-Jensen M, Andersen NT, Herlin T, Stenbøg E. Ultrasonographic measurements of joint cartilage thickness in healthy children: age- and sex-related standard reference values. J Rheumatol. 2010;37:2595–601.
4. Collado P, Naredo E, Calvo C, Crespo M. Assessment of the joint recesses and tendon sheaths in healthy children by high resolution B-mode and power Doppler sonography. Clin Exp Rheumatol. 2007;25:915–21.
5. Roth J, Jousse-Joulin S, Magni-Manzoni S, et al.; Outcome Measures in Rheumatology Ultrasound Group. Definitions for the sonographic features of joints in healthy children. Arthritis Care Res (Hoboken). 2015;67:136–42.
6. Windschall D, Collado P, Vojinovic J, et al.; OMERACT Paediatric Ultrasound Subtask Force. Age-related vascularization and ossification of joints in children: an international pilot study to test multi-observer ultrasound reliability. Arthritis Care Res (Hoboken). 2017. https://doi.org/10.1002/acr.23335.
7. Collado P, Vojinovic J, Nieto JC, et al.; Omeract Ultrasound Pediatric Group. Toward standardized musculoskeletal ultrasound in pediatric rheumatology: normal age-related ultrasound findings. Arthritis Care Res (Hoboken). 2016;68:348–56.
8. Magni-Manzoni S. Ultrasound measurement of cartilage thickness in childhood arthritis – target the tissue, tailor the technique. J Rheumatol. 2015;42(3):360–2.
9. Lin CD, Nazarian LN, O'Kane PL, et al. Advantages of real-time spatial compound sonography of the musculoskeletal system versus conventional sonography. AJR Am J Roentgenol. 2002;171: 1629–31.
10. Claudon M, Tranquart F, Evans DH, et al. Advances in ultrasound. Eur Radiol. 2002;12:7–18.
11. Whittingham TA. An overview of digital technology in ultrasonic imaging. Eur Radiol. 1999;9: 307–11.
12. Rizzatto G. Evolution of ultrasound transducers: 1.5 and 2D arrays. Eur Radiol. 1999;9(Suppl 3):S304–6.
13. Kremkau FW. Doppler color imaging. Principles and instrumentation. Clin Diagn Ultrasound. 1992;27:7–60.
14. Torp-Pedersen ST, Terslev L. Settings and artifacts in colour/power Doppler ultrasound in rheumatology. Ann Rheum Dis. 2008;67:143–9.
15. Whittingham TA. Broadband transducers. Eur Radiol. 1999;9:298–303.
16. Derci LE, Rizzatto G. Technical requirements. In: Bianchi S, Martinoli C, editors. Ultrasound of the musculoskeletal system. Berlin: Springer; 2007. p. 1–16.
17. Van Holsbeeck MT, Introcaso JH. Musculoskeletal ultrasound. 2nd ed. St. Louis: Mosby; 2001.
18. Teefey SA, Middleton WD, Yamaguchi K. Shoulder sonography: state of the art. Radiol Clin N Am. 1999;37:767–85.
19. Brandl H, Gritzky A, Haizinger M. 3D ultrasound: a dedicated system. Eur Radiol. 1999;9:331–3.
20. Wallny TA, Theuerkauf I, Schild RL, Perlick L, Bertelsbeck DS. The three-dimensional ultrasound evaluation of the rotator cuff: an experimental study. Eur J Ultrasound. 2000;11:135–41.
21. Lalitha P, Balaji Reddy MC, Jagannath Reddy K. Musculoskeletal applications of elastography: a pictorial essay of our initial experience. Korean J Radiol. 2011;12:365–75.
22. Rumack CM, Wilson SR, Charboneau JW, Johnson J. Diagnostic ultrasound. 3rd ed. St. Louis: Mosby; 2004.
23. Serafin-Król M, Artur Maliborski A. Diagnostic errors in musculoskeletal ultrasound imaging and how to avoid them. J Ultrason. 2017;17:188–96.

Standardized Musculoskeletal Ultrasound in Pediatric Rheumatology: (normal Age-Related Ultrasound Findings)

2

Paz Collado and Esperanza Naredo

Abbreviations

JIA	Juvenile idiopathic arthritis
MCP II	Second metacarpophalangeal joint
MSUS	Musculoskeletal ultrasound
OMERACT	Outcome Measures in Rheumatology

Introduction

Imaging is among the most rapidly evolving fields within medicine. In the last 30 years, clinical practice has been transformed by the rapid expansion of sophisticated new technologies in that field offering a large range of instruments for better identifying and monitoring rheumatic diseases.

Among the various imaging modalities, musculoskeletal ultrasonography (MSUS) has been shown to be a readily available, reliable, and friendly tool for the assessment of inflammatory disease activity, particularly in children [1–11]. MSUS has demonstrated a higher sensitivity for detecting synovitis and tenosynovitis as compared to clinical examination in children [3–5]. One of the main problems is the lack of standardised procedures for validating this imaging modality before its widespread application. An additional problem is related to the unique anatomy of the growing skeleton in the child that is different from adult. Thus, the simple use of standards established for adults should be taken with caution.

The Outcome Measures in Rheumatology (OMERACT) Ultrasound Task Force is an international collaborative group of experts aiming to investigate the applicability of MSUS in rheumatology and to develop its metric properties for clinical trials. Among the different aspects of MSUS validation, the paediatric field has been considered as one of the main areas. With the aim of improving the validity of MSUS for the diagnosis and management of synovitis in juvenile idiopathic arthritis (JIA), a new subtask force was created. This task force has developed a stepwise process: first, the development and validation, using the Delphi process, of definitions for US findings in healthy children and patients with JIA, and, second, creating a consensus agreement on a precise scanning method in different age groups, with the collection of images showing the sonographic appearance of physiologic vascularisation in several joints [12–16].

P. Collado (✉)
Department of Rheumatology, Transitional Care Clinic, Hospital Universitario Severo Ochoa, Madrid, Spain

E. Naredo
Department of Rheumatology, Bone and Joint Research Unit, Hospital Universitario Fundación Jiménez Díaz, IIS-FJD, UAM, Madrid, Spain
e-mail: enaredo@ser.es

Y. El Miedany (ed.), *Pediatric Musculoskeletal Ultrasonography*,
https://doi.org/10.1007/978-3-030-17824-6_2

Here we describe briefly the main joint components in the healthy child as well as a systematic examination method (i.e. patient position, transducer placement, and joint positioning) for joint in children that can be easily reproducible among different sonographers and US machines.

Joint Components

MSUS examinations in paediatric rheumatology tend to focus mainly on peripheral skeleton, particularly synovial joints. Synovial joints are composed of several tissues, such as the articular bone surface, joint capsule, synovial membrane, and hyaline cartilage. Nevertheless, children differ significantly from adults in their bony anatomy as seen on US image; depending on the age and stage of maturity, their bones will not be completely ossified yet. At birth, the primary ossification centre is present in most of the long bone (diaphysis); meanwhile it is not present in most of the short bones. Throughout the first years, the secondary ossification centres will become apparent in the epiphyseal ends of the long bones [15, 17]. Because children with JIA may have abnormal US findings associated with inflammation and hyperaemia of affected joints, the knowledge of age-related US characteristics of healthy joints of children is essential to avoid misinterpretation.

Definitions for the US appearance of joints in healthy children were successfully developed through a consensus process and validated in practical exercises in two studies carried out by the OMERACT US group [12, 14]. The definitions are shown in Table 2.1.

Table 2.1 The definitions of the components of the paediatric joint detected on B-mode and Doppler US image in healthy children

N.	Component	US definition
1	Hyaline cartilage	A well-defined anechoic structure (with/without bright echos/dots) that is non-compressible. The cartilage surface can be detected as (but does not have to) hyperechoic line
2	Epiphyseal secondary ossification centre	A hyperechoic structure, with irregular or smooth surface within the cartilage – with advancing maturity
3	Joint capsule	A hyperechoic structure, which can (but does not have to) be seen over the bone, cartilage and other intraarticular tissues of joints
4	Normal synovial membrane	Under normal circumstances the thin synovial membrane is undetectable
5	The ossified portion of articular bone	A hyperechoic line. Interruptions in this hyperechoic line might be detected at the growth plate and at the junction of two or more ossification centres
6	Physiological vascularity	Doppler signal(s) in the joint structures: the fat pads and unossified joint structures (i.e. the physis, the hyaline cartilage of epiphysis and the short bones cartilage) at any age during growth
7	Physis	An anechoic unossified structure, intra- or extra-articular according to its anatomical location
8	Fat pad	An intraarticular structure with heterogeneous echotexture (similar to the subcutaneous tissue) which might show vascularity

Given the unique anatomy of the growing skeleton, it was not surprising that the development of those definitions, particularly, those related to the presence of joint Doppler signal, was more difficult to achieve. Since periarticular Doppler signal or that within joints may be a source of uncertainty or misinterpretation for inexperienced sonographers in paediatric MSUS, it seems mandatory to include the definition of physiological vascularity as one more component of the paediatric joint. The interpretation of the Doppler signal in the paediatric joint was the most challenging issues for the investigator group. As a result of the complexity of defining physiological vascularity, several separate statements for Doppler-detected normal joint vascularisation were provided instead of a full definition (Table 2.2).

Despite the fact that ossification is not a structural component of joint, ossification process in the child was an aspect to be taken into account during the development of those definitions. Ossification is an age- and joint-dependent process. A detailed knowledge about sonographic changes in the appearance of physeal and epiphyseal cartilages through the childhood is essential [17, 18]. Moreover, bone landmarks are impor-

Table 2.2 Final statements regarding final definition of physiological vascularity

N.	Definition statement
1	Physiological vascularity can be detected by PD as Doppler signal in the joint structures at any age during growth
2	Physiological intraarticular vascularity can be detected in children within the fat pads and unossified joint structures (i.e. the physis, the cartilage of epiphysis and the short bones cartilage)
3	Detection of physiological vascularity and its intraarticular anatomical position is joint and age (particularly in the youngest children) dependent
4	Ossification grade is age and joint dependent. Ossification centres can be detected with different maturation state due to the skeletal development

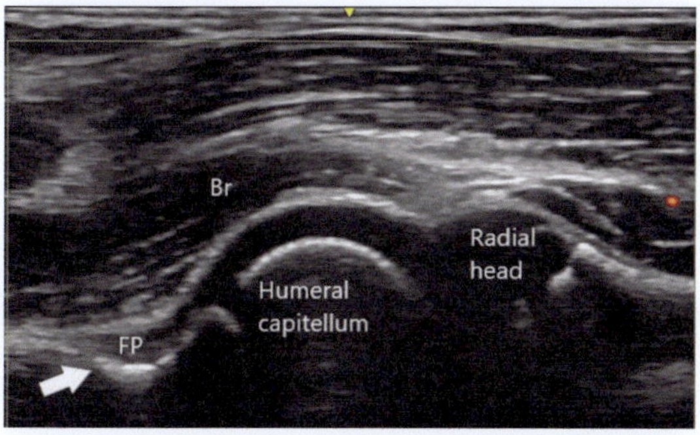

Fig. 2.1 Elbow. Anterior joint recess. Br, brachialis muscle; arrow, anterior coronoid recess; FP, anterior fat pad

tant for proper image acquisition in children even though those are detected as unossified hyaline cartilage (Fig. 2.1).

Standardisation of MSUS

General Comments

High-resolution US equipment is essential for paediatric MSUS work-up. The choice of the transducer depends on the type of examination. Higher-frequency transducers provide better spatial resolution, but these transducers have less penetration depth than a lower-frequency transducer. In children, high-frequency (7.5–18 MHz) linear transducers are generally appropriate for superficial and deeper joints. However, in obese patients, lower-frequency transducer may help the examination. The size of the footprint (the surface area of the transducer in contact with the skin) is also an important factor in the examination technique for paediatric patients. The hockey stick transducer (the smaller footprint) allows better angulations in small joints, particularly in the youngest children, reducing risk of artefacts.

The practical use of colour Doppler/power Doppler is the detection of increased joint and soft tissue perfusion, reflecting usually vascular abnormalities and active inflammation. However, Doppler signals should be carefully considered due to the presence of feeding vessels in growing skeleton as physiological vascularity [14, 15].

Last but not least, image documentation is another important aspect of MSUS. In general, every examination should be carefully documented, particularly descriptions regarding the age-related variations in the growing skeleton. All displayed structures should be documented in a standardised fashion to ensure an optimal reproducibility of these results. The orientation of the transducer in the standardised MS examination must be taken into account when documenting the reports with images. In longitudinal scan, the proximal part of the examined joint should be located on the left side of the screen, whereas the distal part of the joint should be located on the right side of the screen. In transverse scan, the medial/ulnar/tibial structures are usually shown on the left side of the screen, whereas the lateral/radial/fibular structures are shown on the right side of the screen.

US Examination Technique

Over the last years, a huge number of studies focused on paediatric MS conditions have been published, which have described patient positioning and US examination technique used in those studies. To overcome a strong operator dependence and the lack of standardised scanning protocols, the OMERACT US Task Force has recently published a systematic method for US examination of the four most commonly involved joints in JIA, i.e. wrist, second metacarpophalangeal joint (MCP II), knee and ankle joint. Additionally, one reference book published by the authors of this chapter provides information regarding patient positioning and transducer placement, as well as the sonographic appearance of each joint in different age groups [19].

The authors of this chapter have attempted to include the screening protocols considered essential for detecting joint synovitis in the paediatric population, in particular, patients with JIA, based on the clinical findings of JIA and the most common MSUS descriptions published in the literature (Table 2.3).

Table 2.3 Description of standard scans for evaluating the paediatric joint recesses

Joint	Scan approach
Shoulder	[a]*Posterior glenohumeral joint recess* The child is sitting on the parent's lap with the child's hand on their opposite shoulder held by parent (Fig. 2.2) Transducer placed over the posterior aspect of the glenohumeral joint below the outer edge of the spine of the scapula The transverse scanning plane should provide the following anatomic landmarks: 1. Infraspinatus tendon (superficial) 2. The humeral head, posterior labrum and the bony glenoid (deeper)
Elbow	*Anterior joint recess* With the forearm supinated and palm facing upwards, the elbow should be positioned in an extension position over the stretcher or the table Transducer placed over the anterior aspect of the radiocapitellar joint The longitudinal scanning plane should provide the following anatomic landmarks: 1. Coronoid fossa and the humeral capitellum (proximal) 2. Radial head (distal) *Posterior joint recess* With the child lying supine on the stretcher with the child's hand on their opposite shoulder held by parent (Fig. 2.3) Transducer placed cranial to the olecranon, over the triceps tendon and muscle The longitudinal scanning plane should provide the following anatomic landmarks: 1. Triceps tendon and muscle (superficial) 2. The olecranon fossa and the posterior olecranon recess (deeper)
Wrist	*Lateral/midline/medial dorsal*[b] *joint recess* With the palm facing downwards, the wrist should be positioned flat in neutral position Transducer longitudinally placed at the sagittal midline of the wrist with the cranial edge of transducer positioning just distal to the radial diaphysis The longitudinal scanning plane should provide the following anatomic landmarks: 1. Distal end of diaphysis and epiphyseal cartilage of radius (proximal) 2. Dorsal recess of the radiocarpal and midcarpal joints and over them 3. A compartment of the extensor tendons according to the area imaged (i.e. the extensor pollicis longus tendon in lateral [radial] aspect, the extensor digitorum tendon in midline aspect and the extensor carpi ulnaris tendon in medial [ulnar] aspect)
MCP	*Dorsal/lateral*[c]*/volar joint recesses* With the palm facing downwards, laterally, or upwards, the finger should be positioned flat in neutral position Transducer longitudinally placed at the sagittal midline of finger just at the MCP joint (dorsal/lateral/ volar) The longitudinal scanning plane (performed for each approach) should provide the following anatomic landmarks: 1. Head of metacarpal bone (proximal) 2. Base of proximal phalanx (distal)
IFP	*Dorsal/lateral/volar recesses* With the palm facing downwards, laterally, or upwards, the finger should be positioned flat in neutral position Transducer longitudinally placed at the sagittal midline of finger just at the IF joint (dorsal/lateral/volar) The longitudinal scanning plane (performed for each approach) should provide the following anatomic landmarks: 1. Head of proximal phalanx (proximal) 2. Base of medial phalanx (distal)
Hip	*Anterior joint recess* With the child lying supine Transducer in an oblique longitudinal plane over the femoral neck The oblique longitudinal scanning plane should provide the following anatomic landmark: 1. Femoral head 2. Concave bony surface on the femoral neck

Table 2.3 (continued)

Joint	Scan approach
Knee	*Anterior suprapatellar recess* The knees should be flexed around 30° on the examination bed Transducer placed at the sagittal midline of the leg with the caudal edge of transducer positioning just cranial to the superior edge of the patella The longitudinal scanning plane should provide the following anatomic landmarks: 1. Superior edge of patella 2. Distal portion of the femur *Lateral parapatellar recess* The knee should be straightened with the patella lying in a central position over the femoral condyles Transducer placed at the sagittal midline of the leg on the patella and then rotated 90° for transverse scanning The transverse scanning plane should provide the following anatomic landmarks: 1. Superior edge of the patella 2. Femoral condyle *Posterior recess* The post aspect of the knee is examined with the patient prone with knee full-extension to identify the presence of semimembranosus-gastrocnemius bursa in communication to the knee joint Transducer placed transverse over the popliteal fossa and then rotated 90° for longitudinal scanning over the posterior medial knee The longitudinal scanning plane should provide the following anatomic landmarks: 1. Crossing between semimembranosus tendon and the medial head of the gastrocnemius tendon (superficial) 2. Medial femoral condyle (deeper)
Ankle	*Medial/midline/lateral dorsal joint recess*[d] The ankle should be dorsally extended around 120° with sole resting on the examination bed Transducer placed at the sagittal midline of the ankle with the distal end of transducer positioned on the dome of talus The longitudinal scanning plane should provide the following anatomic landmarks: 1. Distal end of tibia (proximal) 2. Talus (distal)
Subtalar[e]	*Lateral joint recess* The sole foot resting on the surface of the examination bed and the ankle bent in slight flexion, and with the forefoot oriented in a slightly inversion, for the lateral approach Transducer placed in the coronal plane along the distal fibula. The transducer is then moved distal and anterior to the lateral malleolus The oblicuo-transverse scanning plane should provide the following anatomic landmarks: 1. Distal end of fibula (proximal) 2. Calcaneus (distal) (Fig. 2.4) *Posterior joint recess* With the child lying prone on the stretcher with the foot out of bed Transducer placed over the Achilles tendon The longitudinal posterior scanning approach should provide the following anatomic landmarks: 1. Inferior posterior facet of the talus (distal) 2. Superior posterior facet of the calcaneus (proximal) (Fig. 2.5)

[a]The glenohumeral joint normally has several recesses that preferentially distend with joint fluid, which include the biceps brachii long head tendon sheath, the posterior glenohumeral joint recess, the subscapularis recess and the axillary recess. A small amount of joint fluid can be seen in the biceps tendon sheath. Thus, an anterior approach of long head of the biceps brachii tendon may be recommended in children. The rotator cuff damage is uncommon in children

[b]As the dorsal approach allows an excellent view of the anechoic/hypoechoic profile of unossified epiphyseal cartilage of bones forming the dorsal recess of radiocarpal and midcarpal joints, the volar approach is not usually included in children

[c]The lateral approach is only possible on the 2nd metacarpophalangeal joint

[d]Medial aspect: the transducer should be longitudinally placed on the tibialis anterior tendon (used as a landmark). Midline aspect: the transducer should be placed at the sagittal midline of the ankle on the extensor hallucis longus and extensor digitorum tendons with the distal end of the transducer positioned on the talar dome (used as a landmark). Lateral aspect: the transducer should be longitudinally placed on the extensor digitorum tendon (used as a landmark)

[e]So far, there is no universal agreement on how to approach the subtalar joint. The authors include the lateral and posterior based on literature and personal view [22]

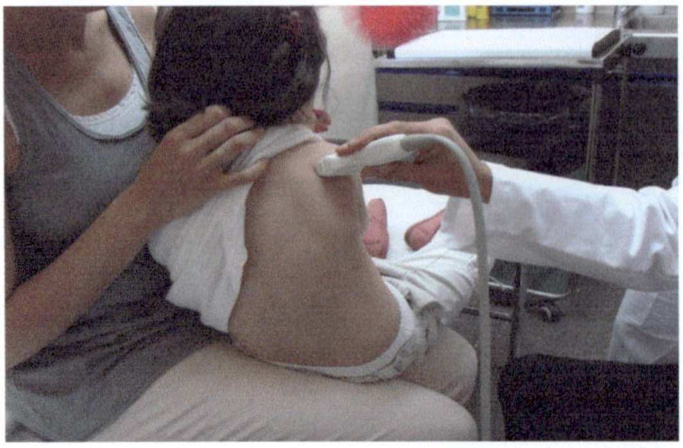

Fig. 2.2 Scan approach of posterior glenohumeral joint recess. The child is sitting on the parent's lap with the child's hand on their opposite shoulder held by parent

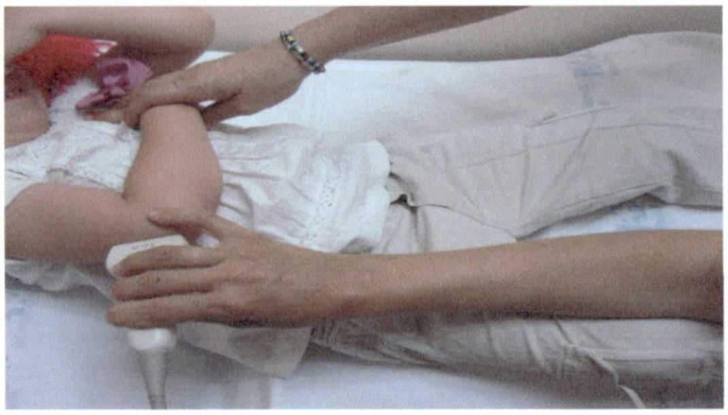

Fig. 2.3 Scan approach of posterior elbow joint recess. The child is lying supine on the stretcher with the child's hand on their opposite shoulder held by parent

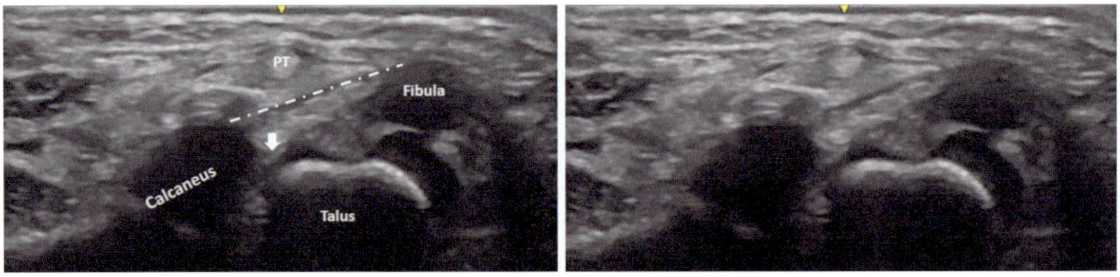

Fig. 2.4 Subtalar. Lateral joint recess. Calcaneofibular ligament (Lig); arrow, joint recess

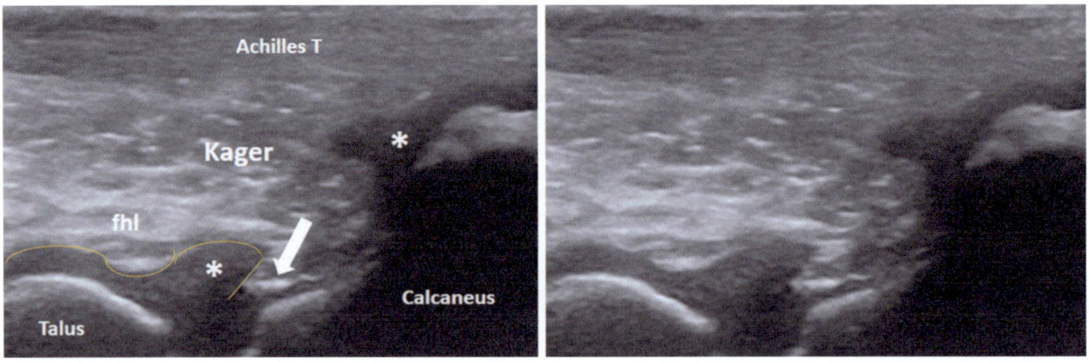

Fig. 2.5 Subtalar. Posterior joint recess. Asterisk, anechoic hyaline cartilage; arrow, joint recess; fhl, flexor hallucis longus muscle

Among extra-articular structures, the entheses have been attracting a growing interest for paediatric rheumatologists working in the field of MSUS imaging. A few detailed descriptions of US-assessed entheseal involvement in JIA patients have been provided. The first study was published by Jousse-Joulin et al. in 2011 [7] followed by the study of Weiss et al. in 2014 and Chauvin et al. in 2015 [20, 21]. The first authors described grey-scale and Doppler US abnormalities of lower limb enthesitis (i.e. quadriceps tendon insertion, proximal and distal patellar tendon insertions, Achilles tendon insertion and plantar fascia insertion on the medial calcaneal tubercle)

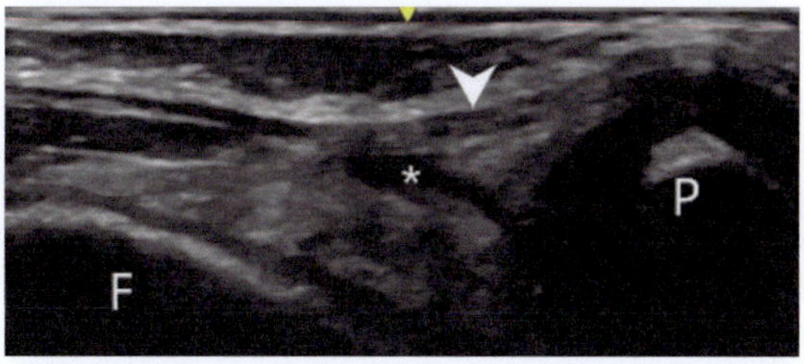

Fig. 2.6 Knee. Anterior parapatellar joint recess. Asterisk, lateral parapatellar recess; arrowhead, patellar retinaculum; F, femur; P, patella

of juvenile spondyloarthritis (JSpA). The second authors studied a wider enthesis spectrum, including several entheses of the upper limbs (common extensor tendon on lateral humerus epicondyle and common tendon flexor on medial humerus epicondyle). The third study established the normal appearance of the entheses in children. However, there is no consensus on which entheses should be evaluated in JIA and what approaches may be used in children yet.

Since children are usually restless, for US examination of the joint recess, the longitudinal axis was the first axis used in nearly all described scanning approaches (with the parapatellar recess being the exception) to identify each structure and image orientation, whereas the short (transverse) axis was usually used to scan tendons. In the knee, the transverse view of the parapatellar recess allows detection of a minimum amount of fluid, which may be not detected by sweeping the transducer from the medial to lateral side of the knee joint, using only the longitudinal suprapatellar approach (Fig. 2.6).

Although the positioning of patient depends on the examined joint and varies according to the experience of different examiners, in the youngest children (e.g. 5 years), it is currently recommended to perform the US examination with the child lying supine/prone on the stretcher, or the child may sit on the parent's lap in order to keep them calm. Whenever possible, in the case of a newborn/baby, it is preferable to scan them while sleeping. The patient position will be detailed in each joint throughout the chapter.

Care should be taken to examine the child for the detection of synovial effusion because of the high ratio of anechoic hyaline cartilage to bone in paediatric joint, which can be mistaken for fluid. Dynamic imaging during joint movement can improve the assessment of synovial fluid. As in adults, pathological findings should be documented in two perpendicular planes. Moreover, joints must be examined in their full length. It is mandatory to place the transducer in the axial plane and sweep it up and down over the dorsal/volar (palmar) of the peripheral joints to visualise as much as possible all joint components.

In general, we examine the child supine with arms placed near the side of the body and palms upward or downward in order to explore the anterior aspect of the elbow and shoulder and the volar and dorsal aspects of the joints of the hands. To explore the posterior aspect of the shoulder, the child is sitting on the parent's lap with the child's hand on their opposite shoulder held by parent. To explore both the knee and ankle, the child is lying in a supine position with the knee in flexion, around 45 degrees, and the foot resting on the surface of the examination bed.

References

1. Colebatch-Bourn AN, Edwards CJ, Collado P, D'Agostino M-A, Hemke R, Jousse-Joulin S, et al. EULAR-PReS points to consider for the use of imaging in the diagnosis and management of juvenile idiopathic arthritis in clinical practice. Ann Rheum Dis. 2015;74:1946–57.
2. Collado P, Jousse-Joulin S, Alcalde M, Naredo E, D'Agostino MA. Is ultrasound a validated imaging tool for the diagnosis and management of synovitis in juvenile idiopathic arthritis? A systematic literature review. Arthritis Care Res (Hoboken). 2012;64:1011–9.
3. Magni-Manzoni S, Epis O, Ravelli A, Klersy C, Visconti C, Lanni S, et al. Comparison of clinical versus ultrasound- determined synovitis in juvenile idiopathic arthritis. Arthritis Rheum. 2009;61:1497–504.
4. Filippou G, Cantarini L, Bertoldi I, Picerno V, Frediani B, Galeazzi M. Ultrasonography vs. clinical examination in children with suspected arthritis. Does it make sense to use poliarticular ultrasonographic screening? Clin Exp Rheumatol. 2011;29:345–50.
5. Pascoli L, Wright S, Mcallister C, Rooney M. Prospective evaluation of clinical and ultrasound findings in ankle disease in juvenile idiopathic arthritis: importance of ankle ultrasound. J Rheumatol. 2010;37:2409–14.

6. Collado P, Naredo E, Calvo C, Gamir ML, Calvo I, Garcia ML, et al. Reduced joint assessment vs comprehensive assessment for ultrasound detection of synovitis in juvenile idiopathic arthritis. Rheumatology (Oxford). 2013;52:1477–84.
7. Jousse-Joulin S, Breton S, Cangemi C, et al. Ultrasonography for detecting enthesitis in juvenile idiopathic arthritis. Arthritis Care Res. 2011;63:849–55.
8. Breton S, Jousse-Joulin S, Cangemi C, et al. Comparison of clinical and ultrasonographic evaluations for peripheral synovitis in juvenile idiopathic arthritis. Semin Arthritis Rheum. 2011;41:272–8.
9. Laurell L, Court-Payen M, Nielsen S, Zak M, Fasth A. Ultrasonography and color Doppler in juvenile idiopathic arthritis: diagnosis and follow-up of ultrasound-guided steroid injection in the wrist region. A descriptive interventional study. Pediatr Rheumatol Online J. 2012;10:11.
10. Laurell L, Court-Payen M, Nielsen S, Zak M, Boesen M, Fasth A. Comparison of ultrasonography with Doppler and MRI for assessment of disease activity in juvenile idiopathic arthritis: a pilot study. Pediatr Rheumatol Online J. 2012;10:2.
11. Pradsgaard DØ, Spannow AH, Heuck C, Herlin T. Decreased cartilage thickness in juvenile idiopathic arthritis assessed by ultrasonography. J Reumatol. 2013;40:1596–603.
12. Roth J, Jousse-Joulin S, Magni-Manzoni S, Rodriguez A, Tzaribachev N, Iagnocco A, et al. Definitions for the sonographic features of joints in healthy children. Arthritis Care Res. 2015;67:136–42.
13. Collado P, Vojinovic J, Nieto JC, Windschall D, Magni-Manzoni S, Bruyn GAW, et al. Toward standardized musculoskeletal ultrasound in pediatric rheumatology: normal age-related ultrasound findings. Arthritis Care Res. 2016;68:348–56.
14. Collado P, Windschall D, Vojinovic J, Magni-Manzoni S, Balin P, Bruyn GAW, et al. OMERACT ultrasound subtask force on pediatric. Amendment of the OMERACT ultrasound definitions of joints' features in healthy children when using the DOPPLER technique. Pediatr Rheumatol Online J. 2018;16(1):23.
15. Windschall D, Collado P, Vojinovic J, Magni-Manzoni S, Balin P, Bruyn GAW, et al. Age-related vascularization and ossification of joints in children: an international pilot study to test multi-observer ultrasound reliability. Arthritis Care Res. 2017; https://doi.org/10.1002/acr.23335.
16. Roth J, Ravagnani V, Backhaus M, Balint P, Bruns A, Bruyn GA, et al. Preliminary definitions for the sonographic features of synovitis in children. Arthritis Care Res. 2017;69:1217–23.
17. Windschall D, Pommerenke M, Haase R. Ultrasound assessment of the skeletal development of the proximal femoral, distal femoral and proximal tibial epiphyses in premature and mature neonates. Ultrasound Med Biol. 2016;42:451–8.
18. Windschall D, Trauzeddel R, Haller M, Krumrey-Langkammerer M, Nimtz-Talaska A, Berendes R, et al. Pediatric musculoskeletal ultrasound: age- and sex-related normal B-mode findings of the knee. Rheumatol Int. 2016;36:1569–77.
19. Collado P, Naredo E. Sonographic images of children's joints. EUROMEDICE, Ediciones Medicas SL: Badalona (Spain); 2007.
20. Weiss PF, Chauvin NA, Klink AJ, et al. Detection of enthesitis in children with enthesitis-related arthritis: dolorimetry compared to ultrasonography. Arthritis Rheumatol. 2014;66:218–27.
21. Chauvin NA, Ho-Fung V, Jaramillo D, et al. Ultrasound of the joints and entheses in healthy children. Pediatr Radiol. 2015;45:1344–54.
22. Lanni S, Bovis F, Ravelli A, Viola S, Magnaguagno F, Pistorio A, et al. Delineating the application of ultrasound in detecting synovial abnormalities of the subtalar joint in juvenile idiopathic arthritis. Arthritis Care Res. 2016;68:1346–53.

FUNDAMENTALS OF MUSCULOSKELETAL Sonoanatomy in adults

3

Ingrid Möller, Maribel Miguel-Pérez, and Yasser El Miedany

Introduction

Anatomy is a basic science of knowledge concerned with the study of the organisms' structure and their parts. The triad of human anatomy, physiology and pharmacology represents the three basic disciplines considered to be most relevant to daily clinical activity by both surgery and medicine healthcare professionals [1]. In the medical profession, anatomy is essential for performing precise physical examination and making a diagnosis, especially in soft tissue alterations, as well as for the interpretation of the images taken on scanning the affected body organ(s). During the last few decades, there has been an explosion of new techniques for imaging anatomy in living patients. Examples range from endoscopy and laparoscopy to ultrasonography, computed tomography and magnetic resonance imaging, together with new technology for three-dimensional visualization. The emergence of these sophisticated imaging techniques has been accompanied by the development of minimally invasive therapy targeted to specific organs and/or sites within them. As a result, knowledge of gross anatomy has become increasingly important, not only to interpret the images that are produced by these sophisticated techniques but also to understand the pathway for targeting therapy to a specific site [2].

Musculoskeletal ultrasonography is an imaging technique that uses high-frequency sound waves to produce detailed pictures of soft tissues, cartilage, bone surfaces and fluid-containing structures. The use of real-time ultrasound guidance has revolutionized the standard musculoskeletal assessment and management practice. Ultrasound is safe, is non-invasive, does not use ionizing radiation and offers dynamic live evaluation of the pathology site. Consequently, ultrasound has not only been shown as a tool useful for clinical rheumatology and orthopaedics standard clinical practice but also in the teaching and learning of anatomy [3]. Naturally, this requires

I. Möller
Unit of Human Anatomy and Embryology, Department of Experimental Pathology and Therapeutic, Faculty of Medicine and Health Sciences (C.Bellvitge), University of Barcelona, Barcelona, Spain

Instituto Poal de Reumatologia, Barcelona, Spain
e-mail: ingrid.moller@ipoal.com

M. Miguel-Pérez (✉)
Unit of Human Anatomy and Embryology, Department of Experimental Pathology and Therapeutic, Faculty of Medicine and Health Sciences (C.Bellvitge), University of Barcelona, Barcelona, Spain
e-mail: mimiguel@ub.edu

Y. El Miedany
Medway Foundation Trust, King's College London, London, Kent, UK

Rheumatology and Rehabilitation, Ain Shams University, Cairo, Egypt
e-mail: drelmiedany@rheumatology4u.com

Y. El Miedany (ed.), *Pediatric Musculoskeletal Ultrasonography*,
https://doi.org/10.1007/978-3-030-17824-6_3

the operating healthcare professionals, who wish to augment own practice and learn techniques complementary to their specialty whether they are rheumatologists, orthopaedic surgeons, interventional radiologists, physiotherapists or occupational therapists to have a very good knowledge of musculoskeletal anatomy [4].

The organization of the human musculoskeletal anatomy is governed by general principles. Basically, it is composed of the bony skeleton, muscles, cartilage, tendons, ligaments, joints, as well as the other connective tissue which supports and binds tissues and organs together. The disposition of these different structures facilitates their ability to endure and achieve maximum performance with the minimum workload and, at the same time, lessen the injury risk and protect the essential elements. Furthermore, understanding the anatomy of the musculoskeletal system involves understanding the functions, biomechanics and interrelationships between the different musculoskeletal structures that span from the subcutaneous tissue to the bone. Correct interpretation of musculoskeletal ultrasound requires thorough knowledge of the normal anatomy and musculoskeletal movements (kinesiology); hence, sonoanatomy plays a vital role for identifying the anatomic details as well as any pathological changes of the involved structures [5]. This chapter will discuss sonoanatomy, the anatomical knowledge necessary to explain the often complex images of musculoskeletal tissue. To serve its intention to consider the aspects of greatest interest to the musculoskeletal system imaging, it has been organized from superficial to deep structures including the fascia for their biomechanical contribution to the musculoskeletal system.

Sonoanatomy of the Locomotor System

The Fascia

The concept of fascia and its role in the musculoskeletal system were reviewed by M. Benjamin [6]. The fascia has been identified as the continuous connective tissue, present throughout the body and capable of transmitting mechanosensitive signals. Its characteristics and the ability of integrating functions make the fascia similar to that of nervous tissue. According to its location and function, the fascia can be stratified into superficial and deep, although, in some locations of the locomotor system, this distinction could be difficult.

The Superficial Fascia Superficial fascia is the lowermost layer of the skin in nearly all of the regions of the body, which blends with the reticular dermis layer [7]. It consists mainly of loose areolar and fatty adipose connective tissue (Figs. 3.1 and 3.2) and is the layer that primarily determines the shape of a body. It also transports blood vessels (Fig. 3.3) and nerves to and from the skin while facilitating movement between it and the underlying tissues. In addition to its subcutaneous presence, superficial

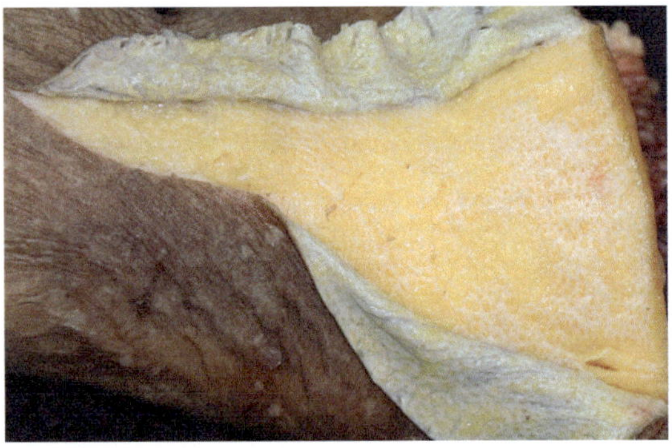

Fig. 3.1 Superficial fascia: the superficial fascia is just under the skin in a dissection of the arm

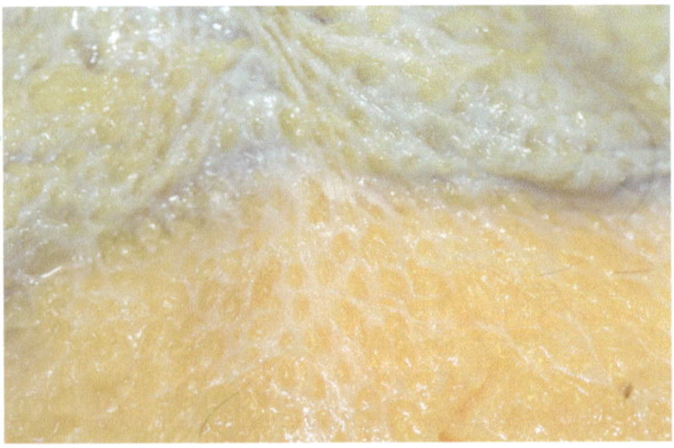

Fig. 3.2 The close relation of the superficial fascia with the skin

fascia surrounds organs and glands and neurovascular bundles and is found at many other locations where it fills otherwise unoccupied space. It serves as a storage medium of fat and water; as a passageway for lymph, nerve and blood vessels; and as a protective padding to cushion and insulate [8, 9]. Due to its viscoelastic properties, superficial fascia can stretch to accommodate the deposition of adipose that accompanies both ordinary and prenatal weight gains. After delivery and weight loss, the superficial fascia slowly reverts to its original level of tension. Superficial fascia gives the skin the ability to slip and then recover its initial position; for example, the fascia presents on the back of the hand or foot. In other locations, it is firmly fixed to deep planes, for example, palm of the hand or sole of the foot (Fig. 3.4a, b), restricting the movement to favour a firm grip function. This might have clinical implications, as in places such as the interphalangeal folds, it attaches directly to the flexor tendon sheaths with the consequent risk of infection when there are puncture wounds at that level (Fig. 3.5).

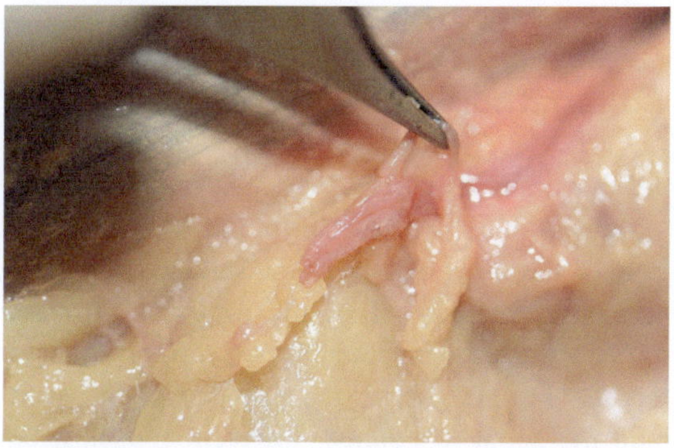

Fig. 3.3 In the superficial dissection of the forearm, it is possible to see a basilic vein (superficial vein) of the upper limb crossing the superficial fascia

The collagen fibres maintain a certain direction in the dermis giving rise to some skin marks called Langer and Kraissl's lines. Langer lines of skin tension, or sometimes called cleavage lines, are topological lines drawn on a map of the human body. They correspond to the natural orientation of collagen fibres in the dermis and are generally parallel to the orientation of the underlying muscle fibres. Langer's lines have relevance to forensic science and the development of surgical techniques. On the other hand, the Kraissl's lines are a set of anatomical skin lines. They differ from Langer's lines in that unlike Langer's lines, which are defined in terms of collagen orientation, Kraissl's lines are the lines of maximum skin tension. While Langer's lines have been defined in cadavers [10], Kraissl's lines have been defined in living individuals as they show the maximum tension of the skin when the muscles contract [11]. On another front, superficial and deep can be combined and be affected jointly in fibromatosis such as Dupuytren's disease or Ledderhose's disease.

The Deep Fascia Deep fascia is a layer of dense fibrous connective tissue which surrounds and "bundles" muscles and tendons of the locomotor system (Fig. 3.6a). It also divides different groups

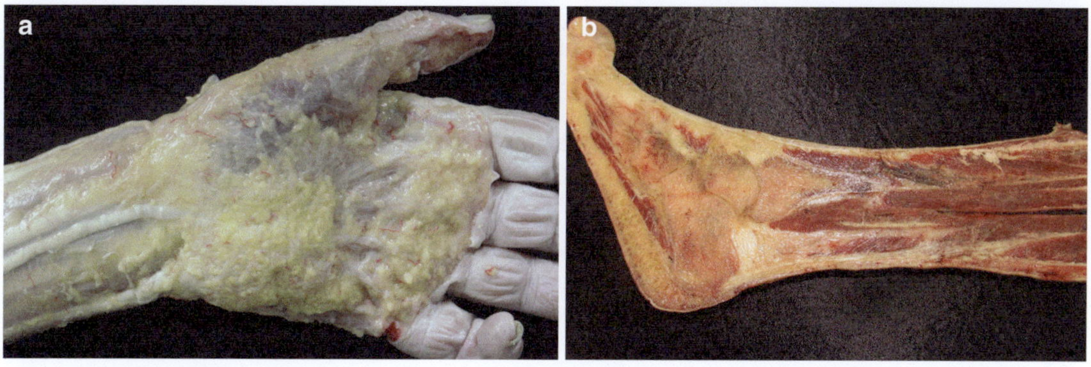

Fig. 3.4 (**a**) In the anterior of the hand, it is possible to recognize the adipose tissue in a very close relation with the palm. (**b**) This sagittal view of the inferior lower shows the adipose tissue in the plant of the foot

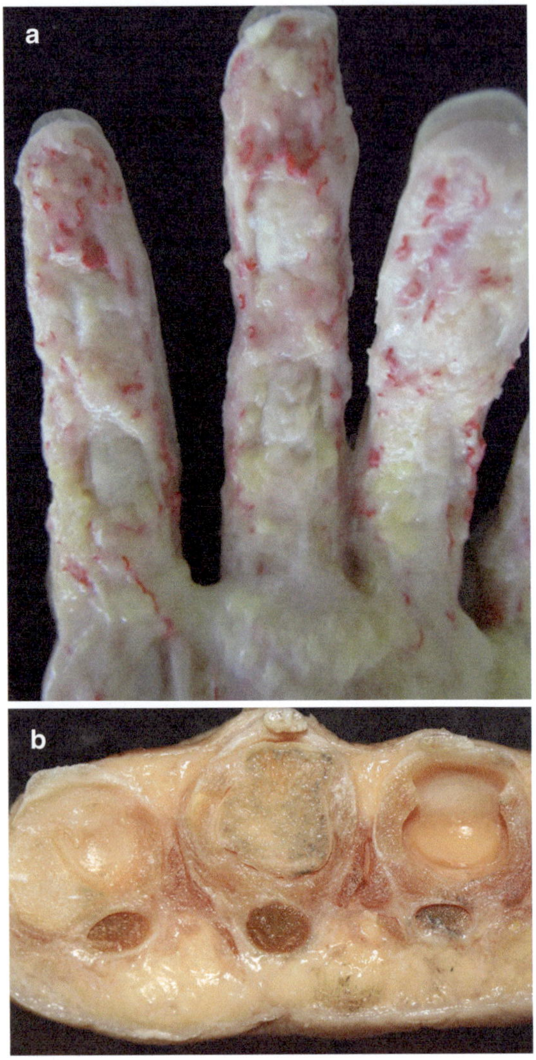

Fig. 3.5 (**a**) Vision of the fingers in the palmar view. The fat attaches directly to the flexor tendon sheaths. (**b**) The transversal cut of a finger shows the close relations of the adipose tissue with the flexor tendon sheaths

of muscles into fascial compartments. This fascia has a high density of elastin fibre that determines its extensibility or resilience [12]. Deep fascia was originally considered to be essentially avascular. However, more recent investigations confirmed a rich presence of thin blood vessels [13]. Deep fascia is also richly supplied with sensory receptors [14]. Examples of deep fascia are fascia lata, fascia cruris, brachial fascia, plantar fascia, thoracolumbar fascia and Buck's fascia. The anatomical distribution of the deep fascia surrounding the muscles under the superficial fascia and dividing the different muscular compartment of the extremities helps them performing their function (Fig. 3.6b).

Traditionally, fasciae were thought of as passive structures that transmit mechanical tension generated by muscular activities or external forces throughout the body. An important function of muscle fasciae is to reduce friction of muscular force. In doing so, fasciae provide a supportive and movable wrapping for nerves and blood vessels as they pass through and between muscles [15]. Fascial tissues are frequently innervated by sensory nerve endings. These include myelinated as well as unmyelinated nerves. Based on this a proprioceptive, nociceptive as well as interoceptive function of fascia has been postulated [16]. Fascial tissues – particularly those with tendinous or aponeurotic properties – are also able to store and release elastic potential energy.

Clinical Implications: Fascia Sonopathology

As our understanding of the anatomy and physiology of these structures expands, the important role of the deep fasciae in the interaction among the different muscles of the limbs has become more apparent. The deep fasciae could be considered to be like a bridge, passing over the joints and the septa to connect different muscles, but recent studies [17] also recognize a primary role in the perception and coordination of movements, due to the unique mechanical properties and dense innervation of these fasciae. Fascia becomes important clinically when it loses stiffness, becomes too stiff or has decreased shearing ability [18]. When inflammatory fasciitis or trauma causes fibrosis and adhesions, fascial tissue fails to differentiate the adjacent structures effectively. This can happen after surgery where the fascia has been incised and healing which includes a scar that traverses the surrounding structures.

Another classic example of the clinical interest of this structure is the fascia of the psoas muscle that originates in T12 vertebrae and from L1 to L5. A localized infection in one of the men-

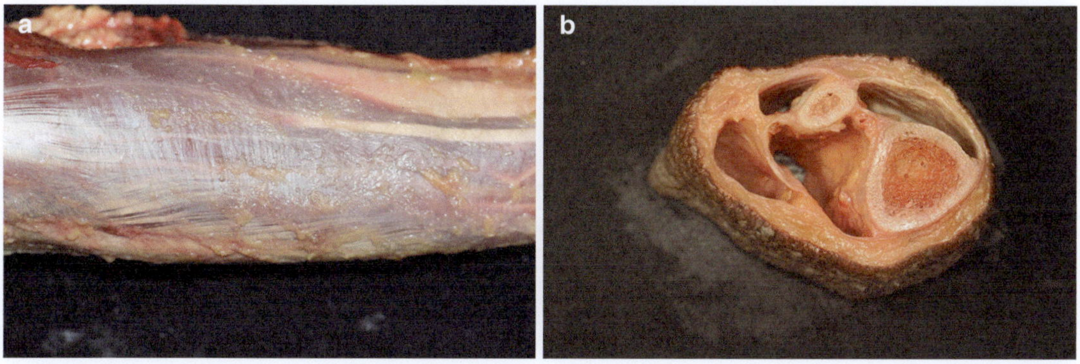

Fig. 3.6 (**a**) The deep fascia under the superficial fascia surrounding the muscles of the anterior area of the forearm. (**b**) This transversal cut of the leg shows the deep fascia how it makes the different compartments for the anterior, lateral and posterior muscles. In the posterior compartment also, there is a different compartment for the superficial and deep muscles

tioned vertebral bodies can appear distal in the inguinal region transmitted via the deep fascia.

Fasciae vary according to their location adapting to the function they perform. These modifications, whether in the superficial or deep fascia, may be of interest when interpreting ultrasound or magnetic resonance imaging of the locomotor system. In certain retinacula, which are adaptations of the deep fasciae, or in the plantar fascia when subjected to significant load, the fibroblasts can present a chondrocytic phenotype transforming into fibrocartilage. This can also happen in tendons subjected to a lot of friction, such as the tibialis posterior at its angulation around the medial malleolus. Similarly, in the sole of the foot or in the palm of the hand, the superficial fascia is mainly formed of fibroadipose tissue to adapt to the pressures suffered by these areas. Modifications of the fibroadipose tissue of the sole of the foot should be taken into account in the differential diagnosis of biomechanical talalgias.

The Retinacula

The retinacula are typically regional specializations of the deep fascia; in particular, they are thickenings of the deep fasciae and, as such, are not separable. They appear as a strong fibrous bundle with a criss-cross arrangement of the collagen fibres. The retinacula have many bone insertions, and these entheses may be fibrocartilaginous. At other points, they can glide over the bones thanks to interposing loose connective tissue between the retinacula and the periosteum. The retinacula are destined to create tunnels that facilitate the sliding and direction to the tendons keeping them in their correct position. It is interesting to know that the tendons located under the retinacula will always have synovial sheaths. When creating closed spaces, they can give pathologies due to entrapment. The classic example is the flexor retinaculum of the wrist (Fig. 3.7a), through which pass not only the flexor tendons of the fingers but also the median nerve. Under the retinaculum, the median nerve can get trapped producing carpal tunnel syndrome (Fig. 3.7b). Another example of functional retinacula is the extensor retinaculum which is formed of sagittal bands located on the dorsum of the hand. It provides stability and protection of the extensor muscles at the distal forearm and avoids the subluxation of the extensor tendons of the fingers (Fig. 3.8a, b) [19]. Similar function is exerted by the pulleys present on the palmar aspect of the hand/fingers which help to avoid the bulging of the flexor tendons of the hands (Fig. 3.9a, b). The retinacula of the wrist, the ankle or the flexor pulleys of the fingers, are composed of three different layers of tissue adapted to their function. These include (1.) a sliding internal surface composed of cells that secrete hyaluronic; (2) an intermediate thicker layer, which supports function, made of collagen fibres, fibroblasts and elastin; and (3) an outer layer, of

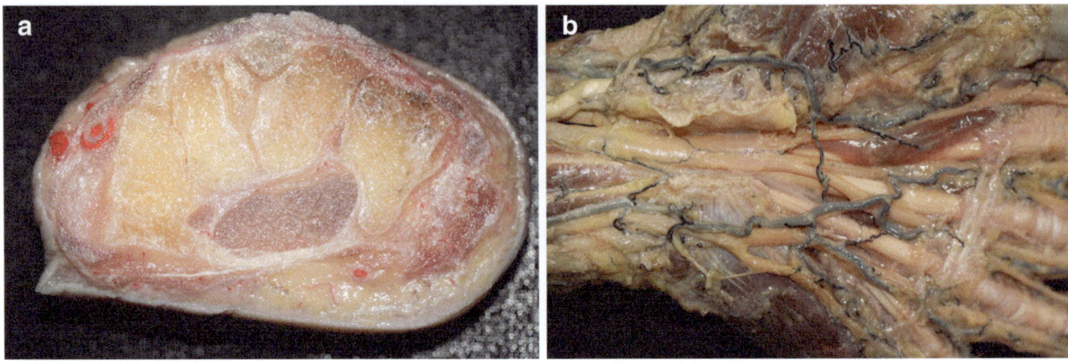

Fig. 3.7 (**a**) The transversal cut of the wrist shows the flexor retinaculum that keeps the flexor digitorum tendons and median nerve. (**b**) The anterior dissection of the hand allows to see the flexor retinaculum that is cut and shows the median nerve as the more superficial structure under it. The nerve seems thicker as consequence of a compression of the retinaculum

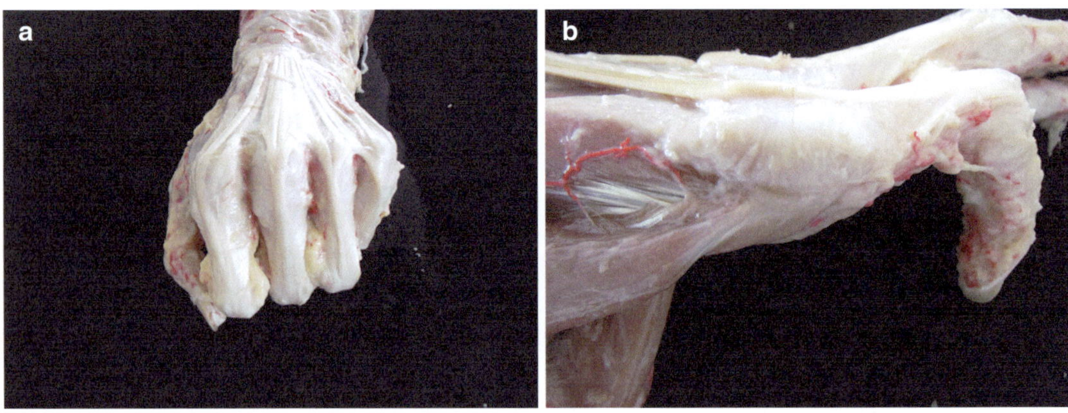

Fig. 3.8 (**a**) In the dorsum of the hand, it is possible to visualize the sagittal bands that keep the extensor tendon. (**b**) The lateral vision of the second finger shows the sagittal bands

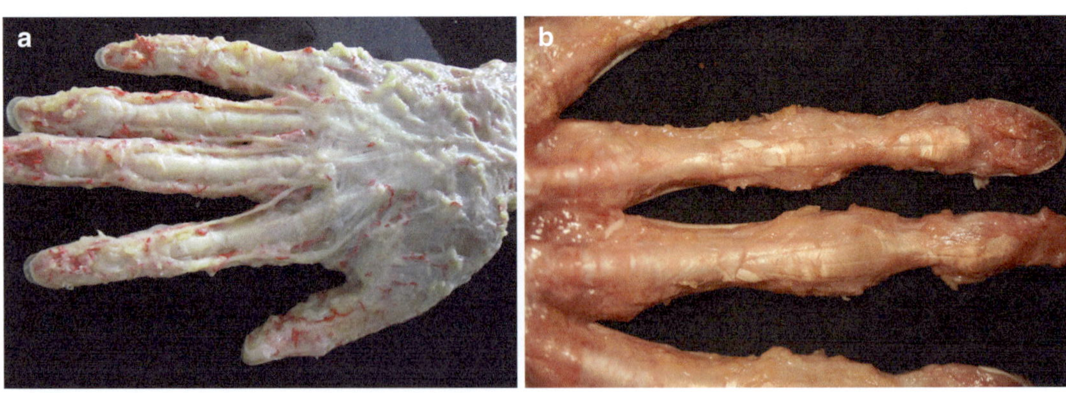

Fig. 3.9 (**a**) The different pulleys are situated in the palmar aspect of the fingers. (**b**) The different pulleys with more detail are situated in the palmar aspect of the fingers

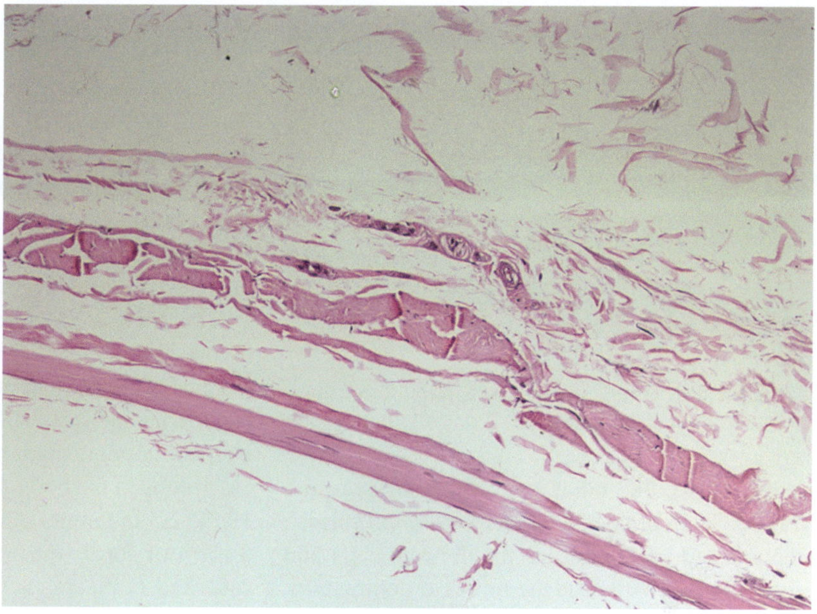

Fig. 3.10 A microscopic vision of the extensor retinaculum of the wrist shows the three different layers of the tissue

loose connective tissue, which contains vascular channels (Fig. 3.10). Variations in both composition and thickness, either of the retinaculum or its content, can generate alterations such as trigger finger or stenosing tenosynovitis.

The Muscles

Skeletal muscle is a type of striated muscle, attached to the skeleton. Skeletal muscles are used to facilitate movement, via contraction, by applying force to bones and joints. They generally contract voluntarily (via nerve stimulation), although they can contract involuntarily. Skeletal muscles have variable functions. They provide mobility, stability and posture to the human body. The basic functional unit of striated muscle tissue is called the sarcomere. Striated muscles can be classified according to their shape, size, direction and function (fast and slow contraction). Stratifying skeletal muscles according to their fibre distribution reveals that there are a number of different muscle shapes within the human body including circular, convergent, parallel, pennate and fusiform (Fig. 3.11). When the alignment of the sarcomeres is oblique with respect to the longitudinal axis of the muscle/tendon, it is called penniform or pennate muscles (Fig. 3.12). These types of muscles generally allow higher force production but smaller range of motion. When a muscle contracts and shortens, the pennation angle increases, which in turn amplifies the muscle shortening velocity and power [20, 21]. The muscle maintains a complex relationship with the neurovascular system, which starts to form as early as the embryonic stages.

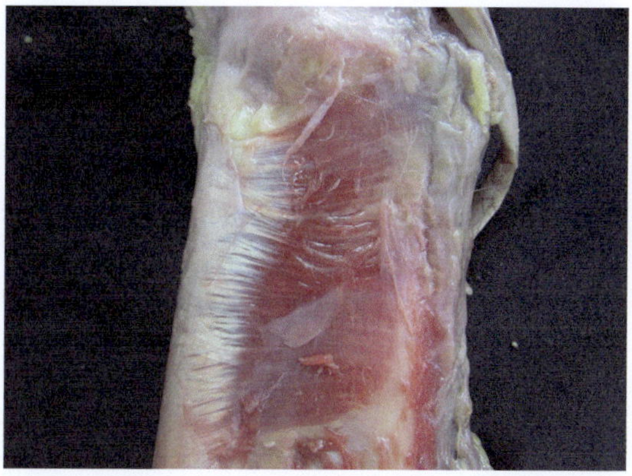

Fig. 3.11 The muscle pronator quadratus, in the anterior and deep area of the forearm, has its name for the quadrangular shape

A whole skeletal muscle is considered an organ of the muscular system. Skeletal muscle

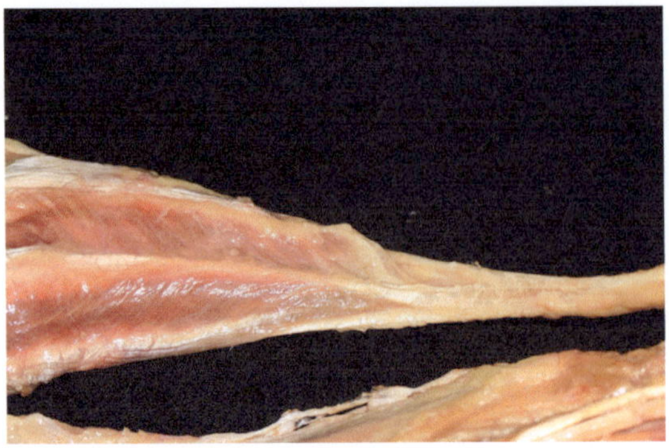

Fig. 3.12 This muscle shows a penniform of this fibres that insert in a central tendon

fibres (cells), like other body cells, are soft and fragile. The connective tissue coverings furnish support and protection for the delicate cells and allow them to withstand the forces of contraction. The coverings also provide pathways for the passage of blood vessels and nerves. The connective tissue associated with muscle tissue is stratified into the endomysium which is the connective tissue that surrounds each muscle fibre (cell); the perimysium which encircles a group of muscle fibres, forming a fascicle; and the epimysium which encircles all the fascicles to form a complete muscle. Commonly, the epimysium, perimysium and endomysium extend beyond the fleshy part of the muscle, the belly, to form a thick rope-like tendon or a broad, flat sheet-like aponeurosis. The tendon and aponeurosis form indirect attachments from muscles to the periosteum of bones or to the connective tissue of other muscles.

The muscle fascia plays an important role in regulating human posture and movements as it acts as force transmitters [22]. Myofascial force transmission is the transmission of muscle force through a continuous cellular matrix of the endomysial facial stroma of the muscle. Intramuscular myofascial force transmission occurs through endomysial-perimysial network and via the epimysium pathways [23]. Epimuscular myofascial force transmission occurs in two ways, namely, intermuscular and extra-muscular pathways. Intermuscular myofascial force transmission occurs through the connective tissues at the interface between the muscle bellies of adjacent muscles. Extra-muscular force transmission occurs between the epimysium of a muscle and an adjacent nonmuscular structure such as matrix supporting nerves and blood vessels and fascia layers, which can connect the borders of the agonistic muscle to the antagonistic and synergistic fibre. Thus, the myofascial force is transmitted between the target muscle and neighbouring muscles and/or extra-muscular tissues.

The myofascial force transmission from the myofascial skeletal system regulates the biomechanics of the human movement via the deep and superficial muscular fascia, which serves as the element of connection between the different muscle groups in the body. Wood Jones highlighted in 1944 [24] the importance of myofascial unions as a form of force transmission to surrounding tissues and compared it with the exoskeleton that non-vertebrate animals possess. In human being, these myofascial unions contribute to create a stable column to maintain the erect position in the lower extremities [25]. Any separation of the muscle fibres and fascial continuity due to any surgical procedures may affect the myofascial force transmission. In this context, when the contractile harmony in the myofascial continuity is disrupted as a result of surgical separation of muscles, movement compensations and altered motor patterns affect the normal biomechanics of the joint, ligaments and other soft tissue structures. In the long run, any such altered myofascial force distribution may lead to a pathological stress or overload to the joints and possibly may cause recurrence of joint pathologies or even affect the outcomes of the musculoskeletal surgeries [26].

The Tendons

Tendons are a type of connective tissue, composed of dense fibrous connective tissue made up primarily of collagenous fibres. The primary cell types of tendons are the spindle-shaped tenocytes (fibrocytes) and tenoblasts (fibroblasts). Tenocytes are mature tendon cells that are found throughout the tendon structure, typically anchored to collagen fibres. Tenoblasts are spindle-shaped immature tendon cells that give rise to tenocytes. The main function of a tendon is to connect skeletal muscles to bones. The tendons transmit mechanical forces from the muscle to the bone to generate movement while controlling the speed at which it is performed.

For each muscle, there will be at least two tendons, proximal and distal, a myotendinous junction and an enthesis (Fig. 3.13). The tendon continues with the periosteal tissue that lines the bone. Many tendons reinforce the joint capsules forming part of it and contributing to its function; an example is the extensor digitorum complex that forms the dorsal capsule of the proximal phalangeal joint (Fig. 3.14a, b). The extensor digitorum complex also shows the functional collaboration that may exist between various muscles-tendons, in this case interossei and lumbricals that join the extensors of the fingers, in addition to reinforcing the capsule of the metacarpophalangeal joint, contributing to its delicate function (Fig. 3.15).

The morphology of the tendon is adapted to its function in such a way that if it exerts a lot of force, it will be short and wide, while if it performs delicate movements as in the fingers, it will be long and slim. Another example, the muscles in the extremities whether upper or lower limbs,

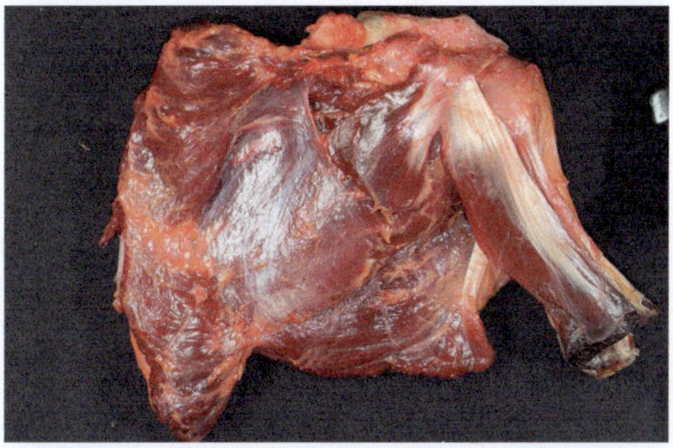

Fig. 3.13 The insertion tendon of the pectoralis minor in the coracoid process (**a**) and the conjunct origin tendon of the coracobrachialis and short head of the biceps brachialis (**b**) as examples of a myotendinous junction and an enthesis

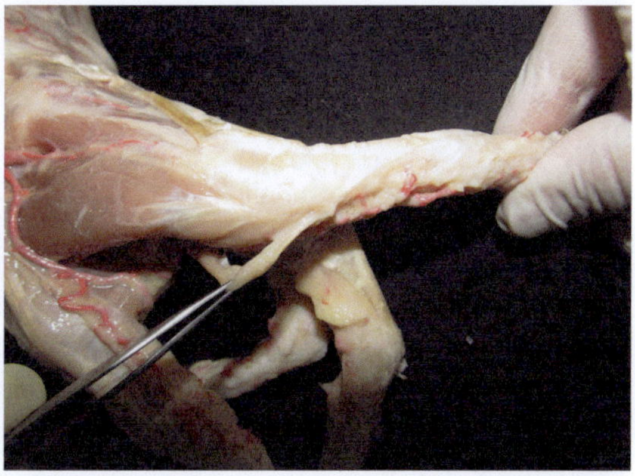

Fig. 3.15 The first posterior interosseous muscle arrives to the insertion reinforcing the capsule of the phalangeal metacarpal join: also it is possible to visualize the first lumbricals tendon that joins the extensors of the fingers

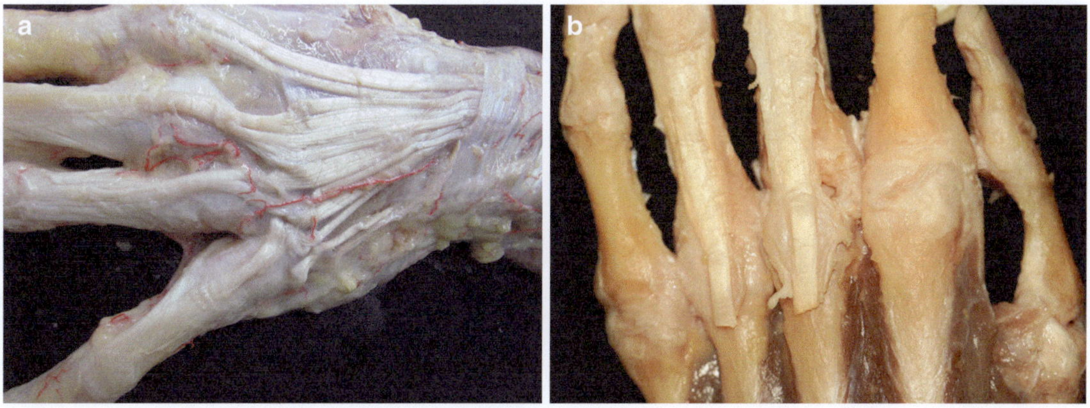

Fig. 3.14 (**a**) The extensor digitorum complex reinforces the dorsal joint capsules in the proximal phalangeal joint. (**b**) This picture shows the importance of the extensor digitorum complex in the dorsal joint capsules in the proximal phalangeal joint of the third and fourth fingers, while the second and fifth fingers are without the extensor tendons

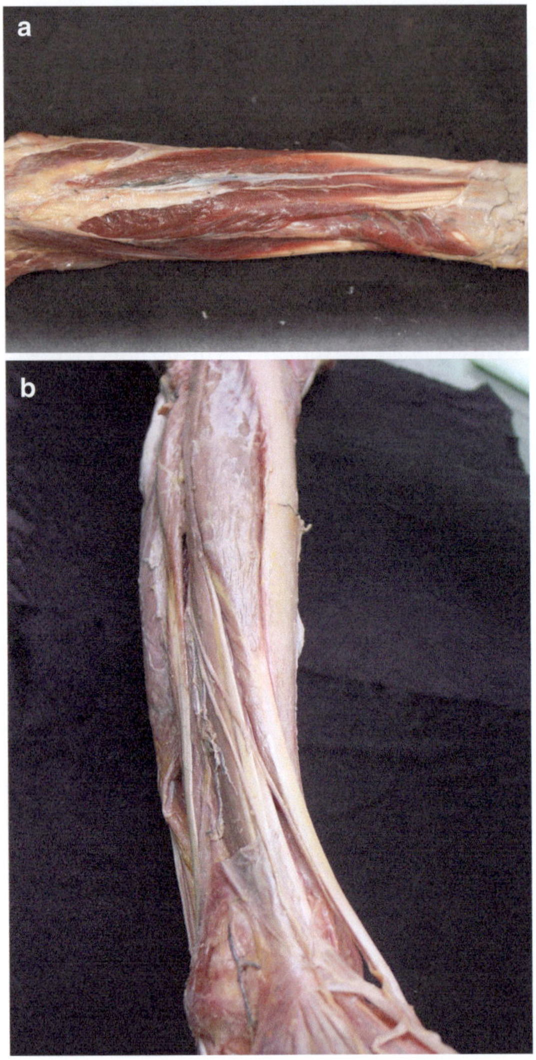

Fig. 3.16 (**a**) The posterior vision of the forearm shows the different posterior muscles and the origin of their tendons before they arrive to the extensor retinaculum. (**b**) The anterior vision of the leg shows the different anterior muscles and the origin of their tendons before they arrive to the extensor retinaculum in the ankle. The tendon of the tibialis anterior muscle has been remove of this retinaculum

gives origin to their tendon before reaching the insertion, for example, "hand/wrist" or "foot/ankle" in order to avoid dysfunctions that may arise if the muscle mass got trapped in a space closed by a retinaculum (Fig. 3.16a, b).

Studying the tendon internal structure reveals that the tendon is made primarily of fibrils which assemble further to form fascicles, which are about 10 mm in length with a diameter of 50–300 μm, and finally into a tendon fibre with a diameter of 100–500 μm [27]. Fascicles are bound by the endotendineum, which is a delicate loose connective tissue containing thin collagen fibrils [28] and elastic fibres [29]. Groups of fascicles are bounded by the epitenon. Filling the interstitia within the fascia where the tendon is located is the paratenon, a fatty areolar tissue [30].

The tendon's internal architecture facilitates movement between the different fascicles of the tendon in different planes. Endotendon is a thin sheath of connective tissue that surrounds each fibre, connects it with neighbouring fibres and facilitates interfascicular displacement while directing the vasculo-nervous bundle. This ability to slide independently between the different fibres and fascicles (bundles of fibres) is an important property of the tendon from the functional point of view and can be damaged in numerous tendon injuries.

The tendons may be surrounded by a synovial sheath or may lack it. Tendons like Achilles are wrapped in the paratenon (Fig. 3.17a, b), loose areolar connective tissue that functions as an elastic cover which allows free movement of the tendon in relation to the surrounding tissues. Others, such as the peroneus, present synovial sheaths intermittently at points where it is more necessary to minimize friction (Fig. 3.18a, b, c). There are also bursae that contribute to reduce friction and facilitate the tendon sliding. In the ageing process or secondary to trauma/microtrauma, the size of the tendon collagen fibres decreases, and as a consequence the tendon volume is smaller [31].

The vascularization of the tendon is less than that of the corresponding muscle (Fig. 3.19a) and is maintained mainly at the level of the myotendinous junction. After penetrating the tendon, the vessels run in parallel to the tendinous fibres and are scarce in the areas where the tendon changes its angulation (Fig. 3.19b, c); examples of this are the tibialis posterior, at the level of the medial malleolus of the ankle or flexor tendons of the fingers when they run under a pulley (Fig. 3.20a, b). In places where the tendon is more ischaemic, there is a greater predisposition to degenerative processes and/or ruptures.

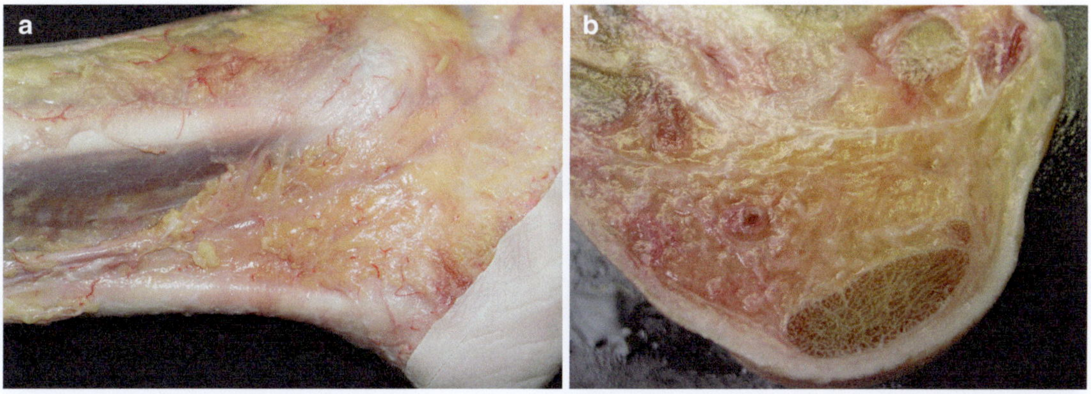

Fig. 3.17 (**a**) In this lateral vision of the ankle and foot, the calcaneal tendon is surrounded by a synovial sheath that is wrapped in the paratenon. (**b**) The calcaneal tendon transverse cut shows the paratenon with a close relation with the tendon

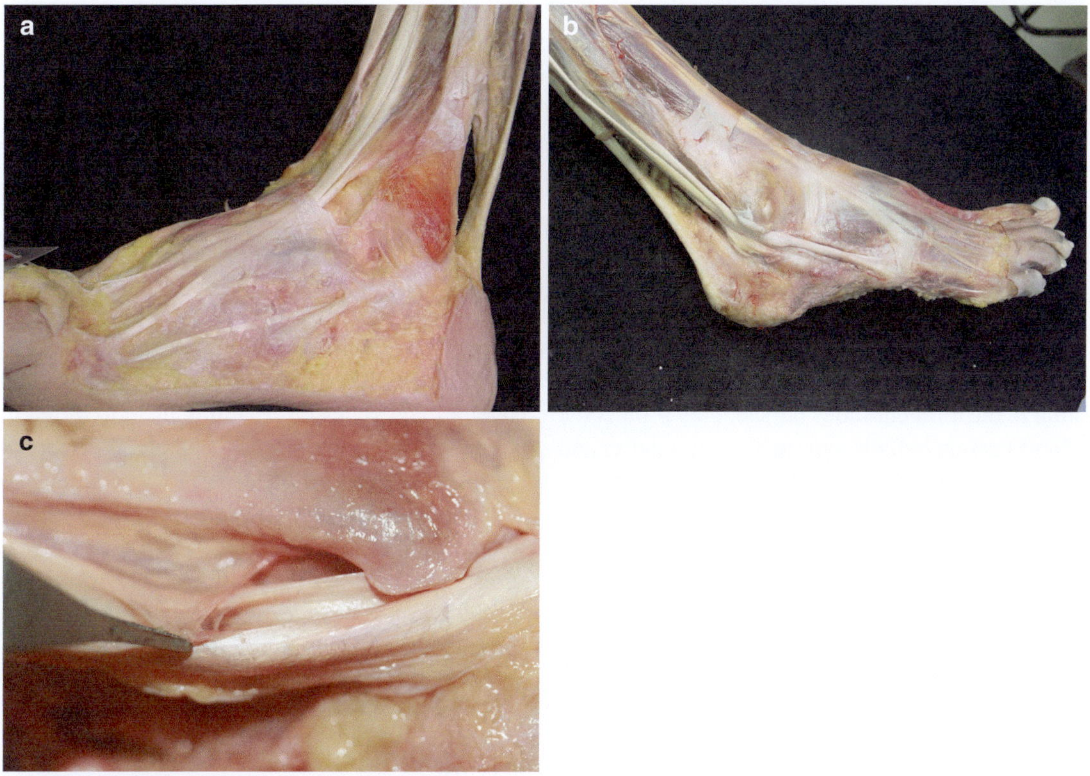

Fig. 3.18 (**a**) The peroneus tendons are fixed by the lateral retinaculum. (**b**) In the lateral retinaculum of the foot, the peroneal tendons are without their sheaths. (**c**) Synovial sheaths of the peroneal tendons in a lateral view: longus peroneus (**a**) and brevis peroneus (**b**) tendons. Lateral malleolus

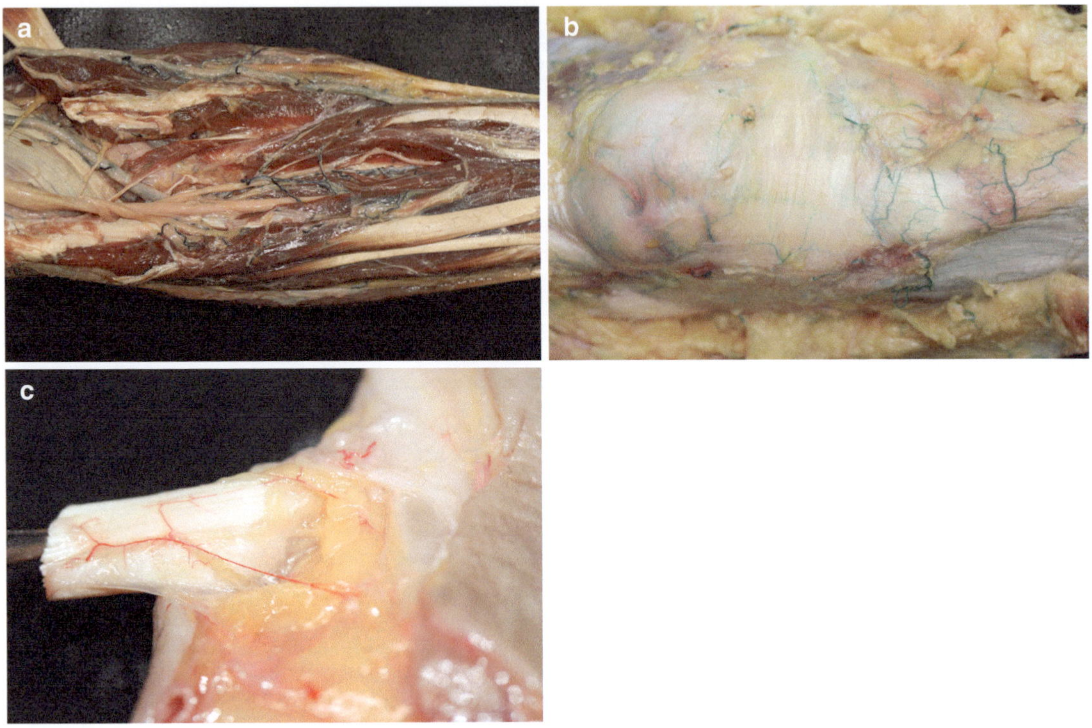

Fig. 3.19 (**a**) The different vessels form the brachial artery (injected with black latex), which arrives in a great number to the anterior muscles of the forearm. (**b**) In this anterior view of the knee, the vessels, injected in green colour, arrive to patellar tendon superficially to supply it. (**c**) This picture shows the thin vessels that arrive parallel to the tendon for the deep area of the tendon of the tibialis posterior

The fat pads associated with the tendons serve several functions: they distribute the synovial fluid in the intratendinous bursae; they protect the blood vessels in their entrance to the tendon and for their content of lymphocytes, granulocytes and macrophages as well as secretion of interleukins, cytokines, growth and adipokines; they act as an immune organ [32].

The Enthesis

The integration of tendon into bone occurs at a specialized interface known as the enthesis. However, enthesis is not limited to mere tendon-bone attachment. In fact, the area of confluence of tissues of different consistencies, such as bone with tendon, capsule, ligament or retinaculum, is called also an enthesis. Furthermore, the enthesis may expand beyond the bone attachment site. To ensure a balanced distribution of forces and a better transmission of the tensile forces generated by muscle cells to the bone, the enthesis can have fascial expansions that link them to different neighbouring structures; for example, the bicipital aponeurosis which, in addition to contributing to the supination function of the biceps brachii, stabilizes it by inserting it into the deep fascia of the forearm in the ulnar region (Fig. 3.21). Similar to the tibialis posterior in the sole of the foot, the semimembranosus muscle presents multiple attachments located in different sites such as in the posterior capsule of the knee, the proximal/middle third of the tibia, the patella and the femoral condyle. These improve the muscle role as a medial stabilizer of the knee joint (Fig. 3.22). Another example is the rectus femoris which attaches to the ilium, and it is also a flexor of the hip. The origin of the tendons of the rectus femoris, the only part of the quadriceps that crosses two joints, allows the rectus femoris to be not only extensor of the knee but also a flexor of the hip joint; its function

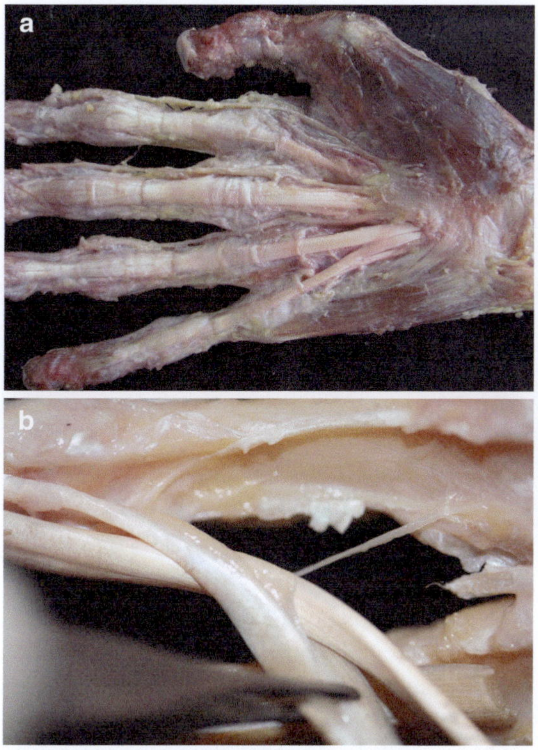

Fig. 3.20 (**a**) Tendons of flexor digitorum superficialis and profundus run under the pulleys of the fingers. No vessels are seen in their surface. (**b**) Presence of the vessels that arrive under the flexor tendons of the fingers. Their pulleys are cut to allow see this vincula

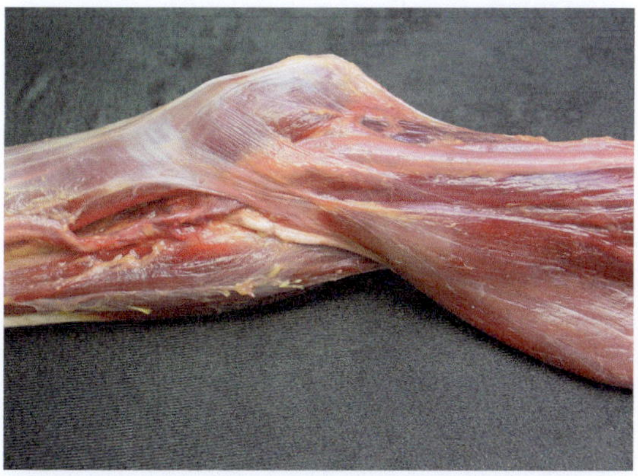

Fig. 3.21 The bicipital aponeurosis that comes from the biceps brachii muscle contributes to the supination function of the biceps brachii muscle

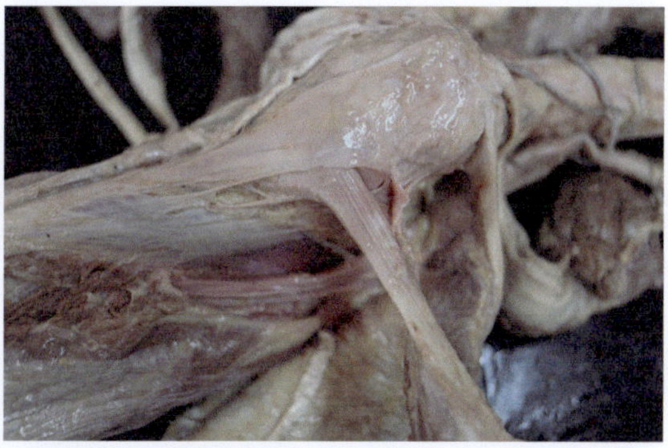

Fig. 3.22 A vision of the several insertions of the semimembranosus muscle in relation with the collateral medial ligament

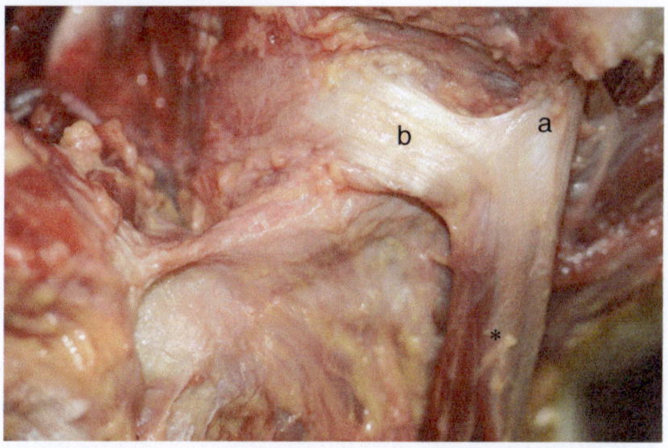

Fig. 3.23 The origin of the rectus femoris muscle has two important tendons: one direct in the anteroinferior iliac spine (a) and another indirect in the acetabulum border (b)

is facilitated by having an enthesis in different directions that would act as vectors of force for each movement (Fig. 3.23). This action is crucial to walking or running as it swings the leg forward into the ensuing step. Both in the clinical evaluation and in the study of the US images, one must bear in mind such potential anatomical complexity and possible sonopathology features.

The enthesis organ concept has attracted the attention for its relevance to the spondyloarthropathies. In principle, an organ is a group of tissues that work together to carry out a shared function. The enthesis organ is composed of the enthesis insertion into the bone along with the adjacent tissues, namely, the fibrocartilage, the adjacent trabecular bone, the bursa and fat pad; the deep fascia can also be integrated, though inconstantly. The entheses are avascular in their fibrocartilaginous components, but in response to pathological stimuli, they can be vascularized (Fig. 3.24).

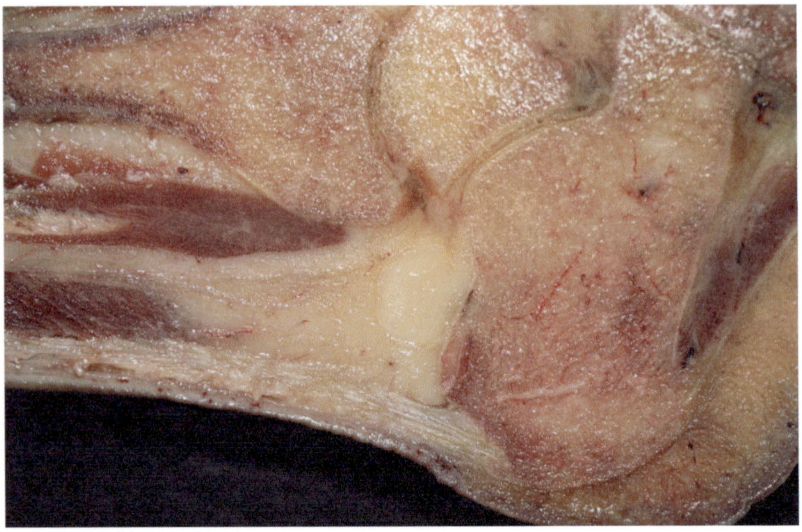

Fig. 3.24 Sagittal cut of the ankle shows the organ of the enthesis of the calcaneal tendon. Notice the fibrocartilage, the adjacent trabecular bone, the bursa and the fat pad

The function of the enthesis organ is to provide a stable anchorage to the skeleton and to minimize damage at the insertion site which is subject to high levels of physical stress; hence, the enthesis organ cushions and protects attachment sites to the bone. Understanding the sonoanatomy of the enthesis organ is a key to understanding the extensive nature of soft tissue swelling or bone abnormalities that accompany diseases of the enthesis [31, 32]. The two interdependent components of the enthesis organ are the tendon attachment to the bone and the adjacent synovial component (e.g. local bursa). The concept of a synovio-entheseal complex and of a "functional enthesis" is complimentary to that of an enthesis organ and also has important implications for understanding enthesitis [33]. The synovio-entheseal complex concept emphasizes the interdependence between synovial membrane and entheses within the enthesis organs. It draws attention to the fact that one component (the enthesis) is prone to microdamage and the other (the synovium) to inflammation. If an enthesis is damaged, any ensuing inflammatory reaction is likely to occur in the synovium [34]. Such morphologically distinct pathological lesions can be identified by imaging techniques such as ultrasound.

Key Points

- Linking sonoanatomy with clinical orientation is essential to understand and identify the possible underlying pathology as well as interpret the locomotor system US images.
- Musculoskeletal tissues generally adapt morphologically to their function and can be modified phenotypically with age, and these findings can be observed by ultrasound.
- The fasciae contribute to the correct function of the locomotor system and constitute an area of interest for the rheumatologist.
- Entheses are anatomically complex structures that can be identified by ultrasound.

References

1. Pabst R. Anatomy curriculum for medical students what can be learned for future curricula from evaluations and questionnaires completed by students, anatomist and clinicians in different countries? Ann Anat. 2009;191:541–6.
2. McCuskey R, Carmichael S, Kirch D. The importance of anatomy in health professions education and the shortage of qualified educators. Acad Med. 2005;80(4):349–51.
3. So S, Patel RM, Orebaugh SL. Ultrasound imaging in medical student education: impact on learn-

ing anatomy and physical diagnosis. Anat Sci Educ. 2017;10(2):176–89.
4. Torralba KD, Villaseñor-Ovies P, Evelyn CM, Koolaee RM, Kalish RA. Teaching of clinical anatomy in rheumatology: a review of methodologies. Clin Rheumatol. 2015;34(7):1157–63.
5. Möller I, Ianta J, Backhaus M, Ohnrdorf S, Bong D, Martinoli C, et al. The 2017 EULAR standardised procedures for ultrasound imaging in rheumatology. Ann Rheum Dis. 2017;0:1–6.
6. Benjamin M. The fascia of the limbs and back – a review. J Anat. 2009;214(1):1–18.
7. Skandalakis JE, Skandalakis PN, Skandalakis LJ, Skandalakis J. Surgical anatomy and technique. 2nd ed. Atlanta: Springer; 2002. p. 1–2. ISBN 0-387-98752-5
8. Paoletti S. The fasciae: anatomy, dysfunction & treatment. Seattle: Eastland Press; 2006. p. 23–4. ISBN 0-939616-53-X
9. Hedley G. The integral anatomy series. Vol. 1: skin and superficial fascia; 2005. https://www.youtube.com/watch?v=K68kC9R7THc&list=PLQRL-lRQd-b5iiox5vBd8kfcXumHMYN2XU.
10. Wilhelmi BJ, Blackwell SJ, Phillips LG. Langer's lines: to use or not to use. Plast Reconstr Surg. 1999;104(1):208–14.
11. Bland KI, Sarr MG, Büchler MW, Csendes A, Garden OJ, Wong J, editors. General surgery: principles and international practice. London: Springer Science & Business Media; 2008.
12. Hedley G. The integral anatomy series vol. 2: deep fascia and muscle (DVD). Integral Anatomy Productions; 2005. Retrieved 17 Jul 2006. https://www.youtube.com/watch?v=cK49wx75FN8.
13. Stecco C. Functional atlas of the human fascial system. Edinburgh: Churchill Livingstone Elsevier; 2015. p. 59. ISBN 978-0-7020-4430-4
14. Schleip R. Fascial plasticity – a new neurobiological explanation: part 1. J Bodyw Mov Ther. 2003;7(1):11–9. https://doi.org/10.1016/S1360-8592(02)00067-0.
15. Faller A, Schuenke M. Color atlas of human body. Stuttgart: Thieme Medical Publishers; 2004. p. 127.
16. Schleip R. Fascia as an organ of communication. In: Schleip R, et al., editors. Fascia – the tensional network of the human body. Edinburgh: Elsevier; 2012. p. 77–112.
17. Langevin HM, Huijing PA. Communicating about fascia: history, pitfalls, and recommendations. Int J Ther Massage Bodywork. 2009;2(4):3.
18. Klingler W, Velders M, Hoppe K, Pedro M, Schleip R. Clinical relevance of fascial tissue and dysfunctions. Curr Pain Headache Rep. 2014;18(8):439.
19. Klein DM, Katzman BM, Mesa JA, Lipton JF, Caligiuri DA. Histology of the extensor retinaculum of the wrist and the ankle. J Hand Surg Am. 1999;24(4):799–802.
20. Maganaris CN, Baltzopoulos V, Sargeant AJ. In vivo measurements of the triceps surae complex architecture in man: implications for muscle function. J Physiol. 1998;512:603–14.
21. Wakahara T, Kanehisa H, Kawakami Y, Fukunaga T, Yana T. Relationship between muscle architecture and joint performance during concentric contractions in humans. J Appl Biomech. 2013;29:405–12.
22. Schleip R, Klingler W, Lehmann-Horn F. Active fascial contractility: fascia may be able to contract in a smooth muscle-like manner and thereby influence musculoskeletal dynamics. Med Hypotheses. 2005;65(2):273–7.
23. Huijing PA, Baan GC. Myofascial force transmission via extramuscular pathways occurs between antagonistic muscles. Cells Tissues Organs. 2008;188(4):400–14.
24. Wood Jones F. The principles of anatomy as seen in the hand. London: Baillière, Tindall and Cox; 1944a.
25. Wood Jones F. Structure and function as seen in the foot. London: Bailliere, Tindall and Cox; 1944b.
26. Leonard J. Importance of considering myofascial force transmission in musculoskeletal surgeries. J Surg Acad. 2013;3(2):1–3.
27. Fratzl P. Cellulose and collagen: from fibres to tissues. Curr Opin Colloid Interface Sci. 2009;8(1):32–9.
28. Caldini EG, Caldini N, De-Pasquale V, Strocchi R, Guizzardi S, Ruggeri A, Montes GS. Distribution of elastic system fibres in the rat tail tendon and its associated sheaths. Cells Tissues Organs. 1990;139(4):341–8.
29. Grant TM, Thompson MS, Urban J, Yu J. Elastic fibres are broadly distributed in tendon and highly localized around tenocytes. J Anat. 2013;222(6):573–9.
30. Zhang G, Ezura Y, Chervoneva I, Robinson PS, Beason DP, Carine ET, Soslowsky LJ, Iozzo RV, Birk DE. Decorin regulates assembly of collagen fibrils and acquisition of biomechanical properties during tendon development. J Cell Biochem. 2006;98(6):1436–49.
31. Dressler MR, Butler DL, Wenstrup R, Awad HA, Smith F, Boivin GP. A potential mechanism for age-related declines in patellar tendon biomechanics. J Orthop Res. 2002;20:1315–22.
32. Shaw HM, Santer RM, Watson AHD, Benjamin M. Adipose tissue at entheses: the innervation and cell composition of the retromalleolar fat pad associated with the rat Achilles tendon. J Anat. 2007;211:436–43.
33. Benjamin M, McGonagle D. The anatomical basis for disease localisation in seronegative spondyloarthropathy at entheses and related sites. J Anat. 2001;199(Pt 5):503–26.
34. Benjamin M, McGonagle D. The enthesis organ concept and its relevance to the spondyloarthropathies. Adv Exp Med Biol. 2009;649:57–70.

Applied Pediatrics Sonoanatomy

4

Yasser El Miedany, Ingrid Möller,
and Maribel Miguel-Pérez

Introduction

In comparison to the adult's sonoanatomy, plasticity and elasticity are two of the most important characteristics of children's anatomy which are the key points to understand the differences with the anatomy of the adult. The knowledge of the characteristics of pediatric anatomy is a requirement to perform a precise examination and interpretation of the ultrasound images. One of the major differences between the musculoskeletal system of infants and adults is that infants have more bones as compared to adults (a newborn human has about 300 bones) [1]. This has been attributed to the fact that adults' bones fuse together to form single bones as they age. When this happens, the fused bones are counted as one instead of counting them as different ones in the case of young children (ending up with 206 bones) [2]. Another difference between the bones of children and adults is that the musculoskeletal system of young children is composed of cartilage, while that of adults is composed of solid bone tissue. As the aging process takes place, the bones undergo an ossification process which transforms the cartilage into bone. A third difference is the bone structure itself which differs in the children when compared to the adults. The bone structure of children is more flexible as compared to that of aged people. This has been attributed to the large cartilage component in the infants' musculoskeletal system. This may also explain why children's bones tend to fracture differently. Children's bones tend to break along their length, rather than across the shaft. The process of growing the bone structure goes on until the 20s when the bone stops growing reaching the adult age. Besides growing, the children's skeleton is modeling. Bone modeling reflects the reaction of developing bone (i.e., cartilaginous precursor, metaphyses, epiphyses, and articular surfaces) to imposed forces (e.g., decreased or increased density) ensuring optimum strain response and lightness. This section is intended

Y. El Miedany (✉)
Medway Foundation Trust, King's College London, London, Kent, UK

Rheumatology and Rehabilitation, Ain Shams University, Cairo, Egypt

I. Möller
Unit of Human Anatomy and Embryology, Department of Experimental Pathology and Therapeutic, Faculty of Medicine and Health Sciences (C.Bellvitge), University of Barcelona, Barcelona, Spain

Instituto Poal de Reumatologia, Barcelona, Spain

M. Miguel-Pérez
Unit of Human Anatomy and Embryology, Department of Experimental Pathology and Therapeutic, Faculty of Medicine and Health Sciences (C.Bellvitge), University of Barcelona, Barcelona, Spain
e-mail: mimiguel@ub.edu

Y. El Miedany (ed.), *Pediatric Musculoskeletal Ultrasonography*,
https://doi.org/10.1007/978-3-030-17824-6_4

to highlight the structures of greatest interest in children's musculoskeletal ultrasound imaging and describe their differences with respect to the skeletal anatomy of the adult.

Development of the Skeleton in Children-Prenatal: Basic Science

Bones

Throughout fetal development and into childhood growth and development, bone forms on the cartilaginous matrix. Both the cartilaginous and bony tissues are formed from the mesenchyme, an embryonic connective tissue derived from the mesoderm. The mesenchymal cells differentiate into chondroblasts which produce the hyaline cartilage and build the primordial skeleton, a miniature copy of the future skeleton. In the course of development, this hyaline cartilage is replaced by bone tissue. Except for the clavicle and skull bones, the remaining parts of the skeleton will be formed in part by chondral osteogenesis. The formation of an individual bone is called osteogenesis, while ossification is the term that defines the formation of bone tissue.

There are five types of bones in the human body: long, short, flat, irregular, and sesamoid. Long bones are characterized by a shaft, the diaphysis, that is much longer than its width, and by an epiphysis, a rounded head at each end of the shaft. They are made up mostly of compact bone, with lesser amounts of marrow, located within the medullary cavity, and areas of spongy, cancellous bone at the ends of the bones. Most bones of the limbs, including those of the fingers and toes, are long bones. The exceptions are the eight carpal bones of the wrist, the seven articulating tarsal bones of the ankle, and the sesamoid bone of the kneecap. Long bones such as the clavicle that have a differently shaped shaft or ends are also called modified long bones [3].

The diaphyses of the long bones arise directly from the mesenchyme, the so-called direct or desmal osteogenesis. While the ossification of the diaphysis begins in the eighth week of the embryonic period, the ossification of the bone epiphyses does not start until after the birth except for the distal epiphysis of the femur and proximal of the tibia present at birth (Fig. 4.1). The ossification of the remaining epiphyses occurs through the secondary ossification centers, which are called apophyses. During skeletal maturation, the apophyses in the skeleton are regions where muscles or ligaments are inserted and are biomechanically more unstable in addition to being subject to different types of force mainly tensile forces. In the child it is more frequent to find apophyseal fractures than muscular or ligamentous lesions. Consequently, when the apophyses get subjected to traction forces rather than compressive forces, it can be a point of interest, particularly when it gets inflamed causing pain. An example of this is the anterior tuberosity of the tibial bone that during the development responds to the traction generating a variable amount of fibrocartilage. Repetitive stress or muscle strain can produce apophysitis, a common cause of pediatric pain (Fig. 4.2). The secondary ossification centers ossify predictably according to the age and gender of the individual [4].

The Latin word for bone is os; hence there are many terms that use it as a prefix – such as osseous and osteopathy – whereas all disorders of the endochondral ossification are included in a broader term: osteochondrosis.

On the other hand, most of the short bones of the tarsus and all of the carpus bones are entirely cartilaginous at the time of birth and do not form their own bone ossification center/s until sometime later.

Understanding the bone morphological development helps to understand some of the morphological anomalies that may occur. Example is the development of the foot bones. In the seventh embryonic week, there is still angulation of the foot in relation to the leg, with both feet facing each other, and the foot is in an equine position with respect to the leg. The entire lower limb is in external rotation in this embryonic period. With the internal rotation of the lower extremities, the foot acquires its angular position, although it maintains a marked supination. Equinism (equinus is a condition in which the upward bending

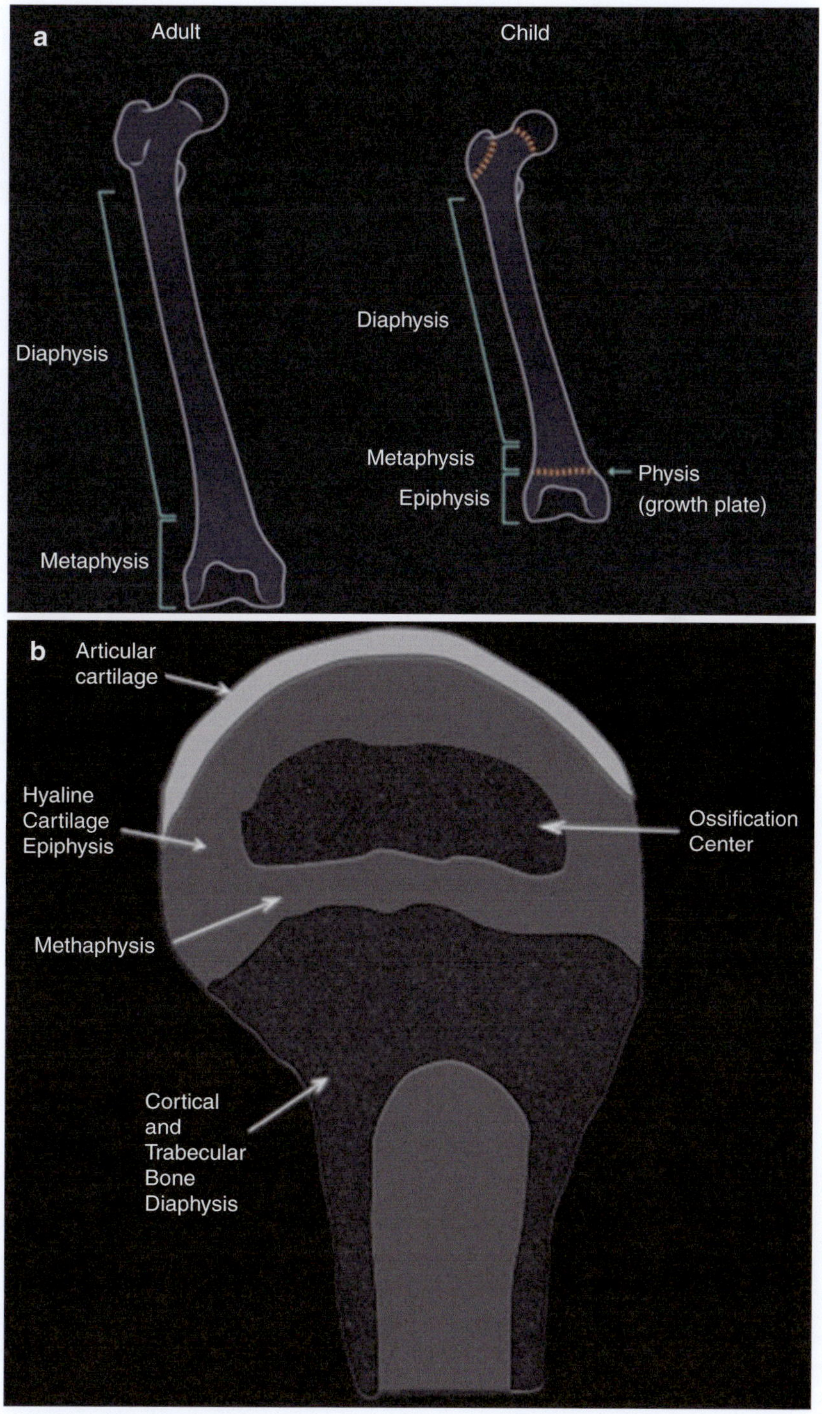

Fig. 4.1 Bone development in children versus adults. Since the growth cartilage contains a high amount of water, it usually appears as anechoic structure. With advancing maturity, the epiphyseal secondary ossification center will appear (**a**). This is seen on musculoskeletal US as hyperechoic stricture with a smooth or irregular surface within the cartilage. (**b**) Schematic structure of the articular end of the bone

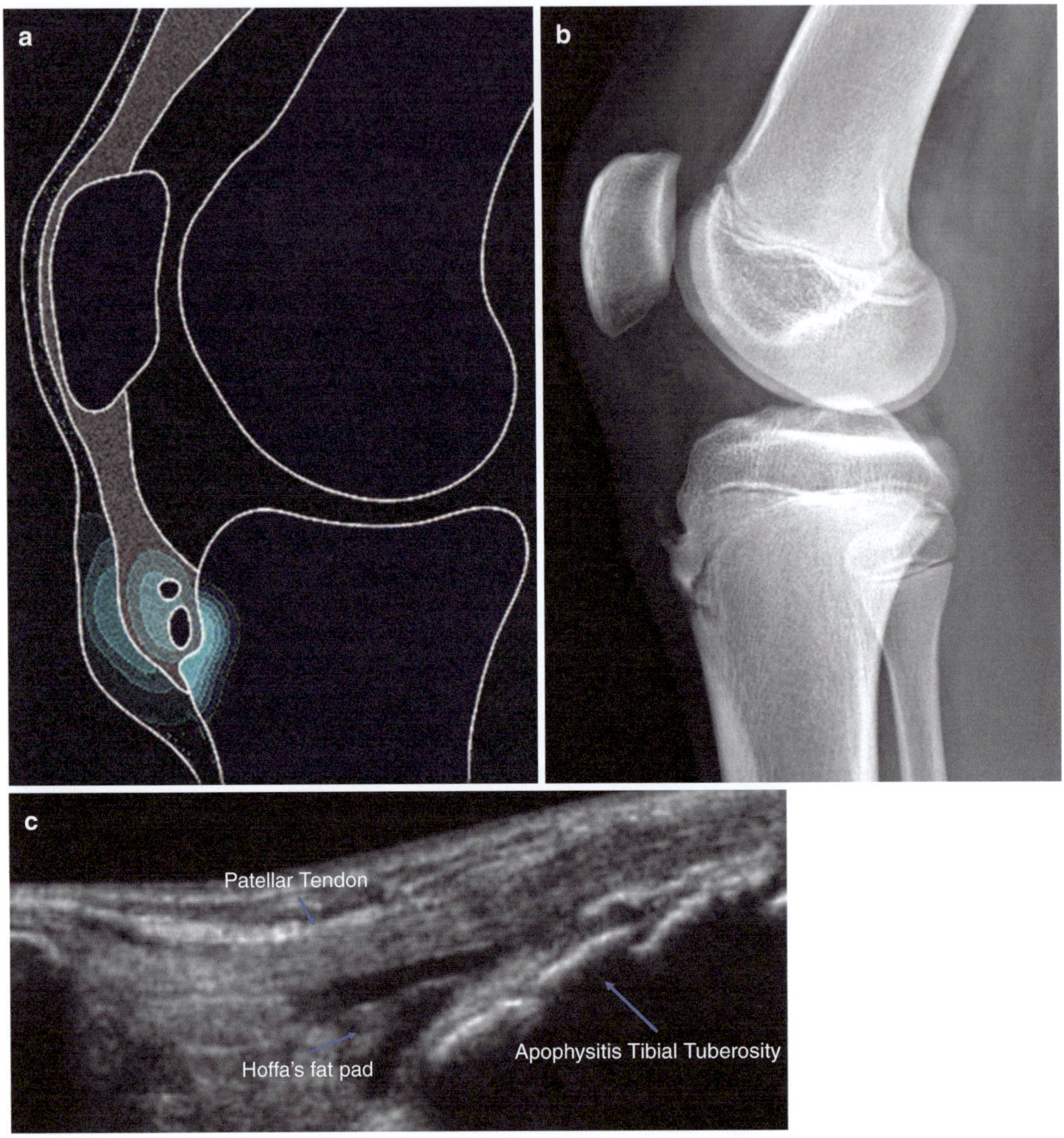

Fig. 4.2 Apophysitis: Osgood-Schlatter disease showing fragmentation of the ossification center. (**a**) Diagram showing the pathology site; (**b**) X-ray knee joint lateral view showing apophysitis of the anterior aspect of the tibial tuberosity; (**c**) longitudinal US scan of the infrapatellar region showing fragmentation of the tibial tuberosity

motion of the ankle joint is limited) is corrected in the fourth month of development, and pronation of the foot is not completed until after birth. Regarding ossification, the forefoot ossifies before the hindfoot.

On another front, in joints such as the hip, development occurs by segmentation, which is the most frequent way. In the hip, the slit and joint cavity are formed from the eighth embryonic week when the joint capsule also develops, initiating the formation of synovial fluid. By week 12, cartilage is formed whose nutrition cannot rely only on the synovial fluid, which is insufficient; hence, blood vessels arise along the cartilaginous ducts, except in the area near the articular slit. This vascularization is not related to the appearance of secondary epiphyseal bone center (Uhthoff). The presence of fat pads within the capsule, visible in joints such as

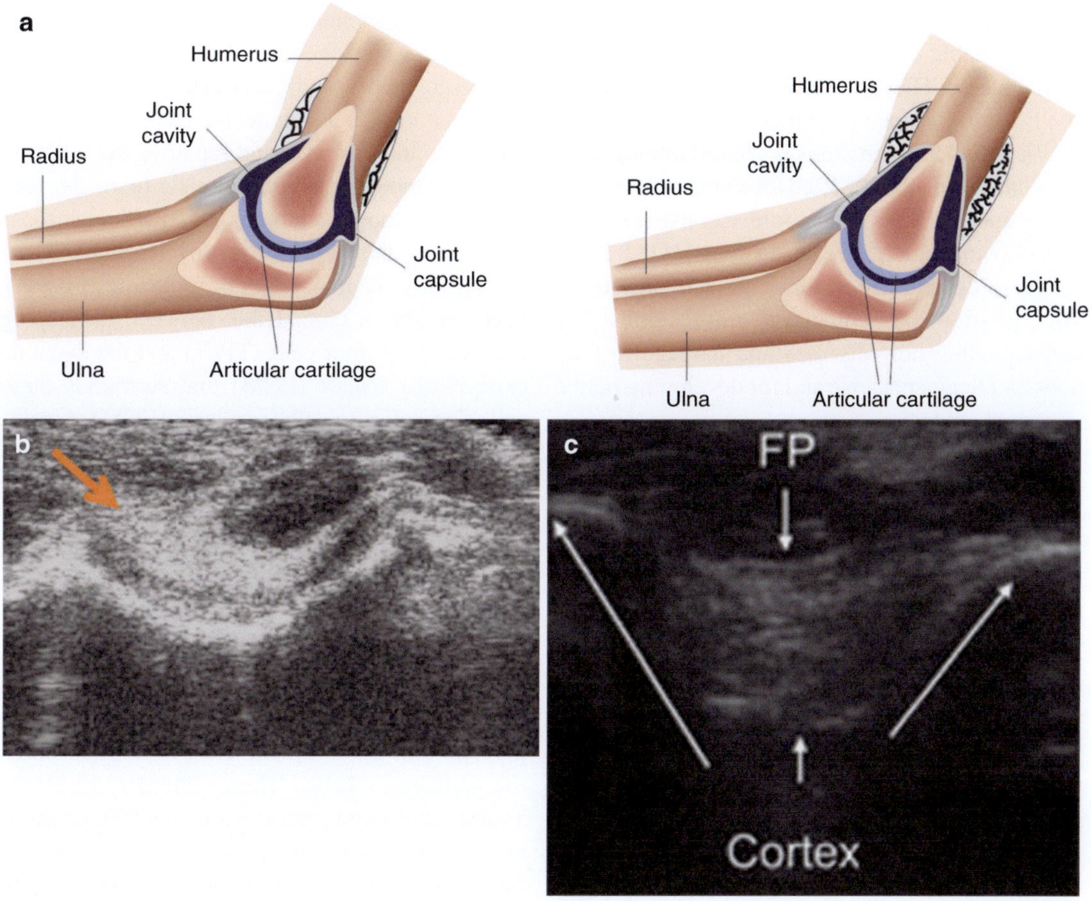

Fig. 4.3 (**a**) Diagram showing the fat pad in the elbow joint. (**b**) US of the elbow joint, transverse views showing normal posterior fat pad. The "sail sign" refers to the posterior fat pad visible on the lateral X-ray. (**c**) Transverse US elbow joint showing elevated posterior fat pad

the elbow or the ankle, is helpful to identify synovitis in children as well as in adult (Fig. 4.3). In patients with synovitis, a displacement of the capsular fat pad can be seen.

Other joints such as sacroiliac or temporomandibular joints develop by sedimentation or approach of two osseous elements initially separated from each other.

Tendons

Tendons and ligaments are connective tissues that transmit mechanical forces between muscles and bones. Tendons attach muscle to skeleton, whereas ligaments attach skeletal elements to each other and stabilize skeletal joints. Vertebrates have evolved a remarkable variety of tendons and ligaments to accommodate their distinct modes of locomotion as well as their dramatic variations in body size and strength. These range from broad sheets to highly elastic cables, such as those of the Achilles tendon and the cruciate ligaments of the knee. Because of their structural roles, injuries to tendons and ligaments are extremely common and often debilitating [5]. Thus, a fundamental question in musculoskeletal biology is how these connective tissue structures develop in the correct locations and acquire the strength necessary to translate contractions of muscles into skeletal movements.

Both tendons and ligaments contain fibroblasts (termed tenocytes and ligamentocytes, respectively) embedded in a unique extracellular matrix

(ECM) that is composed mainly of collagen fibril arrays capable of withstanding incredibly strong tensile forces. These fibrils are cross-linked to one another and wrapped in a tendon sheath (Fig. 4.4) [6, 7]. This basic structure is shared among tendons and ligaments [8–10]. However, each tendon or ligament differs in its precise extracellular matrix composition, size, and strength [11]. How are these differences established? The answer to this question has important implications for understanding how diseases and damage to tendons and ligaments arise and for developing better treatment strategies.

Despite their pivotal roles in musculoskeletal connectivity and functional stability, the mechanisms that control tendon development have received less attention than the processes of myogenesis or skeletogenesis. Only few factors are known to help specify tenocyte progenitor cells (TPCs) at muscle attachments, induce them to differentiate and maintain and repair in the adult [9, 12–14]. Studies in animal models (e.g., fly, fish, chick, and mouse embryos), in particular those focusing on the formation of myotendinous junctions (MTJs; the major sites of force transmission), have revealed a crucial link between developing tenocyte progenitor cells (TPCs) and the dynamic extracellular matrix (ECM) that surrounds these cells. Indeed, extracellular matrix (ECM) proteins (e.g., collagens, laminins, thrombospondins) initially guide myofibers to their sites of attachment but also mediate signaling between tenocyte progenitor cells and muscles, regulate the maturation of myotendinous junctions, and maintain tendons in response to mechanical force [15–17].

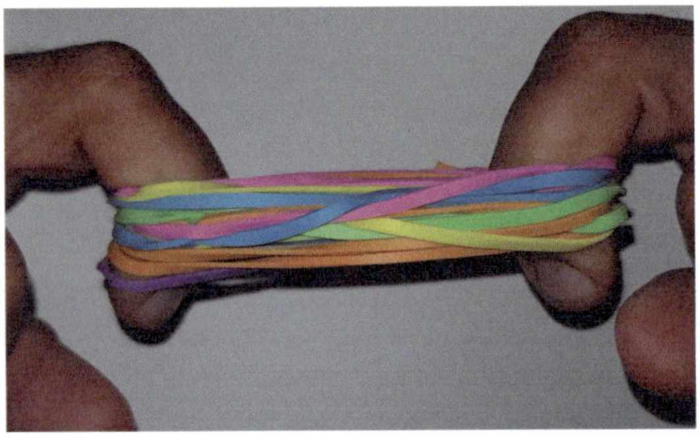

Fig. 4.4 Energetic loading of ligaments and tendons: the anatomical arrangement of muscle and tendon enhances limb versatility and locomotor performance

As myotendinous junctions (MTJs) mature, tenocytes secrete the bulk of the MTJ/tendon ECM, particularly the many proteins and proteoglycans that make up the core functional units, the collagen fibrils. These interact with one another and align into groups of fibrils or fascicles during progressive phases of muscle attachment. This fibrillar organization is essential for tendons to bear the stress of muscle contraction and prevent bone detachment (avulsion fractures) by controlling force distribution (Fig. 4.5)

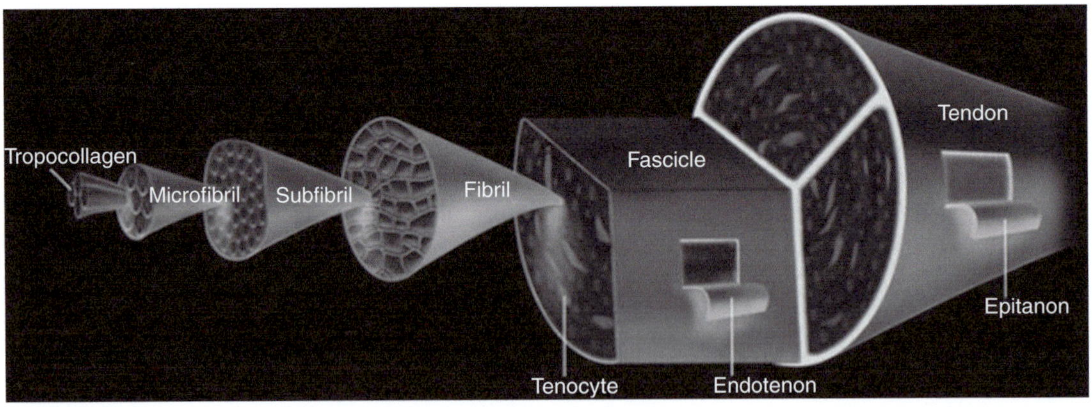

Fig. 4.5 The fibrillar organization of the tendon: the tendon's hierarchical structure begins at the molecular level with tropocollagen. Approximately every five tropocollagen molecules form a microfibril, which then aggregate to create a subfibril. Several subfibrils form a single fibril. Multiple fibrils form a tendon fascicle, and fascicles, separated by the endotenon, join to form the macroscopic tendon. Tendon fibroblasts, or tenocytes, are found on collagen fibers allowing for the regulation of the extracellular environment in response to chemical and mechanical stimuli

[11, 16]. The fibrillar network of proteins includes (1) core force-transmitting, structural collagens (particularly Col1a1, Col1a2, Col2a1, and Col3a1), (2) scaffolding proteins [e.g., Tsp2 (Thbs2), Tsp4, Comp, Lama2], and (3) specialized cross-linking collagens (e.g., Col6a1, Col12a1, Col14a1, and Col22a1) and various cross-linking factors [e.g., Dcn, Fmod, biglycan (Bgn)], which hold fibrils together to distribute forces efficiently and reduce friction [18, 19]. Although the integration of structural collagens into fibrils has been well documented, recent studies have provided insight into the functions of scaffolding proteins and specialized collagens during fibril assembly. These studies suggest that similar to the early extracellular matrix (ECM) at developing MTJs, extracellular matrix proteins of the maturing tendon provide continuous feedback in response to mechanical force [20–23].

In reference to the tendons development and maturation, taking as an example the peroneus longus, the first synovial sheath develops in the plantar aspect of the tendon with its corresponding mesotenon, later developing the synovial sheaths of both peroneal tendons that extend proximally, penetrating into the superior retromalleolar segment [24].

Ligaments and Retinacula

Ligaments are similar to tendons and fasciae as they are all made of connective tissue. The differences in them are in the connections that they make: ligaments connect one bone to another bone, tendons connect muscle to bone, and fasciae connect muscles to other muscles (Fig. 4.6). These are all found in the skeletal system of the human body. Ligaments cannot usually be regenerated naturally.

Ligament most commonly refers to a band of dense regular connective tissue bundles made of collagenous fibers, with bundles protected by dense irregular connective tissue sheaths. Some ligaments limit the mobility of articulations or prevent certain movements altogether. Capsular ligaments are part of the articular capsule that surrounds synovial joints. They act as mechanical reinforcements. Extracapsular ligaments join together in harmony with the other ligaments and provide joint stability. Intracapsular ligaments, which are much less common, also provide stability but permit a far larger range of motion. Cruciate ligaments are paired ligaments in the form of a cross [25].

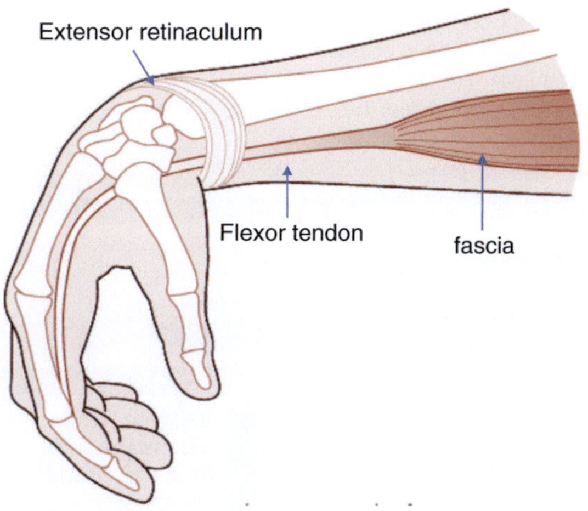

Fig. 4.6 The differences between the ligament, tendon, and fascia: ligaments connect one bone to another bone, tendons connect muscle to bone, and fasciae connect muscles to other muscles. Flexor retinaculum, quadriceps tendon, fascia

Ligaments are viscoelastic. They gradually strain when under tension and return to their original shape when the tension is removed. However, they cannot retain their original shape when extended past a certain point or for a prolonged period of time [26–28]. This is one reason why dislocated joints must be set as quickly as possible: if the ligaments lengthen too much, then the joint will be weakened, becoming prone to future dislocations. Athletes, gymnasts, dancers, and martial artists perform stretching exercises to lengthen their ligaments, making their joints more supple.

The term hypermobility refers to children or adults with more elastic ligaments, allowing their joints to stretch and contort further; this is sometimes still called double-jointedness. The consequence of a broken ligament can be instability of the joint. Not all broken ligaments need surgery, but, if surgery is needed to stabilize the joint, the broken ligament can be repaired. Scar tissue may prevent this. If it is not possible to fix the broken

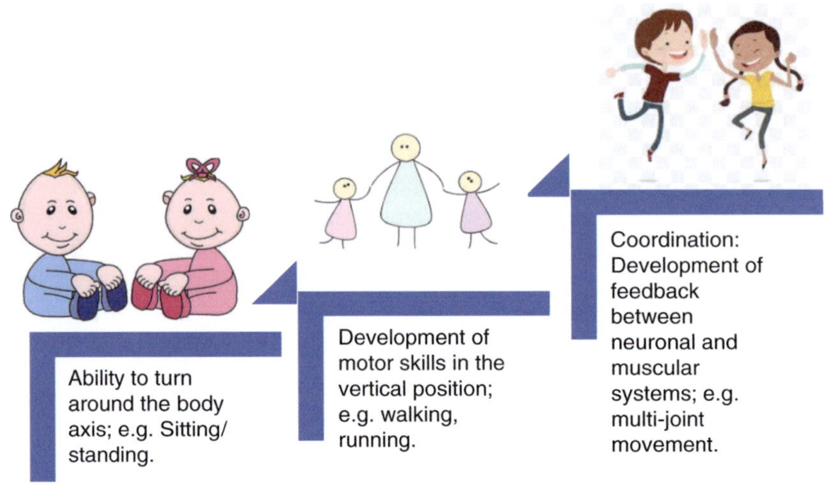

Fig. 4.7 Diagram showing the three phases of motor skills development. Phase 1, ability to turn around the body axis; phase 2, development of motor skills in the vertical axis; and phase 3, coordination accuracy of multi-joint movements such as stand or jump on one leg

ligament, other procedures such as the Brunelli procedure can correct the instability. Instability of a joint can over time lead to wear of the cartilage and eventually to osteoarthritis.

Muscles and Nerves

The skeletal and muscular systems are very closely linked; hence they are often referred to as the musculoskeletal system. In pediatrics, milestones of child development are typically related to the development of motor skills. Therefore, the assessment of motor performance serves as a useful measure for the evaluation of brain development in the first year of life. For example, typical milestones are the ability to turn around the body axis at the age of 3–7 months, sitting at 5–10 months and standing freely at 10–17 months [20]. In contrast to the first year of life, the next steps of the human development are characterized by the development of motor skills in the vertical position (walking, running, jumping, etc.) [29].

Thereby, the development of motor skills needs permanent feedback between neuronal (CNS and peripheral nerves) and muscular components (skeletal element, tendon, and skeletal muscle) of the motor system. For example, a 4-year-old child is usually able to stand on one leg, whereas a 2-year-old child is not. This is due to better motor skills rather than increased muscle power. Thus, the accuracy of multi-joint movements depends markedly on the developmental stage of a child, which should tremendously influence the assessment of muscle force and power [30] (Fig. 4.7).

Most skeletal muscles develop before birth, and almost all remaining muscles are formed by the end of the first year of life. Increase in the size of muscles is due to an increase in the diameter of the muscle fibers; and muscles increase in length as well as width in order to grow with the skeleton. Not all embryonic muscle fibers persist, as many fail to establish themselves as viable units of muscle and ultimately perish.

The composition of muscle varies with age. During fetal development, muscle fibers contain to a great deal more water and intercellular matrix. After birth, both of these structures reduce as the cells grow in size by accumulating cytoplasm. Muscle fibrils remain constant in their diameter; as the muscle grows, fibrils increase in length, hence, growing at that their ends.

The growth of the connective tissue element of a muscle is maximal in the vicinity of the junction of the tendon with the muscle. After birth, mitotic structures in the skeletal muscle do not appear within the structure of the muscle fibers, but in the undifferentiated cells outside them. These are described as "satellite cells." Interestingly, there are sex differences in the number of muscle fibers found in the muscles of girls and boys. The number of muscle fibers found in the gluteal muscles of boys increases 14-fold between birth and maturity. However, in girls it is estimated that the increase is in the order of tenfold. Furthermore,

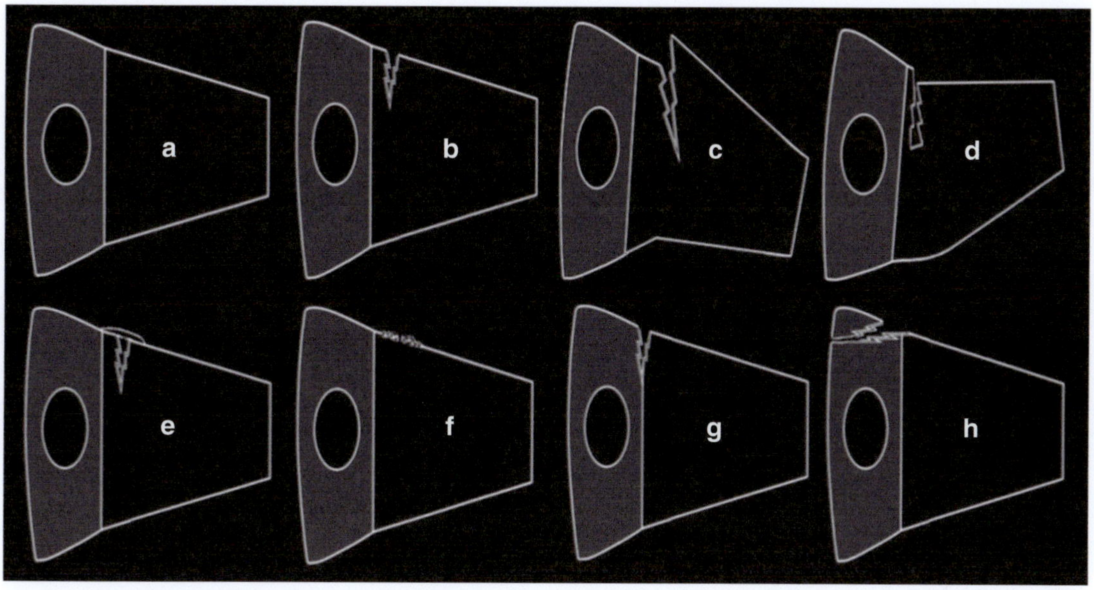

Fig. 4.8 Fracture in pediatric bones: summarized diagram of US findings of occult fractures: (**a**) normal; (**b**) non-displaced (hairline) fracture; (**c**) minimally displaced fracture with step-off deformity; (**d**) impact fracture with step-off deformity; (**e**) fracture with double-line cortex; F, fracture with diffuse irregularity of bone surface; G, growth plate fracture; and H, avulsion fracture. The pediatric bone has a periosteal layer thicker than in adult providing different functions: it prevents bony displacement and has a relevant role in the children's skeletal remodeling

muscle fibers attain a maximum diameter in girls at approximately 10 years of age, but not until approximately 14 years in boys.

Maximal muscle strength is usually attained between 25 and 30 years of age, after which there is a gradual decline in the speed and power of muscles. The muscles of the upper body, particularly those of the head, trunk, and upper limbs, are relatively heavier in the infant due to the relatively poor development of the lower limbs. The respiratory muscles and the muscles associated with facial expression are well developed at term to facilitate vital functioning of breathing and suckling [31].

The Peculiarities of Bone in Development

Imaging

Basically, children's bones are substantially different than adults. Infants start off with a skeleton made of cartilage that matures into calcified bone during the early years of development. This explains why during the first few weeks of life, ultrasounds are frequently used to examine children's bones instead of X-rays. As children grow and develop, their bones have a softer structure than adults. The softer characteristic allows their bones to fracture or break in different ways than adult bones do (Fig. 4.8).

In comparison to adults, the main characters of children's bones are the presence of growth plates in children's bones, the continuous modification, and the vascularization.

These impact on the ways doctors treat and care for injuries as well as bone and joint disorders in children [32].

Bone Ossification

Ossification is a landmark in children's skeletal anatomy, making a key difference between the children and adult musculoskeletal systems. The long bone, more accessible from a musculoskeletal ultrasound point of view, is made up of three different regions, two of them cartilaginous, the epiphysis and the physis, and the third is the osseous diaphysis whose terminal ends constitute

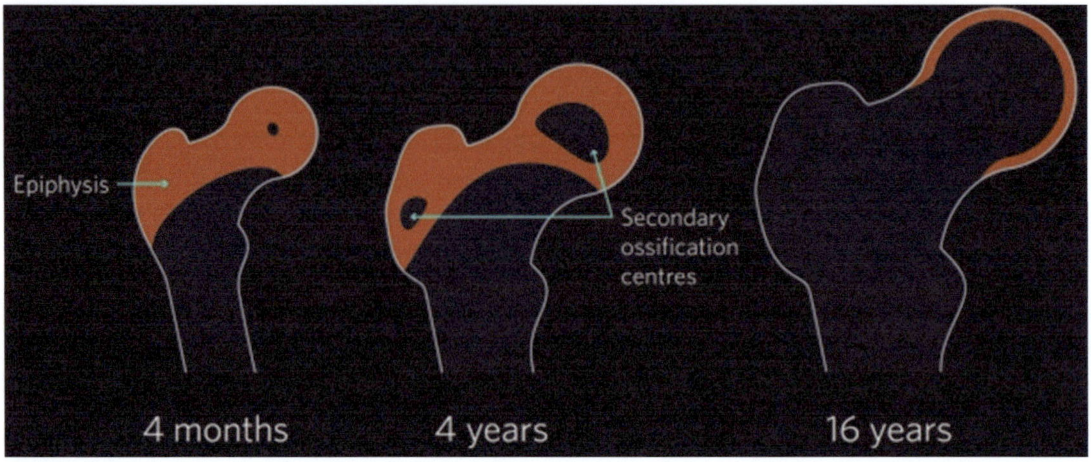

Fig. 4.9 Ossification of the head of the femur: ossification of the ischium, ilium, pubis, femoral shaft, and distal femoral epiphysis occurs before birth. The femoral head ossifies between the second and eighth postnatal months and fuses with the neck between 15 and 21 years in boys and 1 year earlier in girls

the metaphysis (Fig. 4.9). The long bone maturity is achieved throughout an endochondral ossification process, the formation of bone from a cartilaginous anlage. The orientation of collagen fibers in the growing immature bone is characteristic: transphyseal and perichondral are longitudinal and perichondral ring and metaphyseal bone circumferential, whereas epiphyseal are radial. The tensile strengths transmitted by the collagen fibers have a decisive morphological influence on the development of immature bone; its interruption whatever the cause, traumatic or chemical, can lead to pathological consequences altering the morphology of the bone [33, 34].

Growth Plates

Children's growth plates are the center for bone growth. Growth plates consist of developing cartilage tissue near the end of long bones. Bones grow from the ends where the growth plates are located. Fractures can occur within and near the growth plates. These require different types of treatment compared to similar injuries in adults to avoid later problems with growth. At times the growth of a bone near a fracture can even assist in the bone healing and correcting the fracture which adds to differences in treating kids versus adults.

The Epiphysis

The epiphysis is connected with the metaphysis throughout mammillary processes and the periosteum (Fig. 4.10). The mammillary processes are small interdigitations of cartilage present in a variable number extending into the metaphyseal bone and contributing to the intrinsic stability of the physis against shearing forces. The cartilaginous epiphysis of the long bone is responsible for increasing in length; it can be considered as a secondary ossification center that appears at various ages to be able to determine the skeletal age although the sequence of ossification can vary according to different sources.

The Physis

The key difference between the child's bone and that of an adult is the presence of a physis. The growth plate, or physis, is the translucent, cartilaginous disc separating the epiphysis from the metaphysis and is responsible for longitudinal growth of long bones (Fig. 4.11).

The cells of the physis are arranged in columns or layers described as the germinal or resting layer, the proliferative zone, the hypertrophic zone, and the zone of provisional calcification (Fig. 4.10). The proliferative zone is where the chondrocytes undergo rapid division by mitosis and is the most metabolically active zone. Osteoblasts use the chondrocyte columns as a scaffold for ossification in the zone of provisional calcification.

The hypertrophic zone is the weakest because it lacks both collagen and calcified tissue.

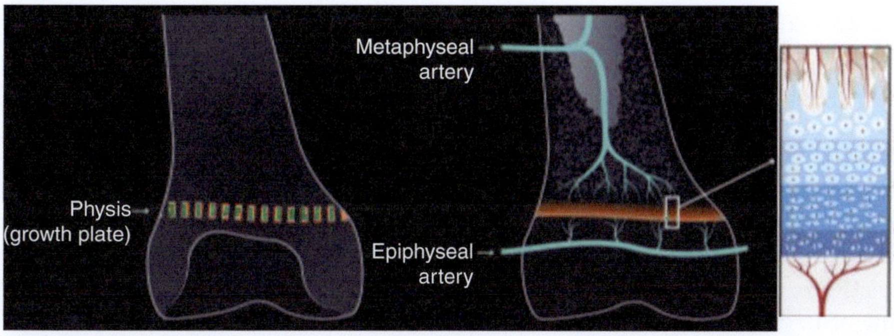

Fig. 4.10 The junction between the epiphyses and metaphyses: the growth plate, or physis, is the translucent, cartilaginous disc separating the epiphysis from the metaphysis and is responsible for longitudinal growth of long bones. The cells of the physis are arranged in columns or layers described as the germinal or resting layer, the proliferative zone, the hypertrophic zone, and the zone of provisional calcification. The proliferative zone is where the chondrocytes undergo rapid division by mitosis and is the most metabolically active zone. Osteoblasts use the chondrocyte columns as a scaffold for ossification in the zone of provisional calcification. The hypertrophic zone is the weakest because it lacks both collagen and calcified tissue. Most physeal separations occur through this layer because it is less able to resist shearing stress

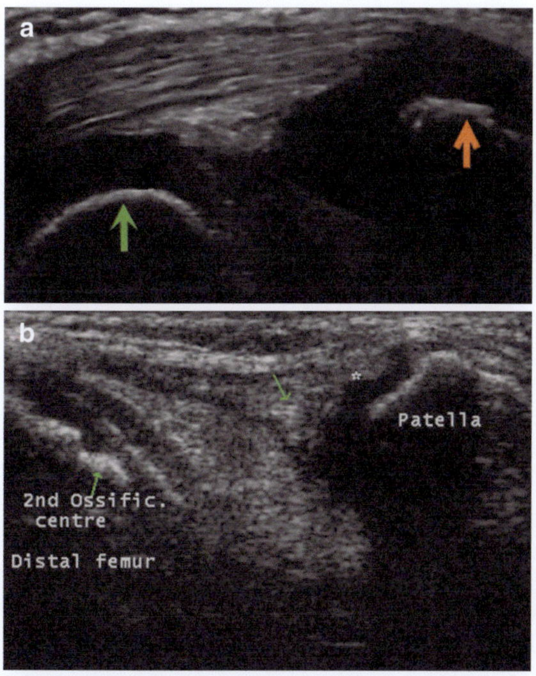

Fig. 4.11 Transverse ultrasound scan of parapatellar knee recess. The image provides anatomic information on the following structures: suprapatellar recess, superior edge of the patella, and distal end of the femur. (**a**) A 7-year-old child's knee joint: the image also depicts the patella as an unossified structure located anterior to the distal epiphysis of the femoral condyle. (**b**) A 13-year-old boy's knee joint: epiphyseal cartilage of the femoral condyle and the patella decrease during the growth of the child

Most physeal separations occur through this layer because it is less able to resist shearing stress. Around the knee, the stresses are high, and in order to resist shear, the physis interdigitates with surrounding bone in what are known as mammillary bodies. This anatomic arrangement locks the physis solidly. If it does sustain a shear injury, there is a higher chance of developing a bony bar across the physis and subsequent growth arrest.

A basic principle of physiology indicates that the more metabolically active, the more it is susceptible to injury. Therefore, the growing plates are the most vulnerable to damage particularly when they are actively growing as in prepubertal and pubertal age. However, there is no evidence to associate growth pains with ossification process. In rickets the hypertrophic zone cannot be replaced by osseous tissue with failure of the vessel invasion from the metaphysis.

The growth plates, or physis, are visible on virtually all images obtained in skeletally immature children. The physis is relatively thick in infancy and childhood; the physis vascularity decreases with age as the marrow undergoes a transformation from hematopoietic vascularized marrow to fatty marrow. An injury at the physis level can generate grown arrest. The epiphysiodesis is the normal replacement of the physis during the adolescence, beginning earlier in females than in males; it means a complete exchange from cartilaginous tissue to bone tissue; the characteristic line formed at this level can be evidenced radiologically in some anatomical locations in the adult.

There is a specialized region surrounding the physis in the zone of proliferation, the zone of Ranvier containing mesenchymal tissue, epiphyseal and physeal cartilage, fibrovascular tissue, and the osseous ring of Lacroix which acts as a peripheral mechanical restrain of the physis. This region may have a radiographic step-off appearance because it does not grow continuously. The appositional grow of the physis occurs primarily from the zone of Ranvier and limits the latitudinal development of the physis.

The Metaphysis

The metaphyses (singular: metaphysis) are the narrow portion of a long bone between the epiphysis and the diaphysis. It contains the growth plate, the part of the bone that grows during childhood, and as it grows it ossifies near the diaphysis and the epiphyses (Fig. 4.12). The metaphysis may be divided anatomically into three components based on tissue content: a cartilaginous component (epiphyseal plate), a bony component (metaphysis), and a fibrous component surrounding the periphery of the plate. The part of the metaphysis where the calcified cartilage becomes vascularized is called "primary spongiosa bone"; osteoblasts can be identified lining up on the calcified cartilage. When no calcified cartilage is present, the trabeculae are named "secondary spongiosa bone." The metaphysis is responsible for bone formation and remodeling and vascular invasion; in principle, it is a region with intense osteoblastic activity and the location where the greatest bone remodeling takes place.

The Vascularization

Vascular supply of long bones depends on several points of inflow, which feed complex sinusoidal networks within the bone. These in turn drain to various channels through all surfaces of the bone except that covered by articular cartilage. One or two main diaphyseal nutrient arteries enter the shaft obliquely through one or two nutrient foramina leading to nutrient canals. Their sites of entry and angulation are almost constant and characteristically directed away from the growing epiphysis. Except for a few with double or no foramina, 90% of long bones have a single nutrient foramen in the middle third of the shaft. The nutrient arteries divide into ascending and descending branches in the medullary cavity, dividing into smaller rami. Near the epiphysis they anastomose with the metaphyseal and epiphyseal arteries (Fig. 4.13). Metaphyseal arteries

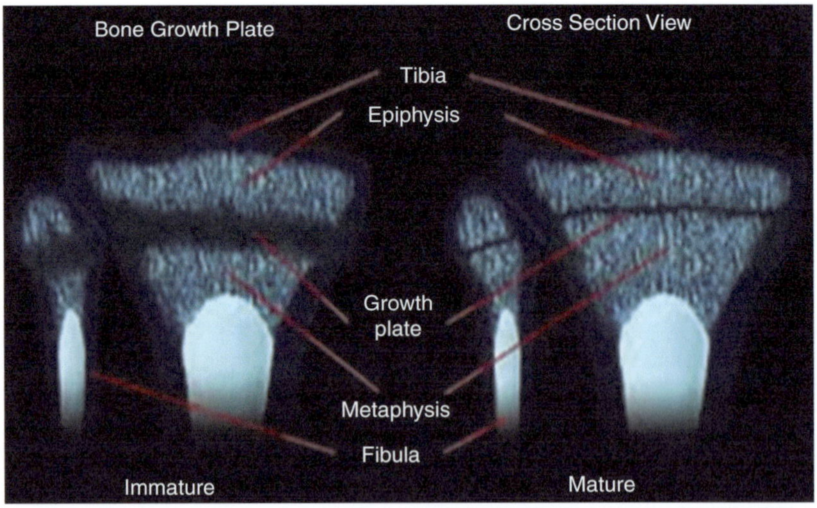

Fig. 4.12 Growth plate: the epiphyseal plate is the area of growth in a long bone. It is a layer of hyaline cartilage where ossification occurs in immature bones. On the epiphyseal side of the epiphyseal plate, cartilage is formed. On the diaphyseal side, cartilage is ossified, and the diaphysis grows in length

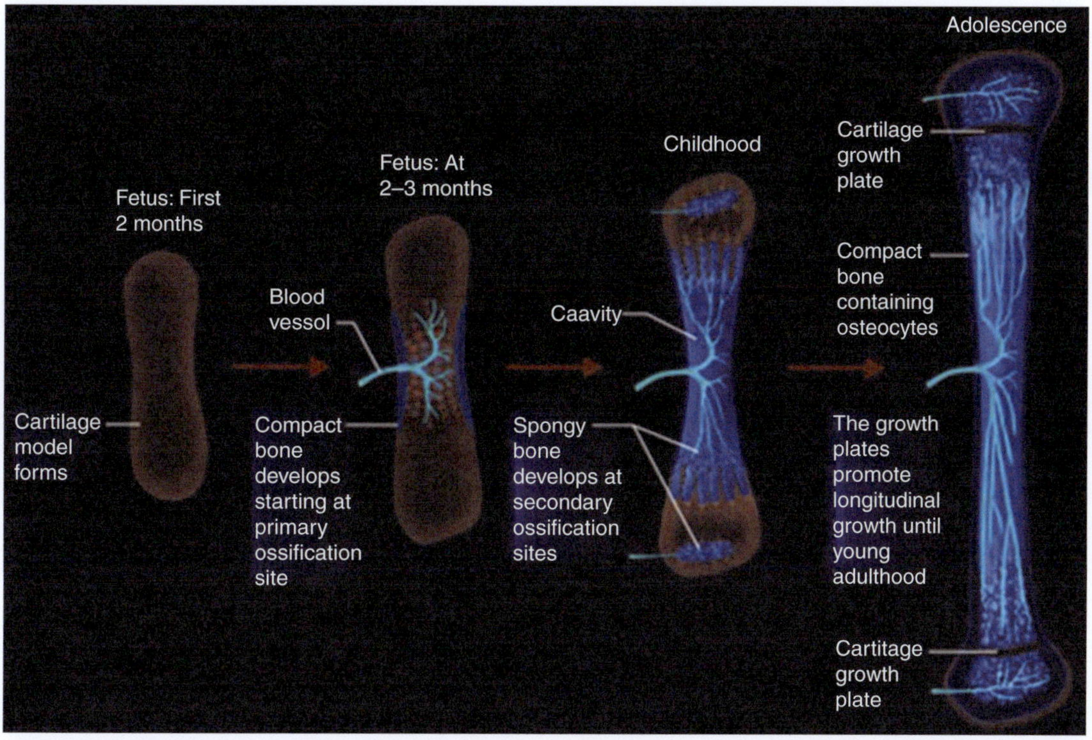

Fig. 4.13 Bone development and vascularization: the vasculature in bone appears to be formed mainly or perhaps even exclusively by angiogenesis. In murine long bones, blood vessels start to invade the cartilage template at embryonic day 13.5–14.5, and vascular growth is largely completed in adolescent and young adult animals. This process of endochondral angiogenesis involves a series of events. First, chondrocytes in the location of the future primary ossification center (POC) cease proliferation, become hypertrophic, and secrete pro-angiogenic factors to stimulate angiogenesis; osteoprogenitors in the POC are also a source of pro-angiogenic factors. Next, blood vessels invade the hypertrophic chondrocytes and form an initial vascular network, which is accompanied by ossification processes. The release of signals by maturing and hypertrophic growth plate chondrocytes at the two ends of the developing long bone further promotes vessel growth and ossification along the longitudinal axis, which leads to the extension of the growing skeletal element. This also involves the formation of distinguishable metaphyseal and diaphyseal capillary networks. Later in development, vessels invade the epiphyseal chondrocytes at the two distal ends of the long bone and thereby initiate secondary ossification center (SOC) formation

are the branches of neighboring systemic vessels. They enter the long bones in the region of the metaphysis. Epiphyseal arteries compose the periarticular vascular arcades formed on nonarticular surfaces of the long bones. The physis receives vessels from the metaphysis, epiphysis, and perichondral region of Ranvier (the ossification groove of Ranvier is a wedge-shaped collection of cells pushing into the reserve and proliferative regions of the growth plate. It also appears to supply cells for the reserve layer, causing mainly an expansion of the diameter of the growth plate). The vessels run through the physis in channels.

In children there is a complex network of intracartilaginous vessels located in a number of vascular canals within the epiphyseal cartilage that will disappear in the adult. The vascular canals contain arterioles, venules, and capillaries in a loose connective tissue bed. The function of the vascular canals is essential to supply nutrients and in the development of the epiphyseal ossification. The mesenchymal tissue within the canal could be a source of chondroblastic cells. The distribution of the canals is not homogeneous, being numerous around the secondary center of ossification and in areas of high cellular turnover, whereas they decrease with age;

hence, the cartilage will be avascular at the end of the growth [35, 36].

In the younger child, the physis is thicker with fewer undulations, and the epiphysis is very vascular with vascular canals visible within; some of the canals are extending from the metaphysis to the epiphysis in children less than 18 months, and then the transphyseal channels regress. The epiphyseal vascular channels increase their size with maturity and may undergo numerous modifications in the inflammatory patient. In the older child, the physis is thinner with more undulations. Differences in the number and size of vascular channels have been seen in children with achondroplasia or in the case of vertical trauma where trans-epiphyseal channels can be affected, creating abnormal bone bridges that affect normal growth. The level of fracture is of prognostic significance in a growing bone having more impact in arresting the growth when they involved active metabolic regions [37].

The growing cartilage anatomy, function, and pathological changes have been best studied by magnetic resonance imaging (MRI) supporting the clinical relevance of the vessel channels. Ischemia of the epiphyseal cartilage during endochondral ossification has been related to the pathogenesis of **osteochondritis dissecans**. Common sites of osteochondritis dissecans include the femoral condyles, talar dome, and capitellum. Consequently, osteochondritis causes thickness loss of articular and epiphyseal cartilage as well as cartilage contour irregularity. The increase of vascularization and the high metabolism of the cartilage make it less frequent to identify osseous erosive changes in the child in relation to the adult [38, 39].

Bone Age

The age of each bone can be deduced from the moment of appearance of its ossification center; the primaries will be generally embryonic. With synostosis (fusion of the epiphysis), the longitudinal growth of the bones of the extremities stops. Skeletal age reflects the state of skeletal maturation that is related to future body size. The progression of ossification in the course of 9 years is well established in the bones of the carpus: the large bone (capitulum) has a nucleus of ossification from the first year, while the pisiform is the last to present it around 9 years of age. In the elbow, the first ossification center to appear is the capitulum (1 year old), whereas the last secondary center to ossify is the lateral epicondyle (10 years old). The sequence is as follows: capitulum (1 year old), radial head and medial epicondyle (5–6 year old), trochlea and olecranon (8–10 year old) and lateral epicondyle (10 year old). Bone age is an indicator of the skeletal and biological maturity of an individual. This is different from chronological age, which is calculated using the date of birth of an individual.

As they grow, children will be "reducing" the bones number in their body by fusing together the variable components of the different bones. The ossification changes vary according to the anatomical region considered and the child's age (Table 4.1). For example, the upper limbs are better developed than the lower limbs in the neonates, whereas the lower limbs may bow due to the imbalance between the medial and the lateral gastrocnemius.

Radiography of the hand and wrist is the commonest modality used to calculate bone age. Automated methods for evaluation of hand and wrist radiographs are also being developed which reduce inter-rater variability compared to manual methods [40]. Nonradiation-based techniques of visualizing hand and wrist bones such as ultrasonography for bone age calculation have been theorized but are not as accurate as radiographic methods. By the age of 18 years, bone age cannot

Table 4.1 Appearance of ossific centers

During intrauterine life (primary)	
Calcaneus center	5th month
Talus center	7th month
Lower end of the femur	8th month
Cuboid and upper end of the tibia	At full term
After birth (secondary)	
Head of the humerus and femur	1st
Lower end of the radius	2nd
It attains 2/3 the breadth of the epiphysis	7 years
Upper end of the radius	6 years
Upper end of the ulna	12 years

be computed from hand and wrist radiographs; therefore the medial end of the clavicle is used for bone age calculation in individuals aged 18–22 years. CT visualization of the clavicle has been extensively studied but requires a high dose of radiation. MRI-based methods are being developed but require more research. Dental age is an alternate form of bone age determination, which also gives an estimate of skeletal maturity. The iliac bone and femoral head have also been studied for computation of bone age, but no standardized methods have yet been generated [41].

There are other measurements guiding in how to calculate the size of different anatomical parts; for example, at the age of 1 year in girls and 1.5 years in boys, the foot acquires half of its adult dimension, reaching maturity at 14 years in girls and 16 years in boys with a lower growth in girls from 12 years. The feet grow parallel to the body more than in relation to the lower extremity so that adult size is acquired first in the foot, then in the long bones, and finally in the stature. Interestingly, in women, the foot can still increase in size during and after pregnancy [42].

At the beginning of mid-puberty, the growth rate increases and then decreases later once the epiphyseal fusion has been achieved, that is, the chondrogenesis of the epiphyseal plate is stopped. There is a trend toward earlier physeal fusion in girls compared with boys although there are no anatomic differences between the physes of boys and girls.

A growing individual develops postural habits that have a multifactorial origin, and the chondro-osseous skeleton adapts as the child grows. Maintaining the upright position is a complex work exerted by numerous joints of the body that must coordinate with the center of gravity at all times and adapt to the variation of external conditions and the voluntary motor action. Multimuscle synergies are involved in maintaining vertical position.

Sonoanatomy of Bones in Children

In contrast to radiography, cartilaginous structures within immature joints and epiphyses are well depicted by US. The chondral epiphysis appears speckled and homogenously hypoechoic to anechoic, is well visualized by US, and can serve as an acoustic window to evaluate deeper tissues.

Musculoskeletal ultrasonography has several advantages on the assessment of the musculoskeletal system. Initially, there are no contraindications to musculoskeletal US. In fact, musculoskeletal ultrasound can offer more detail than an MRI. Musculoskeletal US has also the privilege of being dynamic or movement-related image done in real time. This is also supported by the patients' feedback which enables the treating healthcare professional to pinpoint the source of pain at the time of the image. Furthermore, metal and surgical implants are not contraindications and can be visualized on imaging. Doppler can point the examining rheumatologist in the right direction for an accurate diagnosis. In addition, on US examination, it is possible to compare bilateral structures on the same testing day. Also, long structures (like nerves and muscle) can be viewed in their entirety all in one test.

Applied Sonopathology

Visualization of the Skeletal System

Ultrasound (US) is helpful for the early diagnosis of both soft tissue and bone injuries, in children, resulting in appropriate and timely management. US can be performed in young children without sedation, which is frequently required for MRI to prevent a motion artifact. The high reflectivity of US at the interface between the cortical bone and peri-osseous soft tissues can delineate the bone cortical outline and adjacent soft tissue changes [43]. Knowledge of the sonoanatomy and the possible alterations paves the way to correct identification of the sonopathology and, consequently, make the appropriate diagnosis and treatment decisions. These include:

Fractures Children differ from adults in their sensitivity to ionizing radiation since their bony tissues are proliferative and more susceptible to the harmful effects of X-rays. Single case reports of intrauterine fractures and congenital bone disease such as osteogenesis imperfecta diagnosed by ultrasound were published in the early years of the use of B-mode sonography [44–46].

Ultrasound has been used to demonstrate stress fractures [47] and those of the humerus which have been missed on plain radiographs [48]. Radiologists, traumatologists, and physicians have reported that fractures of the ribs may be demonstrated better by ultrasound than by radiography [49–53]. It has also been used to monitor the formation of callus in fractures of the long bones and during limb lengthening [54].

Growth Plate Physeal distance which was measured in millimeters can be defined as the interval between physis and metaphysis/epiphysis. The physis can be measured using 7.5 MHZ ultrasound probe in lateral, medial, and middle points of the growth plate [55]. When present, an ossification center is seen as a central echogenic focus within the epiphysis that demonstrates posterior acoustic shadowing. Similarly, ossified bone is a highly reflective surface with posterior shadowing that precludes evaluation of deeper structures, such as bone marrow which is a relative limitation of musculoskeletal US.

Bone Erosions Bone is often regarded as a barrier to the use of MSUS in clinical practice. This acoustic shadowing from the overlying bones explains why US is less reliable in detecting intramedullary lesions and those within the centers of larger joints [56, 57]. However, studying the cortical bones in sonographically accessible areas represents one of the great advantages of ultrasonography. On US, bone erosions can be seen as interruption of the smooth, continuous hyperechogenic line corresponding to the bony cortex. Marginal erosions are usually seen in inflammatory arthritic diseases and are identified as crater-like defects in the bony contours along the edges of the articular cartilage (Fig. 4.14). Earlier studies supported the superiority of US over radiography in detection of erosions [58, 59]. Experienced ultrasonographers can identify them nearly as well as MRI and notably with lower cost and more efficiency [60].

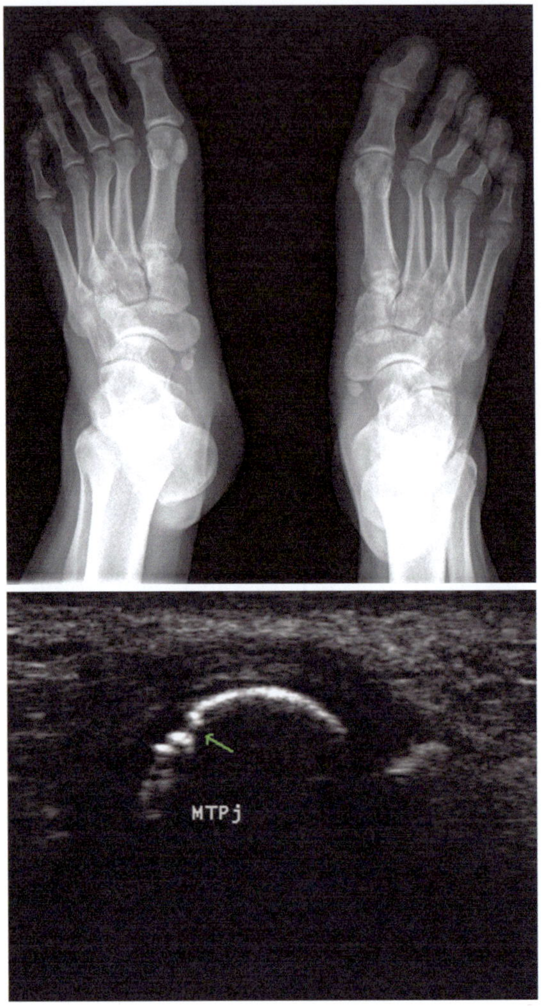

Fig. 4.14 (**a**) X-ray of metatarsophalangeal joints showing erosive inflammatory arthritis. B. Grayscale US longitudinal view of the same foot showing inflammatory synovitis (empty circle) and erosions of the third MTP joint (arrow)

Bone Age Bone age calculated using ultrasound is still in initial stages and needs further refinement. Initial studies carried out using ultrasonography in comparison to the Greulich and Pyle (GP) standard atlas show promising results [61–64]. However, in a few studies, wide discrepancies have also been noted. In order to replace the wrist radiographs, this method needs to be evaluated in multiethnic population with a large sample size.

Quantitative ultrasound (QUS) technology is a radiation-free method currently used for bone

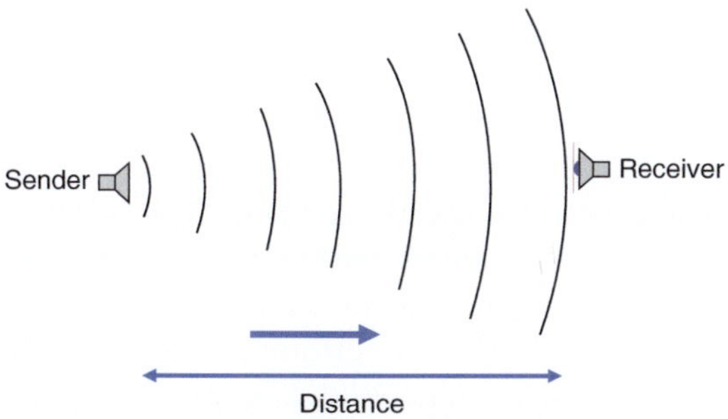

Fig. 4.15 An ultrasound wave is propagated perpendicularly through a medium containing soft tissue and bone, from transmitter (T) to receiver (R). The parameter primarily used in this method is speed of sound (SOS), i.e., time of flight of the ultrasound wave from transmitter to receiver, over the distance (DIS) between the transmitter and receiver. The quantitative US device measures two parameters: speed of propagation through bone of inaudible high frequency waves of a short ultrasound pulse (m/sec) and US attenuation. Ultrasound attenuation is the decay of sound propagation, defined as the reduction in amplitude of the ultrasound beam as a function of distance through a medium. When dealing with attenuation in bone and cartilage as media, both physical processes, which are complicated modalities, have to be taken into account. In addition, the medium length and attenuation coefficient, the frequency of the ultrasound beam, and the structure and viscosity of the bone need to be considered. These parameters are called the attenuation factor

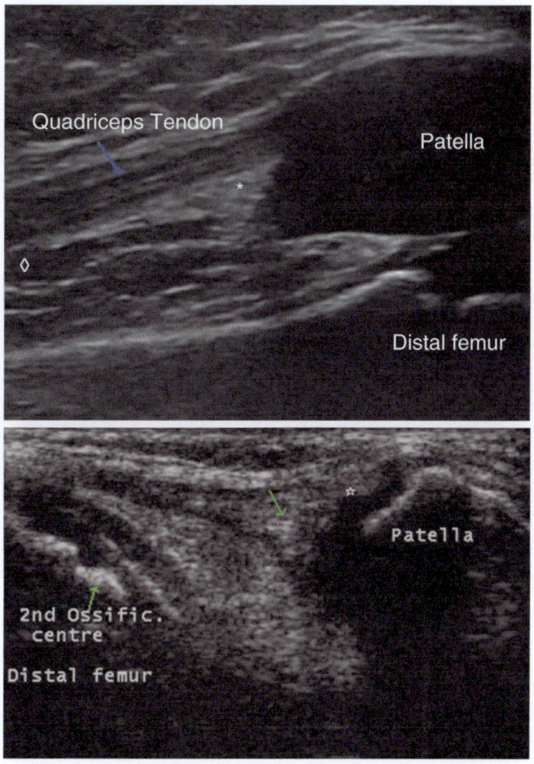

Fig. 4.16 Standardized longitudinal ultrasound examination of the knee joint, showing a longitudinal scan on B-mode for the suprapatellar recess of a 6-year-old boy, with 30°–40° flexion of the knee. The image provides anatomic information on the following structures: suprapatellar recess "◊", superior edge of the patella, fat pad "*", distal insertion of quadriceps tendon, and distal end of the femur. The patella appears as an unossified structure located anterior to the distal epiphysis of the femoral condyle. Epiphyseal cartilage of the femoral condyle and the patella decrease during the growth of the child, (**b**) longitudinal knee scan of a 13-year old child. Secondary ossification centre can be seen at the end of the femur. A minimum fluid may be detected as a normal US finding

composition assessment, measuring the speed of sound (SOS) of US waves propagating along a specific bone distance (DIS) (Fig. 4.15). BonAge is an ultrasound device which includes an ultrasound probe connected to a main unit for calculation of bone age. The method uses two transducers, one that produces ultrasonic waves with a frequency of 750 kHz directed at the epiphysis of distal end of ulna and radius, whereas the other acts as a receiver. The entire process takes about 5 minutes in which 11 cycles of measurement are completed to provide accurate results. A skeletal age is computed using information obtained from demographics of the subject and the ultrasound results [65].

Cartilage

In children, US imaging has been shown to be a sensitive modality to detect alterations in the articular cartilage. It allows direct visualization of articular cartilage that is normally seen as an anechoic structure with a smooth outline over the bone surfaces (Fig. 4.16). Cartilage edema or loss may be seen in inflammatory arthritic diseases according to the level of the condition [66].

In a cohort of healthy children of different ages, the reliability of the assessment of cartilage thickness with US has been demonstrated by Spannow et al. [67]. The authors found a good intra- and interobserver agreement both in large and small joints, using ultrasonographic standard

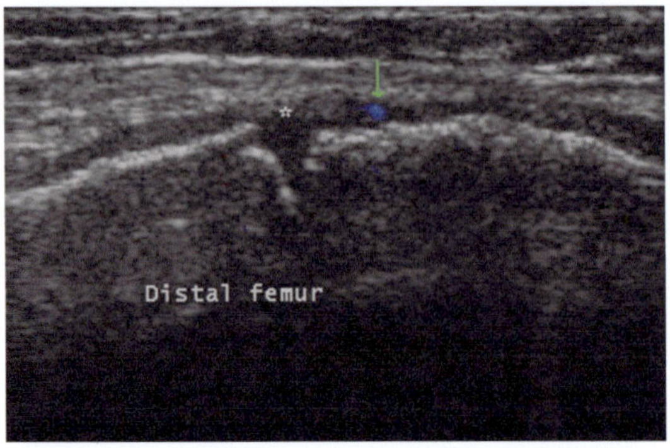

Fig. 4.17 The presence of juxta-articular flow at color Doppler examination in the growing child may either represent normal flow of the well-vascularized cartilage of the epiphysis or can be nutrient vessel. Longitudinal scan of the knee joint lateral view, showing the growth place "*" as well as of juxta-articular normal flow (arrow) of the growth plate

scans according to EULAR guidelines (Fig. 4.17) [67]. Mean cartilage thickness scores as reported in Spannow et al. work were: hip 2.59 ± 0.41, knee 3.67 ± 0.64, ankle 1.08 ± 0.31, MCP 1.52 ± 0.27, and PIP 0.73 ± 0.15 mm. Furthermore, Moller et al. [68] have demonstrated that direct visualization and quantification of cartilage in MCP and PIP joints by using MSUS is objective, reliable, and valid. They have suggested its use for diagnostic purposes in rheumatoid patients.

The presence of juxta-articular flow at color Doppler examination in the growing child may either represent normal flow of the well-vascularized cartilage of the epiphysis or synovial hyperemia indicating inflammation. Flow in the cartilage (Fig. 4.17) probably indicates normal cartilaginous flow in contrast to flow inside the synovium which probably indicates hyperemia [69].

Cartilage edema in early stages of JIA can be detected sonographically as thickening of the articular cartilage. Chronic inflammation of the cartilage results in permanent damage to the articular surface. This is observed sonographically as blurring of the articular surface. Continued destruction of the cartilage due to rheumatoid disease is seen as pitting of the articular surface and measurable thinning of the cartilage. Cartilage loss is better detected than on plain films especially in young children with thick epiphyseal cartilage and at the early stages of the disease [70, 71].

Synovial Membrane

The synovial membrane is an important connective tissue lining the inner surface of the joint capsule, tendon sheath, and bursa. Therefore, it is essential to understand the pathogenesis and the pathological changes seen in inflammatory synovium in order to perform a complete scan of the synovial joints. With US, synovial hypertrophy is detected as solid, non-compressible, hypoechoic tissue in connection to joint lines or surrounding tendons [57]. In children, detection is more challenging than in adults as the synovial tissue is often difficult to distinguish from the hypoechoic cartilage of epiphyses (Fig. 4.18a). To avoid diagnostic errors, it is therefore important to have good knowledge of the age-dependent normal US appearance of each joint.

In inflammatory arthritis, as in any other inflammatory arthritis, the synovium undergoes significant changes leading to the formation of a mass of synovial tissue. This is the result of edema, multiple redundant folds, and villae. The presence of joint, bursal, or tendon sheath effusion is used as an excellent, indirect correlate of synovial inflammation. Further, its presence (as an anechoic structure) technically enables a better visualization of the synovial thickening, proliferation, and villous formation during MSUS imaging (Fig. 4.18b) [72].

Musculoskeletal US offers the advantage of dynamic soft tissue examination (Fig. 4.19). In the absence of an effusion, synovitis is diagnosed by the presence of an abnormally thickened hypoechoic region, usually measured in a standard plane with reference to an established normal range or to the contralateral normal joint. Therefore, US can easily detect significant degrees of synovitis which is not determined by clinical examination [73, 74] and can reliably discriminate inflammatory and noninflammatory joint disease. Moreover, the detection of subclinical synovitis may also lead to re-evaluation of the clinical classification of arthritis as oligoarticular or polyarticular. Table (2) shows the definition for synovitis on ultrasonography (US) in children as reported by Roth et al. [75, 76].

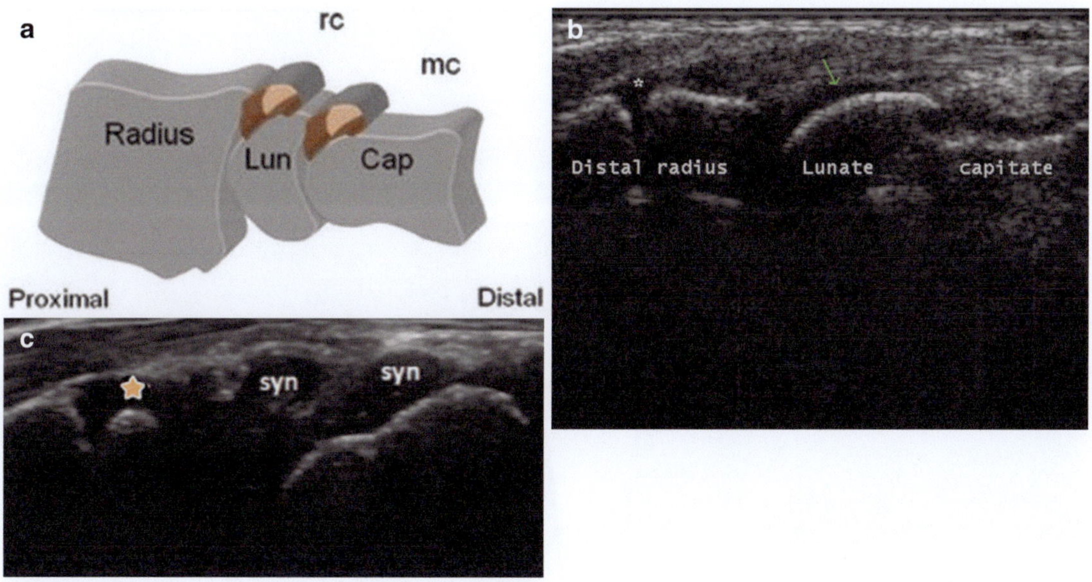

Fig. 4.18 (**a**) Diagram showing the recesses of the wrist joint. (**b**) Longitudinal US scan of the wrist joint in a normal 13-year-old child, (**c**) longitudinal US of the wrist joint of a 12-year-old child with inflammatory arthritis. "*": growth plate and overlying cartilage

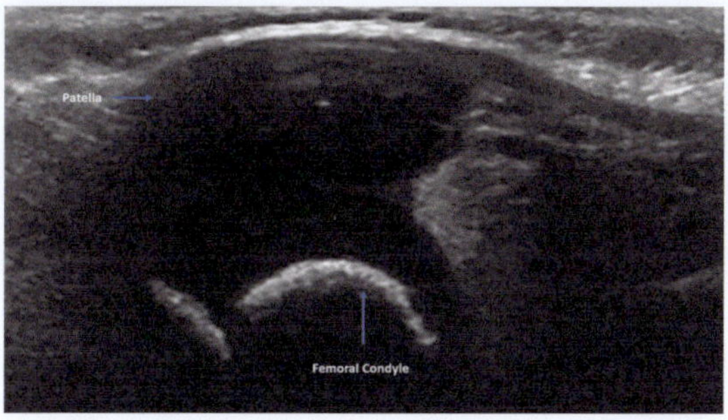

Fig. 4.19 (**a**) Transverse US scan of an 8-month-old child's knee joint showing effusion in the suprapatellar bursa. The effusion can be seen under the unossified patella. Surfaces of the growth cartilage of patella and femur are visible as hyperechoic lines (interface sign) allowing to identify the fluid. Dynamic examination would prove that effusion is compressible and displaceable tissue, whereas the epiphyseal cartilage is not. Similarly, synovial membrane is not compressible in contrast with joint effusion. Enhanced vascularity can be seen in the inflamed synovial membrane

Evaluation has been enhanced with power Doppler setting which depicts the increased vascularity of the hypertrophied synovium by demonstrating microvascular flow. The Doppler signal can distinguish between active and inactive synovitis, correlating to clinical and laboratory data [69, 77, 78], MRI [79], and histology as well [80]. Power Doppler also shows promise in evaluating the amount and the activity of pannus in JIA, as proliferative synovium, which is extremely vascular, shows high-power Doppler signal [81].

Fat Pad

Small masses of fat are enveloped by the fibers of the joint capsule, which separate the fat pads from the synovial lining, making the fat pads intracapsular and extra-synovial in location (Fig. 4.20). This anatomic arrangement is the basis for understanding the role of fat pad in the development of inflammation at the joint level [82, 83]. The Outcome Measures in Rheumatology (OMERACT) US Pediatric Task Force was formed to standardize the use of US in juvenile arthritis. It has developed preliminary B-mode US definitions (or grayscale US definitions) for joint components in healthy children (Table 4.2) [75], as well as a standardized US scanning procedure specifically adapted to children [84]. Besides unossified cartilage, fat pads, particularly in the knee and ankle joints, can show Doppler signal (physiological vascularity) [85].

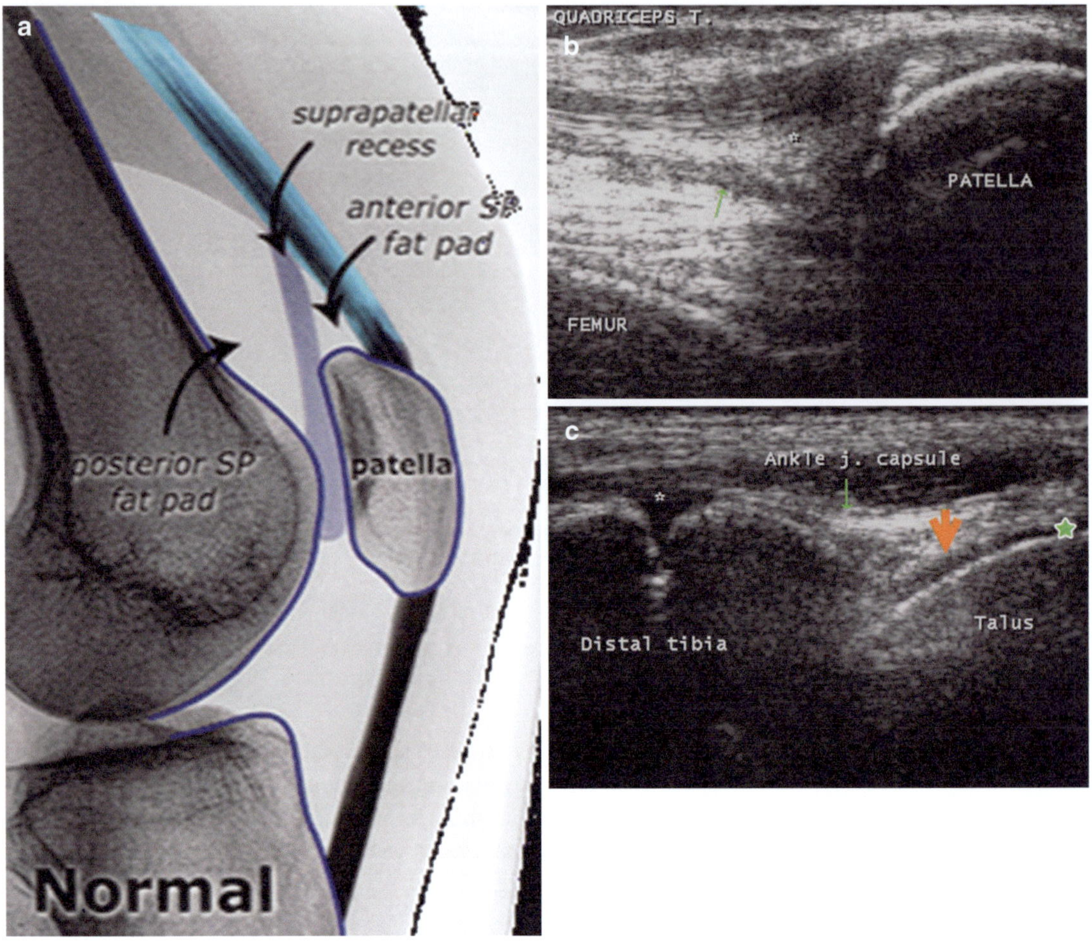

Fig. 4.20 Knee joint, ankle joint fat pad. (**a**) Diagram showing the suprapatellar recess as well as anterior and posterior suprapatellar fat pad. (**b**) Longitudinal US scan of a 13-year-old child showing the suprapatellar recess (arrow) and the anterior fat pad (asterisk). (**c**) Ankle joint longitudinal view: the joint capsule in the tibiotalar joint as a fibrillar structure along the joint. The intracapsular fat (orange arrow). In addition, the metaphyseal growth area of the distal tibia is shown (asterisk)

The fat pad sign: In 1954, Norell described the "fat pad sign" for the first time. This refers to the radiological visualization of the elbow fatty tissue. The fat pads can be evaluated on the lateral flexed view of the elbow. It is important that the view is a true lateral. If not, abnormal fat pads can be missed.

- The anterior fat pad is located in the coronoid fossa. A narrow anterior fat pad is a normal finding on the lateral view.
- The anterior fat pad can be displaced up and out by fluid in the elbow joint, creating the "sail sign." This usually indicates a fracture in children in the setting of an injury.
- The posterior fat pad is located in the olecranon fossa on the lateral view. It should not be visible under normal circumstances. Fluid in the elbow joint can displace the fat pad up and out making it visible on the lateral view. If the posterior fat pad is visible, it suggests a fracture in the setting of an injury.

Table 4.2 Definition for the sonographic features of joints in healthy children versus those with inflammatory synovitis [75, 76]

Definitions for the sonographic features of joints in healthy children	Definitions for the sonographic features of synovitis in children
The hyaline cartilage will present as a well-defined anechoic structure (with/without bright echoes/dots) that is non-compressible. The cartilage surface can (but does not have to) be detected as a hyperechoic line	Definition for synovitis on ultrasonography (US) in children
With advancing maturity, the epiphyseal secondary ossification center will appear as a hyperechoic structure, with a smooth or irregular surface within the cartilage	Synovitis detection by US in children includes the assessment of B-mode and Doppler mode findings
Normal joint capsule: a hyperechoic structure which can (but does not have to) be seen over bone, cartilage, and other intra-articular tissue of the joint	Synovitis can be detected on the bases of B-mode findings alone. Synovitis cannot be detected based on power/color Doppler alone
Normal synovial membrane: under normal circumstances, the thin synovial membrane is undetectable	B-mode findings include synovial effusion and synovial hypertrophy
The ossified portion of articular bone is detected as a hyperechoic line. Interruption of this hyperechoic line may be detected at the growth place and at the junction of two or more ossification centers	Synovial effusion is defined as an abnormal, intra-articular, anechoic, or hypoechoic material that is displaceable
	Synovial hypertrophy is defined as an abnormal, intra-articular, hypoechoic material that is non-displaceable
	Power/color Doppler signals must be detected within synovial hypertrophy to be considered as a sign of synovitis

The fat pad sign is invaluable in assessing for the presence of an intra-articular pathology or fracture (Fig. 4.21). Any process resulting in joint effusion may also demonstrate an abnormal fat pad sign. In addition to intra-articular fractures, increased intracapsular fluid is also seen in several conditions which can produce the abnormal fat pad sign, e.g., toxic synovitis, septic arthritis, hemoarthrosis, juvenile idiopathic arthritis, osteomyelitis of the distal humeral physis, and secondary septic joint. In these instances, history and clinical examination in addition to laboratory results (full blood count, ESR, CRP) will guide the provider in determining whether to treat the condition as an occult fracture or continue workup for other pathology.

Muscles and Tendons

Ultrasound imaging is a useful technique for visualizing normal and pathological skeletal muscle tissue [86, 87]. With ultrasonography, it is possible to study muscular morphology in a non-invasive manner, without exposure to ionizing radiation [88]. Using ultrasound imaging, normal muscle tissue appears as a structure with low echo intensity. Muscle tissue is divided by echogenic sheets of perimysial connective tissue, which give it a speckled appearance. The boundaries of the muscle are clearly visible, as the epimysium surrounding the muscle is a highly reflective structure. In normal subjects, the bone echo is strong and distinct. The subcutaneous fat has low echo intensity. In the subcutaneous tissue, several echogenic septa of connective tissue may be visible (Fig. 4.22a, b) [89, 90].

Measurement of muscle thickness, ratio of muscle thickness to subcutaneous fat thickness, and echo intensity with ultrasonography can be performed easily in children and can be used to identify different pathologies. Echo intensities can be increased by neuromuscular disorders, such as Duchenne muscular dystrophy, spinal

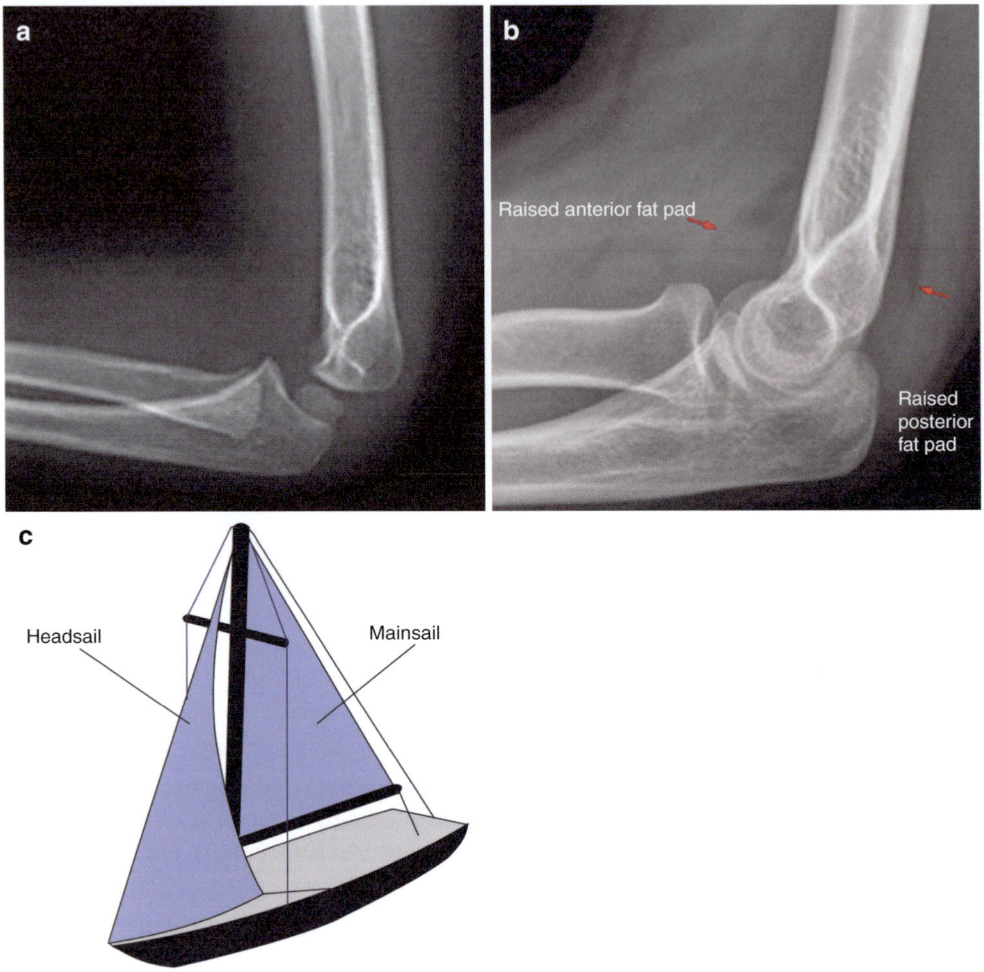

Fig. 4.21 (**a**) X-ray lateral view of normal elbow. (**b**) X-ray lateral view of the elbow showing the displaced anterior and posterior fat pads (sail sign) caused by un-displaced radial head fracture. (**c**) Picture of a sail

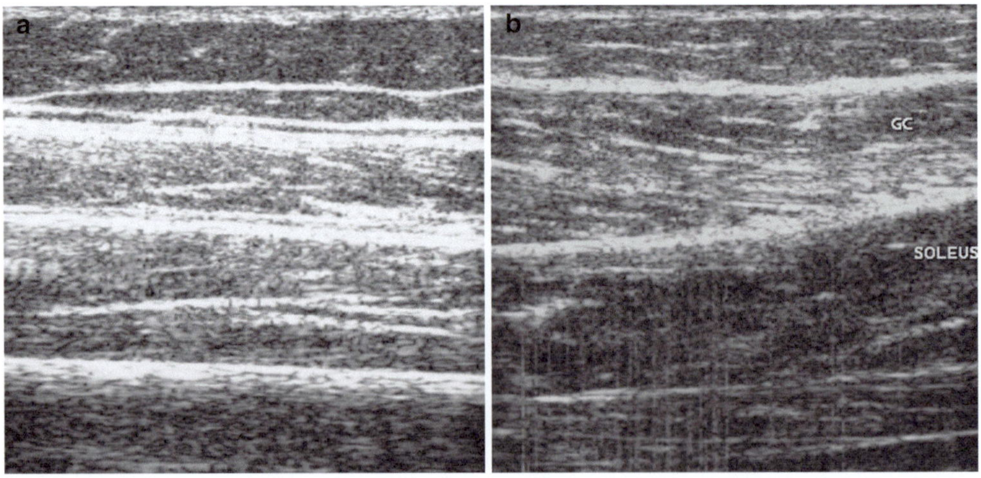

Fig. 4.22 (**a**) Longitudinal US scan of the thigh showing the rectus femoris muscle and underneath is the vastus intermedius muscle architecture. (**b**) Longitudinal US scan of the calf muscles showing the distinct sonographic pattern of the gastrocnemius (GC) and soleus muscles

muscle atrophy, and congenital myopathies, because muscular architecture is disrupted by muscle cell replacement with fat and connective tissue [91]. Neuropathies are often associated with atrophy, which can be detected by measuring the muscle thickness. The ratio of muscle thickness to subcutaneous fat thickness can be helpful in detecting specific neuromuscular disorders. For example, previous studies have shown that one of the distinguishing features of spinal muscle atrophy is muscle atrophy and an increase of subcutaneous fat thickness, which result in a decreased ratio [87, 92].

During ultrasonographic imaging, it is important to keep certain conditions constant in order to assure that individual measurements can be compared with one another. These conditions are the exact site of measurement, the position of the child, the muscle relaxation, the pressure exerted on the skin by the transducer, the correct position of the transducer in a transverse plane, and the system settings [93–95].

In contrast to the muscles which appear uniformly hypoechoic with interspersed hyperechoic fibroadipose septa and fascia, tendons and ligaments are uniformly hyperechoic with fibrils internal echotexture [55]. As in adults, synovial membranes that line synovial joints, bursae, and tendon sheaths (tenosynovium) should be less than or equal to 1 mm to 2 mm in thickness if visualized sonographically. Enthesitis (inflammation at the site of attachment of ligaments or tendons to bone) is the main pathology in patients with spondyloarthritis. Enthesitis is most commonly present at the insertions of the Achilles tendon, the plantar fascia, and the patellar and quadriceps tendons (Fig. 4.23). Soft tissue swelling, localized osteopenia, bone erosions, or spurs are commonly observed.

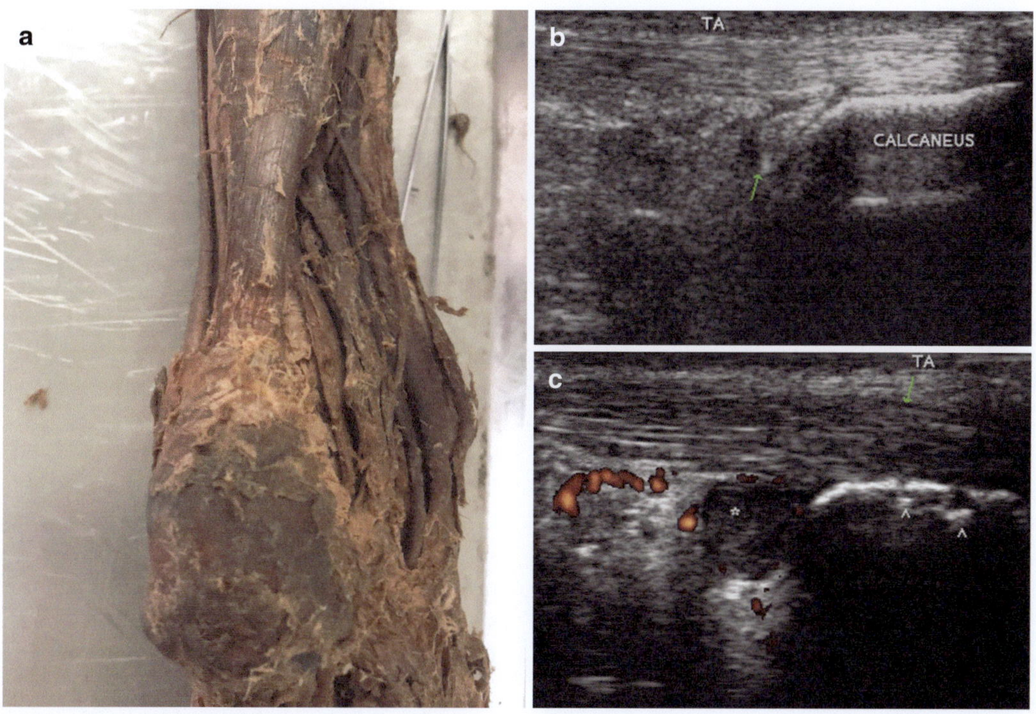

Fig. 4.23 (**a**) Picture of an ankle depicting the distinct areas of tendoachilles insertion into the calcaneus bone. (**b**) Longitudinal US scan of the tendoachilles in a 13-year-old child showing the tendoachilles and its attachment to the calcaneus bone. The pre-Achilles fat pad (Kager's triangle) [arrow] is visible in the form of a well-defined triangle anterior to the tendoachilles and posterior to the tibia. (**c**) Distinctive patterns of enthesitis detected by ultrasound (US) examination in B-mode combined with power Doppler in psoriatic arthritis patients. Abnormal vascularization associated with marked swelling and decreased echogenicity of the enthesis at the cortical junction can be seen, as well as erosions of the calcaneus (arrow heads). Tendon thickness at the level of the enthesis (arrow) is 7.2 mm associated with a retrocalcaneal bursa with enhanced vascularity in a psoriatic patient. TA, Achilles tendon; ∗, retrocalcaneal bursa; arrow heads, erosions. Tendoachilles sonoanatomy, US, enthesitis

Power Doppler

The OMERACT US Pediatric Task Force has published their suggested definitions of B-mode US findings of the healthy joint [96], standardization of US scanning in children, and definitions for the US appearance of synovitis in children [97] (Table 4.3). Five sites have been included in the OMERACT preliminary definitions: the hyaline cartilage, the epiphyseal secondary ossification center, the normal joint capsule, the normal synovial membrane, and the ossified portion of articular bone [96].

Given the unique anatomy of the growing child, the presence of joint Doppler signals in the pediatric population is expected in normal children. Several studies have shown that Doppler signal within joints is detectable in healthy children [84, 98]. This has been attributed to that fact that normal growth and ossification in the developing skeleton are intimately related to the vascularity of the unossified epiphyseal and physeal cartilage [99, 100]. At that point, some obstacles have been found (i.e., the features of this imaging modality, operator dependent linked to both personal factor (expert or trainee) and equipment, and the unclear terminology that is used to refer to physis, also known as "the growth plate" or "the epiphyseal growth plate") [99–101].

Table 4.3 Definitions of joints' features in healthy children when using the Doppler technique [85]

Physiological vascularity can be detected by PD as Doppler signal in the joint structures at any age during growth
Physiological intra-articular vascularity can be detected in children within the fat pads and unossified joint structures (i.e., the physis, the cartilage of epiphysis, and the short bones cartilage)
Detection of physiological vascularity and its intra-articular anatomical position is joint- and age (particularly in the youngest children) dependent
Physis can be detected in children as an anechoic unossified structure, intra- or extraarticular, according to its anatomical location
Fat pad can be detected as an intra-articular structure with heterogeneous echotexture (similar to the subcutaneous tissue) which might show vascularity
In different age groups of children, due to the skeletal development, ossification centers can be detected with different maturation states
Ossification grade is age- and joint-dependent

A study published by Collado and colleagues [85] defined physiological vascularity (normal Doppler signal) as follows: 1) Doppler signal within the pediatric healthy joint can be detected as physiological vascularity of the unossified epiphyseal and physeal cartilage (physis is not detectable in the fully ossified bone of an adolescent) and the fat pads at any age during the growth, but since synovial membrane is undetectable under normal circumstances, any Doppler signal observed in a synovial thickening should be considered an abnormality. 2) Fat pad tissue can be present as an intra-articular structure, in a proper anatomical location, with heterogeneous echogenicity (similar to the US appearance of fat in the tissues below the skin) which might show Doppler signal.

Applied Sonoanatomy in Pediatrics

Standardized Sonoanatomy Assessment

In addition to limited knowledge of sonographic anatomy in healthy children, operator knowledge of how to conduct an MSUS examination has affected the validity of this imaging technique. Consequently, it is crucial to set up a standardized US examination method, particularly in the pediatric population. Development of standardized scanning methods is important to obtain valid US images in children. Although for US examinations, the transducer is usually placed first in the sagittal plane, the parasagittal planes were revealed to be important for a more comprehensive evaluation of the joint [75]. Similarly, identifying defined visible reference points for each scanning approach helps to minimize the operator dependency factor and make the scanning method reproducible and easy to learn regardless of the children age. The predefined scanning approaches provided essential information about blood flow (feeding vessels), as well as anatomic bone reference points within the joints explored (knee, ankle, wrist, and second MCP), showing that the theoretically agreed musculoskeletal ultrasonography definitions on normal joint structures in children are consistent when applied in practice for acquiring images [84]. Figures 4.24, 4.25, 4.26, and 4.27 show standardized US scans for the ankle, knee, wrist, and second MCP joints.

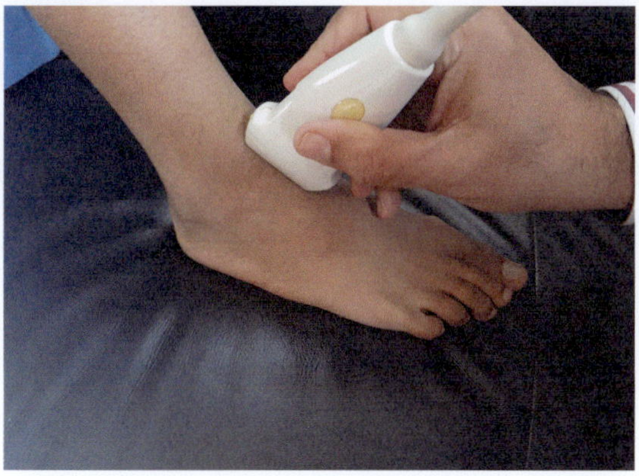

Fig. 4.24 Ankle joint: standardized longitudinal ultrasound examination of the ankle joint. The ankle is dorsally extended 120° with the sole resting on the examination table. The transducer is placed at the sagittal position of the ankle, with the distal end of the transducer positioned on the dome of the talus. Knee joint: Fig. 4.25b. Sagittal ultrasound scan of parapatellar knee recess, with the knee joint in full extension in a 13-year-old child. The image provides anatomic information about the recess, the epiphyseal cartilage of the patella, the patellar retinaculum, and the femoral condyle. The patellar retinaculum is lying anterior to the lateral recess

OMERACT Definitions and Scoring System

Following described methodology, OMERACT US pediatric subtask force recently finalized several important studies. In 2014, the subgroup first published definitions of the five anatomical components of the joints in healthy children [75]. There were two main limitation of this first pioneer work: (a) assessment of

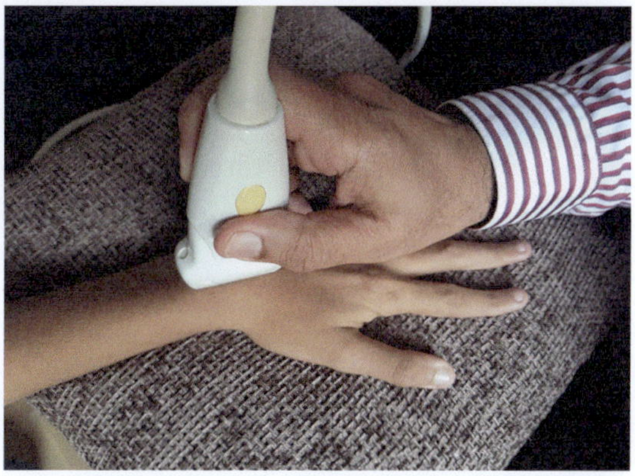

Fig. 4.26 Wrist joint: the standard US examination of the wrist begins with evaluation of its dorsal aspect, followed by the palmar one. Depending on the specific clinical presentation, US images can be obtained in different positions of the wrist (flexion and extension, radial and ulnar deviation, pronation, and supination), with the patient seated in front of the examiner

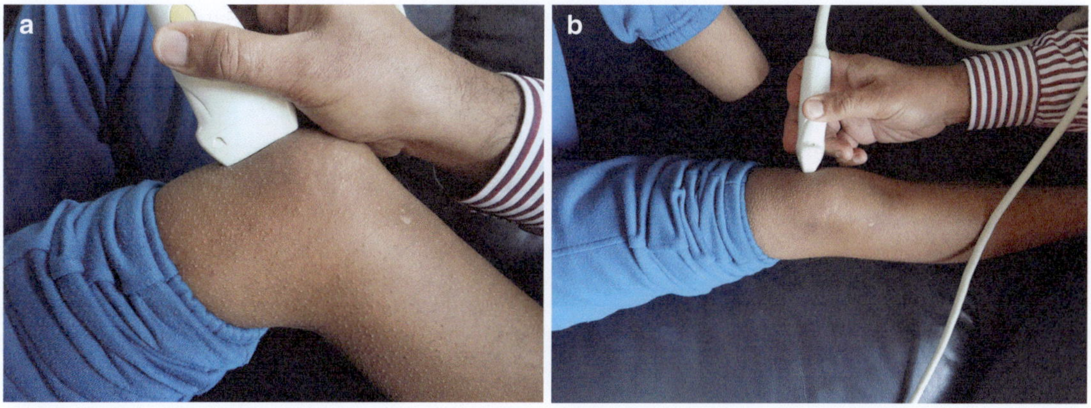

Fig. 4.25 (**a**) Standardized longitudinal US scan of the knee joint: showing a longitudinal scan on B-mode for the suprapatellar recess, with 30°–40° flexion of the knee. The transducer is placed at the sagittal midline of the leg, with the distal end of the transducer positioned just cranial to the superior edge of the patella. The image provides anatomic information on the following structures: suprapatellar recess, superior edge of the patella, distal insertion of quadriceps tendon, and distal end of the femur. (**b**) Transverse US scan of parapatellar knee recess, with the knee joint in full extension in a 13-year old child. The image provides anatomic information about the recess, the epiphyseal cartilage of the patella, the patellar retinaculum, and the femoral condyle

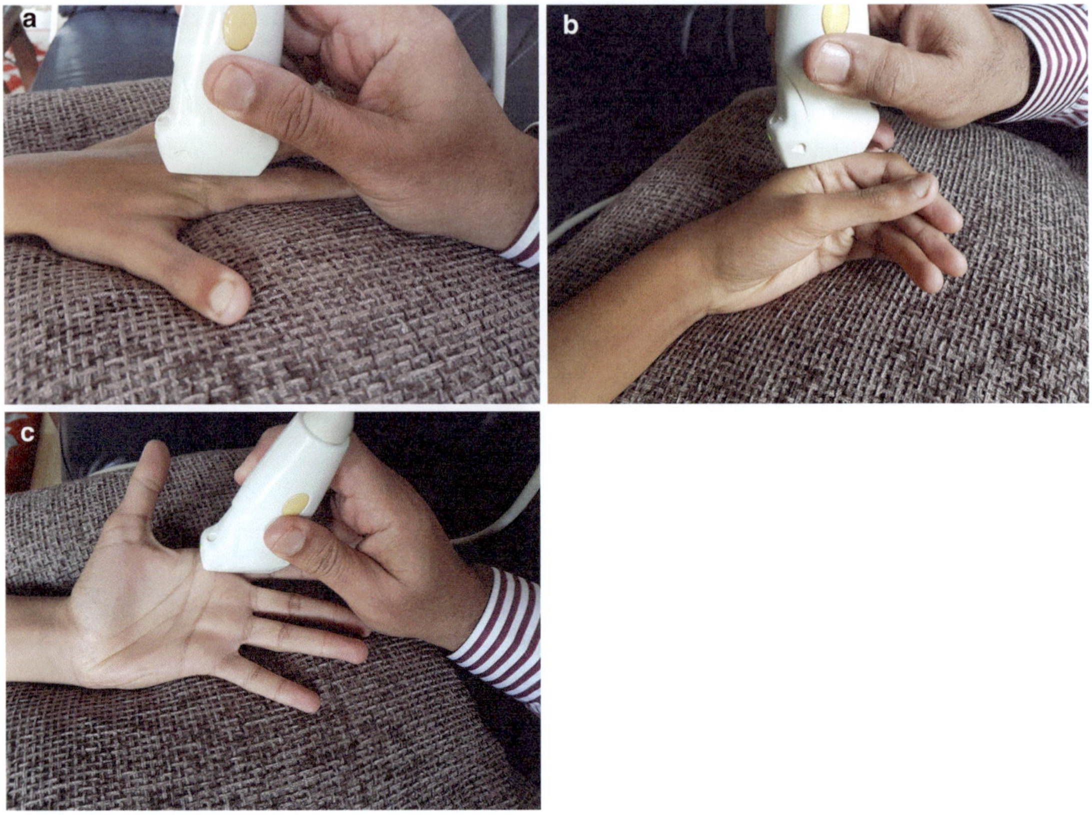

Fig. 4.27 MCP joints: the finger is examined with the palm facing downward, laterally, or upward. The transducer is longitudinally placed at the sagittal midline of the MCP joint, showing dorsal (**a**), lateral (**b**), and volar approaches (**c**). The proximal end of the transducer is positioned at the head of the metacarpal bone and the distal end at the proximal phalanx bone

the joint components on B-mode (or gray scale, GS) without using Doppler technique and (b) some anatomical structures specifically present during childhood were not defined (such as fat pad and cartilaginous structures present in physis and epiphysis). That is why in a subsequent Delphi survey, the OMERACT group provided amendment of the definitions for the US features of the joints in healthy children covering fat pad, vascularization, ossification, and physis [85]. Additionally, the subgroup worked on standardization of the image acquisition for different joints and published recommendations for the four most frequently affected joints in JIA (knee, wrist, ankle, and metacarpophalangeal joint) [84] (Figs. 4.24, 4.25, 4.26, and 4.27 detailed above). The study showed good comparability of images obtained by all examiners despite usage of different US machines; additionally, standard scanning image acquisition was reproducible regardless of child's age.

Due to the age-related differences in normal US findings in healthy children, the group focused on the presence of physiological vascularization and ossification. Multi-observer reliability exercise study in children with different age groups found out that according to specific joint and age up to 3, solitary PD signals can be detected within the joint due to the physiological vascularization in different age groups localized predominantly in the specific anatomic positions (the fat pad, the epiphysis, the physis, and the short bone cartilage). Additionally, the same study resulted in ossification grade definitions in children (Fig. 4.28) [101].

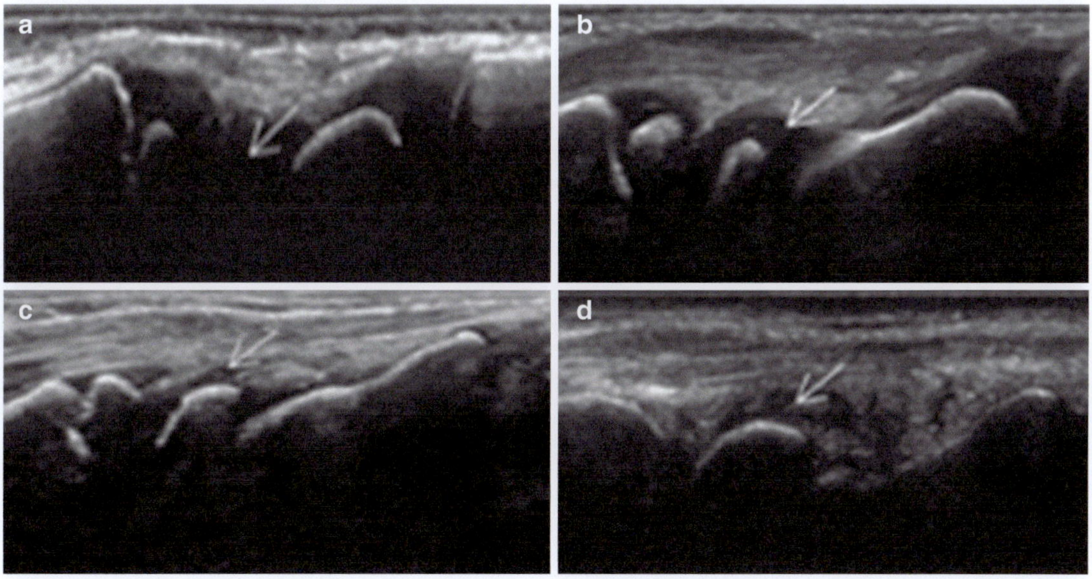

Fig. 4.28 Semiquantitative US score for evaluating skeletal ossification (lunate bone is used in the figure as an example). (**a**) Ossification grade (0), non-ossified epiphyseal bone, short bones or patella. (**b**) Ossification grade (1), small ossification centers, dominant cartilage, visible growth plate. (**c**) Ossification grade (2), large ossification centers, thin cartilage visible growth plate. (**d**) Ossification grade (3): complete ossification

In parallel, using Delphi consensus methodology and still image, the exercise group developed preliminary definitions for synovitis (Fig. 4.29). A subsequent JIA patient-based exercise with intra- and interobserver reliability study resulted in a development of a scoring system for B-mode and power Doppler grading of synovitis components to be used as a measure of synovitis activity [102]. Reliability exercise proposed 0–3 semiquantitative B-mode and color power/Doppler US definitions for synovial components and grading (Table 4.4). The proposed synovitis grading for children showed to be reliable, while the next step should be to test sensitivity to change in order to possibly be used as an outcome tool in JIA.

The Future

US technology continues to evolve in a variety of different directions. Elastography, a measure of tissue stiffness, may be of particular interest in studying nerve and muscle disease. The use of this technique has been primarily for differentiating tumor from healthy tissue, particularly in fat-laden tissue like the breast. However, it is conceivable that the technique could be informative about a variety of conditions that alter the stiffness of the muscles, either via histologic change such as myopathic disorder or via change in muscle tone and the supportive tissue of muscle as it occurs in movement disorders and spasticity. The real-time and noninvasive nature of this technique makes it particularly attractive for research. Furthermore, the potential for 3D and 4D US imaging may have some role in furthering neuromuscular research [103, 104].

In conclusion, musculoskeletal ultrasonography (US) has been shown to be a reliable, widely available, and child-friendly technique in the routine practice. US is a practical and dynamic imaging modality that is suitable for examination of children of all ages. Musculoskeletal US is most commonly used in the assessment of soft tissue disease or detection of fluid collection. It can also be used to visualize musculoskeletal structures, such as muscle, fascia, tendon, paratenon, ligament, synovium/capsule, hyaline and costal cartilage, fibrocartilage, nerve as well as bone

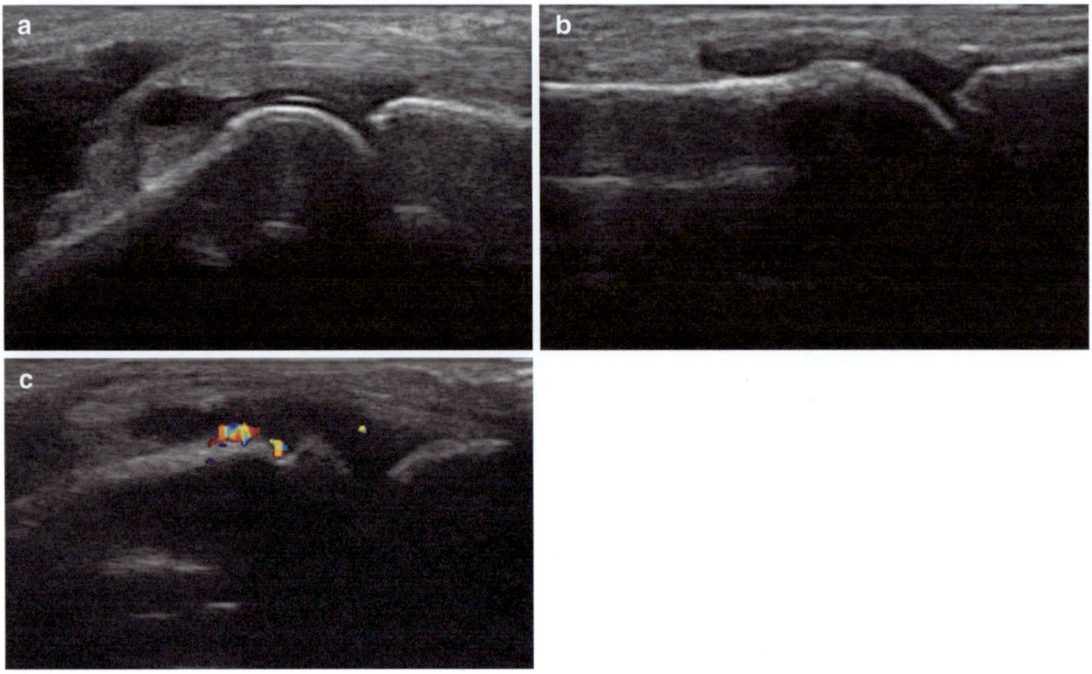

Fig. 4.29 OMERACT preliminary definition for synovitis. Overarching principle: synovitis detection by US in children includes the assessment of B-mode and Doppler mode findings. Synovitis can be detected based on the B-mode findings alone. Synovitis cannot be detected based on power Doppler findings alone. (1) Synovial hypertrophy is defined as an abnormal, intra-articular, hypoechoic material that is not displaceable. (2) Synovial effusion is defined as an abnormal, intra-articular anechoic, or hypoechoic material that is displaceable. (3) Power Doppler signals must be detected within the synovial hypertrophy to be considered as a sign of synovitis. (**a**) Longitudinal scan of the second MCP joint: B-mode findings comprise synovial hypertrophy. (**b**) Synovitis and effusion. (**c**) Power Doppler of the second MCP joint showing enhanced vascularity. (1) Synovial hypertrophy is defined as an abnormal, intra-articular, hypoechoic material that is not displaceable. (2) Synovial effusion is defined as an abnormal, intra-articular anechoic or hypoechoic material that is displaceable. (3) Power Doppler signals must be detected within the synovial hypertrophy to be considered as a sign of synovitis

Table 4.4 Ultrasonography definitions for synovitis grading in children

Grade	B-mode (gray scale)	Power Doppler/Color Doppler
0	No signs of synovial effusion or synovial hypertrophy (i.e., no joint recess enlargement/capsular distension)	Absence of color/power Doppler signal within synovial hypertrophy with or without detection of normal physiological Doppler signals
1	Synovial effusion/synovial hypertrophy that leads to mild change of the joint recess appearance (i.e., mild joint recess enlargement/capsular distention)	Detection of up to three single Doppler signals within the area of synovial hypertrophy with or without normal physiological Doppler signal
2	Synovial effusion/synovial hypertrophy that leads to moderate change of the joint recess appearance (i.e., moderate joint recess enlargement/capsular distention)	Detection of more than three single Doppler signals but less than 30% of the area of synovial hypertrophy with or without normal physiological Doppler signals
3	Synovial effusion/synovial hypertrophy that leads to severe change of the joint recess appearance (i.e., severe joint recess enlargement/capsular distention)	Detection of Doppler signals at more than 30% of the area of synovial hypertrophy with or without normal physiological Doppler signals

surfaces. However, US waves cannot penetrate into bone; therefore, imaging of intrabone disease is not possible. US can also be used for guidance of aspiration, biopsy, and injection treatment. In this regard, when compared with the (already established) role of US in the daily practice of adult musculoskeletal medicine, it is time for pediatric rheumatologists to start to use US as well.

References

1. Steele, D. Gentry; Claud A. Bramblett (1988). The anatomy and biology of the human skeleton. College Station: Texas A&M University Press; 1988. p. 4. ISBN 0-89096-300-2.
2. Marshall Cavendish Mammal anatomy: an illustrated guide. New York: Marshall Cavendish. 2010. p. 129. ISBN 9780761478829.
3. Clarke B. Normal bone anatomy and physiology. Clin J Am Soc Nephrol. 2008;3 https://doi.org/10.2215/CJN.04151206.
4. Haines RW. The evolution of epiphyses and of endochondral bone. Biol Rev. 1942;17:267–92.
5. Subramanian A, Schilling TF. Tendon development and musculoskeletal assembly: emerging roles for the extracellular matrix. Development. 2015;142:4191–204. https://doi.org/10.1242/dev.114777.
6. Banos CC, Thomas AH, Kuo CK. Collagen fibrillogenesis in tendon development: current models and regulation of fibril assembly. Birth Defects Res C Embryo Today. 2008;84:228–44.
7. Kannus P, Jozsa L, Järvinen TAH, Järvinen TLN, Kvist M, Natri A, Järvinen M. Location and distribution of non-collagenous matrix proteins in musculoskeletal tissues of rat. Histochem J. 1998;30:799–810.
8. Juneja SC, Veillette C. Defects in tendon, ligament, and enthesis in response to genetic alterations in key proteoglycans and glycoproteins: a review. Arthritis. 2013;2013:154812.
9. Yang G, Rothrauff BB, Tuan RS. Tendon and ligament regeneration and repair: clinical relevance and developmental paradigm. Birth Defects Res C Embryo Today. 2013;99:203–22.
10. Sugimoto Y, Takimoto A, Akiyama H, Kist R, Scherer G, Nakamura T, Hiraki Y, Shukunami C. Scx+/Sox9+ progenitors contribute to the establishment of the junction between cartilage and tendon/ligament. Development. 2013;140:2280–8.
11. Birch HL, Thorpe CT, Rumian AP. Specialization of extracellular matrix for function in tendons and ligaments. Muscles Ligaments Tendons J. 2013;3:12–22.
12. Aslan H, Kimelman-Bleich N, Pelled G, Gazit D. Molecular targets for tendon neoformation. J Clin Invest. 2008;118:439–44.
13. Huang AH, Lu HH, Schweitzer R. Molecular regulation of tendon cell fate during development. J Orthop Res. 2015;33:800–12.
14. Schweitzer R, Zelzer E, Volk T. Connecting muscles to tendons: tendons and musculoskeletal development in flies and vertebrates. Development. 2010;137:2807–17.
15. Kjaer M. Role of extracellular matrix in adaptation of tendon and skeletal muscle to mechanical loading. Physiol Rev. 2004;84:649–98.
16. Schwartz AG, Lipner JH, Pasteris JD, Genin GM, Thomopoulos S. Muscle loading is necessary for the formation of a functional tendon enthesis. Bone. 2013;55:44–51.
17. Snow CJ, Henry CA. Dynamic formation of microenvironments at the myotendinous junction correlates with muscle fiber morphogenesis in zebrafish. Gene Expr Patterns. 2009;9:37–42.
18. Wang JH-C, Guo Q, Li B. Tendon biomechanics and mechanobiology – a minireview of basic concepts and recent advancements. J Hand Ther. 2012;25:133–41.
19. Dunkman AA, Buckley MR, Mienaltowski MJ, Adams SM, Thomas SJ, Satchell L, Kumar A, Pathmanathan L, Beason DP, Iozzo RV, et al. Decorin expression is important for age-related changes in tendon structure and mechanical properties. Matrix Biol. 2013;32:3–13.
20. Wall ME, Banes AJ. Early responses to mechanical load in tendon: role for calcium signaling, gap junctions and intercellular communication. J Musculoskelet Neuronal Interact. 2005;5:70–84.
21. Zhang J, Wang JHC. Mechanobiological response of tendon stem cells: implications of tendon homeostasis and pathogenesis of tendinopathy. J Orthop Res. 2010;28:639–43.
22. Popov C, Burggraf M, Kreja L, Ignatius A, Schieker M, Docheva D. Mechanical stimulation of human tendon stem/progenitor cells results in upregulation of matrix proteins, integrins and MMPs, and activation of p38 and ERK1/2 kinases. BMC Mol Biol. 2015;16:1219. https://doi.org/10.1186/s12867-015-0036-6.
23. Choi WJ, Park MS, Park KH, Courneya J-P, Cho JS, Schon LC, Lee JW. Comparative analysis of gene expression in normal and degenerative human tendon cells: effects of cyclic strain. Foot Ankle Int. 2014;35:1045–56.
24. Lucien M. Note sur le developpement des coulisses fibreuses et les gaines sinoviales annexées aux péroniers láteraux. Comptes Rendus Assoc Anat. 1908:148.
25. Tozer S, Duprez D. Tendon and ligament: development, repair and disease. Birth Defects Res C Embryo Today. 2005;75:226–36.

26. Hauser RA, Dolan EE, Phillips HJ, Newlin AC, Moore RE, Woldin BA. Ligament injury and healing: a review of current clinical diagnostics and therapeutics. Open Rehabil J. 2013;6(1):5.
27. Beau A. Recherches sur le developpement et la constitution morphologiques de lárticulation du cou-du pied chez l'homme. Arch Anat Histol Embryol. 1939;26:205.
28. Lucien M. Notes dur le developpement du ligament annulaire anterieur du tarse. Comptes rendus Hebd. Soc Biol. 1908;2:253.
29. Kakebeke TH, von Siebenthal K, Largo RH. Movement quality in pre-term infants prior to term. Biol Neonate. 1998;73:145–54.
30. Fricke O, Schoenau E. Examining the developing skeletal muscle: why, what and how? J Musculoskelet Neuronal Interact. 2005;5(3):225–31.
31. Chamley C, Carson P, Randall D, Sandwell M. Developmental anatomy and physiology of children: a practical approach. Edinburgh: Elsevier Churchill Livingston; 2005. p. 83–84. https://books.google.co.uk/books?id=WyWJ7c5Wi4kC&pg=PA83&lpg=PA83&dq=anatomy+of+child+skeletal+muscles&source=bl&ots=drS21ARmE9&sig=6mSN2dXSjn-B6YblLxIcPnTwKBM&hl=en&sa=X&ved=0ahUKEwjrqOS72YjcAhWDasAKHTQ6B_U4FBDoAQg6MAQ#v=onepage&q=anatomy%20of%20child%20skeletal%20muscles&f=false. Accessed 5 July 2018.
32. Hydorn C, Cooper J. Pediatric orthopedics versus adult orthopedics. Orthostreams. 2014. https://orthostreams.com/2014/09/pediatric-orthopedics-versus-adult-orthopedics/. Accessed 5 July 2018.
33. Coffey J. Pediatric XRay Diagnosis, vol. 2. 6th ed. Chicago: Year Book Medical Publishers; 1972. p. 884.
34. Pasturet G. Traité dÁnatomie Humaine, vol 2. Membres superieur et inferieur. Paris: Masson et Cie; 1951. p. 627–629.
35. Gruber HE, Lachman RS, Rimoin DL. Quantitative histology of cartilage vascular canals in the human rib: findings in normal neonates and children and in achondrogenesis II-hypochondrogenesis. J Anat. 1990;173:69–75.
36. Wilsman NJ, Van Sickle DC. Cartilage canals, their morphology, and distribution. Anat Rec. 1972;173:79–93.
37. Thapa M, Iyer R, Khanna P, Chew F. MRI of pediatric patients: part 1, normal and abnormal cartilage. AJR Am J Roentgenol. 2012;198:W450–5.
38. Jaramillo D, Villegas-Medina OL, Doty DK, et al. Age-related vascular changes in the epiphysis, physis, and metaphysis: normal findings on gadolinium-enhanced MRI of piglets. AJR. 2004;182:353–60.
39. Kolb A, Robinson S, Stelzeneder D et al. Vessel architecture in human knee cartilage in children: an in vivo susceptibility-weighted imaging study at 7 T. Eur Radiol. 2017. https://doi.org/10.1007/s00330-017-5290-1.
40. Martin DD, Wit JM, Hochberg Z, Sävendahl L, van Rijn RR, Fricke O, et al. The use of bone age in clinical practice – part 1. Horm Res Paediatr. 2011;76:1–9.
41. Mughal AM, Hassan N, Ahmed A. Bone age assessment methods: A critical review. Pak J Med Sci. 2014;30(1):211–5.
42. Blais MM, Green WR, Anderson M. Lengths of growing foot. J Bone Joints Surg Am. 1956;38:998.
43. Hübner U, Schlicht W, Outzen S, Barthel M, Halsband H. Ultrasound in the diagnosis of fractures in children. J Bone Joint Surg (Br). 2000;82-B:1170–3.
44. Filly RA, Golbus MS. Ultrasonography of the normal and pathologic fetal skeleton. Radiol Clin N Am. 1982;20:311–23.
45. Ghosh A, Woo JS, Wan CW, Wong VC. Simple ultrasonic diagnosis of osteogenesis imperfecta type II in early second trimester. Prenat Diagn. 1984;4:235–40.
46. Pearsall AW, Larkin JJ, Raasch W. Intrauterine femur fracture. Orthopedics. 1992;15:947–50.
47. Howard CB, Lieberman N, Mozes G, Nyska M. Stress fracture detected sonographically. AJR Am J Roentgenol. 1992;159:1350–1.
48. Patten RM, Mack LA, Wang KY, Lingel J. Nondisplaced fractures of the greater tuberosity of the humerus: sonographic detection. Radiology. 1992;182:201–4.
49. Battistelli JM, Anselem B. Echography in injuries of costal cartilages. J Radiol. 1993;74:409–12.
50. Bitschnau R, Gehmacher O, Kopf A, Scheier M, Mathis G. Ultrasound diagnosis of rib and sternum fractures. Ultraschall Med. 1997;18:158–61.
51. Mariacher-Gehler S, Michel BA. Sonography: a simple way to visualize rib fractures. AJR Am J Roentgenol. 1994;163:1268.
52. Martino F, Laforgia R, Rizzo A, et al. The echographic assessment of traumatic rib lesions. Radiol Med. 1997;94:166–9.
53. Smeets AJ, Robben SG, Meradji M. Sonographically detected costochondral dislocation in an abused child: a new sonographic sign to the radiological spectrum of child abuse. Pediatr Radiol. 1990;20:566–7.
54. Leitgeb N, Bodenteich A, Schweighofer F, Fellinger M. Ultrasonic diagnosis of fractures. Ultraschall Med. 1990;11:206–9.
55. Xu H, Shao H, Wang L, Jin J, Wang J. A methodological comparison between ultrasound and X-ray evaluations of bone age. J Sports Sci. 2008;6:27.
56. Malattia C, Damasio MB, Magnaguagno F, Pistorio A, Valle M, Martinoli C, Viola S, Buoncompagni A, Loy A, Ravelli A, Tomà P, Martini A. Magnetic resonance imaging, ultrasonography, and conventional radiography in the assessment of bone erosions in juvenile idiopathic arthritis. Arthritis Rheum. 2008;59:1764–72.
57. Wakefield RJ, O'Connor PJ, Conaghan PG, McGonagle D, Hensor EM, Gibbon WW, Brown C, Emery P. Finger tendon disease in untreated early

rheumatoid arthritis: a comparison of ultrasound and magnetic resonance imaging. Arthritis Rheum. 2007;57:1158–64.

58. Funck-Brentano T, Etchepare F, Joulin SJ, et al. Benefits of ultrasonography in the management of early arthritis: a crosssectional study of baseline data from the ESPOIR cohort. Rheumatology (Oxford). 2009;48:1515–9.
59. Scheel AK, Hermann KG, Ohrndorf S, et al. Prospective 7 year follow up imaging study comparing radiography, ultrasonography, and magnetic resonance imaging in rheumatoid arthritis finger joints. Ann Rheum Dis. 2006;65:595–600.
60. Szkudlarek M, Narvestad E, Klarlund M, et al. Ultrasonography of the metatarsophalangeal joints in rheumatoid arthritis comparison with magnetic resonance imaging, conventional radiography, and clinical examination. Arthritis Rheum. 2004;50:2103–12.
61. Seol J, Callahan M. Pediatric ultrasound. In: Paltiel H, editors. Philadelphia: Elsevier; 2013. p. 459–477. https://books.google.co.uk/books?id=cfYRAAAAQBAJ&pg=PA459&lpg=PA459&dq=ultrasound+of+tendons+and+ligaments+in+children&source=bl&ots=m_4S7m9ivO&sig=DQnObzRB7EMTsC2StpGDxthvRYc&hl=en&sa=X&ved=0ahUKEwjt0cy474ncAhXmAsAKHeD4BBE4HhDoAQg7MAM#v=onepage&q=ultrasound%20of%20tendons%20and%20ligaments%20in%20children&f=false. Accessed 6 July 2018.
62. Mentzel H-J, Vilser C, Eulenstein M, Schwartz T, Vogt S, Bottcher J, et al. Assessment of skeletal age at the wrist in children with a new ultrasound device. Pediatr Radiol. 2005;35(4):429–33. https://doi.org/10.1007/s00247-004-1385-3. [PubMed].
63. Zadik Z, Bistrizer T, Tsoref L, Schwartz T, Yaniv I. A novel method for assessing bone age using ultrasound. Prague: Europediatrics; [cited 2012 Oct 19]. Available from: http://www.sunlightnet.com/international/html/BAZadik2003.pdf
64. Shimura N, Koyama S, Arisaka O, Imataka M, Sato K, Matsuura M. Assessment of measurement of children's bone age ultrasonically with sunlight BonAge. Clin Pediatr Endocrinol. 2005;14(Suppl 24):17–20.
65. Khan KM, Miller BS, Hoggard E, Somani A, Sarafoglou K. Application of ultrasound for bone age estimation in clinical practice. J Pediatr. 2009;154(2):243–7. https://doi.org/10.1016/j.jpeds.2008.08.018.
66. Damasio MB, Malattia C, Martini A, Tomà P. Synovial and inflammatory diseases in childhood: role of new imaging modalities in the assessment of patients with juvenile idiopathic arthritis. Pediatr Radiol. 2010;40:985–98. https://doi.org/10.1007/s00247-010-1612-z.
67. Spannow AH, Stenboeg E, Pfeiffer-Jensen M, Herlin T. Ultrasound measurement of joint cartilage thickness in large and small joints in healthy children: a clinical pilot study assessing observer variability. Pediatr Rheumatol Online J. 2007;2:5–3.
68. Möller B, Bonel H, Rotzetter M, Villiger PM, Ziswiler HR. Measuring finger joint cartilage by ultrasound as a promising alternative to conventional radiograph imaging. Arthritis Rheum. 2009;61:435–41. https://doi.org/10.1002/art.24424.
69. Shahin AA, el-Mofty SA, el-Sheikh EA, Hafez HA, Ragab OM. Power Doppler sonography in the evaluation and follow-up of knee involvement in patients with juvenile idiopathic arthritis. Z Rheumatol. 2001;60:148–55.
70. Buchmann RF, Jaramillo D. Imaging of articular disorders in children. Radiol Clin N Am. 2004;42:151–68.
71. Tok F, Demirkaya E, Özçakar L. Musculoskeletal ultrasound in pediatric rheumatology. Pediatr Rheumatol Online J. 2011;9:25.
72. Kane D, Grassi W, Sturrock R, Balint PV. Musculoskeletal ultrasound--a state of the art review in rheumatology. Part 2: clinical indications for musculoskeletal ultrasound in rheumatology. Rheumatology (Oxford). 2004;43:829–38.
73. Grassi W. Clinical evaluation versus ultrasonography: who is the winner? [editorial]. J Rheumatol. 2003;30:908–9.
74. Karim Z, Wakefield RJ, Conaghan PG, Lawson CA, Goh E, Quinn MA, et al. The impact of ultrasonography on diagnosis and management of patients with musculoskeletal conditions. Arthritis Rheum. 2001;44:2932–3.
75. Roth J, Jousse-Joulin S, Magni-Manzoni S, Rodriguez A, Tzaribachev N, Iagnocco A, et al. Definitions for the sonographic features of joints in healthy children. Arthritis Care Res. 2015;67:136–42.
76. Roth J, Ravagnani V, Backhaus M, Balint P, Alessandra Bruns GA, Bruyn PC, De La Cruz L, Guillaume-czitrom S, Herlin T, Hernandez C, et al. Preliminary Definitions for the Sonographic Features of Synovitis in Children. Arthritis Care Res. 2017;69(8):1217–23.
77. Naredo E, Bonilla G, Gamero F, Uson J, Carmona L, Laffon A. Assessment of inflammatory activity in rheumatoid arthritis: a comparative study of clinical evaluation with grey scale and power Doppler ultrasonography. Ann Rheum Dis. 2005;64:375–81.
78. Karmazyn B, Bowyer SL, Schmidt KM, Ballinger SH, Buckwalter K, Beam TT, Ying J. US findings of metacarpophalangeal joints in children with idiopathic juvenile arthritis. Pediatr Radiol. 2007;37:475–82.
79. Szkudlarek M, Court-Payen M, Strandberg C, Klarlund M, Klausen T, Ostergaard M. Power Doppler ultrasonography for assessment of synovitis in the metacarpophalangeal joints of patients with rheumatoid arthritis: a comparison with dynamic magnetic resonance imaging. Arthritis Rheum. 2001;44:2018–23.
80. Walther M, Harms H, Krenn V, Radke S, Faehndrich TP, Gohlke F. Correlation of power Doppler sonog-

raphy with vascularity of the synovial tissue of the knee joint in patients with osteoarthritis and rheumatoid arthritis. Arthritis Rheum. 2001;44:331–8.
81. Lamer S, Sebag GH. MRI and ultrasound in children with juvenile chronic arthritis. Eur J Radiol. 2000;33:85–93.
82. Caspar-Bauguil S, Cousin B, Galinier A, Segafredo C, Nibbelink M, Andre M, et al. Adipose tissues as an ancestral immune organ: site-specific change in obesity. FEBS Lett. 2005;579:3487–92.
83. Šenolt L. Adipokines: role in local and systemic inflammation of rheumatic diseases. Expert Rev Clin Immunol. 2017;13(1):1–3.
84. Collado P, Vojinovic J, Nieto JC, Windschall D, Magni-Manzoni S, Bruyn GAW, et al. Toward standardized musculoskeletal ultrasound in pediatric rheumatology: normal age-related ultrasound findings. Arthritis Care Res. 2016;68:348–56.
85. Collado P, Windschall D, Vojinovic J, et al. Amendment of the OMERACT ultrasound definitions of joints' features in healthy children when using the DOPPLER technique. Pediatr Rheumatol Online J. 2018;16:23.
86. Heckmatt JZ, Leeman S, Dubowitz V. Ultrasound imaging in the diagnosis of muscle disease. J Pediatr. 1982;101:656–60.
87. Heckmatt JZ, Pier N, Dubowitz V. Assessment of quadriceps femoris muscle atrophy and hypertrophy in neuromuscular disease in children. J Clin Ultrasound. 1988;16:177–81.
88. Heckmatt JZ, Pier N, Dubowitz V. Measurement of quadriceps muscle thickness and subcutaneaous tissue thickness in normal children by real-time ultrasound imaging. J Clin Ultrasound. 1988;16: 171–6.
89. Lamminen A, Jääskeläinen J, Rapola J, Suramo I. High-frequency ultrasonography of skeletal muscle in children with neuromuscular disease. J Ultrasound Med. 1988;7:505–9.
90. Reimers CD, Kellner H. Muscle ultrasound. In: Fleckenstein JL, Crues JV, Reimers CD, editors. Muscle imaging in health and disease. New York: Springer; 1996. p. 13–20.
91. Heckmatt JZ, Dubowitz V. Diagnostic advantage of needle muscle biopsy and ultrasound imaging in the detection of focal pathology in a girl with limb girdle dystrophy. Muscle Nerve. 1985;8:705–9.
92. Schmidt R, Voit T. Ultrasound measurement of quadriceps muscle in the first year of life. Neuropediatrics. 1992;24:36–42.
93. Heckmatt JZ, Dubowitz V, Leeman S. Detection of pathological change in dystrophic muscle with B-scan ultrasound imaging. Lancet. 1980;1: 1389–90.
94. Zuberi SM, Matta N, Nawaz S, Stephenson JBP, McWilliam RC, Hollman A. Muscle ultrasound in the assessment of suspected neuromuscular disease in childhood. Neuromuscul Disord. 1999;9: 203–7.
95. SCHOLTEN RR, PILLEN S, VERRIPS A, ZWARTS MJ. Quantitative ultrasonography of skeletal muscles in children: Normal values. Muscle Nerve. 2003;27:693–8.
96. Collado P, Windschall D, Vojinovic J, Magni-Manzoni S, Balint P, Bruyn GAW, Hernandez-Diaz C, Nieto JC, Ravagnani V, Tzaribachev N, Iagnocco A, D'Agostino MA, Naredo E. Amendment of the OMERACT ultrasound definitions of joints' features in healthy children when using the DOPPLER. Pediatr Rheumatol Online J. 2018;16:23–30.
97. Floyd WE, Zaleske DJ, Schiller AL, Trahan C, Mankin HJ. Vascular events associated with the appearance of the secondary center of ossification in the murine distal femoral epiphysis. J Bone Joint Surg Am. 1987;69:185–90.
98. Bearcroft P, Berman L, Robinson A, Butler G. Vascularity of the neonatal femoral head: in vivo demonstration with power Doppler US. Radiology. 1996;200:209–11. https://doi.org/10.1148/radiology.200.1.8657911. [PubMed] [Cross Ref].
99. Shapiro F. Epiphyseal and Physeal cartilage vascularization: a light microscopic and Tritiated thymidine autoradiographic study of cartilage canals in newborn and young postnatal rabbit bone. Anat Rec. 1998;252:140–8. https://doi.org/10.1002/(SICI)1097-0185(199809)252:1<140::AID-AR12>3.0.CO;2-O.
100. Varich LJ, Laor T, Jaramillo D. Normal maturation of the distal femoralepiphyseal cartilage: age-related changes at MR imaging. Radiology. 2000;214:705–9. https://doi.org/10.1148/radiology.214.3.r00mr20705.
101. Windschall D, Collado P, Vojinovic J, Magni-Manzoni S, Balint P, Bruyn G, Hernandez-Diaz C, Carlos Nieto J, Ravagnani V, Tzaribachev N, Iagnocco A, D'Agostino MA, Naredo E. On behalf of the OMERACT paediatric ultrasound subtask force. Age-related vascularization and ossification of joints in children: an international pilot study to test multi-observer ultrasound reliability. Arthritis Care Res (Hoboken). 2017; https://doi.org/10.1002/acr.23335.
102. Vojinovic J, Magni-Manzoni S, Collado P, Windschall D, Ravagnani V, Hernandez-Diaz C, Nieto Gonzales JC, Malattia C, Tzaribachev N, Susic G, Damjanov N, Czitrom SG, Herlin T, Lanni S, et al. Ultrasonography definitions for synovitis grading in children: the omeract pediatric ultrasound task force. Ann Rheum Dis. 2017;76:1015.
103. Ho-Fung VM, Jaramillo D. Cartilage imaging in children: current indications, magnetic resonance imaging techniques, and imaging findings. Radiol Clin N Am. 2013;51:689–702.
104. Walker F. Future directions in neuromuscular ultrasound, Chapter 13. In: Walker F, Cartwright M, editors. Neuromuscular ultrasound. Philadelphia: Elsevier; 2011. p. 177–86.

Spectrum of US pathology: Tissue pathology and clinical application

5

Jeimylo C. de Castro

Introduction

When examining a patient with musculoskeletal conditions among pediatric age group, it is important to start with a thorough history and physical examination. There is a need to assess the areas that will be relevant to the diagnosis and to determine if there is a need for imaging modalities that can help to ascertain the diagnosis. With this principle in mind, musculoskeletal ultrasound will serve as an extension of the physical examination. Ultrasound examination provides an excellent opportunity for patient education and to explain the rationale for therapy [1].

However, with the developing bone structures, the interpretation of findings may vary and may be very challenging. Other modalities may still be used including radiographs and MRI scans to complement or even to use it for specific conditions, like when looking for structural abnormalities. But with the use of ultrasound, one can monitor the changes and development of the musculoskeletal structures and functionally also monitor the activity of the joints [2–4]. Unique to the ultrasound is its ability to visualize the hyaline cartilage profile in the epiphyses, imaging of the entheses and the dynamic imaging capability. It has inherent advantages of allowing contralateral examination and doing targeted and guided procedures both in the diagnosis and management of diseases [1]. US is the primary imaging modality in some pediatric MSK conditions like infant hip in developmental dysplasia (DDH), hip joint effusion, epiphyseal trauma, and evaluation of the neonatal spine. US is the modality of choice in infants with DDH, both in the initial evaluation and posttreatment follow-up [5].

And as can be seen in the clinical setting, children can easily adapt and are at ease with the scanning of the joints while seeing the images in the monitor. But there is still a lot to be learned in pediatric musculoskeletal ultrasound. Although in the last decade, there is an abundance of studies, there is still a lack of data and standardization in many aspects, and careful interpretation must be made. Even among professionals the challenge of imaging with pediatric musculoskeletal ultrasound also exists [6]. The developing anatomy of children when seen in the ultrasound with its varying degrees of non-ossified cartilaginous and vascular structures, irregular ossification centers, and presence of Doppler signals should be taken into consideration when imaging these patients [5, 7].

J. C. de Castro (✉)
Physical Medicine and Rehabilitation Department, The Medical City-South Luzon, Santa Rosa, Laguna, Philippines

SMARTMD Center for Non-Surgical Pain Interventions, Makati City, Philippines

Y. El Miedany (ed.), *Pediatric Musculoskeletal Ultrasonography*,
https://doi.org/10.1007/978-3-030-17824-6_5

Preparation and Techniques

Proper positioning of the patient is part of the preparation when doing ultrasound for pediatric patients so that areas of interest can easily be scanned and visualized while at the same time the comfort of the child is well addressed. The parents will usually be around to provide additional comfort during the procedure (Fig. 5.1).

Superficial structures of the hands and feet may be visualized by using a standoff gel; otherwise the regular gel or even a warm gel could be used [8]. Resolution is optimized by using a linear high-frequency 7.5–15 MHz transducer [8]. Higher frequency may be required for superficial structures. And for deep structures like the hip, it may be necessary to use a low-frequency transducer. One should at first penetrate to bone for a maximum field of view and then back off to the appropriate depth of interest so as not to miss any deeper lesions [6]. Side-to-side comparisons using a split screen function to help confirm an abnormality on the side being complained about may be used. An extended field of view may be used to show large, continuous areas of anatomy in order to see the full extent of the lesions [6, 8].

Color and power Doppler techniques are used to characterize the inflammation that may exist in the joint and the synovium. It is possible to see some vascularization in the ossification centers in developing bones [7].

Cartilage

Imaging of the epiphyseal cartilage shows a distinct homogenously hypo- to anechoic band adjacent to the hyperechoic ossifying epiphyses [9–14]. Epiphyseal and articular cartilage can hardly be differentiated except with the use of MRI. With skeletal maturation and progressive endochondral ossification, the thickness of epiphyseal cartilage decreases, a change that is readily apparent on sonography [14]. In the study of Chauvin et al., the apophyseal cartilage appeared moderately hypoechoic at most sites in the youngest children and transitioned to increasing echogenicity as the child neared skeletal maturity (Fig. 5.2). Also, the cartilage thickness at all decreases with advancing age and varied with gender [15]. Jousse-Joulin et al. have seen similar findings in their study and that apophyseal cartilage thickness likewise decreases with age and is lower in thickness among girls. The secondary ossification center is visible by ultrasound as young as 2 years old. They have also noted a majority of children in different age groups showing a wavy bone-cartilage interface with relative hypoechogenicity. Most of the apophyseal cartilage was no longer visible in children between 8 and 15 years old except for the remaining 33% of children [15]. Ultrasound among healthy children consistently showed greater cartilage thickness in boys in all ages and at all sites [9]. During growth, the cartilage is gradually replaced by the ossification centers of the patella, tuberosity apophysis,

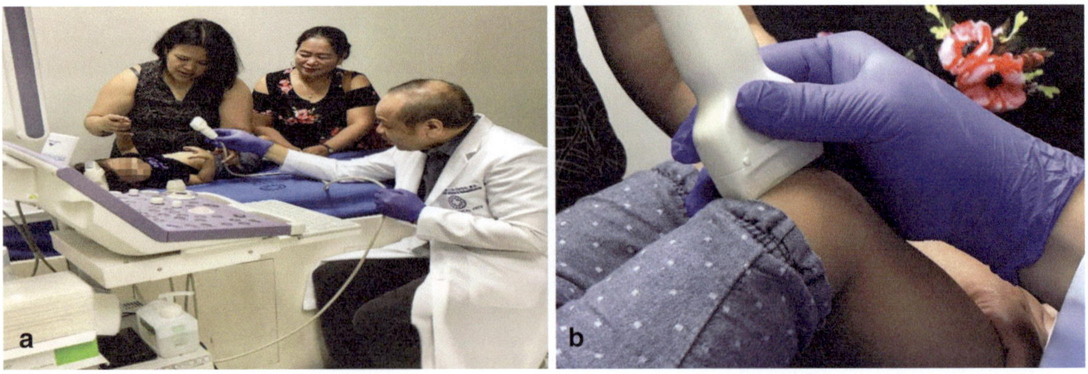

Fig. 5.1 Parents are usually around (**a**) to ad comfort during the ultrasound examination to enable the child (**b**) to adapt to the probe of the ultrasound machine

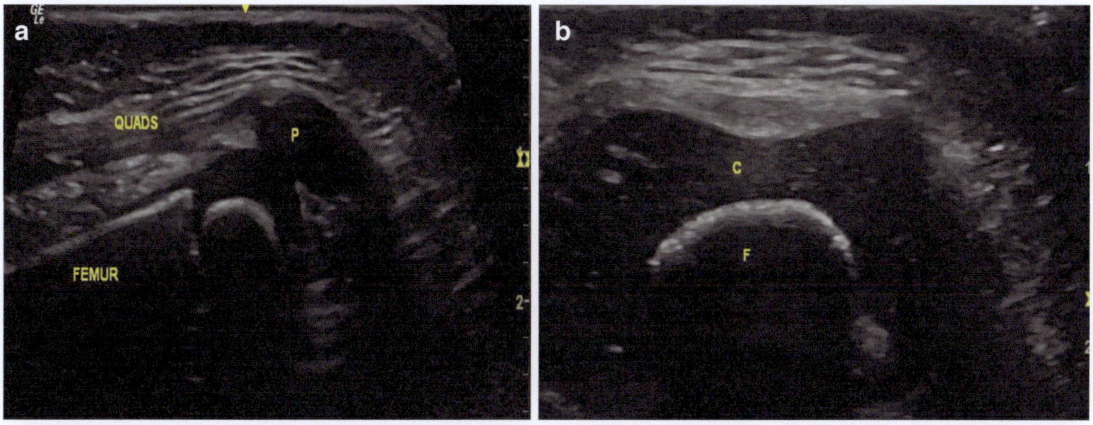

Fig. 5.2 (**a**) Longitudinal view of the knee showing the cartilage thickness of an 8-year-old child showing the cartilage thickness of the knee relative to the bone and the tendon. (**b**) Transverse view of the knee in full-flexion position showing the cartilage thickness. P patella, F femur, C cartilage

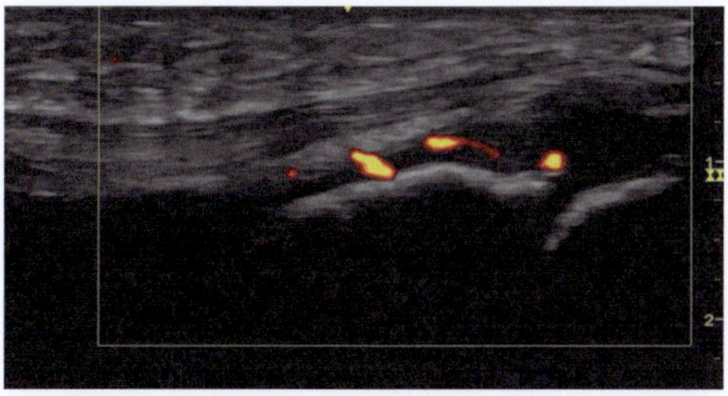

Fig. 5.3 Longitudinal view of the knee of a normal 8-year-old with Doppler examination. Some degree of flow which signifies vascularization is considered normal

and the calcaneal apophysis [15]. Secondary ossification centers will usually appear hyperechoic with the normal cartilage appearing homogenously anechoic [9, 13, 14]. Depending on the joints, the epiphyseal cartilage thickness varies from one joint to the other [13, 14]. Further, fibrocartilage can also be seen in the apophyseal regions of the joint and appears as a structure with a punctate, homogeneous echogenicity [16–18].

Doppler examination of the cartilage may show some degree of flow which may signify normal vascularization of the epiphyseal cartilage instead of hyperemia in the synovium especially among younger healthy children [19, 20] (Fig. 5.3). Cartilage or apophyseal cartilaginous vascularization was apparent in younger age group and disappeared as ossification progressed during growth [15]. Furthermore, cartilage vascularity was seen only when the cartilage appeared moderately hypoechoic [20].

Pradsgaard et al. from the same group of investigators compared ultrasound and MRI measurements of distal femoral cartilage thickness in children with JIA. They identified the intercondylar notch as the best site to assess cartilage thickness, because of its easier assessment and lower variability on MSUS as compared to MRI [21]. Some authors, however, suggest that the normal contour of the cartilage would be more discriminative than the actual measurement of the cartilage thickness when assessing pathologies in the joint [22].

Joint cartilage is a known target in inflammatory arthritis. In the past, radiograph is used for early detection of cartilage damage. The occurrence of cartilage loss in children with juvenile idiopathic arthritis (JIA) represents, therefore, an early indicator of joint damage and raises the need to intensify therapy before irreversible structural changes develop [23]. Loss of ultrasound-detected cartilage in "key sites" of the joints may represent an early marker of damage in JIA [24]. Some authors described this as a blurring of the articular surface [10]. Spannow and coworkers measured cartilage thickness with ultrasound in joints of patients with juvenile idiopathic arthritis (JIA), and compared the findings with those obtained in healthy children. Of note, cartilage thickness in joints of patients with JIA was significantly lower than in the healthy cohort, regardless of whether the examined joints have been previously affected by arthritis [25]. With chronic destruction of the cartilage, it will show pitting of the articular surface and thinning of the cartilage [26].

Bone Erosions

Early onset of bone erosions has been linked to poor prognosis and has been associated with the presence of synovitis and higher risk of progressive disease in rheumatoid arthritis [27–29]. Radiographically, bone erosions do not show changes until 30% of the bones are damaged [30]. With musculoskeletal ultrasound, the detection of bone erosions in early rheumatoid arthritis is seven times more [31]. MRI scans are twice as sensitive than ultrasound for detecting bone marrow edema and bone erosions and are more evident among patients with less than three years duration of disease. Furthermore, MRI findings precede any detectable radiographic bone erosions. Thus, in the study of Malattia et al., the greater sensitivity of the MRI scans to detect bone erosions could be leverage for patients who need aggressive therapy and with a greater tendency for progression [32].

Ultrasound characterizes bone erosions in two perpendicular planes and is defined as provided by the Outcome Measures in Rheumatoid Arthritis Clinical Trials (OMERACT) study group [31, 33]. Bone erosion is defined here as a discontinuity of the bone surface visible in two perpendicular planes [34]. Erosions smaller than 1 mm are not considered and are classified according to the bone involved (metacarpus or metatarsus), their topography (dorsal, volar, or lateral quadrants), and their extent (unifocal, multifocal, or massive). The fifth metatarsal head was the most frequently involved site in terms of bone erosion and its lateral quadrant the one where the greatest number of bone erosions was found, while the first metatarsal head has the highest number of bone erosion occurrence in the early rheumatoid arthritis [35]. In longstanding rheumatoid arthritis patients, the second metacarpal was the most frequently involved site in terms of bone erosion occurrence [35]. Caution must be observed with individuals showing prominent anatomical necks, [36] from vascular bone channels [35] or that with osteoarthritic changes [34] as these may be prone for misinterpretation. Among pediatric patients, the epiphyseal plates may be confused with erosions since the developing bone in that area is usually irregular. Thus, careful considerations must be exercised when imaging these patients [31, 34]. In patients with gout, bone erosions occur mostly on the first metatarsal head, especially on the medial aspect, and are frequently multifocal [37].

In the study by Dohn et al., ultrasound showed an overall moderate sensitivity of 44% and a very high specificity of 95% for US-detected erosions when using CT as the reference method. However, except for the wrist, the sensitivity improved considerably to 71% when only areas with good ultrasound accessibility were included [38].

No scoring systems have been standardized for bone erosions. All scoring systems have been designed to assess erosive changes semi-quantitatively [31, 32, 39–41]. The present study compares different ultrasound erosions scores and these systems are described by Szkudlarek and the ScUSSe (scoring by ultrasound structural erosion) system [39, 42] (Fig. 5.4). The systems agree on larger erosions, whereas the smallest (Szkudlarek grade 1) were not scored by the ScUSSe system [40]. However, majority (86%) of these (Szkudlarek grade 1) erosions were supported by CT scans, thus proving the reliability of using ultrasound even for subtle bone changes and for assessment of the base of proximal phalanges where even images of two perpendicular planes could be very challenging [40]. Interobserver reliability of 91% in the study of Szkudlarek has been reported for bone erosion detection [39].

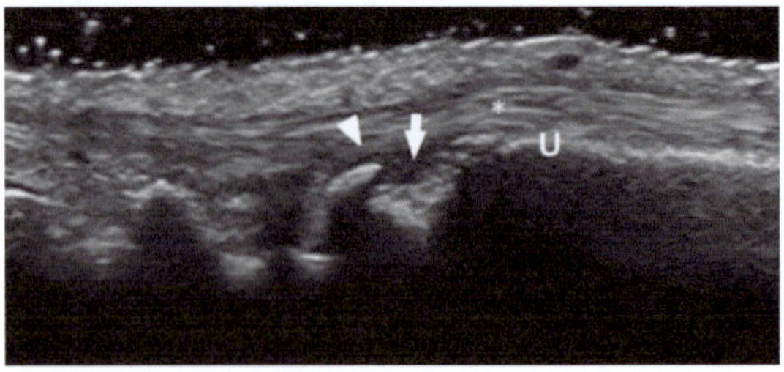

Fig. 5.4 A longitudinal view of the ulna with bone erosions. U, distal ulnar styloid; ∗extensor carpi ulnaris tendon; arrow, with grade 2 ScUSSe scoring; and arrowhead, hook-shaped deformity

Ultrasound is a promising tool for detecting bone erosions in rheumatoid arthritis. The main limitation though is the small acoustic window and the inaccessibility of some structures like the wrist. It is always helpful though to use it side by side with MRI scans to validate the existence of a bone erosions especially in very challenging cases [34–38].

Synovitis

Synovitis as defined by OMERACT is an abnormal hypoechoic intra-articular tissue that is non-displaceable and poorly compressible and that may exhibit a Doppler signal [34]. Synovial fluid on the other hand is an abnormal hypoechoic to anechoic intra-articular material that is displaceable and compressible but does not exhibit a Doppler signal [34, 43] (Fig. 5.5).

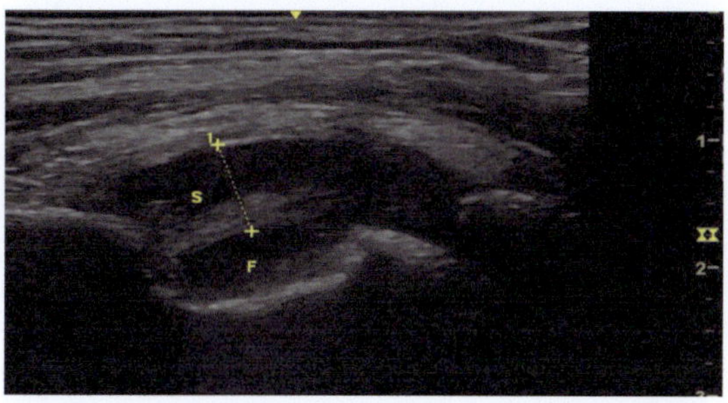

Fig. 5.5 Longitudinal view of a synovial hypertrophy at the level of the anterior elbow joint in a patient diagnosed with rheumatoid arthritis with no sign of active hyperemia. S synovial hypertrophy, F synovial fluid

This also has to be differentiated with synovial hypertrophy which is a swelling of the synovial lining which is non-displaceable and poorly compressible and with no active hyperemia. Therefore, synovitis by ultrasound refer to an abnormally thickened, hypoechoic, intra-articular tissue that is poorly compressible and can demonstrate increased Doppler signals or hyperemia [34, 39, 43]. These definitions by OMERACT would still be adapted by pediatric rheumatology as modifications, validations, and development are still being worked on.

Studies have shown that musculoskeletal ultrasound has been shown to be better than clinical examination in the assessment of synovitis [39, 44, 45]. When differentiating synovitis from synovial hypertrophy or even fluid, it is important not to apply too much pressure on the structures being evaluated as the pressure may compress the flow of the fluid especially when using a color or power Doppler (Fig. 5.6). Distention of the synovium using B-Mode may illustrate abnormalities as well indicating synovitis. A generous amount of gel can be used with a very minimal amount of pressure when imaging suspected synovial abnormalities.

Under normal circumstances, the synovium of the joint is barely visible in ultrasound. Like any inflammatory joint diseases, as in juvenile idiopathic arthritis (JIA), significant changes occur in the synovium leading to the formation of edema, villi, debris, and fluid. Effusions may accompany these findings that may be found in the bursae, tendon sheaths, and the joint itself

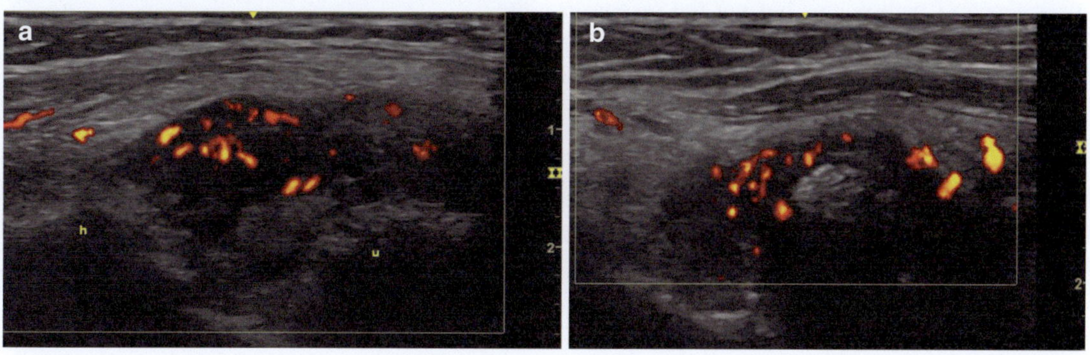

Fig. 5.6 (**a**) Longitudinal view of the elbow showing Doppler flow or signal in a patient diagnosed with rheumatoid arthritis. (**b**) Longitudinal view of the elbow when applying light pressure showing Doppler flow (synovitis). H distal humerus, U proximal ulna

and appear in the ultrasound as anechoic images [10, 46]. To differentiate effusion from synovial hypertrophy, it is helpful to apply minimal pressure where effusion is displaceable and synovial hypertrophy is not [34, 43]. In children, detection of synovial changes may be difficult due to the peculiar presence of hypoechoic cartilage of the epiphyses. It is therefore important to have a good knowledge of age-dependent normal appearance of ultrasound in each joint among this group of patients [10].

Doppler ultrasound is very helpful in demonstrating the increased blood flow in true synovitis. It aids in the diagnosis of any inflammatory activity that may be associated in an abnormal joint effusion. The color Doppler (mean frequency shift) provides qualitative direction of flow and relative velocities, while the power Doppler (power of the Doppler shift) displays the detected blood pool and thus is very sensitive to flow regardless of the velocity or direction of flow [47]. A proliferative and inflamed synovium will usually show high power Doppler signal as well as detect the amount and activity of the pannus in JIA [48]. To some extent, subclinical synovitis can also be detected, although its significance is not yet clear at this point [49].

Synovitis can be monitored by different scoring systems using Doppler activity based on the synovial hypertrophy and the degree of inflammatory activity. There are qualitative, semiquantitative, or quantitative scoring systems. The qualitative scoring systems are used to guide the physicians and patients to evaluate the presence or absence of pathologies but not the responses that can be seen after the treatment. In contrast, the semiquantitative and quantitative Doppler scoring systems, which are correlated with MRI scan findings, monitor the changes identified during medications and therapy [50, 51]. To properly identify the region of interest (ROI) being investigated and monitored, the Doppler box should cover the whole joints and structures to capture all flow information. Newer scoring systems created by the EULAR-OMERACT group have developed a standardized EULAR-OMERACT combined scoring system taking both power Doppler (PD) and synovial hypertrophy (SH) components into account in the evaluation of synovitis of multiple RA joints, which is highly reliable when applied in scanning patients [52]. Further, a Global EULAR-OMERACT Synovial Scoring System may be available for clinical trials and routine care in RA patients with an optimal reduced joint set for scoring synovitis [52]. This consensus-based scoring system hopefully will improve responsiveness and increase the uptake of ultrasound in RA clinical trials [52].

Enthesitis

The integration of tendon to bone occurs at a specialized interface known as the enthesis. It is also defined as the area where tendon, ligament, fascia, and joint capsule insert into the bone and act to transmit tensile load from soft tissues to bone [53]. Two types of entheses are present and are classified depending on the type of tissue at the skeletal attachment site. There is the dense fibrous connective tissue and the fibrocartilage. The fibrous connective tissue is similar to the tendon midsubstance and directly attaches to the bone or periosteum through a fibrous tissue. Fibrocartilaginous enthesis, on the other hand, attaches to the bone through a layer of fibrocartilage transitioning from the fibrous tissue to the bone. Majority of the enthesis in the human body is fibrocartilage, an example of which are the rotator cuffs and Achilles tendon [53–56] (Fig. 5.7).

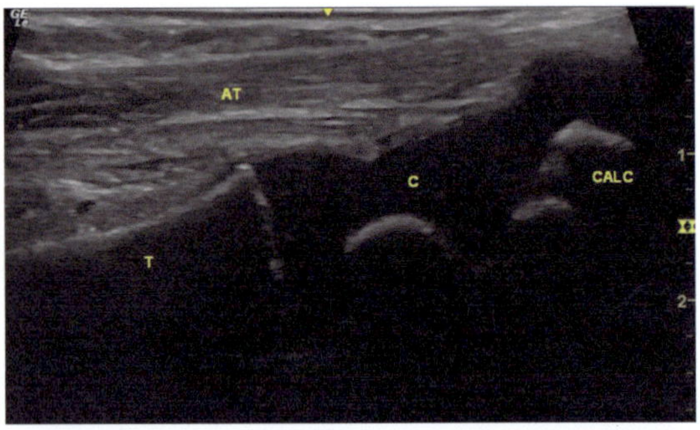

Fig. 5.7 Longitudinal view of the posterior ankle showing the relationship of the Achilles tendon and its insertion at the posterior calcaneal area of an 8-year-old child. AT Achilles tendon, T tibia, C cartilage, Calc immature calcaneal bone

Fibrocartilage entheses are prone to overuse injuries as the insertion angle changes are greater [53, 56]. In the literature, the fibrous and fibrocartilage enthesis may be referred to as "periosteal-diaphyseal" and "chondroapophyseal" or "indirect" and "direct," respectively. The "indirect" attachment is through the periosteum or bone in the metaphyses and diaphysis of the long bones during appositional growth, while the "direct" is through the four transitional layers of the fibrocartilage enthesis in the epiphyses and apophyses [53, 56, 57]. Four anatomic zones of the fibrocartilage enthesis are identified. These are the zone 1, connective tissue (collagen III); zone 2, uncalcified fibrocartilage (proteoglycan aggrecan with collagen); zone 3, calcified fibrocartilage (fibrochondrocytes and predominantly type II collagen); and zone 4 (osteocytes, osteoblasts, and osteoclasts, type I collagen), subchondral bone, which is the site of tendon attachment to bone. Between zone 2 and zone 3 is the tidemark, the basophilic demarcation between calcified and uncalcified fibrocartilage representing between soft and hard tissues [53–57]. This surface reduces the risk of damage to soft tissues during movement [58]. These different layers of the enthesis are indistinguishable sonographically. In fact, the body of the tendon or ligament appears as a normal continuity of the enthesis by ultrasound.

A thorough knowledge of the development of enthesis in children is very important in order to differentiate the normal from pathologic findings. Depending on the age of children, the entheses is mostly composed of the hypo- to anechoic appearance of hyaline cartilage and fibrocartilage rather than the hyperechoic osseous insertion [59]. Study has shown that entheseal thickness increases with age and weight has the strongest correlation and more often boys have thicker enthesis than girls [60]. Power Doppler signal has also been shown to be present at the perientheseal areas as the apophyseal physis closes which may result from physiological stress changes among healthy children during the peripubertal age [20]. With these findings, caution must be exercised when imaging children and thus making a diagnosis of enthesitis.

Enthesitis is a central feature of adult spondyloarthropathies (SpA). And ultrasound has been proven to be very useful and sensitive in the detection of enthesitis and serves as an extension of physical examination in diagnosing enthesopathy [61]. It has also been found out in one study in psoriatic arthritis that ultrasound can detect subclinical entheseal involvement independent of clinical examination and symptoms [62]. With the help of power Doppler ultrasound, neovascularization and subclinical inflammation can detect the increased blood flow found in enthesitis [61].

The most common clinical manifestation of enthesitis in children includes localized pain, tenderness, or swelling over the enthesis. Ultrasound as an extension to physical examination shows increased power Doppler signal, enthesophytes, erosion or cortical irregularities, calcifications or fibrous scar formation, tendon, ligament or capsular thickening and hypoechogenecity [63]. It has also an ability to distinguish enthesitis from possible non-flammatory causes of pain [64]. Among children, ultrasound can detect subclinical enthesitis in patients with juvenile idiopathic arthritis-enthesitis-related arthritis (JIA-ERA) as defined by the International League Against Rheumatism (ILAR). The most commonly affected joints are the sacroiliacs, knees, ankles, and hips. Other joints such as the feet and toes may be involved as well [65]. And the most commonly involved entheses in children with inflammatory joint diseases, as in juvenile idiopathic arthritis, are, in decreasing order, the plantar fascia, Achilles tendon attachment, tibial tuberosity attachment of the patellar ligament, and the patellar attachment of the patellar ligament [15, 66]. Ultrasound is a useful, cost-effective, and safe diagnostic tool in the workup of children with JIA-ERA and for following enthesitis response to treatment [67, 68].

A scoring system for enthesitis in spondyloarthropathy was developed by Balint and colleagues in 2002 comparing ultrasonography with clinical examination, the Glasgow ultrasound enthesitis scoring system (GUESS). GUESS was designed to assess five areas in the lower limb: superior pole of the patella-quadriceps tendon enthesis; inferior

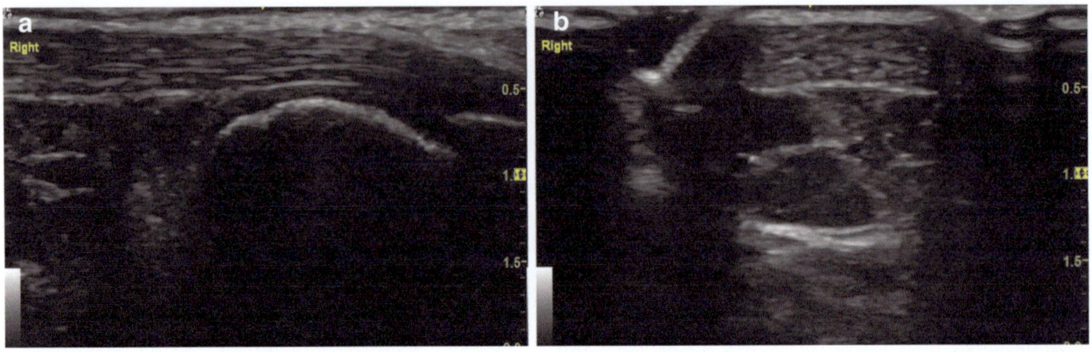

Fig. 5.8 (**a**) Longitudinal view of the tendon of a 9-year-old child over the Achilles tendon insertion at the calcaneus. Notice the hyperechoic, fibrillary linear echoes. (**b**) Transverse view of the Achilles tendon showing the punctated echotexture

pole of the patella-proximal patellar ligament enthesis; tibial tuberosity-distal patellar ligament enthesis; superior pole of the calcaneus-Achilles tendon enthesis; and inferior pole of the calcaneus-plantar aponeurosis enthesis. Except for findings that ultrasound can detect subclinical enthesitis, this scoring system was unable to detect differences for monitoring therapy [69].

Other scoring systems include MASEI (Madrid sonographic enthesitis index) which assesses grayscale and Doppler ultrasound including the assessment of bursa [70]. The Spanish enthesitis index (SEI) also uses grayscale abnormalities at the patient level [71]. These two scoring systems are global enthesitis indices. The D'Agostino System detects Doppler ultrasound and grayscale abnormalities and weighted to the magnitude of Doppler signal and presence of structural damage. This is similar to MASEI as both systems are applied at the enthesis level [72]. There is a need of consensus as to what system is ideal for a given ultrasound finding.

Tendon

Among the musculoskeletal structures, none is more challenging than the tendon sonographically because of the presence of anisotropy which for beginners may affect the interpretation. It usually occurs when the ultrasound beam is not perpendicular with the tendon or ligament [73]. Normal tendon architecture among children by ultrasound showed slightly hyperechoic fibrillary linear echoes extending up to the insertion site on longitudinal view and reticular, punctated echotexture on transverse view (Fig. 5.8).

Chauvin et al. noted that it is not uncommon though to see some perientheseal tendon vascularity during power Doppler examination among healthy children aged 10–13 years old in the absence of any tenderness such that its presence should not be misconstrued as pathological unlike that of adults. This finding was seen among peri-pubertal population and may be due to physiological stress changes as the apophyseal physis closes [20]. Tendon vascularity (intra-entheseal) on the other hand was seen among children between the ages of 4 and 9 years old especially at the quadriceps tendon [20]. Thus, tendon vascularity may be a normal finding in younger children, and peritendinous vascularity may be seen among children nearing apophyseal closure [20].

Tendon thickness is another aspect that seemed interesting among healthy developing children. Tendon thickness was found to have a linear relationship with age [20, 74] but not with gender and showed a consistently increased thickness after puberty [15]. They have observed different insertional patterns of tendon when taking measurements of different tendons. For example, common flexor tendon, patellar tendon, and plantar fascia slightly flared as they attached to the insertion site, while the common extensor, quadriceps, and Achilles tendons slightly tapered at the entheses. However, they have noted that tendon measurements have limited primary diagnostic significance for screening children with tendon pathology unless it is used for following children with established enthesitis-related arthropathy noting the baseline measurements and follow-up measurements on the same child [20].

Tendon pathology in the presence of pain is referred to as tendinopathy. Tendon pathology with or without pain is the term used in the clinical setting [75–79]. Tendon injury is diagnosed in ultrasound as hypoechoic areas or high-grade vascularity irrespective of the clinical diagnosis. Tendinitis was originally used for the term referring to painful and inflamed tendons. However, biochemical, histopathological, and molecular papers have shown rare and limited inflammation as a component of the tendon pathology, thus showing a non-inflammatory tendinosis [79, 80]. Tendinopathy is thus a clinical diagnosis with or without pathology on ultrasound [75].

With tendinosis, there is a hypoechoic swelling of the tendon with loss of the normal fibrillary pattern [81]. There is a wide range of findings that can be seen in tendon inflammation which includes loss of fibrillary architecture, focal or diffuse tendon thickening, focal and extended hypoechoic areas, irregular and ill-defined borders, microruptures, and peritendinous inflammatory edema. In chronic tendon inflammation, there is a loss of the normal sharply defined tendon margin [81]. The most common cause of tendinosis and tenosynovitis among pediatric patients is juvenile rheumatoid arthritis. It can also be seen with overuse injuries or connective tissue disease. Overuse syndrome can eventually lead to inflammation of the tendon and the tendon sheath. Tenosynovitis is defined as abnormal or anechoic material with or without fluid inside the tendon sheath and with possible signs of Doppler signal in orthogonal planes [34]. Further, tenosynovitis is characterized by tendon sheath widening, loss of the normal fibrillary architecture, irregularity of the tendon margin, peritendinous edema, diffuse or focal hypoechoic area inside the tendon, diffuse or focal tendon thickening, and discontinuity of the tendon. Tendon sheath widening is an early sign of rheumatoid arthritis [82]. Power Doppler ultrasound signal may be seen inside the tendon, in the tendon sheath and surrounding soft tissues. Chronic tenosynovitis may show similar findings to acute tenosynovitis. The tendon sheath in chronic tenosynovitis, however, may show nonhomogeneous or hyperechoic material with or without increased vascularity by Doppler ultrasound. The tendon may also show intratendinous calcifications which may be seen in chronic or degenerative tendinopathy associated with endocrine or metabolic diseases [81].

In children, injuries at the tendon affect the apophysis, which is a growth center at the osteotendinous junction. Apophyseal injuries, referred to also as apophysitis, are common especially during the developmental stage. They are however different from injuries at the entheses in adults [75]. Tendinopathy involving the patellar tendon and Achilles tendon has been reported early in life [75]. Tendon load is one of the factors tending to cause this type of injuries [75].

Tendon tears are classified as partial or complete. Minimal partial tendon tears are common in rheumatic diseases. Sonographically, partial tears showed variable hypoechoic areas with associated tendon interruption, and the defects are filled with either fluid, blood, or fat. Complete tendon tear is easily detected with its edges retracted and curled up. Its free ends may move in a pool of fluid, usually termed as "bell-clapper sign." Tendons with synovial sheath may show an "empty sheath sign" [81].

Ligaments, like tendons appear as a hyperechoic fibrillary linear structure. It appears in the ultrasound as a hypoechoic disruption of the normal hyperechoic fibrillary echotexture in a ligamental injury. In contrast to physeal fractures which cause subperiosteal hemorrhage, ligamentous trauma typically results in extraperiosteal hematoma [83].

Muscle

Muscle ultrasound is an established, inexpensive, highly available, painless, and non-sedation-requiring-imaging modality used for screening

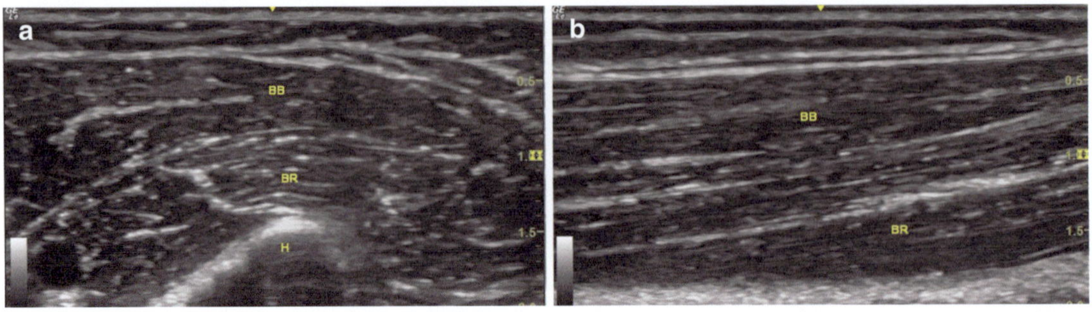

Fig. 5.9 (**a**) Longitudinal view of the muscle of a normal 10-year-old boy at the arm. (**b**) Transverse view of the muscle showing the normal hypoechoic pattern of the muscle and the hyperechoic fibroadipose septa. BB biceps brachii, BR brachialis, H humerus. (Courtesy of Rafael Bennett de Castro)

children with suspected muscle disease and injuries that can be used together with muscle biopsy for pathological confirmation [84]. It is becoming an increasingly important tool for the detection of neuromuscular pathologies [85]. Normal muscles appear uniformly hypoechoic with interspersed hyperechoic fibroadipose septa and fascia in longitudinal ultrasound view. In short-axis view, the muscle has a speckled appearance because of reflections of perimysial connective tissue which is echogenic [83, 86] (Fig. 5.9).

Muscle injuries are classified as strains, tears, or hematomas [87]. Whereas strains result from overuse or overstretching, muscle tears are caused by intense contraction against a firm resistance. Ultrasound findings of muscle strain include diffuse hyperechogenecity in the muscle substance with small hematoma collection or disruption of muscle fibers. Injury does not go beyond the muscle surface [83, 87]. Muscle tear or complete fiber disruption is a full thickness tear of the muscle fibers with the defect extending to the surface of the muscle with associated retraction and hematoma at the site of the tear. Dynamic scanning can help show the size of the retracted fibers. Typically, hematoma appears as a mixed echogenicity mass without increased vascularity. Strains and tears may show increased flow on color Doppler [83, 87].

Muscle ultrasound is a very reliable and useful tool in assessing and detecting neuromuscular disorders and myopathies. Muscle ultrasound has a positive predictive value of 91% and a negative predictive value of 86% in detecting neuromuscular disorders [86]. For patients above 3 years old, the negative predictive value is about 95%, and for those below 3 years old, false negative results were found due to few structural changes noted in the early stage of neuromuscular disorders [86]. Measurements of muscle thickness by ultrasound can be objectively used in assessing neuromuscular disorders and muscle diseases [88–92]. Neuromuscular disorders or myopathies will appear hyperechoic on ultrasound due to the replacement of muscles with fat and fibrosis, although in the early stages of these conditions as the bulk of the muscle tissue is still normal, it is very difficult to distinguish the abnormality by ultrasound [91–95]. The same holds true for metabolic myopathies which have little structural abnormality that can be seen by ultrasound [86]. In neuromuscular disorders, such as muscular dystrophies and spinal muscular atrophy, the muscle fascicles are likewise replaced by fat and connective tissue and with increased number of perimysial septa [87]. Sensitivity of about 67% to 81% is observed when visualizing muscle by ultrasound [94, 96].

Pillen and colleagues made a study distinguishing neurogenic disorders from myopathies using muscle ultrasound. Neurogenic disorders were found to have high echogenic intensity in the legs than in the arms, whereas myopathic disorders reveal an equal distribution of echogenic intensity in the arms and legs. This study showed a positive predictive value of 86% and a negative predictive value of 84% [97]. Recently, they found out that fibrillations and muscle fasciculations can also be detected by ultrasound. Walker and colleagues have even seen ultrasound to be more sensitive than EMG in detecting fasciculations which may be a key to noninvasively identify this electrical activity [98, 99].

With all these developments, muscle ultrasound can be a useful modality in screening children with possible neuromuscular disorders. It can also be used to identify sites for muscle biopsy and even guide the injection site procedures. Additional information regarding muscle fiber injuries can help in determining the type of muscle injuries in a sports trauma [86, 87, 97].

Nerves

Peripheral nerves can be visualized by ultrasound in both children and adults. A high-frequency probe (>10 MHZ) allows good visualization of the internal structure of the peripheral with the typical fascicular or honeycomb-like echotexture in short-axis view. This is characterized by the hypoechoic structures corresponding to the nerve fascicle surrounded by a hyperechoic structure that corresponds to the epineurial layers made up predominantly of fat and connective tissue. In long-axis view, the fascicles are seen as multiple parallel, hypoechogenic bands separated by hyperechogenic internal and external epineurium [100]. Ultrasound images correspond well with histologic studies [100, 101]. Ultrasound is not sensitive enough to visualize endoneurium and perineurium [101] (Fig. 5.10).

Pathologic findings of the peripheral nerve show a hypoechoic enlargement of the peripheral nerve at or proximal to the level of the entrapment, loss of fascicular patterns, increased echogenicity of the distal innervated muscles, and later with decreased muscle size [100, 102]. It has been shown that thickened nerves can be seen in certain hereditary sensory and motor neuropathies [103]. A study by Yiu and colleagues showed an increase in cross-sectional area (CSA) of the peripheral nerve of Charcot-Marie-Tooth type A1 (CMT1A) pediatric patient which is correlated with the severity of the patient. The results of the study have a strong positive linear correlation with age, height, and weight of the patients [104]. The peripheral nerve enlargement of CMT1A is usually uniform up to the level of the nerve roots [105, 106]. In the study of Noto and colleagues, patients with larger CSA in the median and greater auricular nerve may show more marked impairment. The degree of the severity may be determined by the onion-bulb pathological change which is a repetitive demyelination-remyelination event and the proliferation of nerve stroma [106]. Enlarged nerves among children have also been observed in hereditary hypertrophic neuropathies especially Dejerine-Sottas disease and CMT1A. All other types of CMT have larger peripheral nerves but not always especially in demyelinating type of CMT [106]. Focal enlargement of nerves at entrapment site is a characteristic ultrasound finding of hereditary neuropathy with tendency to pressure palsy. Ultrasound is usually studied

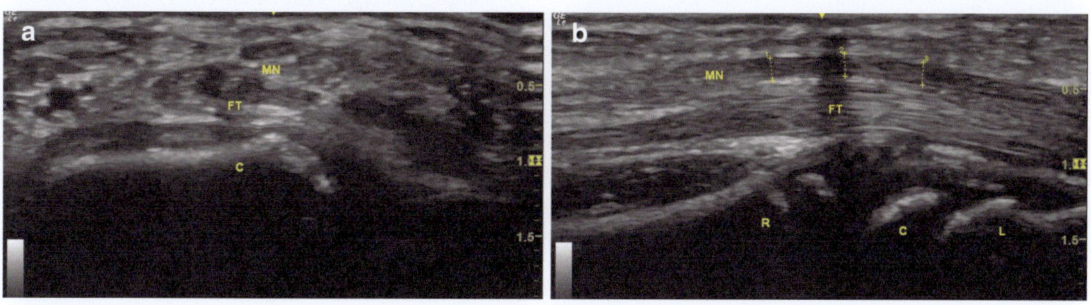

Fig. 5.10 (**a**). Transverse view of the median nerve at the carpal tunnel inlet of an 8-year-old child with the typical hypoechoic nerve fascicles and underneath it lies the hyperechoic flexor tendons. (**b**) Longitudinal view of the median nerve with the hypoechoic nerve fascicles with the flexor tendons below it. MN median nerve, FT flexor tendons, C carpal bones (**a**), R radius, C capitate, L lunate. (Courtesy of Zarah Francine de Castro)

together with nerve conduction studies for classification and diagnosis [105]. There is a significant negative correlation between the CSAs of median nerve and the motor conduction velocity in the corresponding segment. The decrease in motor conduction velocity in CMT1A reflects the functional aspect of a pathologic myelin with corresponding increase in the CSA over time [106]. Children as young as 3 years old may present with enlarged and palpable median nerve at the elbow approximating the pencil size. Nerve hypertrophy has also been reported in Hansen's disease, chronic inflammatory demyelinating neuropathy, nerve tumors, and certain focal nerve lesions [107].

Other interesting findings in children regarding nerve pathology include ulnar nerve instability in the medial elbow. In the study by Erez and colleagues, they found 27.5% with subluxating ulnar nerve and 9.8% with dislocating ulnar nerve. This finding is usually bilateral and is associated with ligamentous laxity and is mostly found between 6- and 10-year-old patients [108]. Ultrasound imaging of the peripheral nerves is also useful for postoperative surgical care and decision-making especially for those cases presenting with weakness and paralysis after a surgical procedure. Typically, careful watchful waiting and neurophysiologic studies are made when no recovery is seen in 4 months. Lee and colleagues made a study where ultrasound was used immediately to guide in the decision-making postoperatively and identify patients who would benefit from early surgical intervention [109, 110].

The use of ultrasound for children knows no bounds. Although there are paucity of studies and the literature is still sparse, the developments that are now available for its use are very promising. Ultrasound provides many advantages not only for diagnostic purposes but also for guidance in interventional procedures and for imaging without sedation and with no radiation exposure. Structures previously visualized can be monitored before, during, and after a treatment. Dynamic and Doppler capabilities are available and with the availability of high-resolution ultrasound and even with the use of elastography, we can discover and enhance the techniques that we know ultrasound can be used for specific purposes. However, care must be exercised in interpreting results, and familiarity with age-appropriate images must be considered carefully during the course of ultrasound scanning especially when interpreting pathological conditions.

Even the youths shall faint and be weary, and the young men shall utterly fall: But they that wait upon the Lord shall renew their strength; they shall mount up with wings as eagles; they shall run, and not be weary; they shall walk, and not faint. (Isaiah 40:30, 31)

References

1. Patil P, Dasgupta B. Role of diagnostic ultrasound in the assessment of musculoskeletal diseases. Ther Adv Musculoskelet Dis. 2012;4(5):341–55. https://doi.org/10.1177/1759720X12442112.
2. Smith J, Finnoff JT. Diagnostic and interventional musculoskeletal ultrasound: part 1. Fundam. PM R. 2009;1(1):64–75.
3. Kane D, Balint PV, Sturrock R, Grassi W. Musculoskeletal ultrasound—a state of the art review in rheumatology. Part 1: Current controversies and issues in the development of musculoskeletal ultrasound in rheumatology. Rheumatology. 2004;43(7):823–8.
4. Dias JM, Costa MM, Canhao H, Saraiva F, da Silva JA. Musculoskeletal ultrasound in paediatric rheumatology: a retrospective analysis. Acta Rheumatol Port. 2014;39(4):309–14.
5. Karnik AS, Karnik A, Joshi A. Ultrasound examination of pediatric musculoskeletal diseases and neonatal spine. Indian J Pediatr. 2016;83(6):565–77. https://doi.org/10.1007/s12098-015-1957-2. Epub 2016 Feb 1. Review.
6. DiPietro MA, Leschied JR. Pediatric musculoskeletal ultrasound. Pediatr Radiol. 2017;47:1144–54. https://doi.org/10.1007/s00247-017-3919-5.
7. Roth J, Jousse-Joulin S, Alcalde M, Magni-Manzoni S, Rodriguez A, Tzaribachev N, Iagnocco A, Naredo E, D'Agostino MA, Collado P. OMERACT definitions for the sonographic features of the normal pediatric joint. Arthritis Care Res (Hoboken). 2015;67(1):136–42.
8. Hryhorczuk AL, Restrepo R, Lee EY. Pediatric musculoskeletal ultrasound: practical imaging approach. Am J Roentgenol. 2016;206(5):W62–72.
9. Spannow HA, Stenboeg E, Pfeiffer-Jensen M, Herlin T. Ultrasound measurement of joint cartilage thickness in large and small joints in healthy children: a clinical pilot study assessing observer variability. Pediatr Rheumatol Online J. 2007;5:3. https://doi.org/10.1186/1546-0096-5-3.

10. Tok F, Demirkaya E, Ozcakar L. Musculoskeletal ultrasound in pediatric rheumatology. Pediatr Rheumatol Online J. 2011;9:25. https://doi.org/10.1186/1546-0096-9-25.
11. McCune WJ, Dedrick DK, Aisen AM, MacGuire A. Sonographic evaluation of osteoarthritic femoral condylar cartilage. Correlation with operative findings. Clin Orthop. 1990;254:230–5.
12. Aisen AM, McCune WJ, MacGuire A, et al. Sonographic evaluation of the cartilage of the knee. Radiology. 1984;153:781–4.
13. Grassi W, Lamanna G, Farina A, Cervini C. Sonographic imaging of normal and osteoarthritic cartilage. Semin Arthritis Rheum. 1999;28:398–403.
14. Panghaal V, Janow G, Angela T, Ilowite N, Levin TL. Normal epiphyseal cartilage measurements in the knee in children: an alternative sonographic approach. J Ultrasound Med. 2012;31:49–53.
15. Jousse-Joulin S, Cangemi C, Gerard S, Gestin S, Luc B, Parscau L, Devauchelle-Pensec V, Saraux A. Normal Sonoanatomy of the paediatric entheses including echostructure and vascularization changes during growth. Eur Radiol. 2015;25(2):2143–52.
16. Ogden JA, Hempton RF, Southwick WO. Development of the tibial tuberosity development. Anat Rec. 1974;182:431–46.
17. Pesquer L, Scepi M, Bihan M, et al. Normal ultrasound anatomy of the triangular fibrocartilage of the wrist: a study on cadavers and on healthy subjects. J Clin Ultrasound. 2009;37:194–8.
18. Lee JC, Healy JC. Normal sonographic anatomy of the wrist and hand. Radiographics. 2005;25:1577–90.
19. Shahin AA, el-Moffy SA, el-Shiek EA, Hafez HA, Ragab OM. Power Doppler sonography in the evaluation and follow-up of knee involvement in patients with juvenile idiopathic arthritis. Z Rheumatol. 2001;60:148–55. https://doi.org/10.1007/s003930170063.
20. Chauvin NA, Ho-Fung V, Jaramillo D, Edgar JC, Weiss PF. Ultrasound of the joints and entheses in healthy children. Pediatr Radiol. 2015;45:1344–54.
21. Pradsgaard DO, Fiirgaard B, Spannow AH, Heuck C, Herlin T. Cartilage thickness of the knee joint in juvenile idiopathic arthritis: comparative assessment by ultrasonography and magnetic resonance imaging. J Rheumatol. 2015;42:534–40.
22. Sureda D, Quiroga S, Arnal C, Boronat M, Andreu J, Casas L. Juvenile rheumatoid arthritis of the knee: evaluation with US. Radiology. 1994;190(2):403–6.
23. Magni-Manzoni S. Ultrasound measurement of cartilage thickness in childhood arthritis—Target the tissue, tailor the technique. J Rheumatol. 2015;42(3):369–2.
24. Magni-Manzoni S. Ultrasound in juvenile arthritis. Pediatr Rheumatol. 2016;14:33. https://doi.org/10.1186/s12969-016-0096-2.
25. Pradsgaard DO, Spannow AH, Heuck C, Herlin T. Decreased cartilage thickness in juvenile idiopathic arthritis assessed by ultrasonography. J Rheumatol. 2013;40:1596–603.
26. Buchman RF, Jaramillo D. Imaging of articular disorders in children. Radiol Clin N Am. 2004;42:151–68. https://doi.org/10.1016/S0033-8389(03)00159-3.
27. Magni-Manzoni S, Rossi F, Pistorio A, Temporini F, Viola S, Beluffi G. Prognostic factors for radiographic progression, radiographic damage, and disability in juvenile idiopathic arthritis. Arthritis Rheum. 2003;48:3509–17. https://doi.org/10.1002/art.11337.
28. Conaghan PG, O'Connor P, McGonagle D, et al. Elucidation of the relationship between synovitis and bone damage: a randomized MRI study of individual joints in patients with early RA. Arthritis Rheum. 2003;48:64–7.
29. Ravelli A. Martini a: early predictors of outcome in juvenile idiopathic arthritis. Clin Exp Rheumatol. 2003;21:89–93.
30. Ejbjerg BJ, Vestergaard A, Jacobsen S, Thomsen H, Ostergaard M. Conventional radiography requires a MRI-estimated bone volume loss of 20% to 30% to allow certain detection of bone erosions in rheumatoid arthritis metacarpophalangeal joints. Arthritis Res Ther. 2006;8:R59.
31. Wakefield RJ, Gibbon WW, Conaghan PG, et al. The value of sonography in the detection of bone erosions in patients with rheumatoid arthritis: a comparison with conventional radiography. Arthritis Rheum. 2000;43:2762–70.
32. Malattia C, Damasio MB, Magnaguagno F, Pistorio A, Valle M, Martinolli C, Viola S, Buoncompagni A, Loy A, Ravelli A, Toma P, Martini A. Magnetic resonance imaging, ultrasonography, and conventional radiography in the assessment of bone erosions in juvenile idiopathic arthritis. Arthritis Rheum (Arthritis Care Res). 2008;58(12):1764–72.
33. Ostergaard M, Peterfy C, Conaghan P, McQueen F, Bird P, Ejbjerg BJ, Shnier R, O'Connor P, Klarlund M, Emery P, Genant H, Lassere M, Edmonds J. OMERACT rheumatoid arthritis magnetic resonance imaging studies. Core set of MRI acquisitions, joint pathology definitions and the OMERACT RA-MRI scoring system. J Rheumatol. 2003;30(6):1385–6.
34. Wakefield RJ, Balint PV, Szkudlarek M, et al. Musculoskeletal ultrasound including definitions for ultrasonographic pathology. J Rheumatol. 2005;32:2485–7.
35. Tamas MM, Filippucci E, Becciolini A, Gutierrez M, Di Geso L, Bonfiglioli K, Voulgari PV, Salaffi F, Grassi W. Bone erosions in rheumatoid arthritis: ultrasound findings in the early stages of the disease. Rheumatol. 2014;53(6):1100–7.
36. Boutry N, Larde A, Demondion X, et al. Metacarpophalangeal joints at US in asymptomatic volunteers and cadaveric specimens. Radiology. 2004;232:716–24.
37. Wright SA, Filippucci E, McVeigh C, et al. High-resolution ultrasonography of the first metatarsal phalangeal joint in gout: a controlled study. Ann Rheum Dis. 2007;66:859–64.

38. Dohn UM, Terslev L, Szkudlarek M, Hansen MS, Hetland ML, Hansen A, Madsen OR, Hasselquist M, Moller J, Ostergaard M. Detection, scoring and volume assessment of bone erosions by ultrasonography in rheumatoid arthritis: comparisons with CT. Ann Rheum Dis. 2012; https://doi.org/10.1136/annrheumdis-2011-201114.
39. Szkudlarek M, Court-Payen M, Jacobsen S, et al. Interobserver agreement in ultrasonography of the finger and toe joints in rheumatoid arthritis. Arthritis Rheum. 2003;48:955–62.
40. Døhn UM, Ejbjerg BJ, Hasselquist M, et al. Detection of bone erosions in rheumatoid arthritis wrist joints with magnetic resonance imaging, computed tomography and radiography. Arthritis Res Ther. 2008;10:R25.
41. Gutierrez M, Filippucci E, Ruta S, et al. Inter-observer reliability of high-resolution ultrasonography in the assessment of bone erosions in patients with rheumatoid arthritis: experience of an intensive dedicated training programme. Rheumatology (Oxford). 2011;50:373–80.
42. Sommier JP, Michel-Batot C, Sauliere N, et al. Structural lesions in RA: proposition for a new semi-quantitative score (ScUSSe: scoring by ultrasound structural erosion). Arthritis Rheum. 2006;53:S140.
43. Wakefield RJ, Balint PV, Szkudlarek M, Filippucci E, Backhaus M, D'Agostino MA, Naredo Sanchez E, Iagnocco A, Schmidt WA, Bruyn GAW, Bruyn G, Kane D, O'Connor PJ, Manger B, Joshua F, Koski J, Grassi W, Lassere MND, Swen N, Kainberger F, Klauser A, Ostergaard M, Brown AK, Machold KP, Conaghan PG. OMERACT 7 special interest group. Musculoskeletal ultrasound including definitions for ultrasonographic pathology. J Rheumatol. 2005;32(12):2485–7.
44. Grassi W. Clinical evaluation versus ultrasonography: who is the winner? J Rheumatol. 2003;30:908–9.
45. Kane D, Balint PV, Sturrock RD. Ultrasonography is superior to clinical examination in the detection and localization of knee joint effusion in rheumatoid arthritis. J Rheumatol. 2003;30:966–71.
46. Kane D, Grassi W, Sturrock R, Balint PV. Musculoskeletal ultrasound–a state of the art review in rheumatology. Part 2: clinical indications for musculoskeletal ultrasound in rheumatology. Rheumatology (Oxford). 2004;43:829–38.
47. Rubin JM, Bude RO, Carson PL, et al. Power Doppler US: a potentially useful alternative to mean frequency-based color Doppler US. Radiology. 1994;190:853–6.
48. Lamer S, Sebag GH. MRI and ultrasound in children with juvenile chronic arthritis. Eur J Radiol. 2000;33:85–93.
49. Hanaa S, El-Banna, Nada DW, Hussein MS, Hablas SA, Darwish NF, Abu-Zaid MH, Gadou SE. Role of musculoskeletal ultrasonography in the detection of subclinical synovitis in oligo and polyarticular juvenile idiopathic arthritis in children. Egypt Rheumatol. 2018; https://doi.org/10.1016/j.ejr.2018.05.008.
50. Terslev L, Torp-Pederson S, Qvistgaard E, et al. Estimation of inflammation by Doppler ultrasound: quantitative changes after intra-articular treatment in rheumatoid arthritis. Ann Rheum Dis. 2003;62:1049–53.
51. Newman JS, Laing TJ, McCarthy CJ, Adler RS. Power Doppler sonography of synovitis: assessment of therapeutic response—preliminary observations. Radiology. 1996;198:582–4.
52. Terslev L, Naredo E, Aegerter P, Wakefield RJ, Backhaus M, Balint P, Bruyn GAW, Iagnocco A, Jousse-Joulin A, Schmidt WA, Szkudlarek M, Conaghan PG, Filippucci E, D'Agostino MA. Scoring ultrasound synovitis in rheumatoid arthritis: a EULAR-OMERACT ultrasound taskforce-part 2: reliability and application to multiple joints of a standardised consensus-based scoring system. Rheum Musculoskelet Dis. 2017;3(1):e000427.
53. Benjamin M, Ralphs JR. Entheses—the bony attachments of tendons and ligaments. Ital J Anat Embryol. 2001;106(2 Suppl 1):151–7.
54. Lu HH, Thomopoulos S. Functional attachment of soft tissues to bone: development, healing, and tissue engineering. Annu Rev Biomed Eng. 2013;15:201–26.
55. Benjamin M, Kumai T, Milz S, Boszczyk BM, Boszczyk AA, Ralphs JR. The skeletal attachment of tendons—tendon "en-theses". Comp Biochem Physiol A Mol Integr Physiol. 2002;133(4):931–45.
56. Apostolakos J, Durant TJS, Dwyer CR, Russell RP, Weinreb JH, Alaee F, Beitzel K, McCarthy MB, Cole MP, Mazzocca AD. The Enthesis: a review of the tendon-to-bone insertion. Muscles Ligaments Tendons J. 2014 Jul-Sep;4(3):333–42.
57. Padulo J, Oliva F, Frizziero A, Maffulli N. Muscles, ligaments and tendons journal. Basic principles and recommendations in clinical and field science research. MLTJ. 2013;4:250–2.
58. Angeline ME, Rodeo SA. Biologics in the management of rotator cuff surgery. Clin Sports Med. 2012;31(4):645–63.
59. Benjamin M, Moriggl B, Brenner E, Emery P, McGonagle D, Redman S. The "enthesis organ" concept:why enthesopathies may not present as focal insertional disorders. Arthritis Rheum. 2004;50:3306–13.
60. Lin C, Diab M, Milojevic D. Grey-scale ultrasound findings of lower extremity entheses in healthy children. Pediatr Rheumatol Online J. 2015;13:14.
61. Kehl AS, Corr M, Weisman MH. Enthesitis: new insights into pathogenesis, diagnostic, modalities and treatment. Arthritis Rheum. 2016 Feb;68(2):312–22.
62. Bandinelli F, Prignano F, Bonciani D, Bartoli F, Collaku L, Candelieri A, et al. Ultrasound detects occult entheseal involvement in early psoriatic arthritis independently of clinical features and psoriasis severity. Clin Exp Rheumatol. 2013;31:219–24.

63. Spadaro A, Iagnocco A, Perrotta FM, Modesti M, Scarno A, Valesini G. Clinical and ultrasonography assessment of peripheral enthesitis in ankylosing spondylitis. Rheumatology (Oxford). 2011;50:2080–6.
64. Gmuca A, Weiss PF. Evaluation and treatment of childhood enthesitis-related arthritis. Curr Treatm Opt Rheumatol. 2015;1(4):350–64.
65. Weiss PF, Klink AJ, Behrens EM, et al. Enthesitis in an inception cohort of enthesitis-related arthritis. Arthritis Care Res (Hoboken). 2011;63(9):1307.
66. Burgos-Vargas R, Pacheco-Tena C, Vazquez-Mellado J. A short-term follow-up of enthesitis and arthritis in the active phase of juvenile onset spondyloarthropathy. Clin Exp Rheumatol. 2002;20:727–31.
67. Shenoy S, Agarwal A. Sonologic enthesitis in children with enthesitis-related arthritis. Clin Exp Rheumatol. 2016;34(1):143–7.
68. Aydin SZ, Karadag O, Filippucci E, Atagunduz P, Akdogan A, Kalyoncu U, et al. Monitoring Achilles enthesitis in ankylosing spondylitis during TNF-alpha antagonist therapy: an ultrasound study. Rheumatology (Oxford). 2010;49(3):578–82.
69. Balint PV, Kane D, Wilson H, et al. Ultrasonography of entheseal insertions in the lower limb in spondyloarthropathy. Ann Rheum Dis. 2002;61:905–10.
70. de Miguel E, Cobo T, Munoz-Fernandez S, et al. Validity of enthesis ultrasound assessment in spondyloarthropathy. Ann Rheum Dis. 2008;68(2):169–74.
71. Alcalde M, Acebes JC, Cruz M, et al. A sonographic enthesitic index of lower limbs is a visible tool in the assessment of ankylosing spondylitis. Ann Rheum Dis. 2007;66:1015–9.
72. D'Agostino MA, Said-Nahal R, Hacquard-Bouder C, et al. Assessment of peripheral enthesitis in the spondyloarthropathies by ultrasonography combined with power Doppler: a cross-sectional study. Arthritis Rheum. 2003;48:523–33.
73. Hryzhorczuk AL, Restreppo R, Lee EY. Pediatric musculoskeletal ultrasound: practical imaging approach. Am J Roentgenol. 2016;206(5):W62–72.
74. Grechenig W, Mayr JM, Peicha G, Hammerl R, Schatz B, Grechenig S. Sonoanatomy of the Achilles tendon insertion in children. J Clin Ultrasound. 2004;32:338–43.
75. Simpson M, Rio E, Cook J. At what age do children and adolescents develop lower limb tendon pathology or tendinopathy? A systematic review and meta-analysis. Sports Med. 2016;46:545–57.
76. Cook JL, Purdam CR. Is tendon pathology a continuum? A pathology model to explain the clinical presentation of load-induced tendinopathy. Br J Sports Med. 2009;43(6):409–16.
77. Khan KM, Cook JL, Kannus P, et al. Time to abandon the "tendinitis" myth. BMJ. 2002;324(7338): 626–7.
78. Magnusson SP, Langberg H, Kjaer M. The pathogenesis of tendinopathy: balancing the response to loading. Nat Rev Rheumatol. 2010;6(5): 262–8.
79. Riley G. The pathogenesis of tendinopathy: a molecular perspective. Rheumatology (Oxford). 2004;43(2):131–42.
80. Scott A, Docking S, Vicenzino B, et al. Sports and exercise-related tendinopathies: a review of selected topical issues by participants of the second international scientific tendinopathy symposium (ISTS) Vancouver 2012. Br J Sports Med. 2013;47(9):536–44.
81. Grassi W, Filippucci E, Farina A, Cervini C. Sonography imaging of tendons. Arthritis Rheum. 2000;43:969–76.
82. Collado P, Naredo E, Calvo C. Assessment of the joint recess and tendon sheaths in healthy children by high-resolution B-mode and power Doppler sonography. Clin Exp Rheumatol. 2007;25:915–21.
83. Seol JG, Callahan MJ. Pediatric musculoskeletal ultrasound. Ultrasound Clin. 2013;8(3):459–75.
84. Hwang HE, Hsu TR, Lee YH, Wang HK, Chiou HJ, Niu DM. Muscle ultrasound: a useful tool in newborn screening for infantile onset Pompe disease. Medicine (Baltimore). 2017;96(44):e8415.
85. Brandsma R, Verbeek RJ, Maurits NM, van der Hoeven JH, Brouwer OF, den Dunnen WFA, Burger H, Sival DA. Visual screening of muscle ultrasound images in children. Ultrasound Med Biol. 2014;40(10):2345–51.
86. Pillen S. Skeletal muscle ultrasound. Eur J Translat Myol. 2010;1(4):145–55.
87. Lee JC, Healy J. Sonography of lower limb muscle injury. Am J Roentgenol. 2004;182:341–61.
88. Heckmatt JZ, Pier N, Dubowitz V. Measurement of quadriceps muscle thickness and subcutaneous tissue thickness in normal children by real-time ultrasound imaging. J Clin Ultrasound. 1988;16:171–6.
89. Heckmatt JZ, Pier N, Dubowitz V. Measurement of quadriceps femoris muscle atrophy and hypertrophy in neuromuscular disease in children. J Clin Ultrasound. 1988;16:177–81.
90. Reeves ND, Maganaris CN, Narici MV. Ultrasonographic assessment of human skeletal muscle size. Eur J Appl Physiol. 2004;91:116–8.
91. Reimers CD, Schlotter B, Eicke BM, Witt TN. Calf enlargement in neuromuscular diseases: a quantitative ultrasound study in 350 patients and review of the literature. J Neurol Sci. 1996;143:46–56.
92. Reimers K, Reimers CD, Wagner S, Paetzke I, Pongratz DE. Skeletal muscle sonography: a correlative study of echogenicity and morphology. J Ultrasound Med. 1993;12:73–7.
93. Heckmatt JZ, Dubowitz V, Leeman S. Detection of pathological change in dystrophic muscle with B-scan ultrasound imaging. Lancet. 1980;1:1389–90.
94. Heckmatt JZ, Pier N, Dubowitz V. Real-time ultrasound imaging of muscles. Muscle Nerve. 1988;11:56–65.
95. Pillen S, Tak R, Lammens M, Verrijp K, Arts I, Zwarts M, Van Engelen B, Verrips A. Skeletal muscle ultrasound: correlation between fibrous tissue and echo intensity. Ultrasound Med Biol. 2009;35:443–6.

96. Zuberi SM, Matta N, Nawaz S, Stephenson JB, McWilliam RC, Hollman A. Muscle ultrasound in the assessment of suspected neuromuscular disease in childhood. Neuromuscul Disord. 1999;9: 203–7.
97. Pillen S, Verrips A, van Alfen N, Arts IM, Sie LT, Zwarts MJ. Quantitative skeletal muscle ultrasound: diagnostic value in childhood neuromuscular disease. Neuromuscul Disord. 2007;17:509–16.
98. Walker FO, Donofrio PD, Harpold GJ, Ferrell WG. Sonographic imaging of muscle contraction and fasciculations: a correlation with electromyography. Muscle Nerve. 1990;13:33–9.
99. Pillen S, Nienhuis M, van Dijk JP, Arts IM, van Alfen N, Zwarts MJ. Muscles alive: ultrasound detects fibrillations. Clin Neurophysiol. 2009;120: 932–6.
100. Martinolli C, Bianchi S, Cohen M, et al. Ultrasound of peripheral nerves. J Radiol. 2005;86:1869–78.
101. Silvestri E, Martinolli C, Derchi LE, et al. Echotexture of peripheral nerves: correlation between US and histologic findings and criteria to differentiate tendon. Radiology. 1995;197:291–6.
102. Jacobson JA, Wilson TJ, Yang LJS. Sonography of the common peroneal nerve disorders with clinical correlation. J Ultrasound Med. March 2016;35(4):683–93.
103. Martinoli C, Schenone A, Bianchi S, Mandich P, Caponetto Abbruzzese M, et al. Sonography of the median nerve in Charcot-Marie-tooth disease. AJR Am J Roentgenol. 2002;178:1553–6.
104. Yiu EM, Brockley CR, Lee KJ, Carroll K, de Valle K, Kennedy R, Rao P, Delatycki MB, Ryan MM. Peripheral nerve ultrasound in pediatric Charcot-Marie-Tooth disease type 1A. Neurology. 2015;84(6):552.
105. Noto Y. Ultrasound diagnosis of Charcot-Marie-tooth disease. Brain Nerve. 2014;66(3):237–46.
106. Noto Y, Shiga K, Tsuji Y, Mizuta I, Higuchi Y, Hashiguchi A, Takashima H, Nakagawa M, Mizuno T. Nerve ultrasound depicts peripheral nerve enlargement in patients with genetically distinct Charcot-Marie-Tooth disease. J Neurol Neurosurg Psychiatry. 2014;86(4):378–84.
107. Walker FO, Ouvrier R. Seeing big nerves in small children (Ed). Neurology. 2015;84(6):569
108. Erez O, Khalil JG, Legakis JE, Tweedle J, Kaminski E, Reynolds RA. Ultrasound evaluation of ulnar nerve anatomy in the pediatric population. J Pediatr Orthop. Sept 2012;32(6):641–6.
109. Lee J, Bidwell T, Metcalfe R. Ultrasound in pediatric peripheral nerve injuries: can this affect our surgical decision making? A preliminary report. J Pediatr Orthop. 2013;33(2):152–8.
110. Dohn UM, Ejbjerg BJ, Court-Payen M, Hasselquist M, Narvestad E, Szkudlarek M, Moller JM, Thomsen HS, Ostergaard M. Are bone erosions detected by magnetic resonance imaging and ultrasonography true erosions? A comparison with computed tomography in rheumatoid arthritis metacarpophalangeal joints. Arthritis Res Ther. 2006;8(4):R110. https://doi.org/10.1186/ar1995.

Part II

Individual Anatomic Sites

Upper limb: Shoulder and Arm

6

Clara Malattia, Stefano Lanni, Federico Zaottini, and Carlo Martinoli

Introduction

The shoulder is one of the largest and most complex joints in the body. It has the greatest range of motion providing the upper extremity with the capability of movements in all planes. The spectrum of pathologies potentially affecting the shoulder is quite different in the children age group compared to adults. The rotator cuff pathology, which is the most common complaint by far in adults as a result of degenerative disease, does not occur in children where positional overload, infection, trauma, dysplasia, and inflammatory disorders are most often observed.

C. Malattia (✉)
Clinica Pediatrica e Reumatologia, Istituto Giannina Gaslini, Genoa, Italy

Dipartimento di Neuroscienze, Riabilitazione, Oftalmologia, Genetica e Scienze Materno-Infantili, Università degli studi di Genova, Genoa, Italy
e-mail: ClaraMalattia@gaslini.org

S. Lanni
Reumatologia Pediatrica, Clinica de Marchi, IRCCS Ca' Granda Ospedale Maggiore Policlinico, Milan, Italy
e-mail: stefano.lanni@policlinico.mi.it

F. Zaottini · C. Martinoli
Division of Radiology Ospedale Policlinico San Martino, Genoa, Italy

Department of Health Science, University of Genova, Genoa, Italy
e-mail: carlo.martinoli@unige.it

Ultrasound is a very sensitive and well-tolerated imaging modality to examine the musculoskeletal system. The low-cost, non-invasive nature and lack of exposure to ionizing radiations make this technique well suited for assessing pediatric patients. Ultrasound represents an excellent imaging modality to obtain a comprehensive depiction of the main anatomical structure of the shoulder, including joint recesses, bursae, ligaments, muscles, and tendons [5]. In addition, it allows dynamic scanning during joint motion and muscle contraction and can guide minimally invasive interventional procedures.

A deep knowledge of anatomy and the use of a proper scanning technique are prerequisites to perform an accurate shoulder examination with ultrasound. In this chapter, the ultrasound anatomy and the most common pathologies of the shoulder which are of interest to pediatric rheumatologists will be reviewed. Special emphasis will be placed to distinguish normal anatomy from imaging pitfalls related to skeletal maturation.

Shoulder Anatomy

The shoulder joint complex includes the scapula, the clavicle, and the proximal humerus acting as a single biomechanical unit. These bones articulate with each other to form the glenohumeral, acromioclavicular, and sternoclavicular joints [30].

Y. El Miedany (ed.), *Pediatric Musculoskeletal Ultrasonography*,
https://doi.org/10.1007/978-3-030-17824-6_6

Glenohumeral Joint

The glenohumeral joint is a "ball-and-socket" synovial joint formed by the articular surfaces of the glenoid cavity and the humeral head [3]. The glenoid cavity is smaller than the humeral head and covers only about one-fourth of its convexity. This discrepancy along with the relative laxity of the joint capsule provides wide mobility but makes the joint inherently unstable. A concentric rim of fibrocartilage, the glenoid labrum, increases the size and depth of the glenoid cavity contributing to the stability of the shoulder joint. The articular surfaces of the humeral head and the glenoid fossa are covered by a continuous layer of hyaline cartilage. In the humerus, the articular cartilage invests the convexity of the humeral head until the level of the anatomic neck, where the joint capsule inserts. The fibrous capsule extends from the outer slope of the glenoid rim to the anatomic neck and is lined by synovial membrane. The glenohumeral joint cavity has three main synovial recess: the biceps tendon sheath anteriorly, the subscapularis recess medially, and the axillary pouch inferiorly (Fig. 6.1). The joint capsule has two openings for the passage of the long head of biceps tendon and for the communication with the subscapularis recess. This recess is connected with the joint through an opening located between the superior and middle glenohumeral ligaments (superior subscapularis recess). The long head of the biceps tendon takes its origin from the upper glenoid rim and the supraglenoid tubercle. Its proximal part is intra-articular in location: it has a curvilinear course and reflects over the anterosuperior aspect of the humeral head, between the anterior border of the supraspinatus and the upper edge of the subscapularis. More distally, it descends the arm crossing a groove between the greater and the lesser tuberosity, the so-called intertubercular sulcus. In the bicipital groove, the biceps is surrounded by a synovial sheath as an extension of the synovial lining of the glenohumeral joint. Detection of intrasheath effusion may therefore reflect an underlying joint disease rather than proper tendon pathology [5].

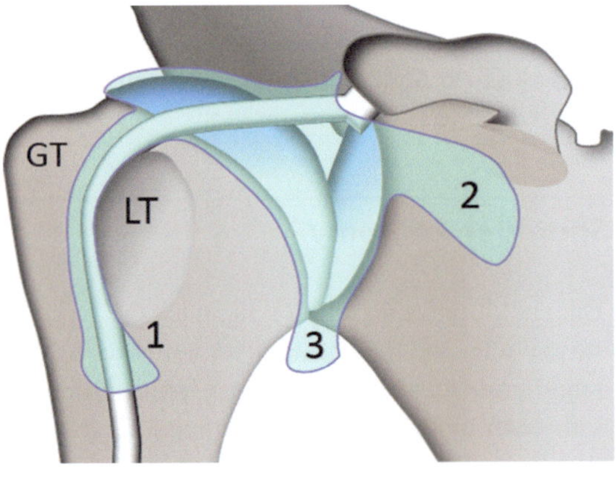

Fig. 6.1 Schematic drawing of the glenohumeral joint cavity. The glenohumeral joint has three main recesses: the biceps tendon sheath (1), the axillary pouch (2), and the subscapular recess (3). GT greater tuberosity, LT lesser tuberosity

Shoulder Ligaments

In the shoulder, five ligaments represent the main sources of passive joint stability (Fig. 6.2).

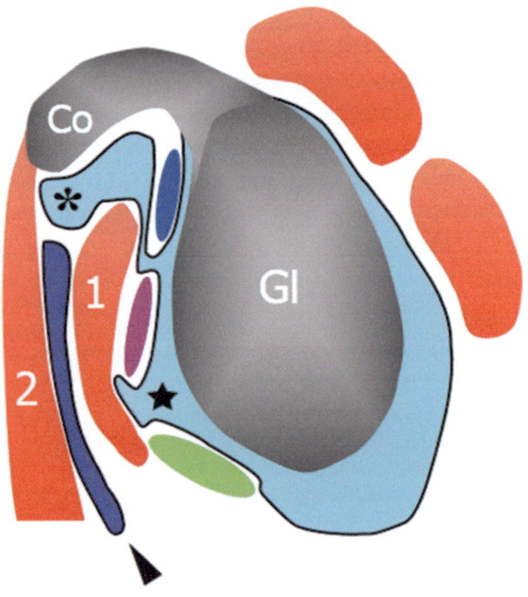

Fig. 6.2 Sagittal view of the glenohumeral joint over the profile of the bony glenoid (Gl) demonstrates the relationship between the superior (brown), middle (purple), and inferior (green) glenohumeral ligaments with the joint cavity (light blue), the subscapularis (1), and the conjoint tendon of the coracobrachialis and short head of the biceps (2). The subscapularis recess (asterisk) appears a small extension of the joint cavity located between the coracoid (Co) and the upper margin of the subscapularis on the anterior aspet of the joint. This recess is separated from the larger subcoracoid bursa (arrowhead) that is an extension of the subacromial subdeltoid bursa

They are the three glenohumeral, the coracohumeral, and the coracoacromial. The superior, middle, and inferior glenohumeral ligaments act to stabilize the anterior aspect of the joint. They arise from the outside slope of the glenoid cavity and attach onto the lesser tuberosity. The coracohumeral ligament supports the superior part of the joint capsule and represents the main stabilizer for the long head of the biceps tendon. It consists two bundles of fibers arising from the coracoid, one (lateral ward) inserting into the greater tuberosity and merging with the joint capsule and the supraspinatus and the other (medial ward) inserting into the lesser tuberosity and the subscapularis. This latter band joins the superior glenohumeral ligament to form the so-called reflection pulley. More distally, the coracohumeral ligament continues as the transverse humeral ligament. This latter ligament bridges over the intertubercular sulcus between the lesser and the greater tuberosity transforming the groove in an osteofibrous tunnel for the long head of the biceps tendon. The coracoacromial ligament joins the acromion and the coracoid, as part of the coracoacromial arch. This structure overlies the shoulder joint, preventing superior displacement of the humeral head [5].

Acromioclavicular Joint and Sternoclavicular Joint

The acromioclavicular joint is a small synovial joint intervening between the medial end of the acromion and the lateral end of the clavicle. Its range of motion is limited. The articular surface of the acromion and the clavicle are invested with hyaline cartilage and are divided by a wedge-shaped disk of fibrocartilage. The joint capsule is attached to the articular margins and reinforced by superior and inferior ligaments.

The sternoclavicular joint is a shallow saddle-shaped joint located between the manubrium of the sternum, the first rib medially and the medial end of clavicle laterally. It represents the only connection between the axial skeleton and the upper extremity. A disk of fibrocartilage splits this joint into medial and lateral cavities, each lined with its own synovial membrane. Costoclavicular and interclavicular ligaments reinforce the joint.

Muscles and Tendons

The muscles around the shoulder may be classified into two groups: intrinsic (i.e., subscapularis, supraspinatus, infraspinatus, teres minor, teres major, and deltoid), which originate and insert on the skeleton of the upper limb, and extrinsic muscles, which join the upper limb with either the spine (i.e., trapezius, latissimus dorsi, levator scapulae, and rhomboid) or the thoracic wall (i.e., serratus anterior, pectoralis minor, and pectoralis major). The rotator cuff consists four muscles that come together as tendons to form a cuff of tissue around the humeral head (Fig. 6.3); it plays an important role as an active stabilizer of the humeral head in the glenoid fossa during

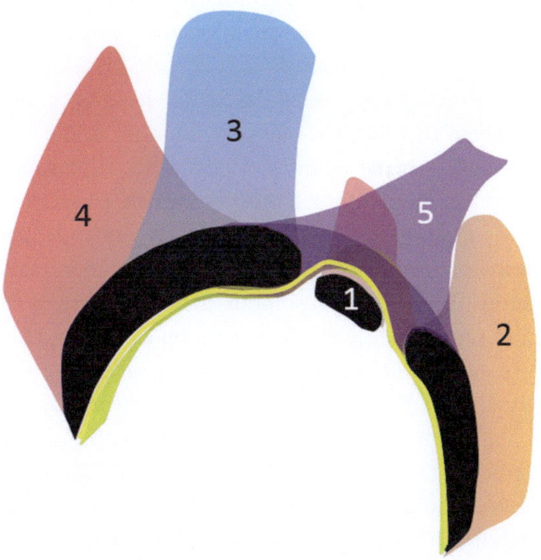

Fig. 6.3 Rotator cuff and biceps tendons. Schematic drawing shows the respective relationships of the long head of the biceps (1), subscapularis (2), supraspinatus (3), and infraspinatus (4) at the level of the humeral head. The supraspinatus and infraspinatus merge in a common flattened tendon. The space located between the anterior border of the supraspinatus and the superior edge of the subscapularis is referred to as the rotator cuff interval. It is roofed by the coracohumeral ligament (5) and houses the long head of the biceps

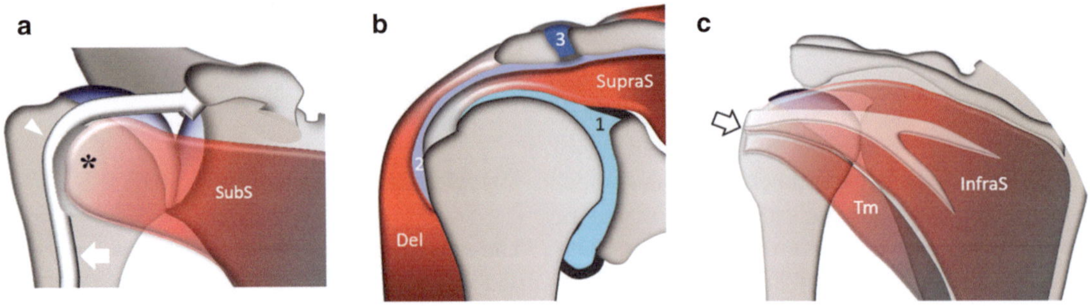

Fig. 6.4 Anatomy of the rotator cuff. (**a**) Anterior view of the shoulder shows the subscapularis (SubS) muscle and tendon inserting into the less tuberosity (asterisk) and the long head of the biceps tendon (arrows) descending the curvature of the humeral head and crossing the intertubercular sulcus (arrowhead). (**b**) Coronal view of the shoulder oriented in the long axis of the supraspinatus tendon (SupraS) demonstrates the extension of glenohumeral joint (1), the subacromial subdeltoid bursa (2), and the acromioclavicular joint (3). The glenohumeral joint cavity extends along the undersurface of the supraspinatus tendon until reaching the anatomic neck (arrowhead) of the humerus. The subacromion subdeltoid bursa lies more superficially, between the supraspinatus and the cover of the deltoid (Del) and the coracoacromioal arch. (**c**) Posterior view of the shoulder shows the infraspinatus (InfraS) and teres minor (Tm) muscles and tendons located inferior to the scapular spine, in the infraspinous fossa of the scapula. Their tendons insert as paired structures into the posterior aspect of the greater tuberosity (arrow)

movements of the arm. The cuff includes the subscapularis, which is placed on the anterior aspect of the shoulder; the supraspinatus, which lies on its superior aspect; and the infraspinatus and teres minor which are located posteriorly (Fig. 6.4). The subscapularis muscle arises from the subscapular fossa; most of its fibers are directed upward and laterally, running under the coracoid on the anterior aspect of the glenohumeral joint, and attach onto the lesser tuberosity. This tendon serves as an adductor and internal rotator of the arm. The supraspinatus muscle stems from the supraspinous fossa of the scapula and runs underneath the acromion and above the glenohumeral joint before inserting on the greater tuberosity. It acts as abductor and internal rotator of the arm. On the posterior shoulder, the infraspinatus muscle originates from the infraspinatus fossa and converges into a large tendon that extends laterally to attach onto the greater tuberosity, just posterior and inferior to the supraspinatus tendon. The smaller teres minor arises from the lateral border of the scapula and inserts into the greater tuberosity, just posterior and inferior to the infraspinatus. The infraspinatus and teres minor muscles act as external rotators of the arm [5]. In addition to the rotator cuff muscles, the intrinsic muscles of the shoulder include the teres major and the deltoid which forms a roof over the rotator cuff tendons and the glenohumeral joint. The deltoid arises from the lateral third of the clavicle, the acromion and the spine of the scapula and attaches on the anterolateral surface of the mid humeral shaft.

Shoulder Bursae

Bursae are synovial lined structures, aiming at reducing friction between tendons and other joint structures during joint movements. Several synovial bursae are found around the shoulder. From the clinical point of view, the most relevant are the subacromial-subdeltoid bursa and the subcoracoid bursa. The subacromial-subdeltoid bursa is a broad synovium-lined structure interposed between the coracoacromial arch and the rotator cuff tendons. It consists of a subacromial and a subdeltoid part. Inferior to the coracoid, the subcoracoid bursa intervenes between the subscapularis and the conjoint tendon of the short head of the biceps and coracobrachialis. This bursa is almost invariably in continuity with the subacromial-subdeltoid bursa and may extend medial to the coracoid. Careful scanning technique is needed to avoid confusion between the subcoracoid bursa and the subscapularis recess.

Peculiarities of the Growing Skeleton

The musculoskeletal is a system that undergoes dramatic changes during growth. At birth, the skeleton is purely chondral and, during the ossification process, cartilage is gradually transformed into bone [18]. A deep knowledge of the evolving patterns of normal skeletal development is mandatory for a correct interpretation of ultrasound images and to avoid misdiagnoses [19]. At full-term birth, the humeral diaphysis, the mid-portion of the clavicle, and the body of the scapula are already ossified, whereas the remaining bones of the shoulder girdle are still chondral. As skeletal maturity progresses, multiple secondary ossification centers arise from the epiphyses and apophyses of the shoulder [37]. The proximal humeral epiphysis exhibits three ossification centers for the humeral head, the greater and the lesser tuberosity. These centers fuse with each other at 3–5 years of age (Table 6.1). The ossification of the humeral head is then completed by the age of thirteen [24]. During skeletal maturation, bone irregularities at the physeal borders are a normal occurrence and should not be mistaken for disease-related bone erosions [7].

The scapula has at least seven secondary ossification centers [23]. The ossification of the glenoid starts with the appearance of the subcoracoid ossification center. This appears as a tongue-like opacity and could be misinterpreted as an avulsion fracture. The inferior two-thirds of the glenoid has several ossification centers that grow and fuse together to form a horseshoe-like complex [17]. Complete fusion occurs by 17–18 years of age. The coracoid starts to ossify at 3 months of age. The first ossification center is located in the center of the coracoid process; the second becomes visible at the base of the coracoid at 8–10 years of age. At birth, the acromion is chondral and shows the footprint of the adult acromion. It consists of up to three ossification centers that ossify and fuse during adolescence. Proximal to distal, these centers include the meta-acromion, mesa-acromion, and pre-acromion, respectively. The failure of fusion of these centers can result in an os acromiale that occurs in approximately 1–8% of patients. The os acromiale is triangular in shape and can articulate with the acromion and the clavicle with a proper articulation. The medial epiphysis of the clavicle starts its ossification at 18 years and fuses with the clavicular metaphysis at 22–25 years of age [25]. Familiarity with the timing, location, and appearance of maturation patterns in the pediatric shoulder is crucial for a correct image interpretation and analysis of findings [14].

Table 6.1 Age of appearance and fusion of the ossification centers in the shoulder girdle

Ossification centers	Age at appearance	Age at fusion
Proximal Humerus		
Humeral head	1–6 months	3–5 years
Greater tuberosity	9–12 months	3–5 years
Lesser tuberosity	12–16 months	3–5 years
Scapula: Glenoid		
Subcoracoid	8–10 years	14–17 years
Centers in the inferior two-thirds of the glenoid	14–15 years	17–18 years
Scapula: Coracoid		
Center of the Coracoid	3 months	15–17 years
Base of the coracoid	8–10 years	15–17 years
Scapula: Acromion		
Acromial secondary ossification centers	14–16 years	18–25 years

Sonoanatomy

Musculoskeletal ultrasound applications are quickly evolving due to improved scanner and transducer technology as well as to an increased awareness of their usefulness among pediatric rheumatologists [21]. Regarding ultrasound technology, a linear array high-frequency (range 10–20 MHz) transducer is required for imaging the shoulder in children. Lower frequencies may occasionally be used to visualize the deep anterior recess of the shoulder in overweight children. Doppler imaging can provide information on regional vessels and tissue microvascular states. When assessing the shoulder with ultrasound, an appropriate patient positioning is crucial to visualize the individual anatomical structures. It has to be comfortable for both patient and examiner in order to reduce the examination time as much as possible. A standardized scanning approach is advisable for obtaining better reproducibility of findings. In our opinion, the technical guidelines issued by the European Society of Musculoskeletal Radiology for adults can perfectly meet the needs for shoulder evaluation in children [2, 4].

Long Head of Biceps Tendon

The standardized examination of the shoulder may start with the evaluation of the long head of biceps tendon, keeping the child seated in front of the examiner. The patient's arm rests on the ipsilateral thigh with elbow flexed at 90° degree and palm upward (Fig. 6.5). The first landmark to identify is the intertubercular sulcus which appears as a groove between the lesser and the greater tuberosities. The appearance of the tuberosities and the sulcus varies with age depending on the degree of skeletal maturation. Placing the probe in a transverse plane over the bicipital groove, the biceps tendon shows a well-defined oval shape. In order to avoid anisotropy, the probe must be kept as perpendicular as possible to the tendon orientation. On the lateral side of the biceps, Doppler imaging may visualize the ascending branch of the anterior circumflex artery. The transverse humeral ligament appears as a thin hyperechoic band bridging over the sulcus. For a complete assessment of the biceps, scanning should be extended upward, to include the intra-articular segment of the tendon as it curves over the convexity of the humeral head, and downward until its myotendinous junction at the level of the pectoralis major tendon (Fig. 6.6a–c). Distal to the humeral tuberosities, the long head lies in front of the proximal humeral metaphysis. It assumes an oblique course, from up down and from anterior to posterior. In this area, a small sheath effusion (e.g., not enough to encircle the tendon) has to be regarded as a normal finding and should not be indicated in the report. Imaging the tendon in the short axis can be enough to screen the status of the biceps. The longitudinal view of the biceps tendon is obtained by rotating the probe ninety degrees clockwise (Fig. 6.7). The long-axis view can also be obtained as a complement of short-axis images to better document abnormal findings.

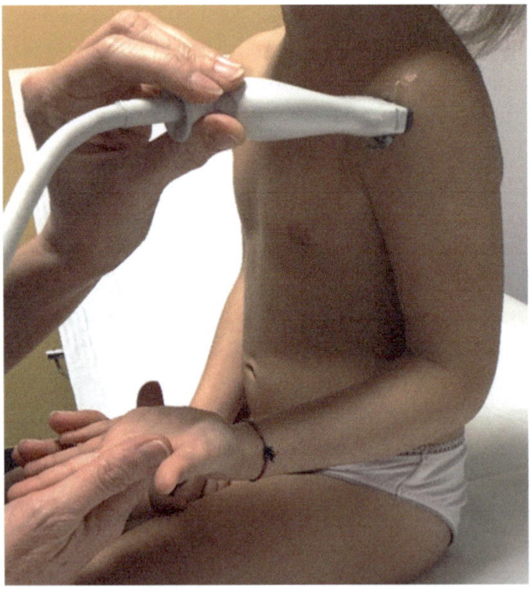

Fig. 6.5 Patient and probe position to examine the long head of the biceps tendon in its short axis

Subscapularis Tendon

The subscapularis is the next tendon to be examined in the cuff after the biceps. The child is invited to rotate the arm externally while keeping the elbow in close contact with the body with supinated hand (Fig. 6.8a). On its long axis, the subscapularis tendon has a convex shape over the curved profile of the humeral head (Fig. 6.8b).

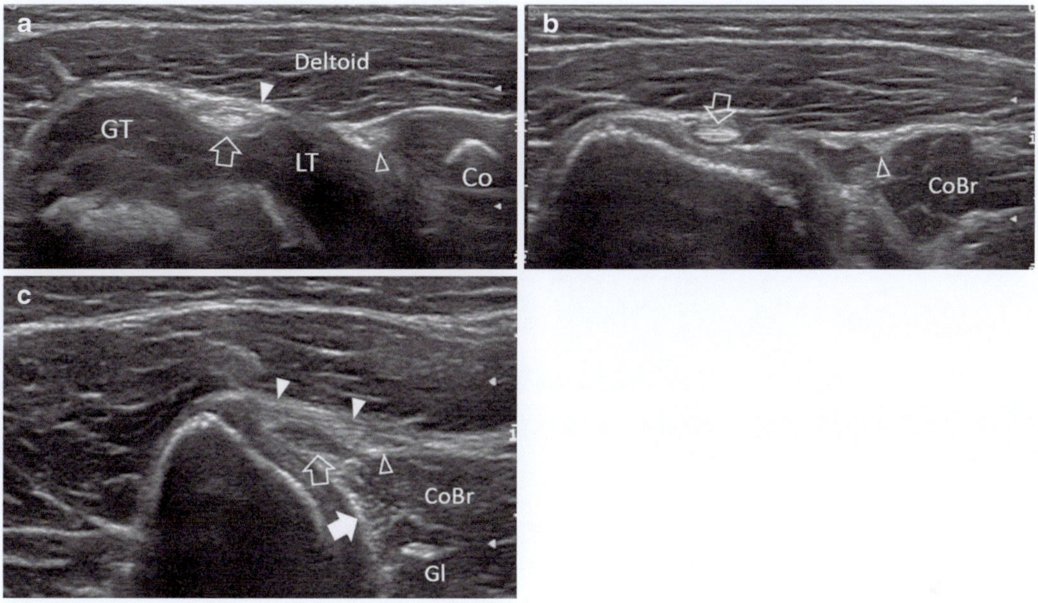

Fig. 6.6 Long head of the biceps tendon examined in the short axis at the level of the (**a**) intertubercular sulcus, (**b**) the most dependent part of its sheath, and (**c**) the musculotendinous junction. In A, the long head of the biceps tendon (void arrow) appears as an oval hyperechogenic image located between the chondral prominences of the greater (GT) and lesser (LT) tuberosities and covered by the transverse humeral ligament (white arrowhead). In C, note the relationship of the myotendinous junction of the biceps with the pectoralis major tendon (white arrowheads). Void arrowhead, short head of the biceps. Co, coracoid (Co). CoBr, coracobrachialis

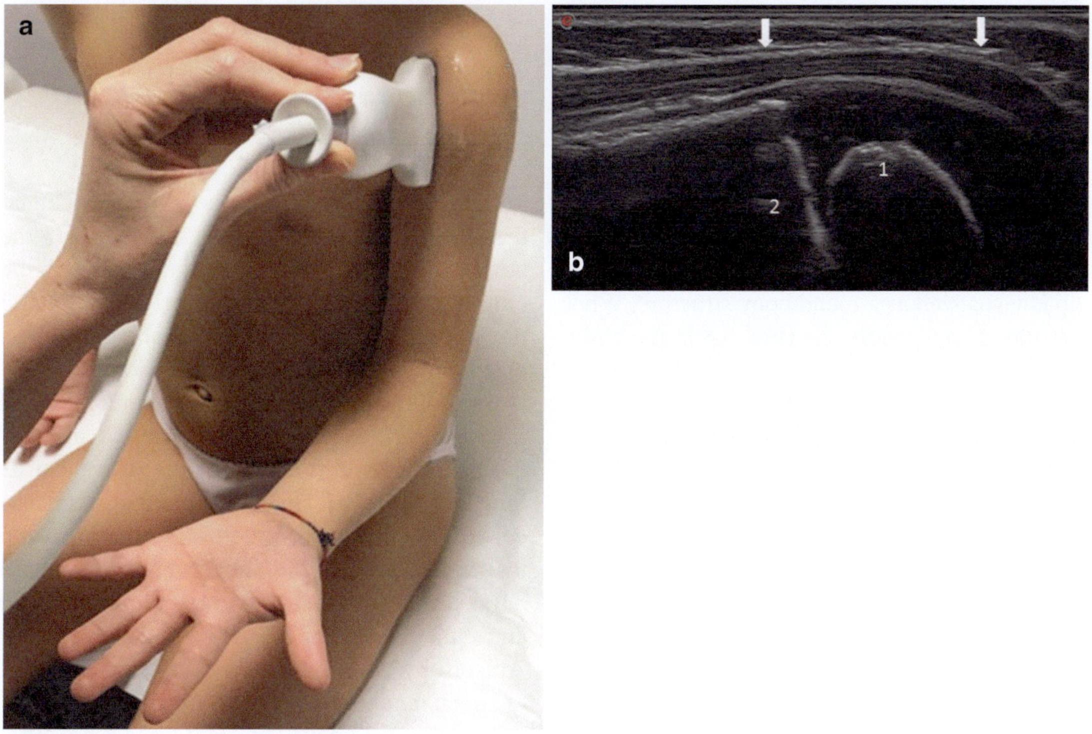

Fig. 6.7 (**a**) Patient and probe position to examine the long head of the biceps tendon in its long axis. (**b**) Long-axis US image of the long head of the biceps brachii tendon (arrows) in a 3-year-old girl. The biceps tendon demonstrates a well-defined fibrillar echotexture made up of multiple parallel linear echoes. 1, humeral head; 2, proximal humeral metaphysis; arrowhead, epiphyseal plate

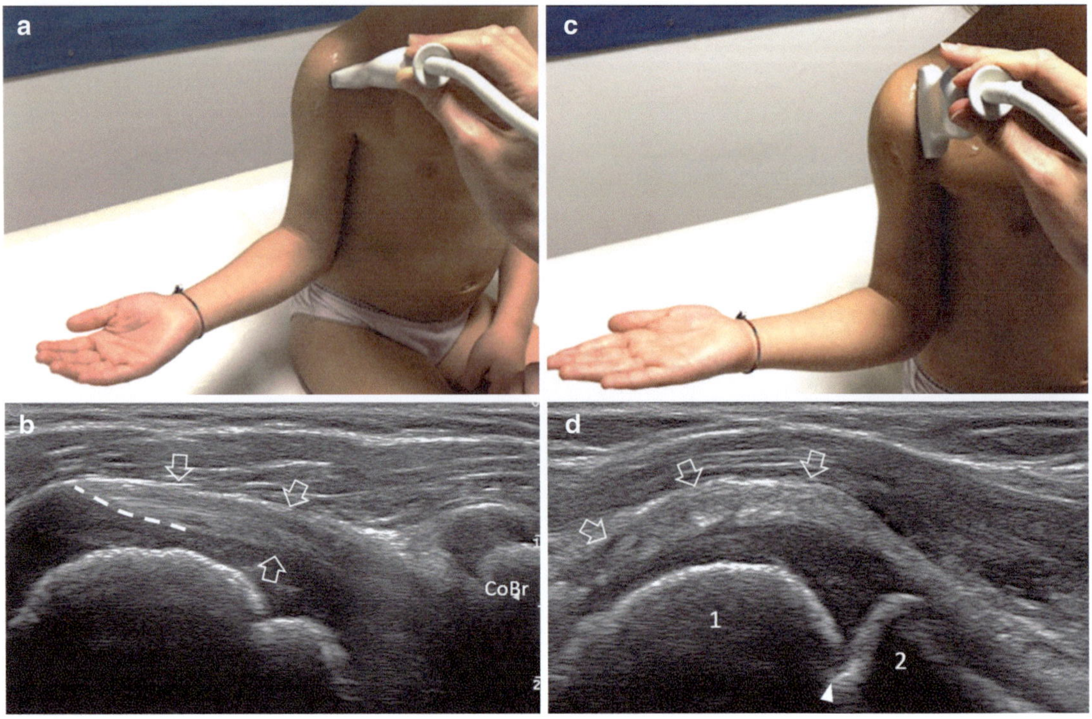

Fig. 6.8 Subscapularis tendon. (**a**) Patient and probe position to examine the subscapularis tendon in its long axis with corresponding (**b**) transverse 12-5 MHz US image over the long axis of the subscapularis tendon (arrows). Note the footprint (dashed line) showing the insertional area of the subscapularis into the lesser tuberosity that looks still chondral. CoBr, conjoint tendon of the short head of the biceps and the coracobrachialis. (**c**) Patient and probe position to examine the subscapularis tendon in its short axis with corresponding (**d**) sagittal 12-5 MHz US image over the short axis of the subscapularis (arrows) shows the multipennate structure of this tendon. Note the nucleus of ossification (1) of the humeral head, the physis (arrowhead), and the metaphysis (2)

The insertion of the subscapularis tendon involves a limited portion of the lesser tuberosity. Shifting the probe medially, the short axis of the coracoid tip is visualized as a round bony structure. When examined on its short axis (Fig. 6.8c), the multipennate structure of the normal subscapularis creates a series of hypoechoic clefts related to muscle fibers interwoven with tendon fascicles that should not be mistaken with tendon tears (Fig. 6.8d).

Supraspinatus Tendon

In neutral position, the supraspinatus tendon is partially masked by the acoustic shadow of the acromion and can only be visualized in its distal part. In order to withdraw the tendon from its bony cover, the patient is invited to extend the arm posteriorly, placing the palm of the hand on the upper part of the iliac wing with the elbow flexed, directed posteriorly and toward the midline (Fig. 6.9a). The probe should be oriented in the long axis of the tendon to visualize simultaneously the convex humeral head invested with cartilage, the anatomic neck of the humerus, and the greater tuberosity. On its long axis, the supraspinatus tendon appears as a convex beak-shaped structure extending deep to the deltoid and the subacromial subdeltoid bursa and superficial to the glenohumeral joint and the articular cartilage (Fig. 6.9b). Anisotropy usually occurs at the insertion of the deep tendon fibers in the area located lateral to the humeral neck. This artifact is a potential mimicker of an articular-sided partial-thickness

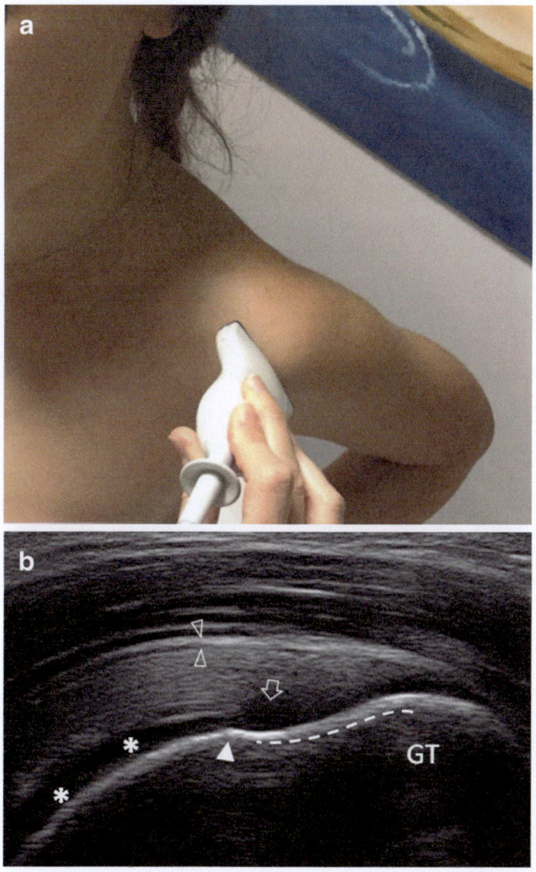

Fig. 6.9 (**a**) Patient and probe position to examine the supraspinatus tendon in its long axis. (**b**) Longitudinal axis of the supraspinatus tendon in a 15-year-old girl. The tendon has a convex beak-like shape. It lies over the hypoechoic cartilage (asterisk) of the humeral head before inserting into the greater tuberosity (GT). Note that the tendon insertion (dashed line) extends from the humeral neck (arrowhead) to the superolateral angle of the greater tuberosity. The articular fibers of the tendon assume a curved diverged course in the preinsertional area, possibly leading to a hypoechoic artifact (empty arrow) related to anisotropy. Between the supraspinatus and the deltoid, the normal subacromial-subdeltoid bursa appears as a thin hypoechoic band (empty headarrows)

tear and can be avoided by gently rocking the probe toward lateral to make the ultrasound beam perpendicular to the tendon fibers. The supraspinatus tendon has also to be examined in its short axis. While the anterior margin of the supraspinatus is clearly delineated, there is no definite separation between the supraspinatus and the infraspinatus due to the interwoven arrangement of these tendons.

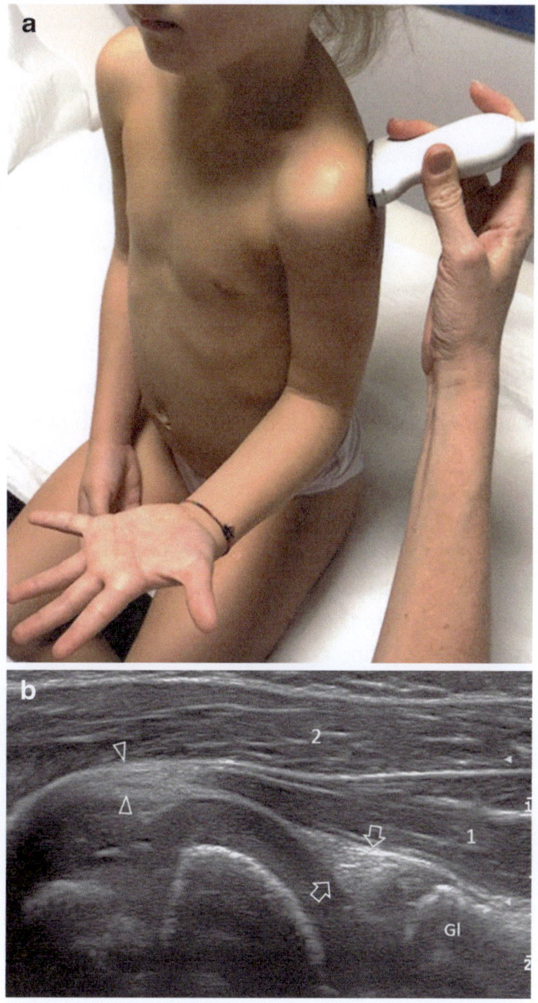

Fig. 6.10 Infraspinatus tendon. (**a**) Probe placement and patient position to examine the external rotators of the shoulder. (**b**) Transverse 12-5 MHz US image over the posterior aspect of the glenohumeral joint obtained from a 3-year-old boy. US image demonstrates the infraspinatus muscle (1) and tendon (arrowheads) examined in their long axis. Note the relationship of the infraspinatus with the deltoid (2) and the posterior glenoid labrum (arrows). The posteriori recess of the glenohumeral joint is located between the humeral head and the posteriori aspect of the bony glenoid (Gl), deep to the infraspinatus tenon, and muscle

Infraspinatus and Teres Minor Tendons

The infraspinatus and teres minor tendons can be examined by placing the probe over the posterior aspect of the shoulder (Fig. 6.10). The forearm should lie on the ipsilateral thigh in a supinated position. The spine of the scapula can be used as a landmark to differentiate the supraspinous from the infraspinous fossa. The infraspinatus and teres minor tendons can be recognized as separate structures arising from the respective muscles and inserting into the greater tuberosity.

Glenohumeral Joint

The glenohumeral joint capsule extends from the outer profile of the glenoid rim to the anatomic neck of the humerus. Ultrasound has high sensitivity to depict even minimal amounts of fluid within the main synovial recesses (i.e., the dependent axillary pouch, the posterior and subscapularis recesses, and the long head of the biceps tendon sheath) of the glenohumeral joint. The posterior recess is examined on transverse planes placing the probe on the posterior aspect of the glenohumeral joint, over the posterior labrum-capsular complex. In its cross section, the fibrocartilaginous labrum appears as a triangular hyperechoic structure with the base directed medially and the apex pointing laterally, capping the bony rim of the glenoid (Fig. 6.10). When synovial hypertrophy/effusion distend the recess, a hypoanechoic area surrounding the tip of the posterior labrum can be observed. Due to the presence of large amounts of anechoic humeral cartilage in younger children, passively assisted movements with internal and external rotation of the arm may make differentiation of effusion/synovium from cartilage more confident by inducing changes in the recess shape. Interventional procedures of needle aspiration or injection can be safely performed to the posterior recess under ultrasound guidance while the patient is seated or prone [26]. The ultrasound evaluation of the anterior recess of the joint is more complex due to its deep location. Fluid distension of this recess can be appreciated on transverse scans as a hypoechoic halo surrounding the anterior labrum. Similarly, the evaluation of the subscapularis recess is challenging due to its small size and location under the coracoid tip. On transverse or sagittal planes, the distension of the subscapularis recess can be appreciated as a small hypoanechoic area located just inferior to the coracoid and superficial to the subscapularis (Fig. 6.11). The small subscapularis recess should not be mistaken for the larger subcoracoid bursa that extends more caudally and does not communicate with the glenohumeral joint.

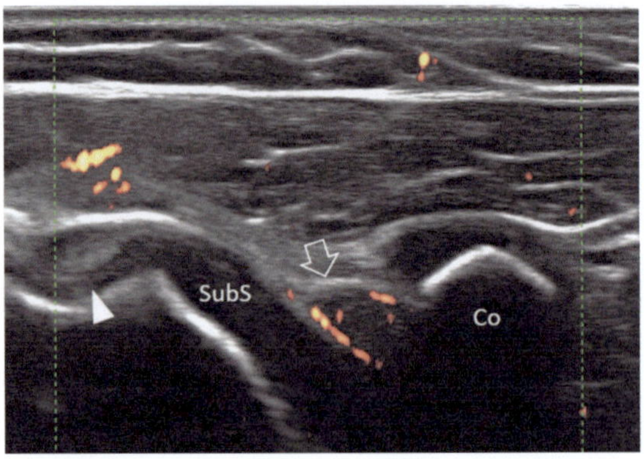

Fig. 6.11 Transverse power Doppler 13-5 MHz US image over the anteromedial space of the shoulder in a 11-year-old girl with juvenile idiopathic arthritis and shoulder involvement. US image shows the subscapularis recess (arrow) distended by hypervascular synovium. Note the relationship of this recess with the subscapularis tendon (SubS) and the coracoid (Co)

The axillary recess of the glenohumeral joint results from a redundant folding of the inferior joint capsule. The examination of this recess can be performed by keeping the patient supine with abducted arm. The probe is placed in a longitudinal plane on the mid-axillary line, oriented in the long axis of the humeral shaft (Fig. 6.12a). This allows the identification of the synovial recess using the humerus head-glenoid complex and the humeral neck as landmarks (Fig. 6.12b). Distension of this recess may extend along the humeral neck. The amount of distension of the axillary recess can be measured in the middle of the humeral surgical neck concavity, where its thickness is maximal. If children cannot abduct the arm due to reduced shoulder mobility, an alternative technique can be carried out in neutral position by sweeping the probe inferior to the posterior recess in a transverse plane. Finally, the biceps tendon sheath can be considered a mere extension of the joint cavity. Sheath effusion secondary to an isolated biceps tendinitis is rare.

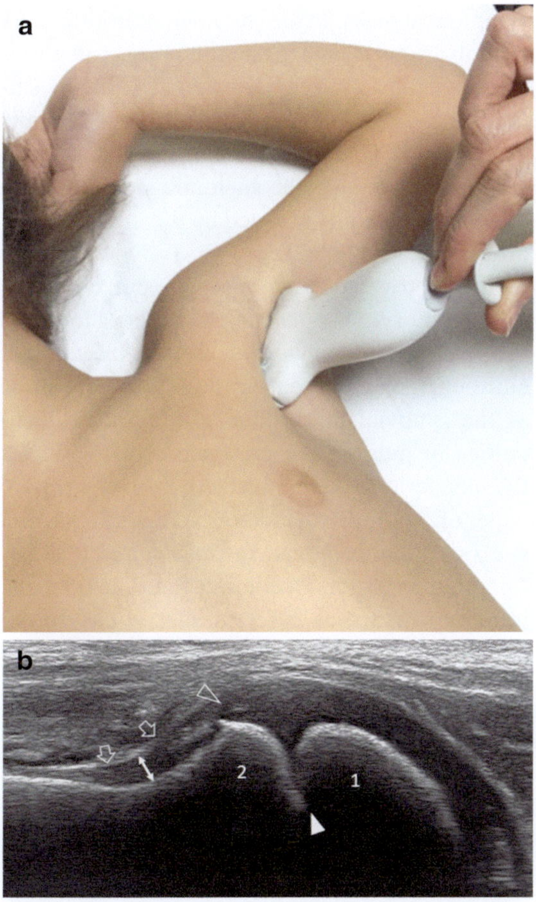

Fig. 6.12 (**a**) Patient and probe position to examine the axillary recess of the glenohumeral joint. The transducer is placed in a longitudinal plane on the mid-axillary line and along the long axis of the humeral shaft. (**b**) Axillary recess of the glenohumeral joint. 1: humeral head; 2: humeral metaphysis; white arrowhead: epiphyseal plate. Distension of the axillary recess can be measured in the middle of the humeral surgical neck concavity, where its thickness is maximal (double-headed arrow)

Subacromial Subdeltoid Bursa

The subacromial subdeltoid bursa is the most extended synovial-lined bursa in the body. Ultrasound can visualize this bursa where it is exposed to the ultrasound beam. The bursal portion located deep to the acromion is not accessible. In normal conditions, the subacromial-subdeltoid bursa is collapsed and appears as a thin hypoechoic band overlying the supraspinatus tendon. In chronic inflammatory condi-

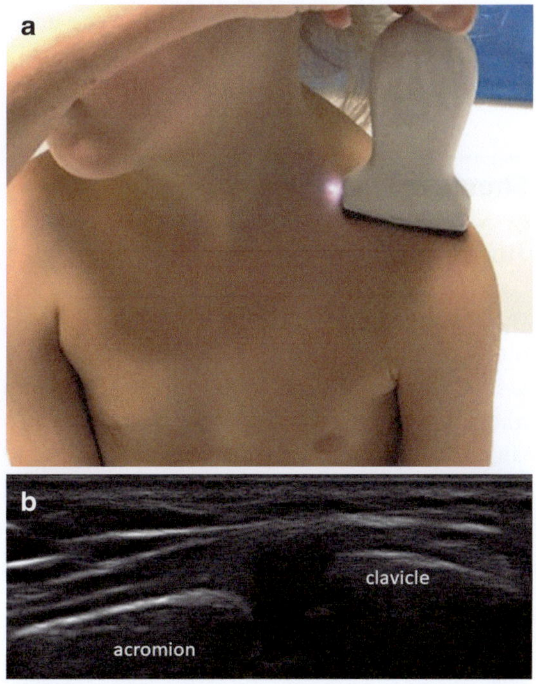

Fig. 6.13 Patient and probe position (**a**) to examine the acromion clavicular joint with corresponding (**b**) US image obtained from a 11-year-old girl

tions, the synovial membrane of the bursa walls may thicken and the cavity may be distended. A careful scanning technique is needed when examining the bursa: an excessive pressure with the probe may squeeze the fluid away from the field of view. With the patient seated, the effusion tends to collect in the most dependent parts of the bursa, along the lateral edge of the greater tuberosity, producing a typical "teardrop" shape.

Acromioclavicular Joint

To examine the acromioclavicular joint, the transducer is placed over the top of the shoulder in a coronal plane (Fig. 6.13). The end of the clavicle rides higher than the acromion and is easily palpable. Once the joint is detected, the probe orientation should be adjusted placing one of its edges over the acromion and the other over the clavicle. Joint distension by hypertrophic synovium/effusion can be appreciated as widening of the joint space or bulging of the superior acromioclavicular ligament and the joint capsule. The internal fibrocartilaginous disk can be seen as a hyperechoic triangle located intra-articularly.

Shoulder Pathology

Juvenile Idiopathic Arthritis

By systematic evaluation of the joint recesses, ultrasound has proved to be a valuable tool for assessment of shoulder involvement in juvenile idiopathic arthritis (JIA). JIA does not represent a single disease form but a diagnosis that applies to all forms of arthritis of unknown origin lasting >6 weeks with onset prior to the 16th year of age [29]. Joint involvement may be either monoarticular or oligoarticular or polyarticular depending on the specific JIA category [28]. All JIA categories have in common a chronic inflammatory process primarily targeting the synovial membrane. In more severe cases, persistence of inflammation may lead to an increased risk of osteochondral damage that is potentially responsible for both short-term and long-term physical disability. Although any joint can potentially be involved, in the oligoarticular forms of JIA large joints such as the knee and the ankle are commonly affected with limping as the leading symptom at onset. In the shoulder, arthritis occurs in polyarticular and systemic-onset categories more often than in oligoarticular JIA. In this setting, ultrasound may be regarded as a valuable extension of physical examination able to provide information on the anatomic structures that are most commonly affected by the inflammatory process [8] (Table 6.2).

It has proved to be very sensitive in detecting inflammatory changes, such as effusion and synovial hypertrophy (Fig. 6.14). In younger children, the epiphyseal cartilage looks anechoic as the synovial fluid, thus creating some difficulties in judging the presence of effusion for the inexperienced examiner. An in-depth knowledge of appropriate anatomic landmarks and analysis of subsynovial fat may make this differentiation easier. Becoming familiar with the joint appearance at different ages is part of the learning curve and a major research focus of the

Table 6.2 Anatomical structures most commonly detectable by shoulder ultrasound in juvenile idiopathic arthritis

Posterior recess of the glenohumeral joint
Axillary recess of the glenohumeral joint
Acromioclavicular joint
Long head of biceps tendon sheath
Subacromial/subdeltoid bursa

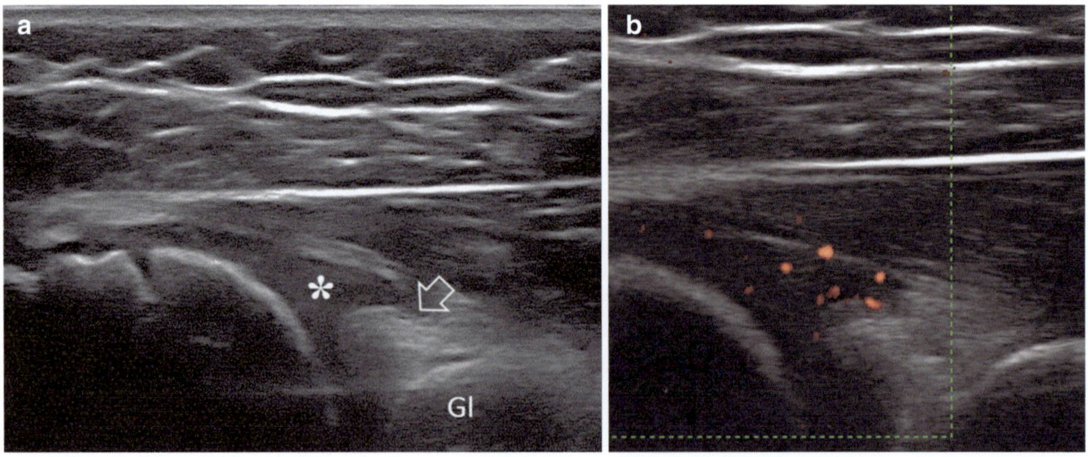

Fig. 6.14 Juvenile idiopathic arthritis. (**a**) Transverse 12-5 MHz US image over the posterior aspect of the shoulder in a 11-year-old child shows the posterior labrum (arrow) inserting into the bony glenoid (Gl) and mild effusion (asterisk) distending the posterior recess of the glenohumeral joint. (**b**) Corresponding power Doppler image reveals signs of hyperemia at the level of the synovial walls of the recess

Outcome Measures in Rheumatology and Clinical Trials (OMERACT) ultrasound special interest group in JIA, which successfully provided ultrasound definitions for the normal pediatric joint [32]. Detailed knowledge of age-related changes of the growing skeleton provides the basis to develop definitions for pathology and support the standardized use of ultrasound in pediatric rheumatology [9, 33]. Although intrinsically inaccurate, the quantitative assessment of synovitis may be attempted by measuring the maximal thickness (i.e., distance between the humeral head and the joint capsule) of the posterior and axillary recesses (Fig. 6.15) [35]. Synovial hyperemia, which is expression of synovial inflammation, can be demonstrated by an increased number and intensity of Doppler blood flow signals. Different from the articular cartilage that is nourished by synovial fluid, the epiphyseal cartilage exhibits a proper vasculature. The cartilage vascularization patterns however show some age- and joint-related variability [36]. The knowledge of the vascular architecture in the immature skeleton is essential for a correct interpretation of the para-articular Doppler signals in JIA patients as detection of blood flow in the growing epiphyseal cartilage is not a disease-specific finding reflecting the only inflammatory process.

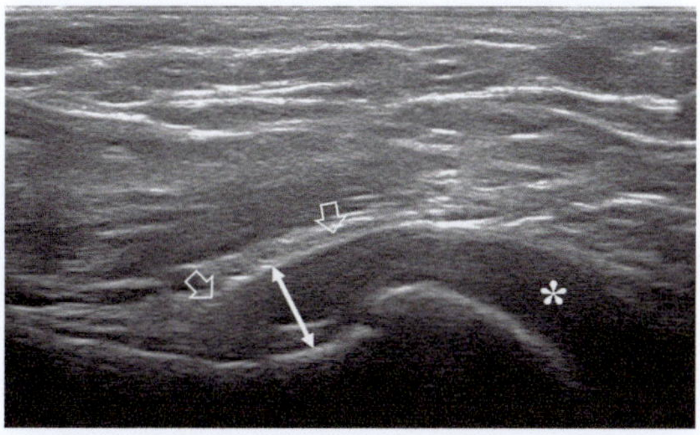

Fig. 6.15 Distension of the axillary recess (double-headed arrow) of the glenohumeral joint in an 11-year-old girl with juvenile idiopathic arthritis and shoulder involvement

As anticipated, in the bicipital groove, the biceps is surrounded by a synovial sheath as an extension of the synovial lining of the glenohumeral joint; in JIA patients with gleno-humeral joint involvement is quite common to detect intrasheath effusion, hyperemia and sheath thickening of the biceps tendon (Fig. 6.16). Hypertrophied synovitis in the subacromial-subdeltoid bursa [34] has been occasionally reported in patients with JIA. Ultrasound is also helpful to evaluate signs of osteochondral damage, such as thinning of the articular cartilage and bone erosions in case of longstanding disease. As the skeletal maturation progresses, the width of joint spaces physiologically decreases, making it difficult to determine whether a decrease in

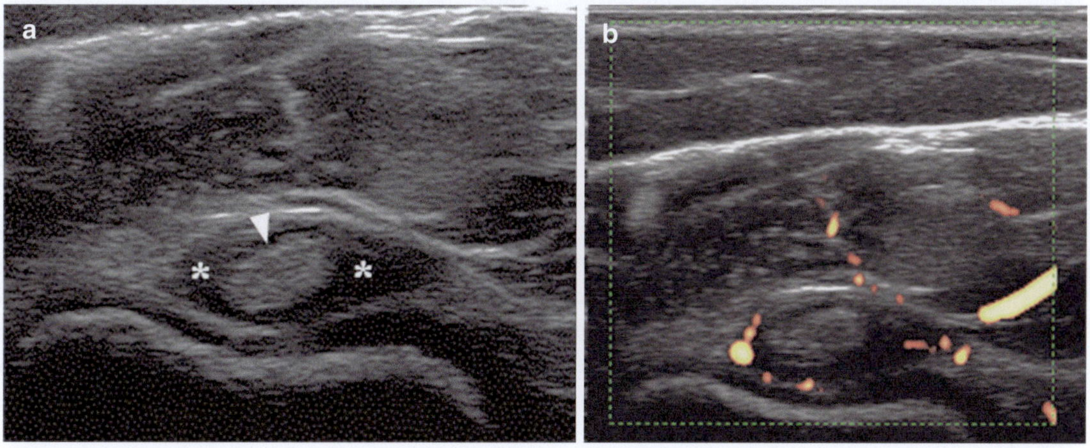

Fig. 6.16 (**a**) Long head of the biceps tendon examined in the short axis (arrowhead) in a 12-year-old girl with juvenile idiopathic arthritis. The sheath of the biceps tendon is distended by fluid (asterisk). Corresponding (**b**) US Power Doppler image shows synovial hyperemia

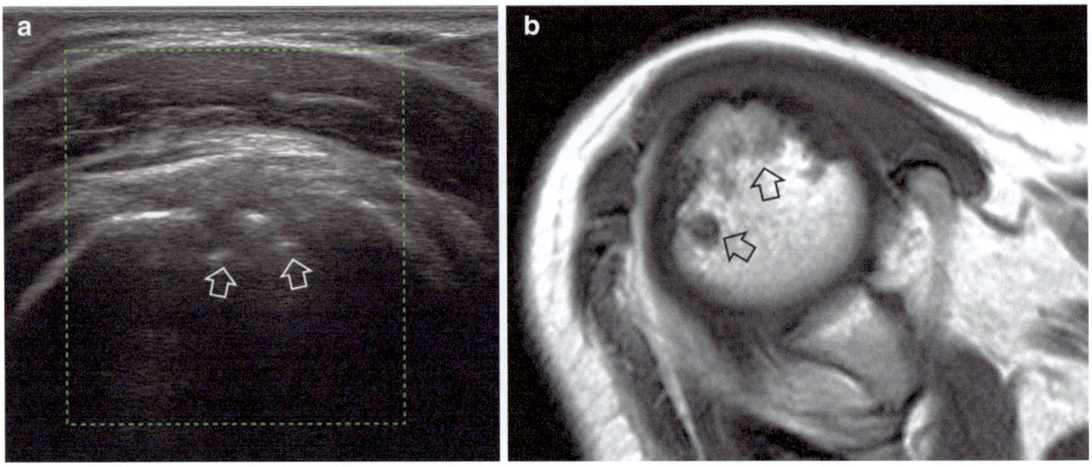

Fig. 6.17 (**a**) Ultrasound image obtained from a 16-year-old-girl with juvenile idiopathic arthritis showing bone erosions (arrows) in the humeral head (H). (**b**) 3D gradient echo T1-weighted MRI sequence confirms the presence of bone erosions in the humeral head

cartilage thickness is part of age-related changes or erosive disease. In chronic advanced disease, ultrasound can visualize bone erosions which appear as well-defined cortical defects filled by hypoechoic synovial pannus (Fig. 6.17a, b) [1].

Septic Arthritis

Glenohumeral joint infection is a severe but relatively uncommon condition in the children age group, accounting for approximately 3–12% of all cases of septic arthritis [20]. It predominantly occurs in very young infants. Since septic arthritis is considered a medical emergency, prompt diagnosis and aggressive treatment are required to avoid permanent joint damage. Fluid distension of the joint cavity, synovial hyperemia, and associated paraarticular soft-tissue changes, including edema, fluid collections, and local hyperemia, are common findings on ultrasound images. Although ultrasound is very sensitive for detection of glenohumeral joint fluid, it does not allow to safely characterize the nature of the effusion and differentiate septic arthritis from other conditions. In many instances, purulent effusions may appear turbid and echogenic, but the infectious nature of an intra-articular effusion cannot be excluded based on echotextural criteria. Limpid and anechoic effusions may in fact be septic in nature. Given these considerations, needle aspiration of the effusion, possibly guided by ultrasound, remains the mandatory key for the diagnosis in suspected infectious disease.

Sports-Related Injuries

The ability of ultrasound to provide depiction of chondral structures and growth plates in young children has opened a new and rewarding option for imaging of traumatic alterations of growing joints. Although there is obvious overlap between sports-related injuries in the pediatric age group and adult population, relevant features can be distinguished in the injury patterns of pediatric patients. These differences are mainly related to the ongoing changes in the immature skeleton and paraarticular structures. It is estimated that ligamentous structures are two to five times stronger than open physes [6]. The disparity in stress resistance between growing bones and adjacent tendons and ligaments predisposes to acute and chronic injuries in children. The shoulder is one of the most common sites of injury in pediatric throwing athletes [27]. The little league shoulder and acromial apophyseosteolysis are examples of common injury patterns restricted to adolescent throwing athletes. The little league shoulder is caused by microtrauma due to repetitive overhead throwing, resulting in disruption of the vascular network located in the medullary bone at the proximal humeral metaphysis [11, 22, 31]. The subsequent defective blood supply impairs the process of ossification of the physis and leads to physeal thickening and irregularity on radiographs and MR images. An early diagnosis is of critical importance for minimizing long-term adverse sequelae such as formation of bone bridges. Specific acute injury patterns affecting pediatric athletes who practice contact sports include physeal fractures of the proximal and distal end of the clavicle (periosteal sleeve fracture) of the proximal humeral physis and the coracoid process.

Clavicle Fracture

Clavicular fractures are a common pediatric injury with an incidence of 5–12/10^4 cases per year [10]. Radiography is the imaging modality of choice to confirm the diagnosis, although ultrasound may be considered a valuable alternative with 95% accuracy [12, 13]. The ability of ultrasound to visualize bones that are partially chondral makes this technique suitable to diagnose clavicle fractures in neonates due to birth trauma [15, 16]. The diagnosis is based on detection of cortical bone discontinuity. Depiction of a callus, hematoma, or paradoxical motion of bone fragments during breath are other relevant diagnostic signs [13].

References

1. Babini JC, Gusis SE, Babini SM, Cocco JA. Superolateral erosions of the humeral head in chronic inflammatory arthropathies. Skelet Radiol. 1992;21:515–7.
2. Backhaus M, Burmester GR, Gerber T, Grassi W, Machold KP, Swen WA, et al. Guidelines for musculoskeletal ultrasound in rheumatology. Ann Rheum Dis. 2001;60:641–9.
3. Balogh B, Frühwald F, Neuhold A, Wicke L, Firbas W. Sonoanatomy of the shoulder. Acta Anat. 1986;126:132–5.
4. Beggs I, Bianchi S, Bueno A, Cohen M, Court-Payen M, Grainger A, Kainberger F, Klauser A, Martinoli C, McNally E, O'Connor PJ, Peetrons P, Reijnierse M, Remplik P, Silvestri E. European society of musculo skeletal radiology: Musculoskeletal ultrasound technical guidelines. Insights Imaging. 2010;1:99–141.
5. Bianchi S, Martinoli C. Ultrasound of the musculoskeletal system: Springer; 2007. ISBN 978-3-540-42267-9.
6. Braithwaite KA, Marshall KW. The skeletally immature and newly mature throwing athlete. Radiol Clin N Am. 2016;54:841–55.
7. Chauvin NA, Jaimes C, Laor T, Jaramillo D. Magnetic resonance imaging of the pediatric shoulder. Magn Reson Imaging Clin N Am. 2012;20:327–47.
8. Colebatch-Bourn AN, Edwards CJ, Collado P, D'Agostino MA, Hemke R, Jousse-Joulin S, Maas M, Martini A, Naredo E, Østergaard M, Rooney M, Tzaribachev N, van Rossum MA, Vojinovic J, Conaghan PG, Malattia C. EULAR-PReS points to consider for the use of imaging in the diagnosis and management of juvenile idiopathic arthritis in clinical practice. Ann Rheum Dis. 2015;74:1946–57.
9. Collado P, Vojinovic J, Nieto JC, Windschall D, Magni-Manzoni S, Bruyn GA, Iagnocco A, D'agostino MA, Naredo E. Omeract ultrasound pediatric group. Toward standardized musculoskeletal ultrasound in pediatric rheumatology: normal age-related ultrasound findings. Arthritis Care Res. 2016;68:348–56.
10. Cross KP, Warkentine FH, Kim IK, Gracely E, Paul RI. Bedside ultrasound diagnosis of clavicle fractures in the pediatric emergency department. Acad Emerg Med. 2010;17:687–93.
11. de la Puente R, Boutin RD, Theodorou DJ, Hooper A, Schweitzer M, Resnick D. Post-traumatic and stress-induced osteolysis of the distal clavicle: MR imaging findings in 17 patients. Skelet Radiol. 1999;28:202208.
12. Eksioglu F, Altinok D, Uslu MM, Gudemez E. Ultrasonographic findings in pediatric fractures. Turk J Pediatr. 2003;45:136–40.
13. Hubner U, Schlicht W, Outzen S, Barthel M, Halsband H. Ultrasound in the diagnosis of fractures in children. J Bone Joint Surg Br. 2000;82:1170–3.
14. Jaramillo D, Kleinman P. Special aspects of musculoskeletal imaging in children. In: Hodler J, Zollikofer CL, Von Schulthess GK, editors. Musculoskeletal diseases 2009–2012. Milan: Springer; 2009. p. 158–65.
15. Katz R, Landman J, Dulitzky F, Bar-Ziv J. Fracture of the clavicle in the newborn. An ultrasound diagnosis. J Ultrasound Med. 1988;7:21–3.
16. Kayser R, Mahlfeld K, Heyde C, Grasshoff H. Ultrasonographic imaging of fractures of the clavicle in newborn infants. J Bone Joint Surg Br. 2003;85:115–6.
17. Kothary S, Rosenberg ZS, Poncinelli LL, Kwong S. Skeletal development of the glenoid and glenoid-coracoid interface in the pediatric population: MRI features. Skelet Radiol. 2014;43:1281–8.
18. Kwong S, Kothary S, Poncinelli LL. Skeletal development of the proximal humerus in the pediatric

population: MRI features. AJR Am J Roentgenol. 2014;202:418–25.
19. Laor T, Jaramillo D. MR imaging insights into skeletal maturation: what is normal? Radiology. 2009;250:28–38.
20. Lossos IS, Yossepowitch O, Kandel L, Yardeni D, Arber N. Septic arthritis of the glenohumeral joint. A report of 11 cases and review of the literature. Medicine (Baltimore). 1998;77:177–87.
21. Malattia C, Rinaldi M, Martini A. The role of imaging in juvenile idiopathic arthritis. Expert Rev Clin Immunol. 2018;14:681–94.
22. Obembe OO, Gaskin CM, Taffoni MJ, Anderson MW. Little Leaguer's shoulder (proximal humeral epiphysiolysis): MRI findings in four boys. Pediatr Radiol. 2007;37:885–9.
23. Ogden JA, Phillips SB. Radiology of postnatal skeletal development. VII. The scapula. Skelet Radiol. 1983;9:157–69.
24. Ogden JA, Conlogue GJ, Jensen J. Radiology of postnatal skeletal development: the proximal humerus. Skelet Radiol. 1978;2:153–60.
25. Ogden JA, Conlogue GJ, Bronson ML. Radiology of postnatal skeletal development. III. The clavicle. Skelet Radiol. 1979;4:196–203.
26. Otjen J, Parnell SE, Menashe S, Thapa MM. Ultrasound-guided joint injections for MR arthrography in pediatric patients: how we do it. Pediatr Radiol. 2015;45:126.
27. Paz DA, Chang GH, Yetto JM Jr, Dwek JR, Chung CB. Upper extremity overuse injuries in pediatric athletes: clinical presentation, imaging findings, and treatment. Clin Imaging. 2015;39:954–64.
28. Petty RE, Southwood TR, Manners P, Baum J, Glass DN, Goldenberg J, He X, Maldonado-Cocco J, Orozco-Alcala J, Prieur AM, Suarez-Almazor ME, Woo P. International league of associations for rheumatology. International league of associations for rheumatology classification of juvenile idiopathic arthritis: second revision, Edmonton, 2001. J Rheumatol. 2004;31:390–2.
29. Ravelli A, Martini A. Juvenile idiopathic arthritis. Lancet. 2007;369:767–78.
30. Rockwood CA, Matsen FA. The shoulder. 4th ed. Philadelphia: Saunders/Elsevier; 2009. p. 12.
31. Roedl JB, Morrison WB, Ciccotti MG, Zoga AC. Acromial apophysiolysis: superior shoulder pain and acromial nonfusion in the young throwing athlete. Radiology. 2015;274:201–9.
32. Roth J, Jousse-Joulin S, Magni-Manzoni S, Rodriguez A, Tzaribachev N, Iagnocco A, Naredo E, D'Agostino MA, Collado P. Outcome measures in rheumatology ultrasound group. Definitions for the sonographic features of joints in healthy children. Arthritis Care Res. 2015;67:136–42.
33. Roth J, Ravagnani V, Backhaus M, Balint P, Bruns A, Bruyn GA, et al. OMERACT ultrasound group. Preliminary definitions for the Sonographic features of synovitis in children. Arthritis Care Res (Hoboken). 2017;69:1217–23.
34. Ruhoy MK, Tucker L, McCauley RG. Hypertrophic bursopathy of the subacromial-subdeltoid bursa in juvenile rheumatoid arthritis: sonographic appearance. Pediatr Radiol. 1996;26:353–5.
35. Trauzeddel R, Windschall D, Trauzeddel RF, Nirschl C, Ganser G, Palm-Beden K, Berendes R, Haller M, Krumrey-Langkammerer M, Nimtz-Talaska A, Schoof P, Lehmann H. Arthrosonographic reference values of the shoulder joint in healthy children and adolescents: a cross-sectional multicentre ultrasound study. Klin Padiatr. 2017;229: 293–301.
36. Windschall D, Collado P, Vojinovic J, Magni-Manzoni S, Balint P, Bruyn GAW, Hernandez-Diaz C, Nieto JC, Ravagnani V, Tzaribachev N, Iagnocco A, D'Agostino MA, Naredo E. OMERACT paediatric ultrasound subtask force. Age-related vascularization and ossification of joints in children: an international pilot study to test multiobserver ultrasound reliability. Arthritis Care Res (Hoboken). 2017; https://doi.org/10.1002/acr.23335.
37. Zember JS, Rosenberg ZS, Kwong S, Kothary SP, Bedoya MA. Normal skeletal maturation and imaging pitfalls in the pediatric shoulder. Radiographics. 2015;35:1108–22.

Elbow and Forearm

7

Waleed A. Hassan and Mohammed A. Mortada

Introduction

The elbow joint is formed of three separate articulations that have one joint capsule. The first is the radiohumeral articulation between the radial head and the capitulum of the humerus. This is a limited ball-and-socket joint, hinge type of synovial joint. Second, the ulno-humeral articulation that forms a hinge joint between the olecranon process of the ulna and the trochlea of the humerus to allow for flexion and extension. The last articulation is the superior radio-ulnar joint, a synovial pivot joint, which allows for pronation and supination [1].

Skeletal growth is the main variation in musculoskeletal ultrasound (MSUS) examination in children compared to adults, as bony landmarks are usually used as reference points during scanning. The main difference points between pediatric and adult MSUS examination include the presence of varying amount of nonossified hyaline cartilage in addition to the articular cartilage which gives much larger cartilage thickness than in adult as well as the presence of secondary ossification centers and growth plates [2] (Fig. 7.1).

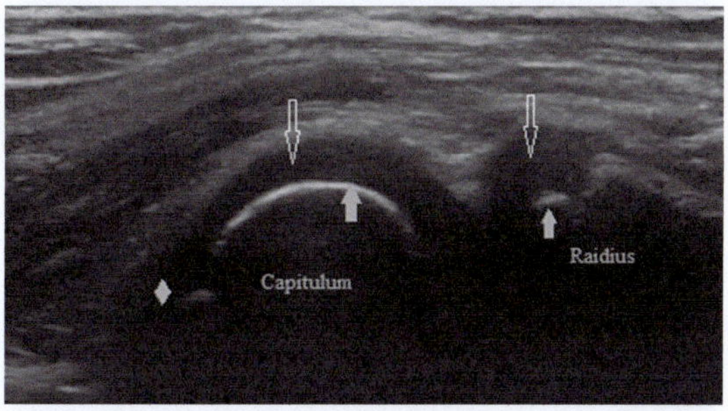

Fig 7.1 Normal ultrasound anatomy in 9-year-old boy showing nonossified cartilage (open arrow), secondary ossification centers of the capitulum and head of radius (gray arrow), and joint recess (diamond)

Secondary Ossification Centers

The elbow joint is completely cartilaginous at birth, and there are six secondary ossification centers (OC) that appear and ossify in a consecutive manner which may vary according to the child's maturity and sex and may even differ between the two extremities. This makes imaging of the contralateral elbow helpful in identification of subtle pathology. Considering the development of secondary ossification centers, "CRITOL" is a mnemonic for the chronologic order of appearance of secondary ossification centers:

W. A. Hassan (✉)
Benha University, Banha, Egypt

M. A. Mortada
Zagazig University, Zagazig, Egypt

Y. El Miedany (ed.), *Pediatric Musculoskeletal Ultrasonography*,
https://doi.org/10.1007/978-3-030-17824-6_7

- C for capitulum, R for radial head
- I for internal (medial) epicondyle, T for trochlea
- O for olecranon, L for lateral epicondyle

Ossification appears first in the capitulum at the age of 1 year, but it can appear as early as 3 months, followed by sequential appearance of other centers with an interval of about 2 years for each center [3].

Displaced fractures of the epicondyle can be easily missed if the normal chronological pattern of the development of secondary ossification centers is not well recognized [4].

The lower epiphysis of the humerus fuses with its shaft at the age of 16–17 years, the upper epiphysis of the ulna fuses with its shaft at the age of 16 years, and the upper epiphysis of the radius fuses with its shaft at the age of 17–18 years [5].

Elbow Joint: Ultrasound Scanning Technique

As most of the structures of interest in the elbow region are superficially located, the use of high-frequency linear probe usually 12–18 MHz is recommended. One of the most important issues in ultrasound examination in children is lack of cooperation during scanning. Many strategies can be used to tackle this challenge such as using warmer gel to avoid the use of the cool gel and use of toys and soft light. Modification of the standard US examination positions to become more comfortable to the child might be needed. For example, we can examine the child while sitting on his/her parent's leg instead of sitting on a chair or lying on examination couch [6].

Probe Orientation

According to EULAR guidelines, the orientation marker of the probe is facing proximally in longitudinal scan and the proximal parts are seen in left side of the screen and distal parts are seen in the right side of the screen. In transverse scan, the orientation marker of the probe is directed to the left side of the examiner [7].

Standard Elbow Scans

MSUS examination of the elbow joint should focus on the area of clinical complaint and any pathological finding should be examined and documented in two perpendicular planes. Complete examination of the elbow joint is according to defined scans [7, 8] and includes evaluation of four compartments:

1. Anterior compartment
2. Lateral compartment
3. Medial compartment
4. Posterior compartment

Anterior Compartment

MSUS examination of the anterior compartment of the elbow focuses on the anterior recess of the elbow joint (Fig. 7.1), the distal biceps tendon, the brachialis muscle, and median nerve. The child sits facing the examiner while the elbow is in full extension and the forearm in supination. The probe should move 5 cm above and 5 cm below the joint [7, 9, 10].

Anterior Longitudinal Humero-Radial Scan

Anatomical landmarks are the capitulum, radial head, radial fossa, and joint capsule. The secondary OC of the capitulum appears at age of 1 year and usually appears as a single smooth center, and the secondary OC of the head of the radius appear at age of 4 years, and it usually begins as oval shaped and later on becomes disk shaped [9]. Shen et al. [11] described the appearance of anterior humero-radial joint in healthy children below 3 years to look like opposing double fists and called it "double-breast." Also Herring et al. [12] described a depression in the distal humerus that is not noticeable till the age of 6 months and then appears more obviously later on. (Fig. 7.2).

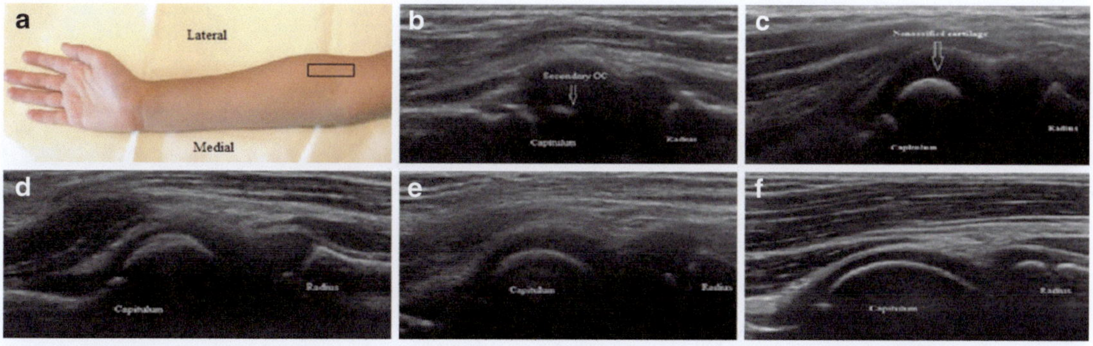

Fig. 7.2 Anterior longitudinal humero-radial scan of different age groups: (**a**) probe position, (**b**) 11 months old, (**c**) 2 years old, (**d**) 5 years old, (**e**) 9 years old, and (**f**) 14 years old

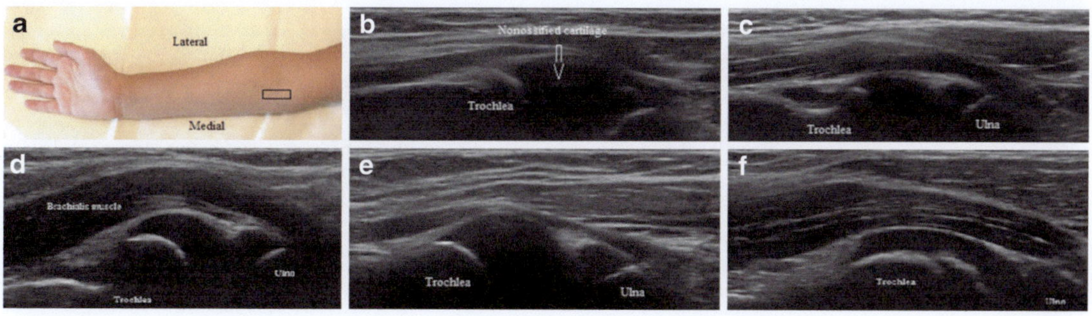

Fig. 7.3 Anterior longitudinal humero-ulnar scan of different age groups: (**a**) probe position, (**b**) 11 months old, (**c**) 2 years old, (**d**) 5 years old, (**e**) 9 years old, and (**f**) 14 years old

Anterior Longitudinal Humero-Ulnar Scan

Anatomical landmarks are the distal humerus, the coronoid fossa, the trochlea, coronoid process, joint capsule, brachialis muscle, and pronator teres muscle. The secondary OC of the trochlea appears at age of 7 years and usually has irregular and fragmented appearance [9]. The coronoid fossa is usually not detectable till 6 months of age and then it becomes noticeable later on, and it contains a triangular hyperechoic pad of fat which is intracapsular but extrasynovial and can be displaced by effusion in the coronoid fossa [12] (Fig. 7.3).

Anterior Transverse Scan

Anatomical landmarks are the capitulum, the trochlea, cartilage, joint capsule, brachialis muscle, brachial artery, median nerve medial to brachial artery, radial nerve between brachialis and brachioradialis, distal biceps, pronator teres medially, and brachioradialis laterally. The lower part of distal biceps tendon is surrounded by extrasynovial paratenon till its insertion in the radial tuberosity, and it is difficult to be visualized due to its deep oblique course. The best technique to find the distal biceps tendon is to locate it first in the transverse plane with the elbow extended and the forearm fully supinated then follow the tendon till insertion while rotating the probe to be oriented sight inferolaterally [13] (Fig. 7.4).

Lateral Compartment

MSUs examination of the lateral compartment of the elbow focuses on the recess of the radiocapitellar joint, the common extensor origin (CEO), the lateral collateral ligament and the radial nerve. The child sits facing the examiner while the elbow in full extension and the forearm in supination. The standard scanning technique of the lateral compartment is longitudinal with proximal end of the probe resting on the lateral

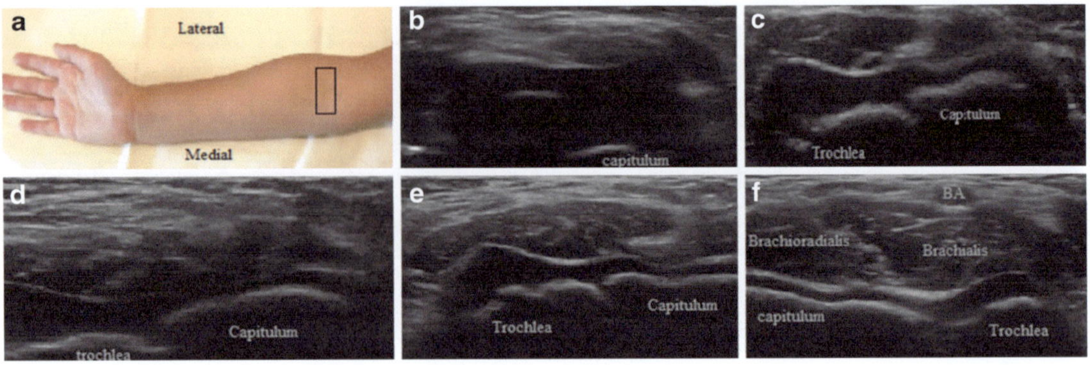

Fig. 7.4 Anterior transverse elbow scan of different age groups: (**a**) probe position, (**b**) 11 months old, (**c**) 2 years old, (**d**) 8 years old, (**e**) 9 years old, and (**f**) 14 years old. BA brachial artery

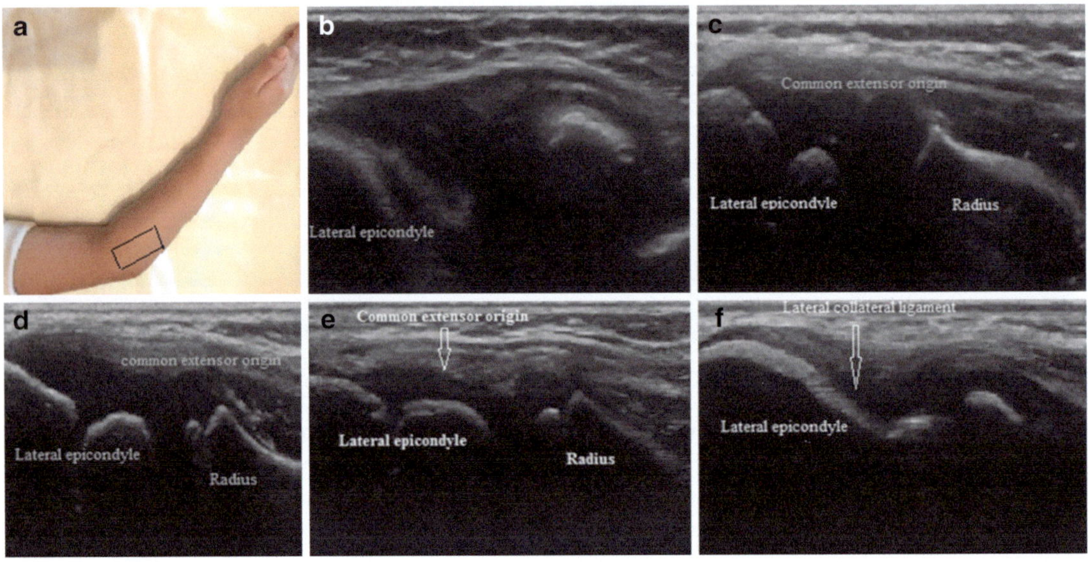

Fig. 7.5 Longitudinal scan of the lateral compartment of the elbow in different age groups: (**a**) probe position, (**b**) 11 months old, (**c**) 2 years old, (**d**) 5 years old, (**e**) 9 years old, and (**f**) 14 years old

epicondyle, and transverse scan is needed to confirm pathological findings [7]. The common extensor origin (CEO) is formed by contribution from extensor carpi radialis brevis, extensor digitorum, extensor digitiminimi, and extensor carpi ulnaris. CEO attaches to the lateral surface of the lateral epicondyle which is considered the main bony landmark in the lateral compartment [12] (Fig. 7.5).

The secondary OC of the lateral epicondyle appears at the age of 10 years and usually appears as a single linear center or multiple centers. This linear center begins peripherally and is separated from the lateral condyle by a relatively wide distance and so, it can be easily misinterpreted as avulsion fracture [9].

Medial Compartment

The child sits facing the examiner while the elbow is extended and the forearm is abducted and supination. MSUS examination of the medial compartment of the elbow focuses on the common flexor origin (CFO), the medial collateral ligament, and medial part of elbow joint [14]. The standard scanning technique of the medial compartment is longitudinal, with proximal end of the probe resting on the medial epicondyle in order to see the hyperechoic bony contour of the medial epicondyle and the articulation between the ulna and the trochlea [7, 15]. Transverse scan is needed to confirm pathological findings.

CFO attaches to the medial epicondyle which constitutes the main bony landmark in the medial compartment. The secondary OC of the medial epicondyle can be seen at age of 5 years and usually appears as a single center [9]. Shen et al. [10] described the appearance of the completely cartilaginous medial epicondyle, distal humerus, and the cubital tunnel in healthy children below 3 years to look like humps of the camel and called it "double-hump sign."

CFO is formed by contribution from flexor carpi radialis, flexor digitorum superficialis, palmaris longus, flexor carpi ulnaris, and pronator teres. With US examination, it appears shorter, more hyperechoic, and easily separated from joint capsule as compared to the CEO [15] (Fig. 7.6).

The medial collateral ligament (MCL) consists of three bands: anterior, oblique, and posterior. With US examination, the anterior band is seen as a hyperechoic fibrillar band between the medial epicondyle and the coronoid process of the ulna deep to the CFO. The anterior band is functionally considered as the main stabilizer against varus stress to the elbow [14]. Ulnar nerve can be visualized by placing the probe transversely between the olecranon and medial condyle.

Posterior Compartment

MSUS examination of the posterior compartment of the elbow focuses on the triceps tendon and muscle, the olecranon fossa, posterior joint recess, and the ulnar nerve in the cubital tunnel [16]. The child sits facing the examiner while the elbow in 90 degrees of flexion and the palm of the hand resting on a table "crabposition." The standard scanning technique of the posterior compartment is longitudinal, with distal end of the probe resting on the olecranon process of the ulna in order to see the hyperechoic bony contour of the olecranon [7, 15]. Transverse scan is needed to confirm pathological findings. Triceps tendon is inserted in the posterior aspect of the superior part of the olecranon process which constitutes the main bony landmark in the posterior compartment. Usually there are two secondary ossification centers of the olecranon process that become visible at age of 9 years, and they may be misinterpreted as a fracture [9].

The olecranon fossa is a depression in the posterior aspect of the distal part of the humerus, and it is filled with hyperechoic fat pad which can be easily displaced in the presence of synovitis or effusion [17]. It is also the favored plane for recognition of intra-articular loose bodies [14].

Triceps muscle is formed of three heads: long, medial, and lateral heads. It has a superficial part which is formed from long and lateral heads, and the deep part is formed from medial head, and it appears hypoechoic with ultrasound, while triceps tendon is hyperechoic, and both

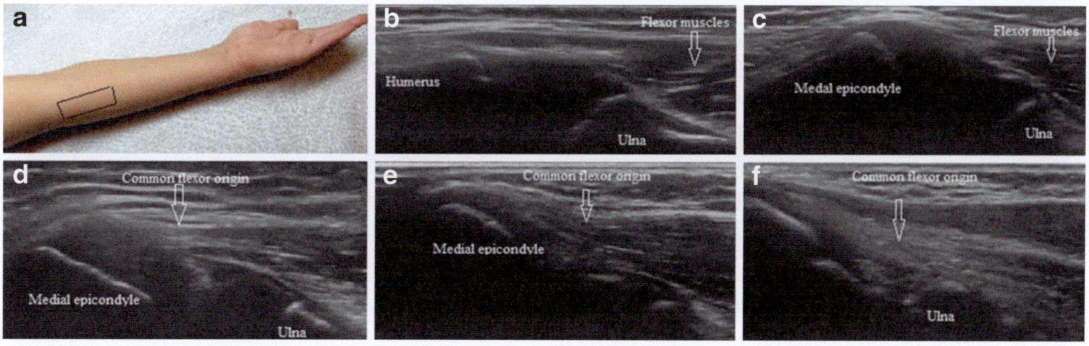

Fig. 7.6 Longitudinal scan of the medial compartment of the elbow in different age groups: (**a**) probe position, (**b**) 11 months old, (**c**) 2 years old, (**d**) 5 years old, (**e**) 9 years old, and (**f**) 14 years old

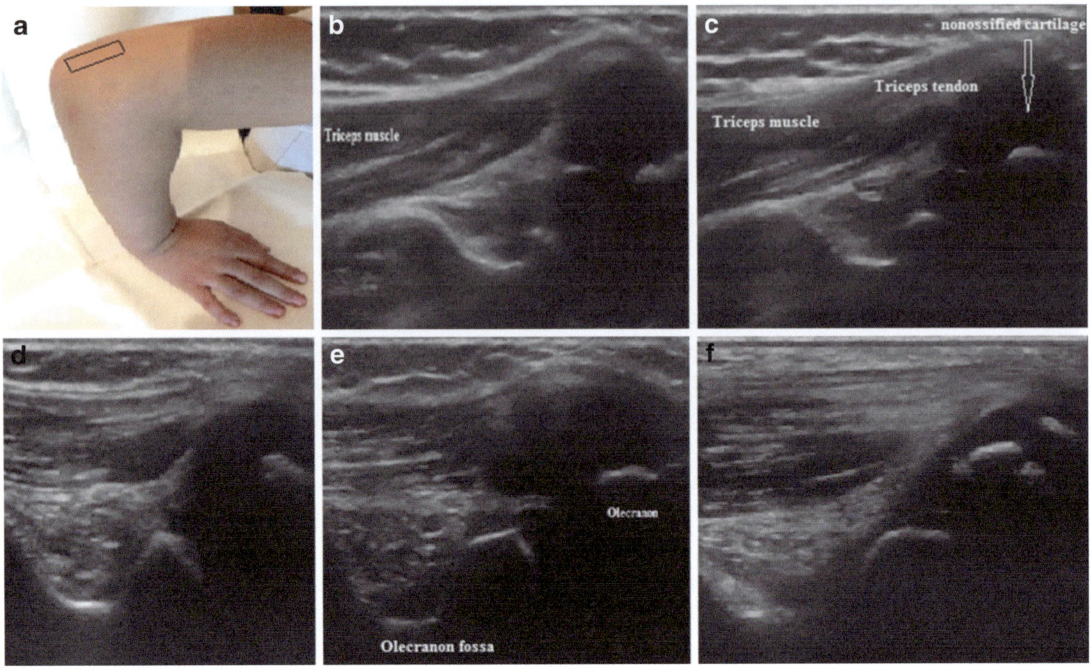

Fig. 7.7 Longitudinal scan of the posterior compartment of the elbow in different age groups: (**a**) probe position, (**b**) 11 months old, (**c**) 2 years old, (**d**) 5 years old, (**e**) 9 years old, and (**f**) 14 years old

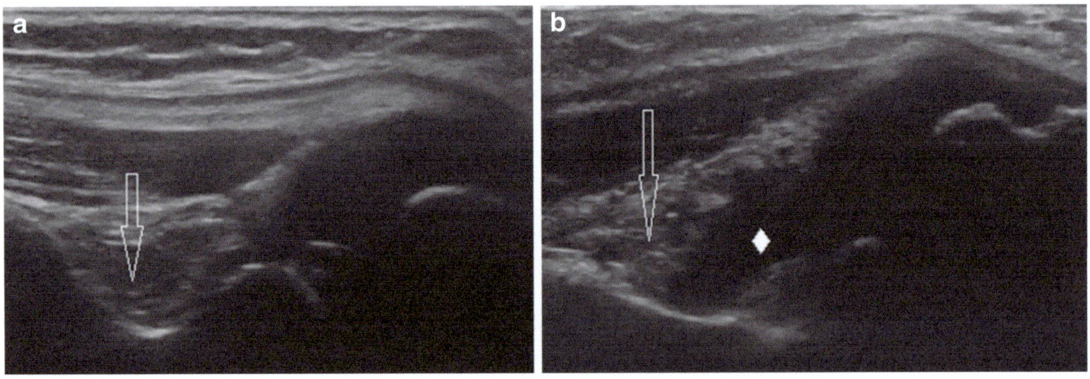

Fig. 7.8 Longitudinal scan of the posterior compartment of the elbow showing posterior fat pad (open arrow) in (**a**) normal position in 13-year-old boy and (**b**) displaced position due to synovitis (diamond) in 7-year-old boy

triceps muscle and tendon are visualized superficial to the olecranon recess of elbow joint [15] (Fig. 7.7).

Another important structure is the posterior fat pad, which has a triangular hyperechoic appearance in longitudinal scanning and lies deep to the triceps tendon in intracapsular but extrasynovial position. This allows for displacement of the fat pad with abnormal synovial collection of fluid as in intra-articular fractures, synovitis, and hemoarthrosis [15] (Fig. 7.8).

Forearm: Anatomy and Examination Technique

The bones of the forearm are the radius and ulna that articulate with each other by the superior and inferior radioulnar joints and are connected to each other with a strong interosseous membrane which divides the forearm into anterior and posterior compartments [18].

Muscle Sonoanatomy

Normal muscles have a characteristic MSUS appearance as they appear hypoechoic interspersed with curvilinear or punctate hyperechoic fibroadipose septa. In longitudinal plane, the probe is parallel to the muscle long axis, and the perimysial connective tissue appears as linear or pennate isoechoic structures, while in transverse plane, the reflection of perimysial connective tissue has a speckled appearance [19]. The epimysium surrounding the muscle appears hyperechoic [20]. The best method to locate the muscles of the forearm with MSUS is to begin their scanning at wrist level as their tendons are separated and simply recognized; then the probe can be easily moved in proximal direction to identify their muscles of origin [21].

Complete examination of the forearm includes evaluation of the anterior and posterior compartments:

Flexor Compartment (Figs. 7.9 and 7.10)
It is thicker than the extensor compartment, which may be related to its antigravity action. It is composed of nine muscles which are arranged into two groups: the superficial and deep group. The flexor compartment is mainly supplied by median nerve.

The superficial group takes origin from the common flexor origin on medial epicondyle, and it includes five muscles that are arranged from lateral to medial as pronator teres, flexor carpi radialis (FCR), flexor digitorum superficialis (FDS), Palmaris longus, and flexor carpi ulnaris (FCU). Deep into these lie two muscles: flexor digitorum profundus (FDP) and flexor pollicis and pronator quadrates (PQ).

The median nerve passes between the two heads of pronator teres and then runs in the middle of the flexor compartment between FDS and FDP muscles, while the ulnar nerve runs in the medial side of the flexor compartment under cover of FCU muscle, and its lower part accompanies the ulnar artery [22].

Extensor Compartment
It is formed of lateral and posterior layers. The posterior layer is further arranged in two groups:

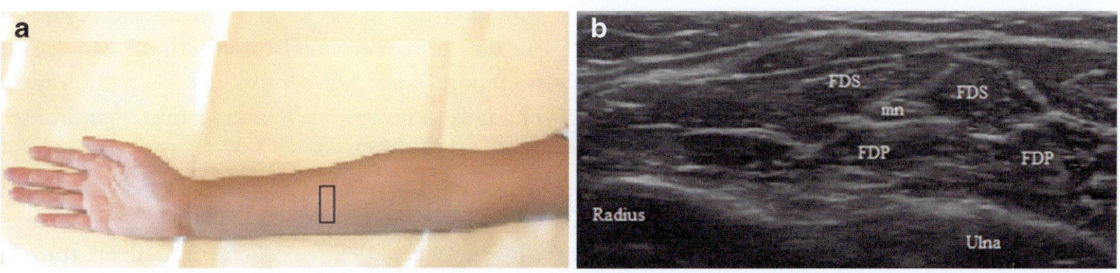

Fig. 7.9 Transverse scan of the middle of flexor compartment of the forearm: (**a**) probe position and (**b**) ultrasound anatomy. FDS flexor digitorum superficialis, FDP flexor digitorum profundus, mn median nerve

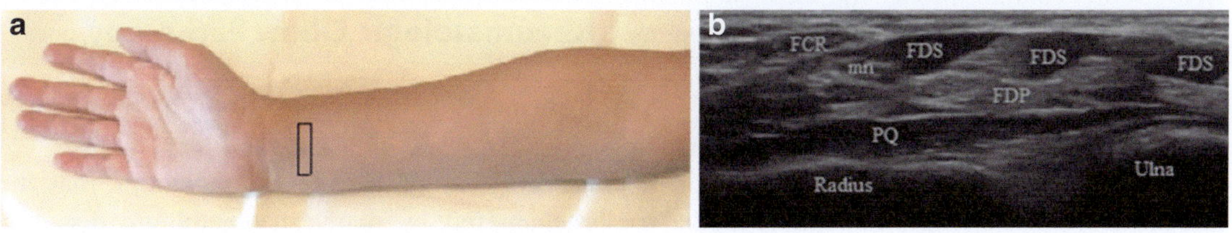

Fig. 7.10 Transverse scan of the distal aspect of flexor compartment of the forearm: (**a**) probe position and (**b**) ultrasound anatomy. FDS flexor digitorum superficialis, FDP flexor digitorum profundus, mn median nerve, PQ pronator quadratus

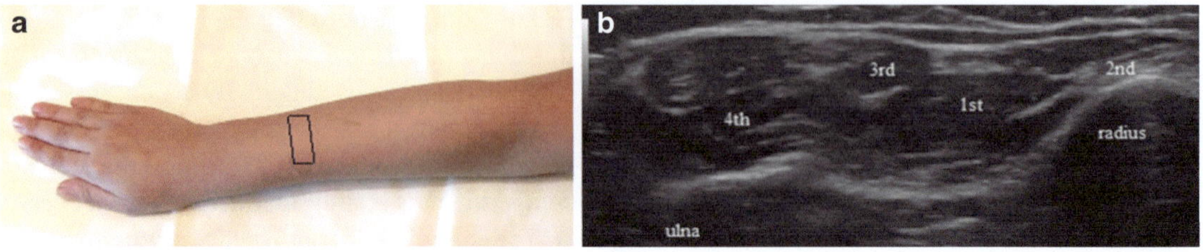

Fig. 7.11 Transverse scan of the extensor aspect of the forearm: (**a**) probe position and (**b**) ultrasound anatomy of the extensor compartments

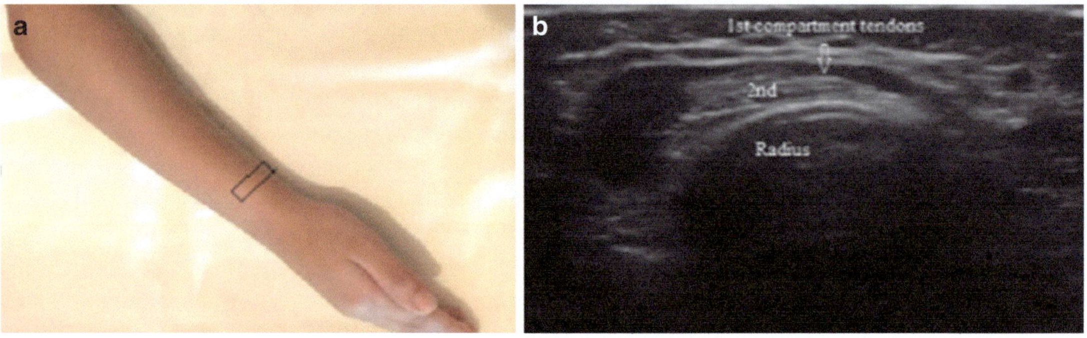

Fig. 7.12 Transverse scan of the area of proximal intersection: (**a**) probe position and (**b**) ultrasound anatomy showing the crossing of the tendons of the first extensor compartment over the tendons of second extensor compartment

the superficial and the deep groups. The extensor compartment is mainly supplied by posterior interosseous nerve which is the motor terminal branch of radial nerve [21].

The lateral group contains extensor carpi radialis longus (ECRL) and brachioradialis muscles, and they take origin from the lateral supracondylar ridge of the humerus. The superficial posterior group contains four muscles: extensor carpi radialis brevis (ECRB), extensor digitorum (ED), extensor digitiminimi (EDM), and extensor carpi ulnaris (ECU). The superficial group takes origin from the common extensor origin (CEO) on lateral epicondyle of the humerus. The deep posterior group contains four muscles: abductor pollicis longus (ABL), extensor pollicis longus (EPL), extensor pollicis brevis (EPB), and extensor indicis [21].

In the proximal part of dorsal forearm, the tendons of ABL and EPB muscles, which constitute the first extensor compartment, lie medial to the tendons of ECRL and ECRL muscles which constitute the second extensor compartment (Fig. 7.11), then tendons of the first extensor compartment cross over the tendons of the second extensor compartment from medial to lateral just proximal to the wrist to form what is known by the term "proximal intersection" which is a common site susceptible for pathological changes known as "intersection syndrome" (Fig. 7.12) [23].

The posterior interosseous nerve passes between the two heads of supinator muscle, then runs between the superficial and deep muscle groups of the extensor compartment, and then passes deep to ED at the level of the wrist [21].

Rheumatologic Elbow Pathology

Synovial Pathology

Elbow joint of infants and juveniles may be encountered by many rheumatologic diseases, such as juvenile chronic arthritis, septic arthritis, and hemophilic arthritis.

Juvenile Idiopathic Arthritis

The diagnosis of JIA remains a clinical one. There are no tests available to confirm or exclude the diagnosis. Hence, an experienced clinician is required to make a diagnosis by defining swollen, tender, or joints with limited range of movements. For the inexperienced, it is sometimes difficult to do this. For the experienced clinician as well, it can pose a challenge [24].

MSUS in JIA is considered particularly useful for its ability to detect subclinical synovitis, to improve the classification of patients in JIA subtypes, for the definition of remission, as guidance to intraarticular corticosteroid injections, and for capturing early articular damage [25].

Elbow joints are commonly affected in JIA especially polyarticular and oligoarticular subtypes.

The use of ultrasonography can be extremely helpful in establishing the presence of an elbow joint effusion or synovitis. Ultrasound has been shown in multiple studies to be more sensitive than clinical examination and radiography in detecting synovitis in the elbow joint in children [26].

According to the OMERACT preliminary definitions for the sonographic features of synovitis in children that was published in 2017 [27], synovitis detection by US in children includes the assessment of B mode and Doppler mode (color and power Doppler). Synovitis could be detected on the basis of B mode alone but not on Doppler mode alone. B mode findings include synovial effusion and synovial hypertrophy. Synovial effusion is defined as abnormal, intra-articular, hypoechoic, or anechoic material that is displaceable (Fig. 7.13). Synovial hypertrophy is defined as abnormal, intra-articular, hypoechoic material that is nondisplaceable (Fig. 7.14). Doppler sig-

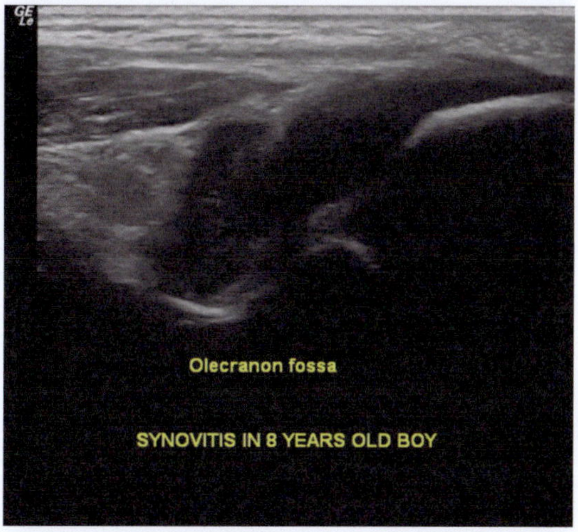

Fig. 7.14 Longitudinal scan of the posterior compartment of the elbow showing synovial hypertrophy; abnormal, intra-articular, hypo echoic material that is nondisplaceable

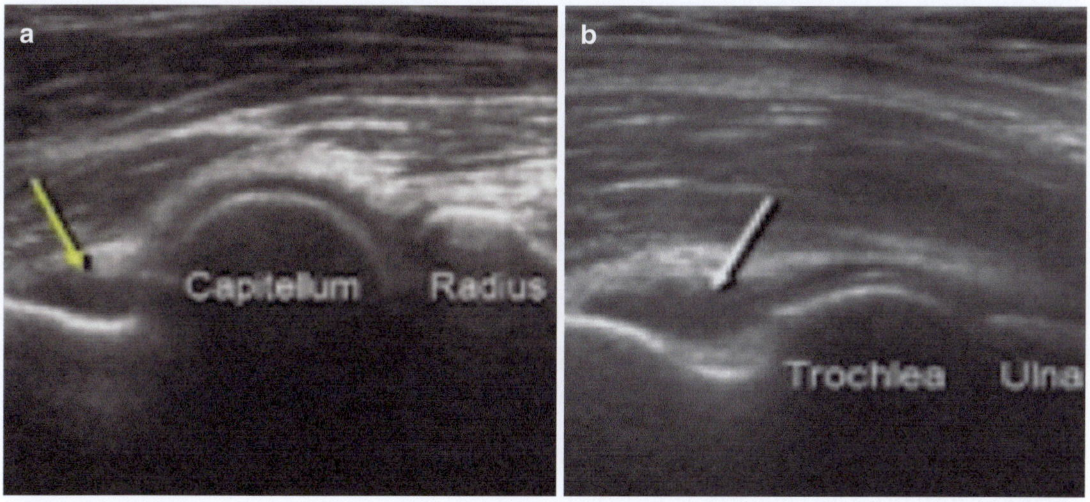

Fig. 7.13 Longitudinal scans of the lateral (**a**) and medial (**b**) compartments of the elbow show mild effusion in both compartments (arrow)

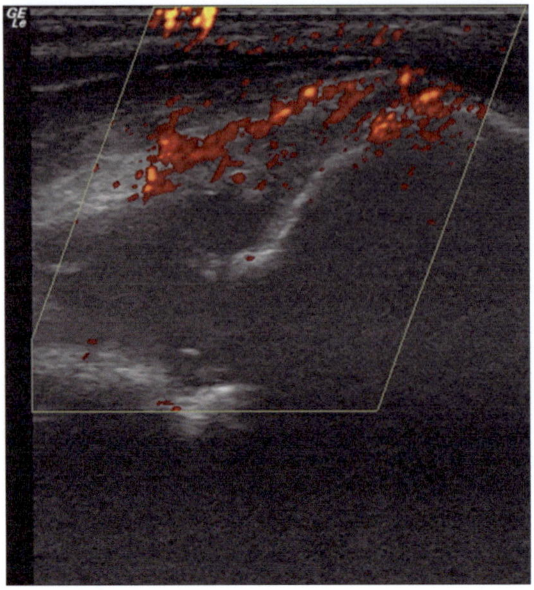

Fig. 7.15 Longitudinal scan of the posterior compartment of the elbow showing Doppler activity

nals must be detected within the synovial hypertrophy to be considered as sign of synovitis.

At the elbow, effusion and synovial hypertrophy are most commonly seen at the lateral or posterior aspect of the joint, although it can be detected anteriorly or medially as well. It should be remembered that effusion up to 1 mL can be seen by US in normal joints [28].

US cannot reliably detect the nature of effusion whether it is inflammatory, infectious, or hemophilic arthropathy. US gives a very good guidance in aspiration of fluid which remains the key for the diagnosis of joint disorder [29].

Doppler ultrasound (either power or color) can be used to detect inflammatory activity in the synovium and is essential in a full ultrasound evaluation of children with inflammatory arthritis (Fig. 7.15).

But it should be stressed that in children, the epiphysis is vascularized and metaphyseal vessels anastomose with epiphyseal vessels through the growth plate. Vascularization in this area can be physiologically detected by MSUS in healthy children. According to the definition of US-detected synovitis in children by OMERACT, pathological Doppler signals should be detected in an area of synovial hyperplasia/hypertrophy detected on B mode [27].

Septic Arthritis

Acute monoarthritis due to infection (septic arthritis) in infants and children particularly can have potentially serious consequences and is considered a rheumatological emergency and should be diagnosed within hours to avoid a disastrous outcome, which can lead to joint destruction.

While septic arthritis is relatively frequent in infancy, septic arthritis of the elbow in children is rare [30].

In a recent study of 12 children with septic arthritis, *S. aureus* was the most common pathogen. Diagnosis is often delayed with common presentations including a sudden onset of the pain and joint discomfort, and in most cases, inflammatory markers were elevated (ESR > 40 mm/h, CRP > 2 mg/dL) [31].

None of the clinical findings are highly sensitive or specific for septic arthritis. US may help in differential diagnosis.

The US hallmarks of septic arthritis are articular effusion with inhomogeneous echogenicity, synovial thickening, and frequently synovial hypervascularity upon power Doppler US [32].

In a study of another 12 children with suspected septic arthritis of the elbow, all children were studied with plain-film radiography and ultrasound. Joint effusion was seen by sonography in six patients, four of whom underwent ultrasound-guided joint aspiration, confirming the diagnosis of septic arthritis in two patients and excluding it in two. Of nine patients whose plain films showed only soft tissue swelling, seven had one or more significant findings with sonography: joint effusion (without fat pad elevation on lateral plain films) in three patients, periosteal reaction in two, and epitrochlear mass in three. Sonography confirmed soft tissue swelling alone in two patients, thus excluding the diagnosis of septic arthritis and obviating unnecessary attempts at joint aspiration [33].

It should be emphasized that US cannot reliably confirm septic arthritis and still the golden standard is aspiration and analysis of synovial fluid, the intervention that US could give an excellent guidance.

Hemophilic Arthropathy

Hemophilia is an X-linked recessive bleeding disorder in which circulating levels of coagulation factors are lacking, resulting in a propensity toward bleeding [34].

Intra-articular hemorrhages are a hallmark of hemophilia and may lead a cascade of cytokine elaboration and inflammatory-mediated changes, which ultimately result in cartilage loss and arthropathy. Diarthrodial joints, such as the knee, elbow, and ankle, are most commonly affected [35].

Gray-scale ultrasound can detect the presence of intra-articular fluid, synovial hypertrophy, and hemosiderin deposition and cartilage breakdowns. Ultrasound is also useful in identifying heterotopic calcifications, bursal hemorrhage, and inter- or intramuscular hemorrhage [36].

Recent bleeding appears echogenic, related to the high reflectivity of fresh blood. Later, 48–72 hours after the hemorrhagic event, a progressive decrease in the echogenicity occurs, following blood cell lysis, and the effusion gradually becomes anechoic [37].

After several hemarthroses in hemophilic joints, the synovium often appears as a thickened irregular hypoechoic band lying over anechoic hyaline cartilage. In cases of cartilage degeneration, tears may develop in the cartilage, which appears irregular and subchondral cysts may be apparent [38].

Color Doppler images typically show an increase in the blood supply to the synovium as part of the inflammatory process [39].

Poonnoose et al. [34] developed a concordance study between the physical exam using the Hemophilia Joint Health Score (HJHS version 2.0) and the radiological evaluation. They used the Pettersson score for X-rays [40], the tool of the International Prophylaxis Study Group (IPSG score) for the MR, and the corresponding US scale in 55 joints of subjects with severe hemophilia or Von Willebrand disease.

In this cohort, subjects with normal physical exam had soft changes or osteochondral changes on US or MR evaluation; furthermore, 33% of the joints had findings in US or MR, but it did not have pathological changes on X-ray, so a normal X-ray or physical exam does not exclude joint disease in hemophilia.

In a recent expert consensus [41], MSK US evaluation of hemoarthritic joints is indicated in every follow-up in patient with severe MSK symptom and as needed only in patients with no or medium MSK symptoms.

Bursal Pathology

Elbow bursitis, most commonly involving the olecranon bursa, is inflammation of the subcutaneous synovial-lined sac of the bursa overlying the olecranon process at the proximal aspect of the ulna. The bursa cushions the olecranon and reduces friction between it and the skin, especially during movement [39].

The superficial location of the bursa, between the ulna and the skin at the posterior tip of the elbow, makes it susceptible to inflammation from acute or repetitive trauma. Less commonly, inflammation results from infection (septic bursitis) or as a part of juvenile chronic arthritis.

In normal elbow joint, the olecranon bursa of the posterior elbow should not be able to be readily visualized on ultrasound [42].

In inflamed bursas, the use of ultrasonography has been shown to be extremely effective in the diagnosis of olecranon bursitis and other soft-tissue lesions in the olecranon area by rapidly demonstrating the presence of effusions, synovial proliferation, loose bodies, increased blood flow consistent with inflammation, tendonitis with calcifications, and other indications of bursitis [43].

Visualization of an enlarged olecranon bursa is best performed with the elbow in extension with minimal probe pressure and/or use of a thick layer of gel, since even slight pressure from the probe can displace fluid away from the transducer.

Thin bursal walls and anechoic fluid are typically seen on ultrasound of olecranon bursitis [43].

Ultrasound cannot detect reliably the cause of inflamed bursa, but bursal fluid of heterogeneous and hyperechoic features may suggest septic causes.

Aspiration and synovial analysis remain the gold standard for diagnosis of septic bursitis [44]. Ultrasonography may guide aspiration of fluid for a diagnostic purpose. Also, US can guide injection of corticosteroid as a local therapy.

Tendon and Ligament Pathology

The pediatric and adolescent elbow is subject to both acute and chronic overuse injuries affecting tendons and ligaments. Also, tendons and entheses may be subjected to inflammatory changes in many subtypes of juvenile chronic arthritis.

Pulled Elbow

Nursemaid elbow, also known as "radial head subluxation" or simply "pulled elbow," is the most common upper limb injury in children under the age of 6 [45]. In children younger than 5 years, the annular ligament is relatively loose, allowing the radial head to be pulled through it when acute traction is suddenly placed on a pronated forearm (which is the usual position of the forearm when a child is being pulled along by an adult). Although the annular ligament becomes transiently interposed between the radial head and capitellum, this movement does not cause recognizable widening of the radiocapitellar joint. Therefore, elbow radiographic findings are normal in a pulled elbow.

Diagnosis of pulled elbow usually depends on a history, such as passive traction by parents, and on physical examinations. But patients with pulled elbow are too young to get an exact history from and to perform definite physical examination on. For this reason, misdiagnosis of a fracture as a pulled elbow may be possible [46].

Ultrasound could be used to confirm pulled elbow in terms of reducing unnecessary radiation, especially when the mechanism of injury is not evident or physical examination seems inconclusive. Moreover, ultrasound could be performed with the patient's arm in a neutral position, which could minimize unrecognized complications such as occult fractures. It is easy to compare the ultrasonographic picture of the pulled elbow with the normal contra lateral elbow. Besides, it is useful for the detection of thickening and sometimes annular ligament tear, dislocations of radial head, as well as measuring the distance between radial head and capitellum when the forearm is rotated inward. Ultrasonography can be used as a tool to measure progress and result of recurrent dislocation of the bone during treatment.

Ultrasound findings in pulled elbow include increased echogenicity of the joint space compared with the healthy limb due to slipped annular ligament and expansion of radiocapitellar distance to 2 or more millimeters. Minagawa reported 32 cases of pulled elbow in his sonographic study of the anterior surface of the radiohumeral joint in the long axis, where the muscle originating from annular ligament forms a J-shape with the annular ligament trapped in the radiohumeral joint. He termed this finding as the "J-sign." He reported that sensitivity, specificity, and accuracy of ultrasonography in the diagnosis of J-shaped low resonance imaging were 100% for three abovementioned factors [47, 48].

Medial Epicondyle Apophysitis/Little League Elbow Syndrome

Little league elbow (LLE) syndrome is a valgus overload or overstress injury to the medial elbow that occurs as a result of repetitive throwing motions.

Little league elbow syndrome occurs most commonly in pitchers, but it is also seen in catchers. This condition can also occur in other overhead or throwing sports, such as tennis and football. Diagnosis depends on history of specific-sport-related injury and clinical examination [49].

Sonography can confirm the diagnosis. Sonographic findings includes but not limited to medial epicondylar fragmentation and osteochondritis dissecans of the capitellum [50].

Enthesitis

Enthesitis-related arthritis represents 20% of juvenile inflammatory arthritis categories. Entheses inflammation is the characteristic feature of this category. Typically, enthesitis is more common in lower limb, but in upper limb enthesitis of triceps tendon is commonly detected [51]. Adult definition of enthesitis is used in juvenile patients without change, it includes abnormal hypoechoic (loss of normal fibrillar architecture) and/or thickened tendon or ligament as its bone attachment (may contain hyperechoic foci consistent with calcification) seen in two perpendicular planes that may exhibit a Doppler signal and/or bony changes such as enthesophytes, erosions, or irregularities [52].

It should be noted that in children, tendons and ligaments attach to layers of fibrocartilage and hypoechoic cartilage covering the secondary ossification center of the bone, and it should not be mistaken as a pathological finding.

Additionally, normal Doppler signals could be detected within the nonossified apophysis and epiphyseal cartilage [53].

Bone Lesions

Ultrasonography has a major role in identifying bony lesions in children and juvenile patients with elbow pain. US can reliably help in the diagnosis of fractures and detection of erosions in inflammatory arthritis.

Fractures Around Elbow

Elbow fractures are the most common type of fractures in children. There are multiple types of elbow fractures (supracondylar, condylar, olecranon, radial head) which all cause effusion of the elbow joint [54].

In many cases, it is difficult to obtain a reliable history of trauma especially in infants. So, fractures should be excluded in all children presenting with elbow pain even if there is no obvious history of trauma.

Elbow-associated fractures have a limited potential of spontaneous correction; hence, an exact diagnosis is mandatory. The majority (70%) of clinical suspects of a fracture ends up with a contusion diagnosis and the radiation exposure can be avoided with ultrasound screening [55].

Ultrasonography is highly sensitive for elbow fractures, and a negative ultrasound may reduce the need for radiographs in children with elbow injuries. Of 130 patients (mean age, 7.5 years), 43 (33%) had a radiograph result positive for fracture. Rabiner et al. found a positive elbow ultrasound had a sensitivity of 98% and a specificity of 70% [56].

One of the most important ultrasonographic signs of elbow fracture is positive SOFA (Sonographic Fat-pad) sign, which refers to the displacement of posterior olecranon fat pad due to the presence of joint effusion [57].

SOFA is detected in a single dorsal axial view which visualizes the fossa olecrani; the elbow is flexed 70–90 °. In case of any doubt, the contralateral side may be examined.

It is of utmost importance to understand the developmental anatomy of the pediatric elbow which helps in the detection of an injury when the pattern is altered. For example, the medial epicondyle usually ossifies prior to the trochlea. Therefore, if the medial epicondyle is not seen in its expected location and a single ossicle is seen beneath the medial aspect of the distal humeral metaphysis, the ossicle should be interpreted as an avulsed medial epicondyle that is entrapped in the joint rather than a normal trochlea [58].

Erosions

Erosions of the bony structures of the elbow joint can be found in children with juvenile inflammatory arthritis. Erosions of the elbow joint, as in other joint regions, appear as a discontinuity of the normally smooth bone contour; often with the appearance of a "bite" taken out of the bone. Bone erosions or apparent defects should be documented on ultrasound in two perpendicular planes in order to distinguish true erosions from bony surface irregularity [51].

An important consideration is to differentiate between pathological erosions and the physiological physis (or growth plate) that appeared in US as a discontinuity of cortical bone in the oldest children and physiological irregularities visualized by US in some ossification centers [59].

Nerve Pathology

The use of ultrasound in nerve imaging has proven useful in the elbow region, particularly for the imaging of pathology involving the ulnar nerve.

Subluxation of the ulnar nerve out of its normal anatomic location in the ulnar groove can be a normal variant or pathologic when it is accompanied by symptoms such as paresthesias, dysesthesias, or muscle weakness. Dynamic scanning with ultrasound during elbow flexion and extension can show translocation of the ulnar nerve over the medial epicondyle in cases of subluxation. Ulnar nerve instability has been reported in up to 17% of children. Accurate assessment is important to achieve because of potential nerve complications that can arise from treatment of common pediatric fractures, including supracondylar humerus fractures. Patients with ligamentous laxity are more likely to possess unstable ulnar nerves. Ultrasound evaluation and assessment of ligamentous laxity are additional tools that can be used to assess elbow anatomy and identify children at risk for iatrogenic nerve injury. Patients aged between 6 and 10 showed the highest rate of dislocating or subluxating nerves [60].

Ulnar nerve entrapment at elbow is not common in pediatric patients, but there are many case reports of cubital tunnel syndrome that occurred in patients with hemophilia or as a complication to fractures [61].

As in adults, swelling or edema of the nerve appears on ultrasound as enlargement and hypoechogenicity of the nerve, with loss of the normal speckled or fascicular nerve pattern proximal to the site of entrapment.

Comparing the affected nerve with the contralateral nonaffected side is very helpful [62].

In conclusion, ultrasonography of elbow in pediatric patients gives a major help in diagnosis of different pathologies. Also, it is a very useful tool in assessment of disease activity and following up of therapy.

References

1. Moore KL, Dalley AF. Clinically oriented anatomy. 5th ed. Philadelphia: Lippincott Williams & Wilkins; 2006.
2. Collado P, Naredo E. Sonographic image of children's joints. Badalona: EUROMEDICE, Ediciones Médicas; 2007b.
3. De Boeck H. Radiology of the elbow in children. Acta Orthop Belg. 1996;62(Suppl 1):34–40.
4. DeFroda SF, Hansen H, Gil JA, Hawari AH, Cruz AI Jr. Radiographic evaluation of common pediatric elbow injuries. Orthop Rev (Pavia). 2017;9(1):7030.
5. Soma DB. Opening the black box: evaluating the pediatric athlete with elbow pain. PM R. 2016;8(3 Suppl):S101–12.
6. Hryhorczuk AL, Restrepo R, Lee EY. Pediatric musculoskeletal ultrasound: practical imaging approach. AJR Am J Roentgenol. 2016;206(5):W62–72.
7. Backhaus M, Burmester GR, Gerber T, Grassi W, Machold KP, Swen WA, Wakefield RJ, Manger B, Working Group for Musculoskeletal Ultrasound in the EULAR Standing Committee on International Clinical Studies including Therapeutic Trials. Guidelines for musculoskeletal ultrasound in rheumatology. Ann Rheum Dis. 2001;60(7):641–9.
8. Gruber G, Konermann W. Sonography of musculoskeletal system: standard scans according guidelines of DEGUM. Weinheim: Chapman & Hall; 1997. German
9. Silverman FN. The bones. In: Silverman FN, editor. Caffey's pediatric X-ray diagnosis. 9th ed. Chicago: Year Book Medical Publishers, Inc; 1985. p. 398–9.
10. Beggs I, Bianchi S, Bueno A, Cohen M, Court-Payen M, Grainger A et al. Musculoskeletal ultrasound technical guidelines. II. Elbow. Eur Soc Musculoskelet Radiol. 2006. http://www.essr.org/html/img/pool/elbow.pdf. Accessed Jan 2012.
11. Shen XT, Zhou ZG, Yu LS, Wu X, Chen XL, Xu Y, et al. Ultrasound assessment ofthe elbow joint in infants and toddlers and its clinical significance. ActaRadiol. 2014;55(6):745–52.
12. Herring JA. Tachdjian's pediatric orthopedics. 3rd ed. Philadelphia: WB Saunders Company; 2002. p. 2121–3.
13. Miller TT, Adler RS. Sonography of tears of the distal biceps tendon. AJR Am J Roentgenol. 2000;175(4):1081–6.
14. Martinoli C, Bianchi S, Zamorani MP, Zunzunegui JL, Derchi LE. Ultrasound of the elbow. Eur J Ultrasound. 2001;14(1):21–7.
15. Konin GP, Nazarian LN, Walz DM. US of the elbow: indications, technique, normal anatomy, and pathologic conditions. Radiographics. 2013;33(4):E125–47.
16. Radunovic G, Vlad V, Micu MC, Nestorova R, Petranova T, Porta F, Iagnocco A. Ultrasound assessment of the elbow. Med Ultrason. 2012;14(2):141–6.
17. Fessell DP, Jacobson JA, Craig J, Habra G, Prasad A, Radliff A, et al. Using sonography to reveal and aspirate joint effusions. AJR Am J Roentgenol. 2000;174(5):1353–62.
18. Price CT, Flynn JM. Management of fractures. In: Morrissey RT, Weinstein SL, editors. Lovell and Winter's Pediatric Orthopaedics. 6th ed. Philadelphia: Lippincott; 2006. p. 1463.
19. Walker FO, Cartwright MS, Wiesler ER, Caress J. Ultrasound of nerve and muscle. Clin Neurophysiol. 2004;115(3):495–507.
20. Pillen S, Alfen NV, Zwarts M. Ultrasound of muscle. In: Cartwright MS, Walker FO, editors. Neuromuscular ultrasound. 1st ed. Philadelphia: Elsevier Saunders; 2011.

21. Precerutti M, Garioni E, Ferrozzi G. Dorsal forearm anatomy: US anatomy pictorial essay. J Ultrasound. 2010;13(2):66–9.
22. Gray H, Williams PL, Bannister LH. Gray's anatomy: the anatomical basis of medicine and surgery. New York: Churchill Livingstone; 1995.
23. Draghi F, Bortolotto C. Intersection syndrome: ultrasound imaging. Skelet Radiol. 2014;43(3):283–7.
24. Prakken B, Albani S, Martini A. Juvenile idiopathic arthritis. Lancet. 2011;377:2138–49.
25. Colebatch-Bourn AN, Edwards CJ, Collado P, D'Agostino MA, Hemke R, Jousse-Joulin S, et al. EULAR-PReS points to consider for the use of imaging in the diagnosis and management of juvenile idiopathic arthritis in clinical practice. Ann Rheum Dis. 2015;74:1946–57. https://doi.org/10.1136/annrheumdis-2015-207892.
26. Lamer S, Sebag GH. MRI and ultrasound in children with juvenile chronic arthritis. Eur J Radiol. 2000;33(2):85–93.
27. Roth J, Jousse-Joulin S, Magni-Manzoni S, Rodriguez A, Tzaribachev N, Iagnocco A, et al. Definitions for the sonographic features of joints in healthy children. Arthritis Care Res. 2015;67:136–42. https://doi.org/10.1002/acr.22410.
28. De Maeseneer M, Jacobson JA, Jaovisidha S, Lenchik L, Ryu KN, Trudell DR, Resnick D. Elbow effusions: distribution of joint fluid with flexion and extension and imaging implications. Investig Radiol. 1998;33(2):117–25.
29. Luukkainen R, Sanila MT, Saltyshev M, Huhtala H, Koski JM. Relationship between clinically detected joint swelling and effusion diagnosed by ultrasonography in elbow joints in patients with rheumatoid arthritis. Clin Rheumatol. 2005;24(3):228–31.
30. Welkon CJ, Long SS, Fisher MC, Alburger PD. Pyogenic arthritis in infants and children: a review of 95 cases. Pediatr Infect Dis. 1986;5(6):669–76.
31. Nduaguba AM, Flynn JM, Sankar WN. Septic arthritis of the elbow in children: clinical presentation and microbiological profile. J Pediatr Orthop. 2016;36(1):75–9.
32. Gordon JE, Huang M, Dobbs M, Luhmann SJ, Szymanski DA, Schoenecker PL. Causes of false-negative ultrasound scans in the diagnosis of septic arthritis of the hip in children. J Pediatr Orthop. 2002;22:312–6.
33. Lim-Dunham JE, Ben-Ami TE, Yousefzadeh DK. Septic arthritis of the elbow in children: the role of sonography. Pediatr Radiol. 1995;25:556.
34. Poonnoose PM, Hilliard P, Doria AS, Keshava SN, Gibikote S, Kavitha ML, et al. Correlating clinical and radiological assessment of joints in haemophilia: results of a cross sectional study. Haemophilia. 2016;22(6):925–33.
35. Schulman S. Mild haemophilia. In: World Federation of Haemophilia, editor. Treatment of haemophilia; 2012. p. 1–10.
36. Knobe K, Berntorp E. Haemophilia and joint disease: pathophysiology, evaluation, and management. J Comorb. 2011;1(1):51–9.
37. Kidder W, Nguyen S, Larios J, Bergstrom J, Ceponis A, von Drygalski A. Point-of-care musculoskeletal ultrasound is critical for the diagnosis of hemarthroses, inflammation and soft tissue abnormalities in adult patients with painful haemophilic arthropathy. Haemophilia. 2015;21(4):530–7.
38. Melchiorre D, Linari S, Innocenti M, Biscoglio I, Toigo M, Cerinic MM, Morfini M. Ultrasound detects joint damage and bleeding in haemophilic arthropathy: a proposal of a score. Haemophilia. 2011;17(1):112–7.
39. Martinoli C, Della Casa Alberighi O, Di Minno G, Graziano E, Molinari AC, Pasta G, et al. Development and definition of a simplified scanning procedure and scoring method for haemophilia early arthropathy detection with ultrasound (HEAD-US). Thromb Haemost. 2013;109:1170–9.
40. Pettersson H, Ahlberg A, Nilsson IM. A radiologic classification of hemophilic arthropathy. Clin Orthop Relat Res. 1980;149:153–9.
41. Seuser A, Djambas Khayat C, Negrier C, Sabbour A, Heijnen L. Evaluation of early musculoskeletal disease in patients with haemophilia: results from an expert consensus. Blood Coagul Fibrinolysis. 2018;29(6):509–20.
42. Draghi F, Danesino GM, de Gautard R, Bianchib S. Ultrasound of the elbow: examination techniques and US appearance of the normal and pathologic joint. J Ultrasound. 2007;10(2):76–84.
43. Blankstein A, Ganel A, Givon U, Mirovski Y, Chechick A. Ultrasonographic findings in patients with olecranon bursitis. Ultraschall Med. 2006;27(6):568–71.
44. Rhyou IH, Park KJ, Kim KC, Lee JH, Kim SY. Endoscopic olecranon bursal resection for olecranon bursitis: a comparative study for septic and aseptic olecranon bursitis. J Hand Surg Asian Pac Vol. 2016;21(2):167–72.
45. Schutzman SA, Teach S. Upper-extremity impairment in young children. Ann Emerg Med. 1995;26(4):474–9.
46. Kraus R, Dongowski N, Szalay G, Schnettler R. Missed elbow fractures misdiagnosed as radial head subluxations. Acta Orthop Belg. 2010;76:312–5.
47. Minagawa H. Diagnostic and interventional musculoskeletal ultrasound. J Jpn Orthop Assoc. 2012;86(11):1057–64.
48. Dohi D. Confirmed specific ultrasonographic findings of pulled elbow. J Pediatr Orthop. 2013;33(8):829–31.
49. Benjamin HJ, Briner WW Jr. Little league elbow. Clin J Sport Med. 2005;15(1):37–40.
50. Harada M, Takahara M, Sasaki J, Mura N, Ito T, Ogino T. Using sonography for the early detection of elbow injuries among young baseball players. AJR Am J Roentgenol. 2006;187(6):1436–41.
51. Fisher C, Ioannou Y, Hall-Craggs M, Sen D. Enthesitis related arthritis; a new era of understanding. Ann Paediatr Rheum. 2012;1:8–16.
52. Wakefield RJ, Balint PV, Szkudlarek M, On behalf of the OMERACT Special Interest Group. The OMERACT 7 Special Interest Group: diagnosed

musculoskeletal ultrasound including definitions for ultrasonographic pathology. J Rheumatol. 2005;32:2485–7.
53. Collado P, Windschall D, Vojinovic J, et al., And on behalf of the OMERACT ultrasound subtask force on pediatric. Amendment of the OMERACT ultrasound definitions of joints' features in healthy children when using the DOPPLER technique. Pediatr Rheumatol Online J. 2018;16:23.
54. Skaggs DL, Flynn JM. Supracondylar fractures of the distal Humerus. In: Beaty JH, Kasser JR, editors. Rockwood and Wilkins' fractures in children. 7th ed. Philadelphia: Wolters Kluwer/Lippincott, Williams & Wilkins; 2010. p. 487–532.
55. Chen L, Baker MD. Novel applications of ultrasound inpediatric emergency medicine. Pediatr Emerg Care. 2007;23(2):115–23.
56. Rabiner JE, Khine H, Avner JR, Friedman LM, Tsung JW. Accuracy of point-of-care ultrasonography for diagnosis of elbow fractures in children. Ann Emerg Med. 2013;61(1):9–17.
57. Eckert K, Ackermann O, Janssen N, et al. Accuracy of the sonographic fat pad sign for primary screening of pediatric elbow fractures: a preliminary study. J Med Ultrason. 2001;41:473–80.
58. Emery KH, Zingula SN, Anton CG, Salisbury SR, Tamai J. Pediatric elbow fractures: a new angle on an old topic. Pediatr Radiol. 2016;46(1):61–6.
59. Malattia C, Damasio MB, Magnaguagno F, Pistorio A, Valle M, Martinoli C, Viola S, Buoncompagni A, Loy A, Ravelli A, Tom ÃP, Martini A. Magnetic resonance imaging, ultrasonography, and conventional radiography in the assessment of bone erosions in juvenile idiopathic arthritis. Arthritis Rheum. 2008;59:1764–7.
60. Erez O, Khalil JG, Legakis JE, Tweedie J, Kaminski E, Reynolds RA. Ultrasound evaluation of ulnar nerve anatomy in the pediatric population. J Pediatr Orthop. 2012;32(6):641–6.
61. Renwick SE, MSJ M. Cubital tunnel syndrome in a child with hemophilia. Hand Surg Am. 1993;18(3):458–61.
62. Yoon JS, Hong SJ, Kim BJ, Kim SJ, Kim JM, Walker FO, Cartwright MS. Ulnar nerve and cubital tunnel ultrasound in ulnar neuropathy at the elbow. Arch Phys Med Rehabil. 2008;89(5):887–9.

Wrist and Hand

8

Daniel Windschall

Introduction

For decades, the ossification centres of the carpal bones have been used to determine the individual bone age of children by X-ray [1, 2]. The development of the skeletal system and the associated different stages of maturity of the ossification nuclei of the carpal bones are visible when performing musculoskeletal ultrasound (MSUS) on paediatric wrists and hands. Os capitate (1–3 months) and os hamate (2–4 months) are the first carpal bones to ossify, followed by os triquetrum (2–3 years), os lunate (2–4 years), os scaphoid, os trapezium, os trapezoid (each 4–6 years) and finally the sesamoid pisiform bone (8–12 years).

MSUS has shown high potential to visualize ossification nuclei in paediatric wrists [3, 4]. Recently, two studies by the paediatric OMERACT Ultrasound Group examined the age-dependent ossification and vascularization status of the wrist and fingers of healthy children [5, 6]. MSUS has a high reliability for grading the ossification status of certain carpal bones, and it also shows age-specific findings in vascularization [5–7]. Particularly in young children, more vessels are detected in the regions of the cartilage and epiphysis [6].

To distinguish between normal physiological findings and pathological abnormalities, it is fundamental to understand age-dependent differences. Especially in very young children, it may be difficult to distinguish between the normal hypoechoic cartilage and a pathologic effusion in cases of inflammatory arthritis [7–9].

The wrists and fingers are susceptible to a variety of rheumatic conditions such as synovitis, tenosynovitis and cortical erosions. Most of these pathologic conditions can be detected and diagnosed in their superficial locations by high-frequency ultrasound with high-resolution images of soft tissue structures and bony surfaces.

For all longitudinal standard views of the wrist, the proximal part of the wrist should be visible on the left side of the images. For the transverse views, the ulna is normally considered medial and is also shown on the left side of the images [10]. The wrist joints include the distal radioulnar joint, the radiocarpal and ulnocarpal joint spaces, the midcarpal joints and the articulations of the carpal bones with the proximal metacarpal bones. The finger joints include the metacarpophalangeal (MCP) joints, the proximal interphalangeal (PIP) joints and the distal interphalangeal (DIP) joints.

D. Windschall (✉)
Pediatric Clinic, Asklepios Hospital Weissenfels, Weissenfels, Germany

University of Halle-Wittenberg, Halle, Germany
e-mail: d.windschall@asklepios.com

Y. El Miedany (ed.), *Pediatric Musculoskeletal Ultrasonography*,
https://doi.org/10.1007/978-3-030-17824-6_8

Standard Scans of the Wrist and Fingers in Children

Dorsal Longitudinal View of the Wrist (Ulnar/Midline/Radial)

A very helpful start point for the paediatric wrist is the longitudinal view in the midline position, which shows the radial epiphysis, os lunate and os capitate. Due to their characteristic bony surfaces, the os lunate and os capitate can be used as anatomic landmarks (Fig. 8.1). The hand and wrist should be placed in a neutral position on a flat surface. From this start point, the transducer should be continuously moved to the ulnar side, showing the ulnocarpal aspect with the os triquetrum and os hamatum (Fig. 8.2). Moving to the radial side, the scan shows the radioscaphoid joint and the midcarpal bones, os trapezium and os trapezoideum (Fig. 8.3). All longitudinal dorsal regions should be examined dynamically with extension and flexion of the wrist joints to detect effusion and tenosynovitis. The extensor tendons run longitudinally along the posterior aspect of the wrist and are protected within synovial sheaths. All six extensor tendon compartments can be seen in the longitudinal view (Fig. 8.4). The differentiation between the extensor compartments is easier in the transverse view of the wrist [10, 11].

Dorsal Transverse View of the Wrist

After the longitudinal scans of the wrist, the transducer should be rotated 90° transversely to show the radioulnar joint. From that start point, the transducer should be moved distally to the midcarpal region. This transverse dorsal scan shows the second, third, fourth and fifth extensor

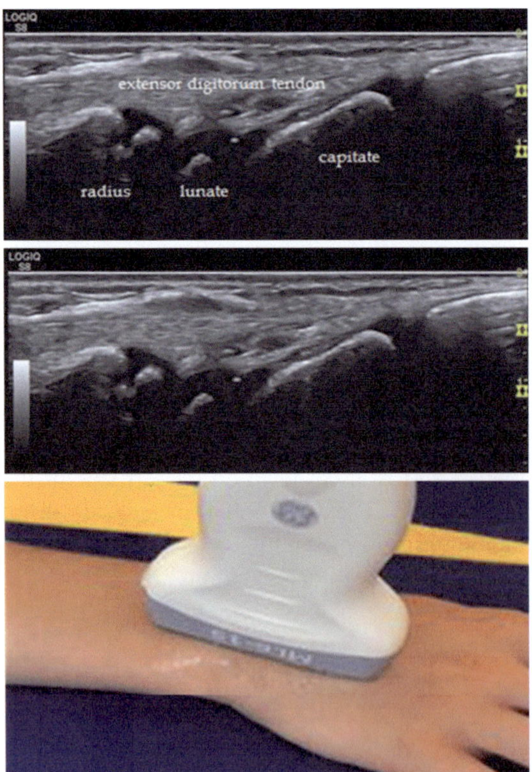

Fig. 8.1 Dorsal longitudinal view of the wrist in the midline position, which shows the radial epiphysis, os lunate and os capitate

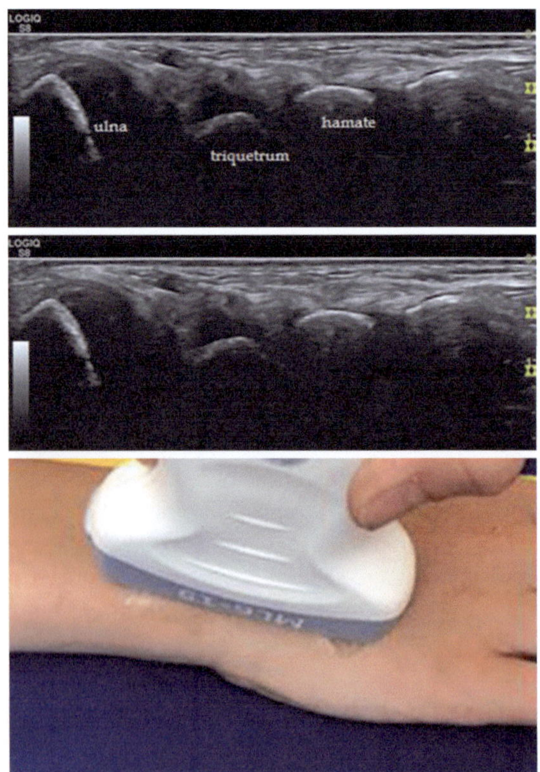

Fig. 8.2 Dorsal longitudinal view of the wrist in the ulnar position, which shows the ulnocarpal aspect with the os triquetrum and os hamate

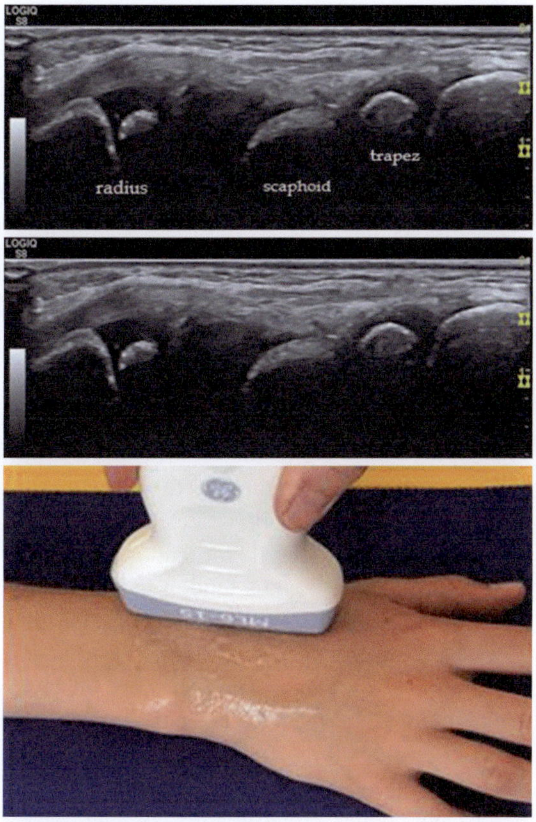

Fig. 8.3 Dorsal longitudinal view of the wrist in the radial position, which shows the radioscaphoid joint and the os trapezium

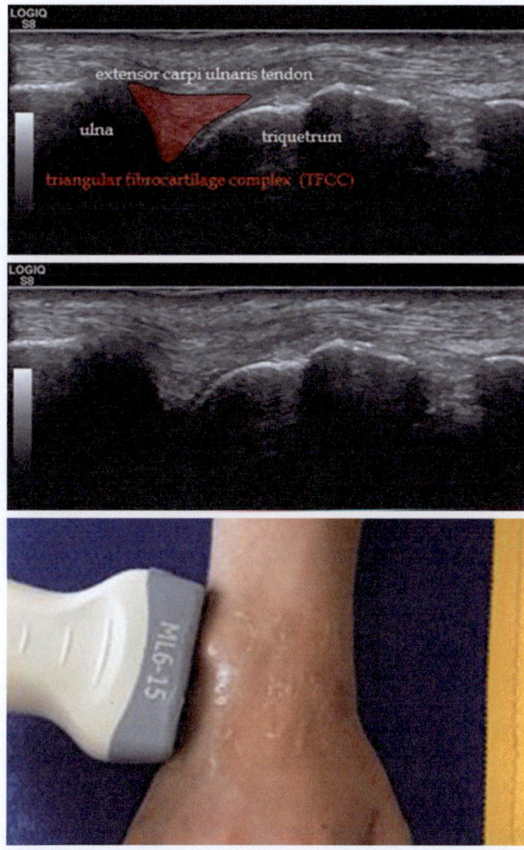

Fig. 8.4 Lateral ulnar longitudinal view of the wrist, which shows the extensor carpi ulnaris tendon above the triangular fibrocartilage complex (TFCC)

tendon compartments (Fig. 8.5). The second and third compartments are separated by the radial tubercle (Lister's tubercle). To obtain the transverse view of the first tendon compartment, the transducer must be moved further to the radial side and shows the tendons of the extensor pollicis brevis and abductor pollicis longus muscles. To obtain the transverse view of the sixth extensor tendon compartment with the extensor carpi ulnaris tendon, the transducer must be moved to the ulnar side.

Anisotropy can help to distinguish between tendons and effusion.

Extensor compartment (1) includes the abductor pollicis longus and extensor pollicis brevis tendons. Extensor compartment (2) contains the extensor carpi radialis longus and carpi radialis brevis tendons. Extensor compartment (3) involves the extensor pollicis longus tendon. The fourth extensor compartment contains the extensor digitorum and extensor indicis tendons, while the fifth extensor compartment contains the extensor digiti minimi tendon. Finally, the sixth extensor compartment protects the extensor carpi ulnaris tendon [10, 11].

Volar Longitudinal View of the Wrist in Children

Analogous to the dorsal side, the transducer start point should be in the volar longitudinal midline, showing the longitudinal plane of the second flexor digitorum tendon and the median nerve. The nerve runs parallel above the tendon and has a hypoechoic and less fibrillar ultrasound pattern (Fig. 8.6).

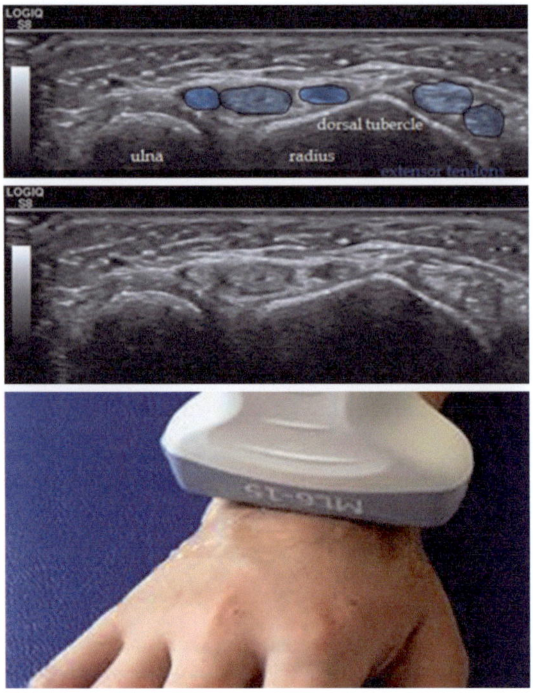

Fig. 8.5 Dorsal transverse scan of the wrist, which shows the second, third, fourth and fifth extensor tendon compartments

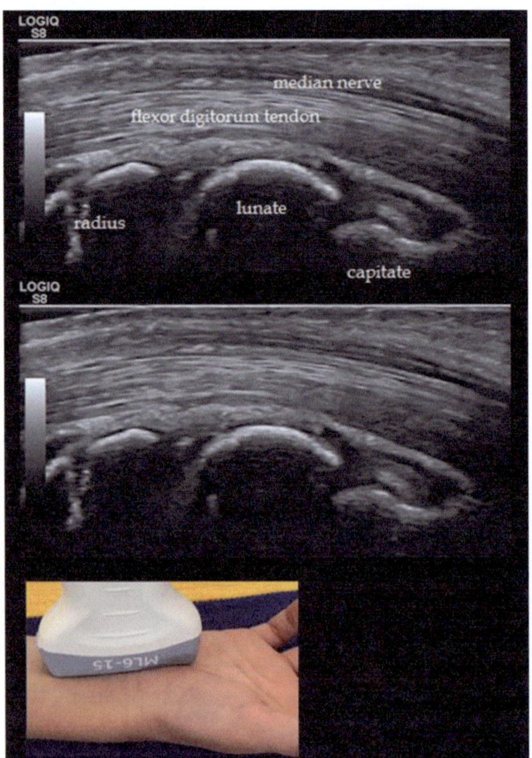

Fig. 8.6 Volar longitudinal view of the wrist, which shows the second flexor digitorum tendon and the median nerve

On dynamic examination, the tendon exhibits stronger movement than the nerve.

Moving from the longitudinal midline to the radial or ulnar side, all flexor tendons can be visualized longitudinally. The volar aspect of the radiocarpal and ulnocarpal joints can be screened for pathologic findings.

Volar Transverse View of the Wrist in Children

The volar transverse view shows all the flexor tendons of the flexor digitorum superficialis and profundus tendons passing through the carpal tunnel. The median nerve can be detected in the radial aspect of the superficial flexor tendons (Fig. 8.7). The flexor pollicis longus tendon has a separate synovial sheath, but also passes through the carpal tunnel. On the ulnar side, the ulnar artery adjacent to the ulnar nerve can be detected above the flexor retinaculum in the space between the os pisiforme and the os hamatum, known as Guyon's canal. The os pisiforme can be used as an anatomic landmark. For better identification of the nerves

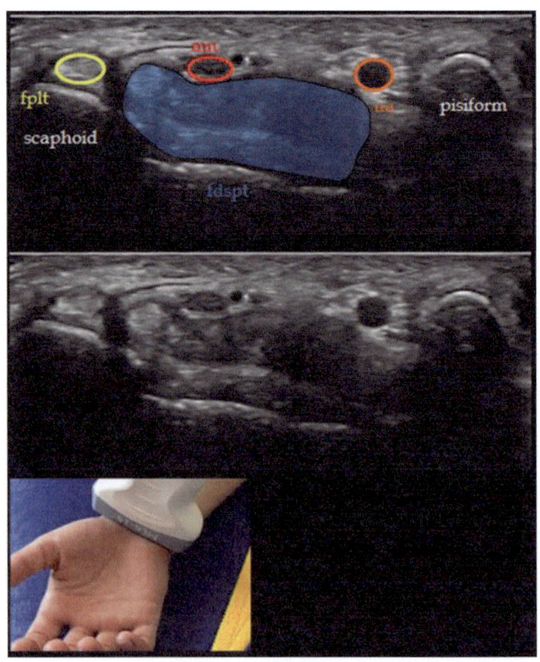

Fig. 8.7 Volar transverse view of the wrist, which shows the flexor digitorum superficialis and profundus tendons (fdspt), the flexor pollicis longus tendon (fplt), the median nerve (mn) and the ulnar artery (ua)

between the tendons, the transducer can be moved to an oblique position to make the hyperechoic tendons hypoechoic by anisotropy [10, 11].

Volar Longitudinal View of the MCP, PIP and DIP Joints

The transducer should be moved longitudinally from the proximal to the distal finger to show the volar longitudinal view of the MCP, PIP and DIP joints. This examination can be done with a high-frequency linear transducer to show more joints in one image or a small linear Hockey-Stick transducer to show each finger joint individually (Fig. 8.8). Thc volar longitudinal view of the fingers shows the flexor tendons crossing the small joint spaces with their thinner anechoic cartilage, depending on age, and subcapsular fat and a small physiological proximal joint recess, especially in the MCP joint. The flexor tendons have superficialis and profundus layers. The superficialis tendon divides at the level of the PIP joint, and the two slips insert along the proximal half of the middle phalanx. The profundus tendon inserts more distally at the base of the distal phalanx. The volar longitudinal view can detect synovialitis in the small finger joints and flexor tenosynovitis of the fingers (Figs. 8.9, 8.10 and 8.11).

Volar Transverse View of the MCP, PIP and DIP Joints

The transverse view helps to confirm flexor tenosynovitis and shows the separation of the superficial and deep flexor tendons at the level of the PIP joint (Fig. 8.12).

Dorsal Longitudinal View of the MCP, PIP and DIP Joints

The patient should have his hand lying on a flat surface in pronation. For a dynamic examination, the fingers can be flexed and extended. From proximal to distal, the MCP, PIP and DIP joints are shown with small joint spaces with thin cartilage, depending on age, and subcapsular fat and a synovial capsule (Figs. 8.13 and 8.14). In smaller children, more anechoic cartilage and an epiphyseal structure with a growth plate are seen on both joint-facing bones. A synovial proximal recess is normally not seen on the dorsal side of the finger joints. The extensor tendons have no synovial sheath and insert with a central band to the middle phalanx and with two lateral slips to

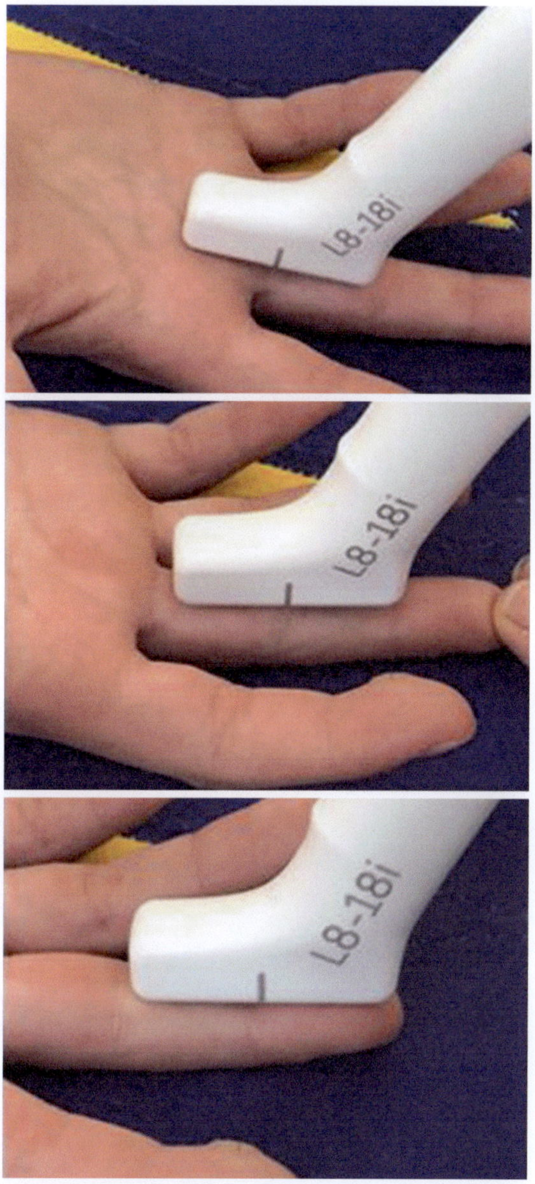

Fig. 8.8 Guiding a small linear Hockey-transducer along the volar aspect of a finger

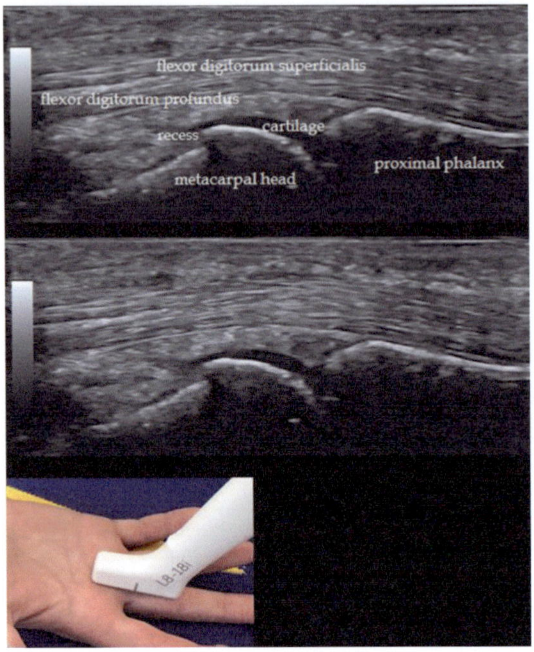

Fig. 8.9 Volar longitudinal view of the MCP joint

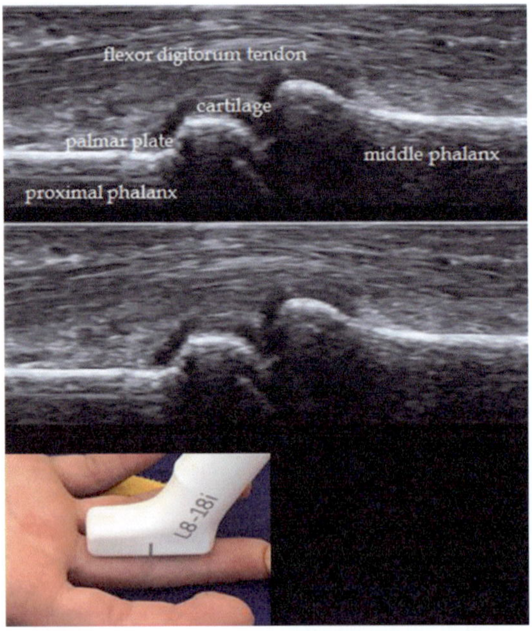

Fig. 8.10 Volar longitudinal view of the PIP joint

the base of the distal phalanx close to the DIP. The dorsal longitudinal view can detect synovialitis in the small finger joints and tenosynovitis of the extensor tendons. In children with rheumatic

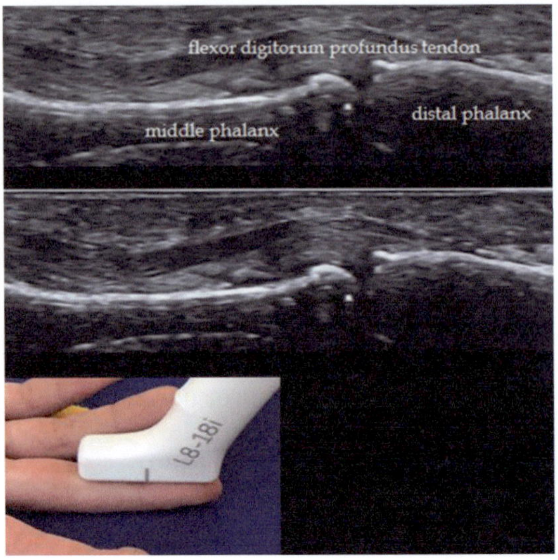

Fig. 8.11 Volar longitudinal view of the DIP joint

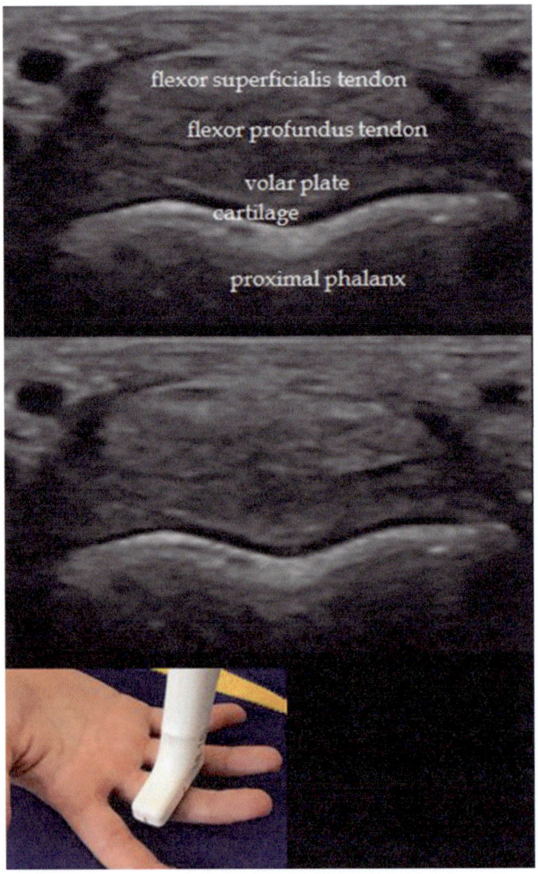

Fig. 8.12 Volar transverse view of the PIP joint, which shows the flexor digitorum superficialis and flexor digitorum profundus tendons

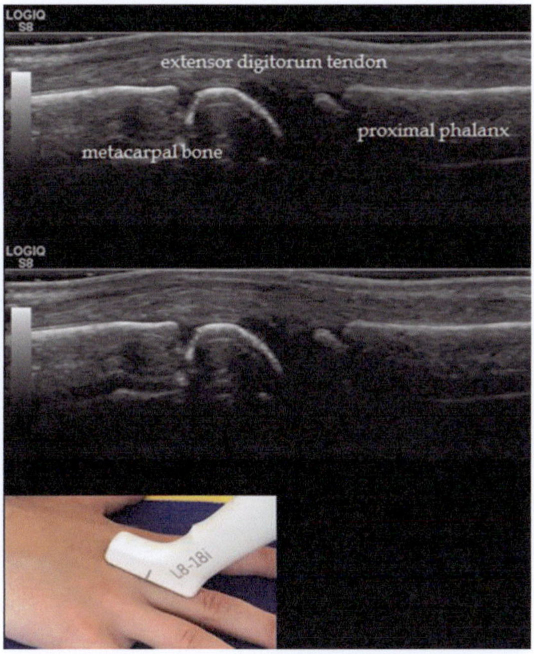

Fig. 8.13 Dorsal longitudinal view of the MCP joint

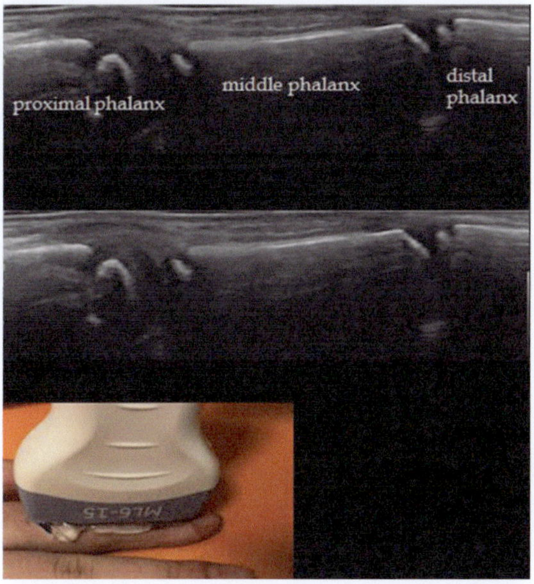

Fig. 8.14 Dorsal longitudinal view of the PIP and DIP joints

arthritis, erosions or cartilage damage of the metacarpal head can sometimes be detected in the dorsal longitudinal view of the MCP by 90°flexion (Fig. 8.15) [10, 11].

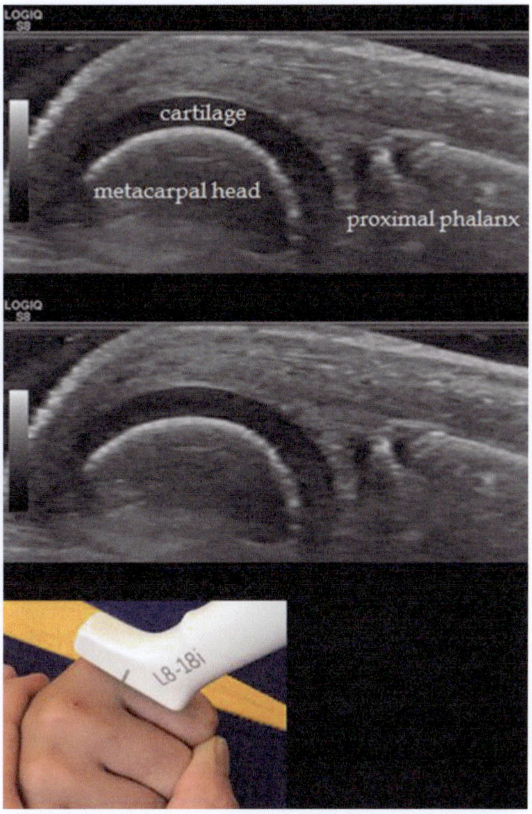

Fig. 8.15 Dorsal longitudinal view of the MCP by 90°flexion

Medial Longitudinal View of the Second MCP Joint and Lateral Longitudinal View of the Fifth MCP Joint

The medial or lateral scanning technique in those two fingers can help in juvenile idiopathic arthritis (JIA) to identify bony erosions at the level of the MCP, PIP or DIP joints (Fig. 8.16).

Age-Specific Findings in the Wrist and Hand

In younger children, the prominent cartilage of the short bones and the epiphyses appears anechoic or hypoechoic (Fig. 8.17) [12, 13]. Particularly, in non-ossified carpal bones, only an anechoic or hypoechoic structure with a well-defined boundary line is seen in ultrasound

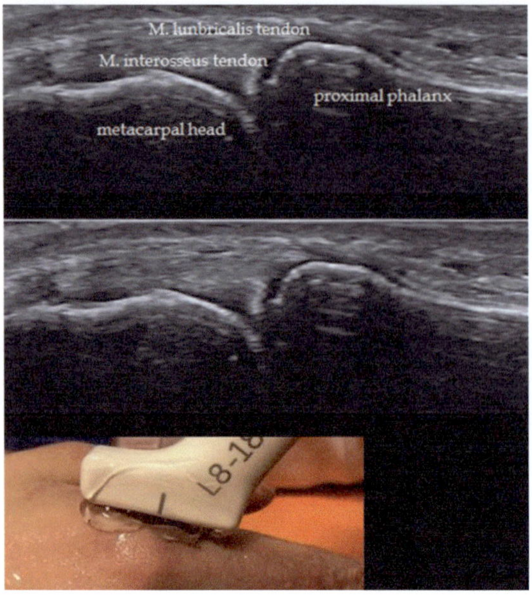

Fig. 8.16 Medial longitudinal view of the second MCP joint

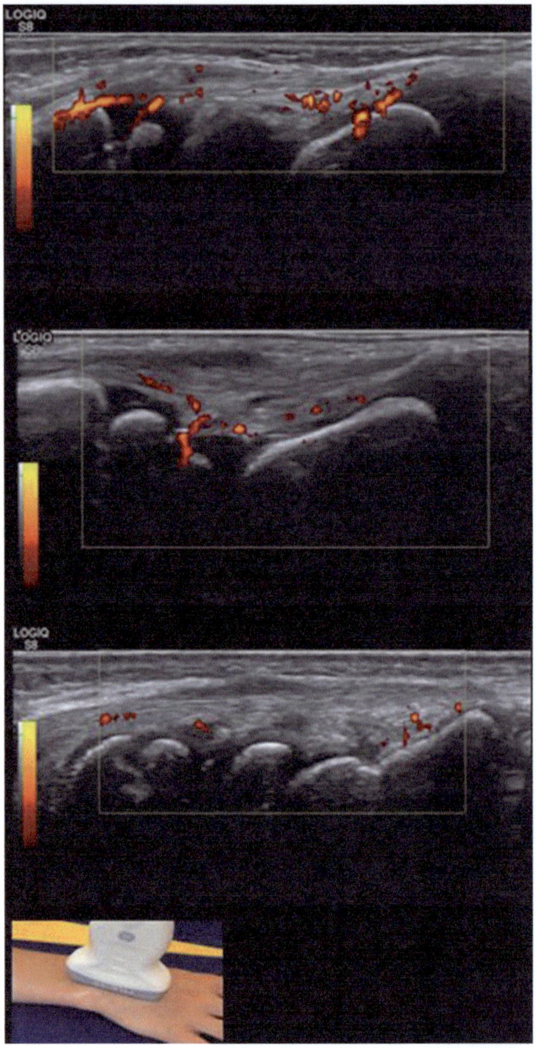

Fig. 8.17 Dorsal longitudinal view of the wrist in the midline position, which shows the radial epiphysis, os lunate and os capitate with normal physiological vessels in three different ages (2, 7 and 17 years)

images of the wrist [9]. Ossification during childhood can be clearly observed by ultrasound in all ages and was shown in a multi-observer ultrasound study to have a high reliability [6]. Other soft tissue structures like muscles, tendons or ligaments show less age-related variability. A typical childhood finding resulting from the incomplete fusion of the primary and secondary ossification centres of the long bones is the anechoic interruption between the metaphysis and epiphysis, which represents the growth plate or physis. A growth plate can be observed at the radiocarpal and ulnocarpal joint space and at the small finger joints.

Recently, normative data for the paediatric wrist was published, describing the radiocarpal and midcarpal joint recesses in healthy children [14]. The dorsal recess of the radiocarpal and midcarpal joints was visible in more than half of healthy children by ultrasound and was perceived as bulging in one out of ten radiocarpal recesses and one out of five midcarpal recesses.

In a recently published study by the paediatric OMERACT Ultrasound Group that aimed to describe age-dependent differences of vascularity, the physiological vascularization in four joint regions was assessed, including the wrist and second MCP of healthy children of different ages. More vessels were seen in the wrist compared with other joints, and the number of vessels was higher in children aged 2–12 years than in those aged 13–16 years [6]. In particular, vessels located at the epiphysis, at the physis and in the small bone cartilage were more frequently detected in children aged 2–12 years. Overall, the epiphysis was the location with the highest number of vessels detected, but this varied depending on the joint. More small bone intra-cartilaginous vessels and fat pad vessels were identified in the wrist joint than in the physis or epiphysis. Most vessels in the second MCP joint were located at the physis or epiphysis.

Wrist and Hand Pathology in Paediatric Rheumatology

Arthritis

Arthritis of the paediatric wrist and fingers is characterized by synovial hypertrophy and effusion. The synovial hypertrophy typically appears hypoechoic compared with subcutaneous fat. The synovial tissue is compressible but not displaceable, and may demonstrate hypervascularization when examined by power Doppler or colour Doppler ultrasound (Figs. 8.18 and 8.19) [15–18]. The synovial hypertrophy can involve all joint recesses in the wrist and fingers (Fig. 8.20). Effusion is characterized by anechoic intra-articular material that is compressible and normally displaceable without any Doppler signals. To distinguish between effusion and anechoic cartilage, the clear hyperechoic boundary line of the cartilage may be helpful. It is important to recognize the normal physiological vascularization in children's wrists and fingers in order to be able to interpret pathologic hypervascularization caused by inflammatory arthritis. Normal vessels can be found in the cartilage and epiphysis of smaller children.

Bone Erosions

Bone erosions can appear with chronic inflammatory arthritis, such as JIA, even in smaller children. A bone erosion is defined as a focal irregularity or discontinuity of the bone surface that has to be seen in two perpendicular planes (Figs. 8.21 and 8.22). It is important that the normal physiological bone irregularities in children, which are caused by ossification and development of the bones, are not misinterpreted as pathologic bone erosions.

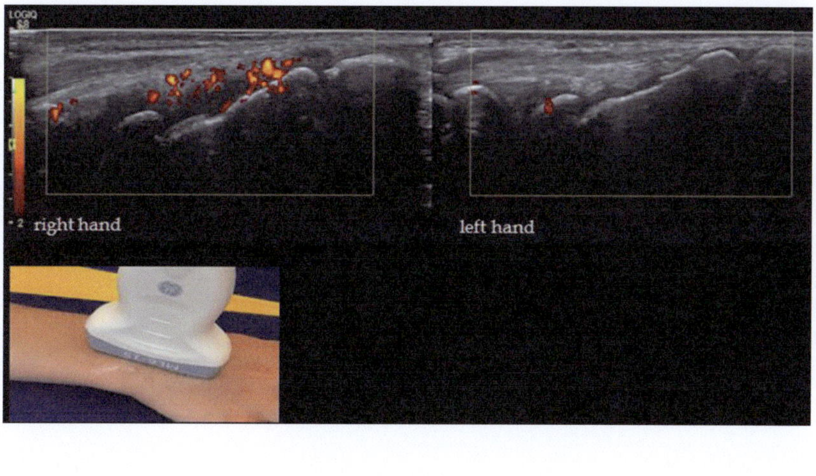

Fig. 8.18 Dorsal longitudinal view of the wrist in the midline position, which shows effusion and synovial hypertrophy in the radiocarpal and midcarpal recess of the right hand. Synovial hypertrophy exhibits hypervascularization above the os capitate. A 9-year-old girl with polyarticular arthritis

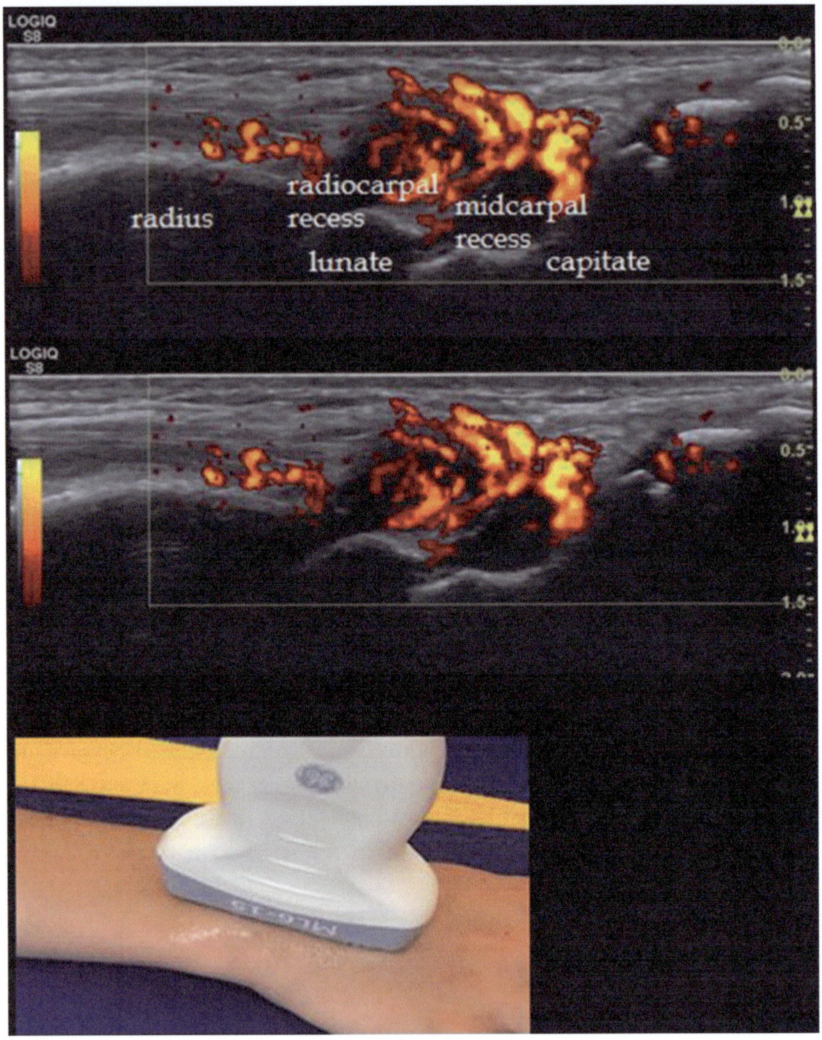

Fig. 8.19 Dorsal longitudinal view of the wrist in the midline position, which shows effusion and high degree synovial hypertrophy, which exhibits strong hypervascularization by power-Doppler. A 16-year-old girl with polyarticular arthritis

Tenosynovitis

Tenosynovitis of the wrist and fingers frequently occurs during the course of JIA and can be clearly detected by ultrasound. Tenosynovitis is characterized by distension of the tendon sheath with anechoic or hypoechoic fluid. It is sometimes combined with synovial hypertrophy within the tendon sheath and thickening of the tendons. The tendons appear hyperechoic within the anechoic fluid and may demonstrate hypervascularization (Figs. 8.23 and 8.24).

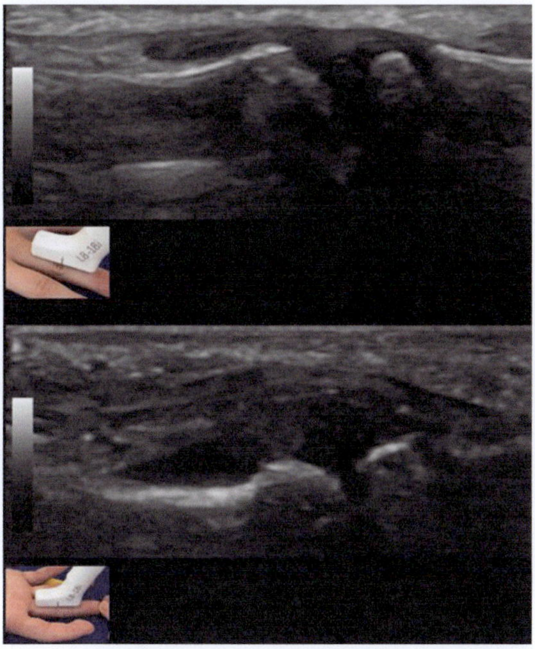

Fig. 8.20 Dorsal and volar longitudinal view of the third PIP joint, showing enlargement of the dorsal and volar joint recess in a 5-year-old girl with oligoarticular arthritis

Enthesitis

Enthesitis of the small finger entheses is characterized by hypoechoic enlargement combined with hypervascularization. Enthesitis occurs in enthesitis-associated arthritis or psoriatic arthritis of JIA. Sometimes, it is associated with overuse in children who play computer games or who use their smartphones for long periods during the day.

Differential Diagnoses and Traumatic Lesions

Ultrasound is an important tool to identify traumatic lesions in the wrist and hands of children, such as fractures, tendon tears or other superficial injuries. A ganglion cyst normally appears as anechoic to hypoechoic material adjacent to a joint or tendon sheath with well-defined margins (Fig. 8.25).

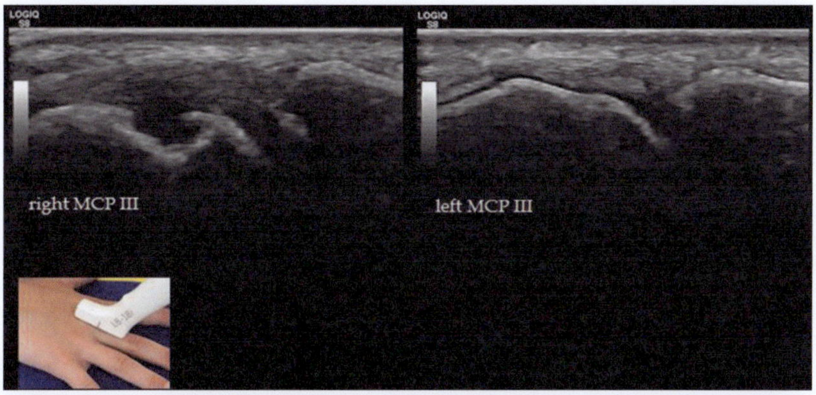

Fig. 8.21 Dorsal longitudinal view of the MCP joint, which shows bone erosion of the third metacarpal head of the right hand in comparison to the healthy side in a 13-year-old girl with extended oligoarthritis

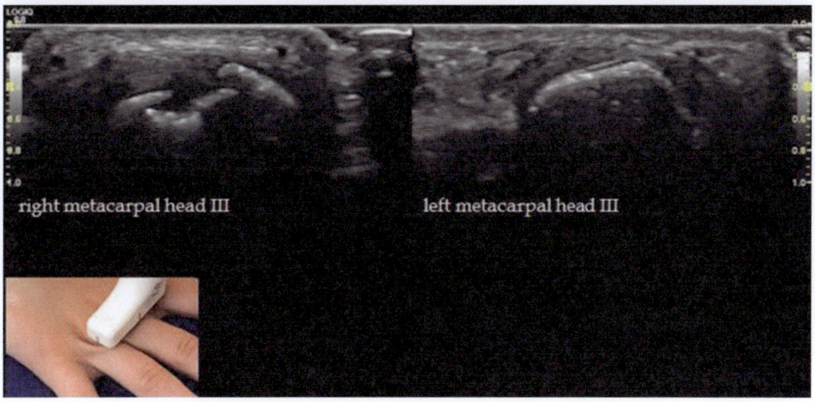

Fig. 8.22 Dorsal transverse view of the MCP joint, which shows bone erosion of the third metacarpal head of the right hand in comparison to the healthy side in a 13-year-old girl with extended oligoarthritis

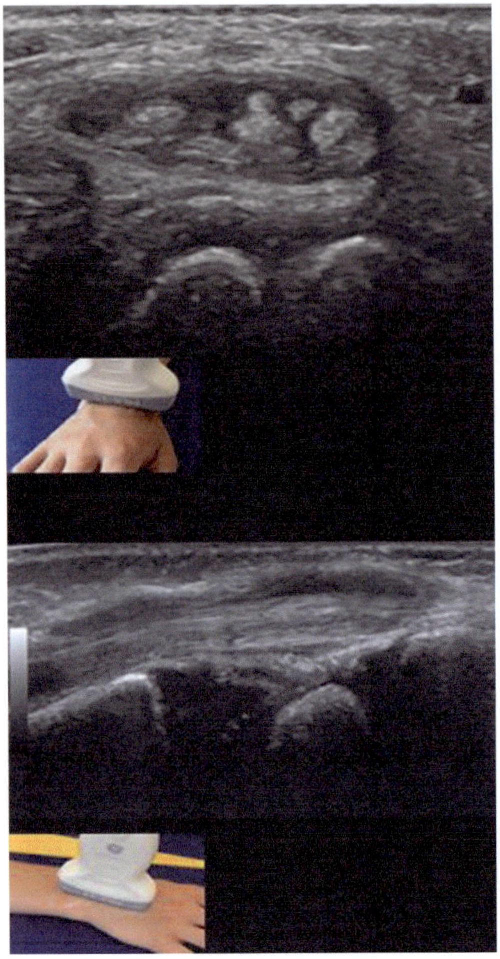

Fig. 8.23 Dorsal transverse and longitudinal view of the wrist in the midline position, which shows tenosynovitis of the extensor tendon sheaths in a 2-year-old girl with oligoarticular arthritis

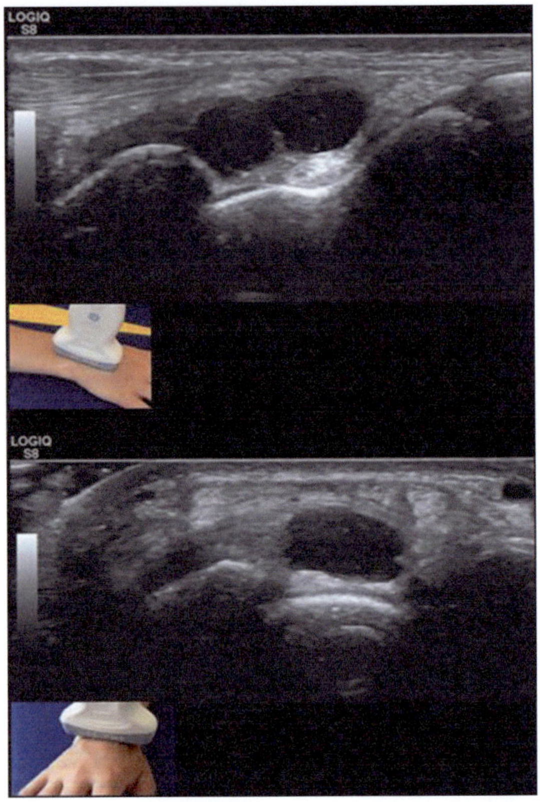

Fig. 8.25 Dorsal longitudinal and transverse view of the wrist in the midline position, which shows a ganglion cyst above the os capitate in a 17-year-old boy with hand pain

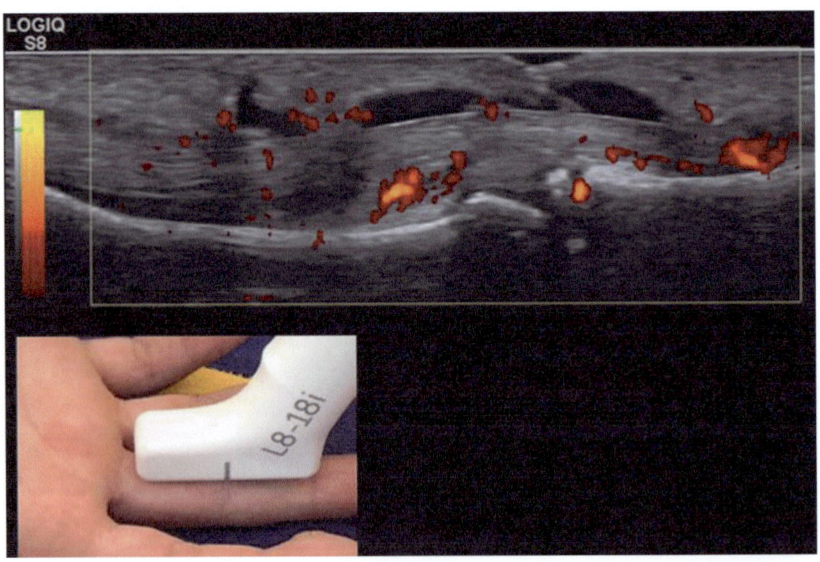

Fig. 8.24 Volar longitudinal view of the fourth finger and PIP joint which shows flexo-tenosynovitis in a 9-year-old girl with oligoarticular arthritis

References

1. Greulich WW, Pyle SI. Radiographic atlas of skeletal development of the hand and wrist. 2nd ed. Stanford: Stanford University Press; 1959.
2. Tanner JM, Whitehouse RH, Marshall WA, Healy MJR, Goldstein H. Assessment of skeletal maturity and prediction of adult height (TW method). 2nd ed. London: Academic Press; 1983.
3. Bilgili Y, Hizel S, Kara SA, et al. Accuracy of skeletal age assessment in children from birth to 6 years of age with the ultrasonographic version of the Greulich-Pyle atlas. J Ultrasound Med. 2003;22:683–90.
4. Wagner UA, Diedrich V, Schmitt O. Determination of skeletal maturity by ultrasound: a preliminary report. Skelet Radiol. 1995;24:417–20.
5. Collado P, Vojinovic J, Nieto JC, Windschall D, Magni Manzoni S, Bruyn GAW, et al., On Behalf of the OMERACT Ultrasound Group. Toward standardized musculoskeletal ultrasound in paediatric rheumatology: normal age-related ultrasound findings. Arthritis Care Res. 2016;68:348–56.
6. Windschall D, Collado P, Vojinovic J, et al. Age-related vascularization and ossification of joints in children: an international pilot study to test multiobserver ultrasound reliability. Arthritis Care Res. 2017. https://doi.org/10.1002/acr.23335.
7. Collado P, Windschall D, Vojinovic J, et al. Amendment of the OMERACT ultrasound definitions of joints' features in healthy children when using the DOPPLER technique. Pediatr Rheumatol Online J. 2018;16:23.
8. Windschall D, Pommerenke M, Haase R. Ultrasound assessment of the skeletal development of the proximal femoral, distal femoral and proximal tibial epiphyses in premature and mature neonates. Ultrasound Med Biol. 2016;42:451–8.
9. Roth J, Jousse-Joulin S, Magni-Manzoni S, Rodriguez A, Tzaribachev N, Iagnocco A, et al., Outcome Measures in Rheumatology Ultrasound Group. Definitions for the sonographic features of joints in healthy children. Arthritis Care Res. 2015;67:136–42.
10. Bruyn GAW, Schmidt WA. Introductory guide to musculoskeletal ultrasound for the rheumatologist. 2nd ed. Houten: Bohn Stafleu van Loghum; 2011.
11. Strunk J. Sonografische Diagnostik in der Rheumatologie. 1st ed. Bremen: UNI-MED Verlag; 2014.
12. Spannow AH, Pfeiffer-Jensen M, Andersen NT, Herlin T, Stenbog E. Ultrasonographic measurements of joint cartilage thickness in healthy children: age- and sex-related standard reference values. J Rheumatol. 2010;37:2595–601.
13. Collado P, Naredo E, Calvo C, Crespo M. Assessment of the joint recesses and tendon sheaths in healthy children by high-resolution B-mode and power Doppler sonography. Clin Exp Rheumatol. 2007;25:915–21.
14. Rosendahl K, Bruserud IS, Oehme N, et al. Normative ultrasound references for the paediatric wrist; dorsal soft tissues. RMD Open. 2018;4:e000642.
15. Wakefield RJ, Balint PV, Szkudlarek M, Filippucci E, Backhaus M, D'Agostino MA, et al., For the OMERACT 7 Special Interest Group. Musculoskeletal ultrasound including definitions for ultrasonographic pathology. J Rheumatol. 2005;32:2485–87.
16. Magni-Manzoni S, Epis O, Ravelli A, Klersy C, Veisconti C, Lanni S, et al. Comparison of clinical versus ultrasound determined synovitis in juvenile idiopathic arthritis. Arthritis Rheum. 2009;61: 1497–504.
17. Roth J, Ravagnani V, Backhaus M, et al. Preliminary definitions for the sonographic features of synovitis in children. Arthritis Care Res. 2017;69:1217–23.
18. Breton S, Jousse-Joulin S, Cangemi C, de Parscau L, Colin D, Bressolette L, et al. Comparison of clinical and ultrasonographic evaluations for peripheral synovitis in juvenile idiopathic arthritis. Semin Arthritis Rheum. 2011;41:272–8.

Lower Limb: Hip and Thigh

9

Mohamed Adel Eltomey and Tomasz Madej

Hip and Thigh Ultrasound

Introduction

The hip joint is a joint in the case of which ultrasonography is particularly useful in children. The sonographic evaluation of developmental dysplasia of the hip (DDH) by Graf is one of the first practical applications of this method in the clinical practice [1]. Currently, hip ultrasound in DDH is a gold standard in the assessment of this pathology at an early developmental stage and is used as a screening tool [2]. The scanning technique, its usefulness and the manner of assessment in DDH are discussed in a separate chapter.

The hip joint is a joint in which ultrasonography is especially significant when inflammation is suspected [3]. The particular value of hip ultrasound is underlined by frequent occurrence of inflammation in the hip joints of children with restricted possibilities to perform a physical examination as well as by unclear clinical signs and the risk that some inflammatory pathologies might have irreversible intra-articular and destructive consequences and lead to osteoarthritis in the future. Owing to high sensitivity, ultrasonography enables early detection of hip joint pathologies and, in selected clinical situations, collection of fluid for analysis. This facilitates aetiopathological diagnosis and implementation of adequate treatment [4].

An increased number of cartilaginous elements in younger children, smaller structures of the musculoskeletal system enabling the application of high-resolution probes of excellent spatial resolution and additionally, the possibility of rapid assessment with no need for sedation are further advantages of this method in the paediatric population and contribute to the fact that it is the preferred tool for the hip joint assessment in terms of inflammation.

Ultrasound is also helpful for hip assessment for other indications: in non-inflammatory pathologies and pathologies involving structures that surround the hip joint, e.g. abnormalities typical of the developmental period associated with apophyseal damage or the presence of focal lesions within the hip joint [5, 6]. In these situations, the usefulness and position of ultrasonography depend on the type of pathology; the most important abnormalities in which US is of particular significance and their typical sonographic images are discussed below.

Owing to the anatomical proximity and overlap of clinical images of certain pathologies, particularly after trauma, thigh ultrasound is

M. A. Eltomey (✉)
Radiology & Imaging Department – Faculty of Medicine, Tanta University, Tanta, Egypt
e-mail: Mohamed.Eltomey@med.tanta.edu.eg

T. Madej
Children's University Hospital, Lublin, Poland
e-mail: tomm74@poczta.onet.pl

Y. El Miedany (ed.), *Pediatric Musculoskeletal Ultrasonography*,
https://doi.org/10.1007/978-3-030-17824-6_9

discussed together with hip US. An example of such a situation is injury to the proximal insertions of thigh muscles located within the pelvis on apophyses that are not fully calcified and have separate secondary ossification nuclei in the developmental period, which results in them being sites of weaker resistance and greater susceptibility to injury.

A discussion on hip and thigh ultrasound starts with the sonoanatomy and scanning technique. This is followed by the presentation of basic normal and abnormal joint images as well as clinical applications and typical pathologies in which ultrasound is used.

Sonoanatomy and Scanning Technique

A hip joint US scan is routinely conducted with linear probes of resolution ranges adjusted to the child's age and size of the joint; high-resolution probes are used in young children, whereas medium-frequency transduces are applied in older children. In patients with a large amount of subcutaneous tissues and deeper location of the hip joints, the application of a convex probe working in a paediatric range (e.g. 9–2 MHz) may be particularly useful.

The scanning technique in hip US differs significantly depending on the purpose of examination, patient's age, clinical information and reported symptoms as well as the mode of examination, either scheduled or urgent.

The scanning technique and image interpretation in the case of developmental dysplasia of the hip are presented in a separate chapter.

In a standard situation, hip US begins from hip joint assessment. Next, periarticular soft tissues undergo evaluation [7].

Hip Joint Scanning Technique

The foundation of proper hip joint assessment is the acquisition of an ultrasound scan in the longitudinal view along the neck of the femur, enabling visualisation of the anterior joint recess (Fig. 9.1). With the patient in the supine position, the transducer is placed almost vertically, distal and medial to the anterior inferior iliac spine. The most significant structure to be visualised is the head of the femur. When it has been found, the transducer should be moved slightly distally so that the site of the femoral head and neck junction is in the centre of the image. The transducer's position should be such that a linear and clearly hyperechogenic outline of the cortical layer of the femoral neck can be obtained. In normal conditions, the cavity of the anterior recess is not distended, and a double layer of the articular capsule, located at the neck outline, is visible – it is the anterior joint recess presenting as a band-like hyperechogenic structure.

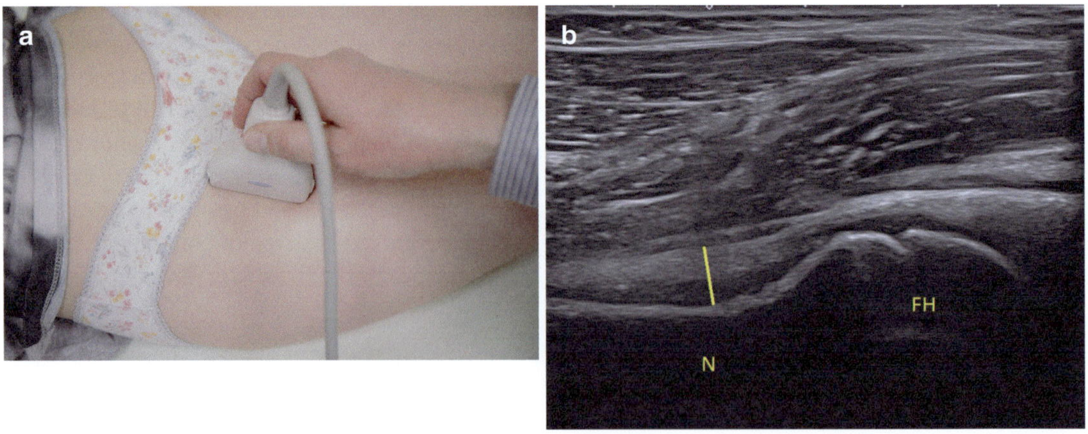

Fig. 9.1 (**a** and **b**) The longitudinal section of the anterior recess of the hip joint showing the joint capsule. Position of the transducer (**a**). Corresponding ultrasound image (**b**). Yellow line, thickness of the hip joint capsule. FH the femoral head, N the femoral neck

A manoeuvre that can improve joint capsule and anterior recess visualisation is the application of light pressure with the distal part of the transducer so that the transducer's head is placed in possibly the most parallel position to the femoral neck; this increases echogenicity of the capsule and facilitates differentiation between a normal image and minor inflammation (Fig. 9.2). This manoeuvre also entails elimination of the phenomenon of anisotropy, which is observed when the joint capsule is positioned obliquely to the scanning surface. The anisotropy artefact is predominant in the ultrasonography of the musculoskeletal system and prevents proper evaluation of its structures [8, 9].

This method of hip joint visualisation is sufficient to assess the joint in terms of the presence of inflammation and to visualise the anterior recess for arthrocentesis in order to collect joint fluid. If joint fluid is to be collected under US guidance, the anterior joint recess must be first visualised in the manner described above. This is followed by insertion of a needle in the long axis of the transducer along the femoral neck from the distal and lateral side. The needle tip is then directed towards the femoral head and neck junction [10].

As for the intra-articular structures assessed in hip US, the following should be evaluated: the outline of the femoral head and its ossification nucleus, the outline and echogenicity of the hyaline cartilage of the proximal epiphysis and the junction of the proximal femoral epiphysis and metaphysis. The examination also shows the acetabular margin and a hyperechogenic triangular structure located at the acetabulum corresponding with the labrum; the most accessible in ultrasound is the anterosuperior part of the labrum.

The hip joints in children can also be examined with the transducer in the lateral longitudinal position in relation to the trochanter region (Fig. 9.3). The probe is positioned more cephalad

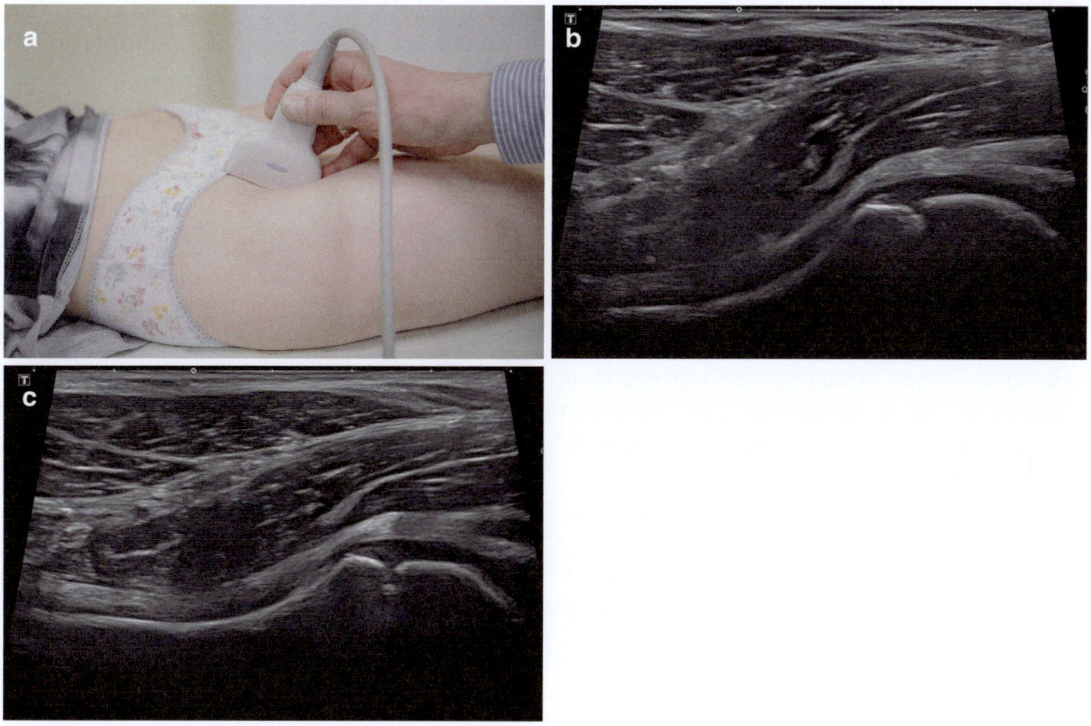

Fig. 9.2 (**a**–**c**) The longitudinal section of the anterior recess gently compressed with the distal part of the transducer (**a**). The recess without applying compression; the echogenicity of the articular capsule is lower due to its oblique position (**b**). Ultrasound image with compression applied by the transducer; the articular capsule is normoechogenic owing to its parallel position in relation to the head of the transducer (**c**)

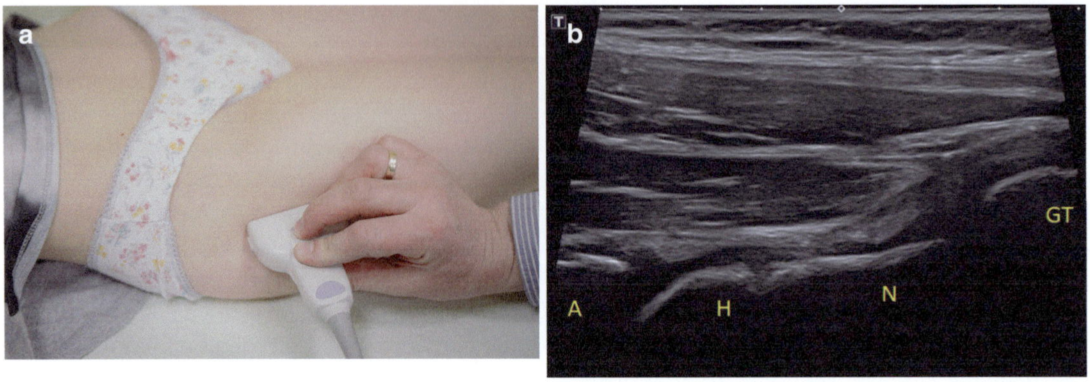

Fig. 9.3 (**a** and **b**) The transducer placed in the lateral longitudinal position in the greater trochanter region to evaluate the hip joint from the lateral side. Position of the transducer (**a**). US appearance (**b**). A the acetabulum, H the femoral head, N the femoral neck, GT the greater tuberosity

than for the assessment of the greater trochanter, with its position being analogous to that in the method of Graf. In this case, the hip joint can be visualised above the trochanter outline. This is a good position for the assessment of the superior aspect of the labrum and the relationship between the femoral head and the acetabulum.

If inflammation in the hip joint is suspected, the contralateral joint should be scanned simultaneously as it helps interpret abnormalities in the involved hip and detect inflammatory signs in the other.

Scanning Technique of the Soft Tissues of the Hip

The hip is conventionally divided into four regions: anterior, medial, lateral and posterior. Each of them contains structures that can be extra-articular sources of clinical signs and symptoms. When examining the hip region in children in the developmental age, particular attention should be paid to apophyses as they are especially prone to injury.

It must be emphasised that when evaluating the hip region in children, it is worth adjusting the pattern of examination to the given clinical case and correlate the sequence of assessed structures with clinical signs and symptoms and sites of the greatest alteration. When inflammation in the hip joint has been ruled out, the suspicious region should be carefully scanned so as to ensure that, if the examination must be shortened due to child's agitation, the most suspicious regions are not examined superficially.

Anterior Hip

The most significant structures to be assessed in the anterior hip include:

- The anterior inferior iliac spine (AIIS) and the straight tendon of the rectus femoris muscle inserting on the AIIS (Fig. 9.4); the insertion of the indirect tendon in the supra-acetabular region of the ilium is rarely a source of pathology [11].
- The anterior superior iliac spine (ASIS) (Fig. 9.5) and the muscle bellies of the sartorius muscle and tensor fasciae latae that attach to it.

The regions of both spines should be visualised in the transverse and longitudinal planes for the assessment of the apophyseal outline which, depending on age, can be completely cartilaginous and anechogenic in the initial stage of life; can assume the form of a small hyperechogenic reflection, often of slightly uneven outlines, located within the cartilaginous apophysis in older children; or can take the form of a clear linear hyperechogenic reflection of an even contour, separated from the remaining bone by a slight space in the outline in adolescents.

In the case of suspected anterior snapping hip, the anterior hip region is critical for examination. A transverse scan at the level of the femoral head helps visualise, in the transverse view, the iliopsoas tendon which in this region is located superficially to the articular capsule. In this view, the snapping of the tendon can be observed in a

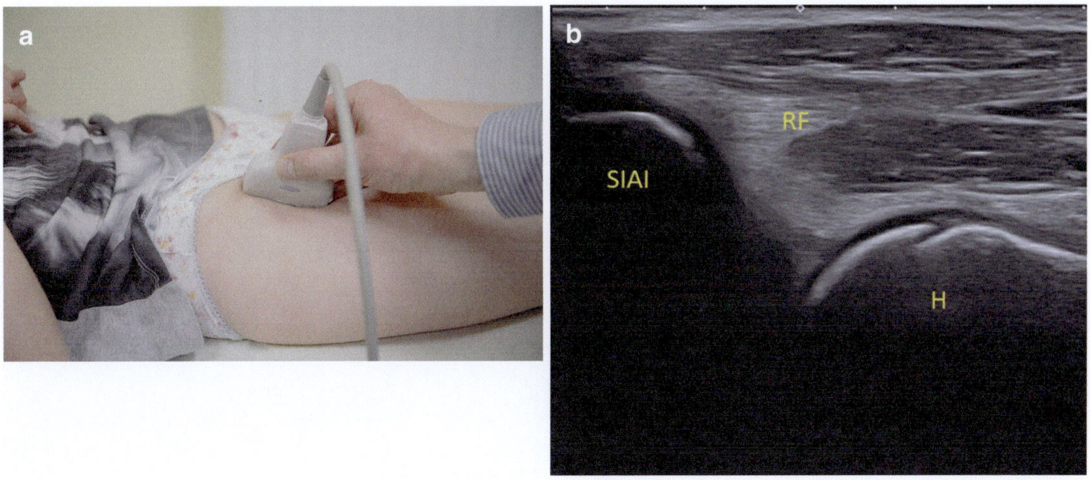

Fig. 9.4 (a and b) The anterior inferior iliac spine (SIAI); longitudinal position of the probe. Position of the transducer (a). Corresponding US image (b). SIAI the anterior inferior iliac spine, RF tendon of the rectus femoris, H the femoral head

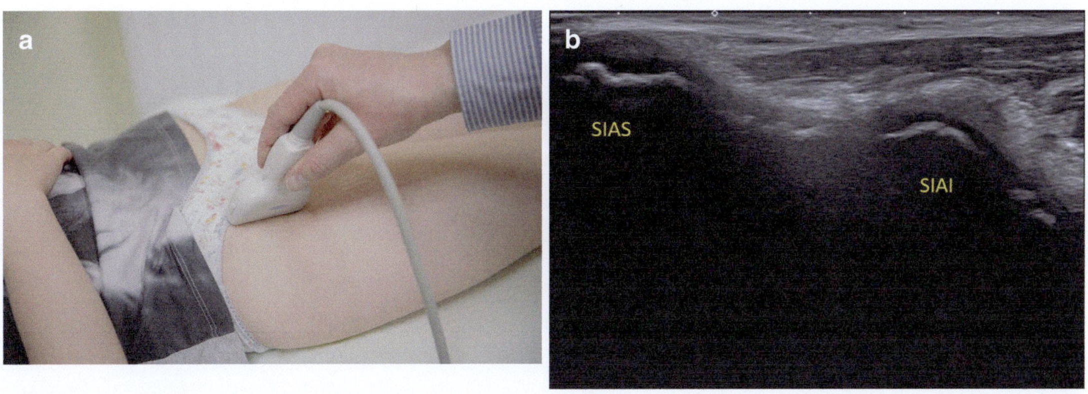

Fig. 9.5 (a and b) The anterior superior iliac spine (SIAS); longitudinal position of the probe. Position of the transducer (a). Corresponding US image (b). SIAS the anterior superior iliac spin, SIAI the anterior inferior iliac spine

dynamic examination during internal and external rotation, thus confirming the pathology.

In the anterior aspect of the hip joint, there is the iliopsoas bursa which can be visualised by transverse probe application, analogous to that in the dynamic assessment of anterior snapping hip. However, the bursa is rarely dilated in paediatric patients.

Medial Hip

The major structure to be assessed in this region is the common adductor muscle enthesis with the pubic bone. For this purpose, the longitudinal view of the pubic bone region should be obtained (Fig. 9.6). It should show the common tendon and proximal parts of stratified adductor muscle bellies (adductor longus, brevis and magnus from the superficial to deep layers). Subsequently, the bellies of these muscles are to be evaluated in the transverse section. Depending on the signs and symptoms reported and the site of the greatest tenderness on palpation, as well as abnormalities seen on the monitor, scanning should encompass an appropriate area.

If the reported symptoms are located in the region of the lesser trochanter, the examination should inspect the distal enthesis of the iliopsoas muscle with the lesser trochanter, which can be

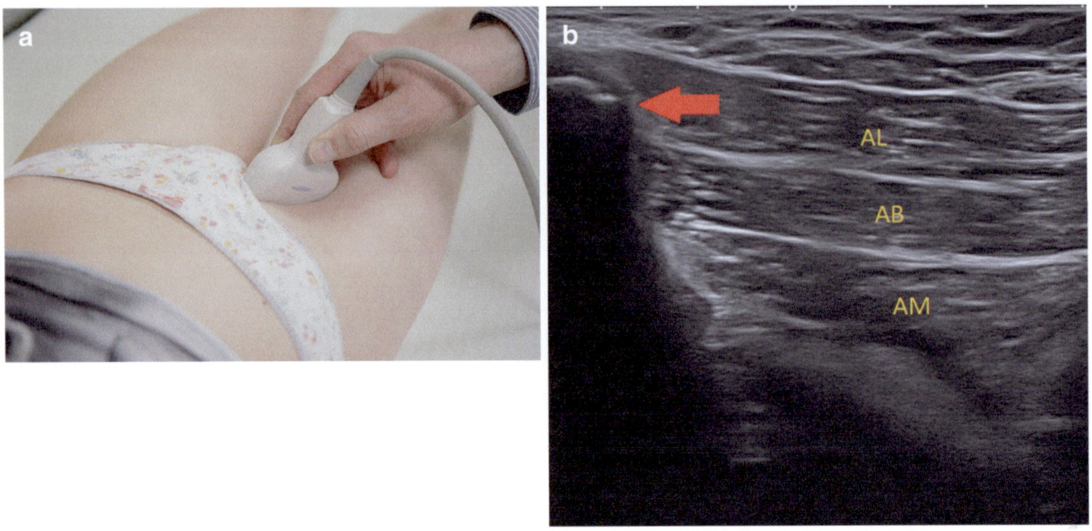

Fig. 9.6 (**a** and **b**) The longitudinal position of the probe from the area of the common insertion of the adductor muscles on the pubic bone. Position of the transducer (**a**). Corresponding US image (**b**). Red arrow, the pubic bone. AL the adductor longus muscle, AB the adductor brevis muscle, AM the adductor magnus muscle

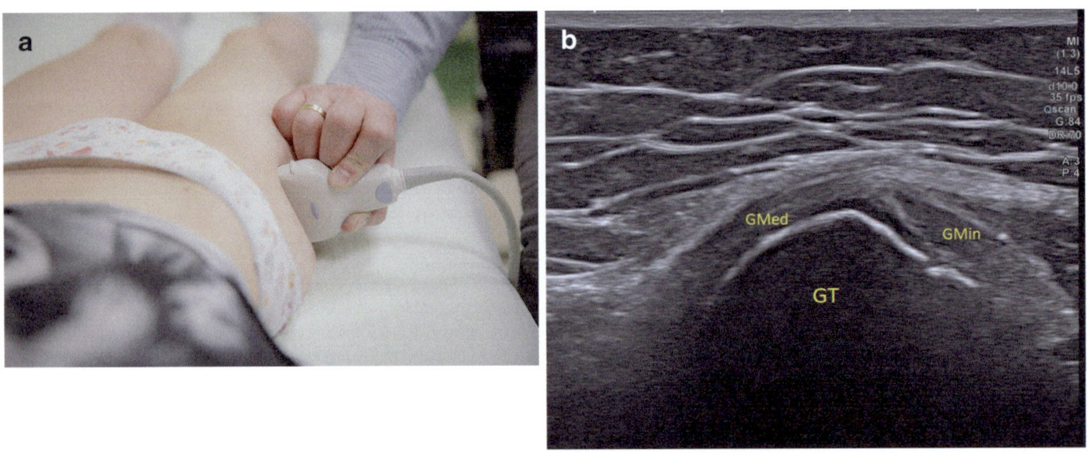

Fig. 9.7 (**a** and **b**) Transverse position of the probe from the area of the greater trochanter. Position of the transducer (**a**). Corresponding US image (**b**). GT the greater trochanter, GMin tendon of the gluteus minimus muscle, GMed tendon of the gluteus medius muscle

seen upon placing the transduced longitudinally in relation to the medial aspect of the hip at the boundary with the thigh, at external rotation, abduction and slight flexion [12].

Lateral Hip

Lateral thigh examination is mainly conducted to assess the greater trochanter and the insertion of the gluteus minimus and medius tendons to the trochanter. Additionally, one may also observe dilated bursae and the iliotibial band running over the trochanter.

The probe is typically applied in the transverse position over the greater trochanter where US shows slight sharpening of the cortical layer of the trochanter, thus separating its anterior surface from the lateral one (Fig. 9.7a, b). The anterior trochanter attaches the gluteus minimus tendon, which, after having been visualised initially in the transverse section, can be also seen in the longitudinal view together with the enthesis after rotating the transducer by 90°. As far as the assessment of the gluteus medius tendon is concerned, the procedure is analogous. However, this tendon is divided into two parts: anterior and posterior. The anterior part inserts on the anterior facet of the lateral trochanter while the posterior part attaches posteriorly and more cephalad.

The evaluation of the greater trochanter region can be made with the patient in the supine position or on the contralateral side. Dynamic assessment of the iliotibial band/gluteus magnus conflict with the greater trochanter for lateral snapping hip is made with the patient in the supine position. One should observe the dislocation of the iliotibial band/gluteus magnus relative to the trochanter during hip rotation or flexion and extension with the transducer placed transversely in relation to the trochanter. Dynamic examination serves for evaluation of whether these structure move freely without obstacles or abnormally with band tension followed by an abrupt snap against the trochanter. This region should also be evaluated in terms of the possible presence of dilated bursae, particularly the trochanteric bursa.

When pain is located on the lateral hip more cephalad to the greater trochanter, the attachment of the proximal gluteus medius to the wing of the ilium should be inspected as the abnormalities might be caused by proximal enthesopathy.

Posterior Hip

The purpose of an ultrasound scan of this region is mainly to assess the proximal insertion of the hamstring muscles and ischial tuberosity. In the patient's prone position, the probe is set transversely over the ischial tuberosity that can be palpated medially on the border of the buttock and thigh (Fig. 9.8). Evaluation involves the outline of the cortical layer of the ischial tuberosity and its inserting tendons. The common enthesis for the semitendinosus and biceps femoris tendons is located more superficially while the enthesis of the semimembranosus tendon can be found deeper. Subsequently, by rotating the probe by 90°, the outlines of the ischial tuberosity and hamstring tendons can be assessed in the longitudinal section (Fig. 9.9).

Somewhat lateral to the ischial tuberosity, there is the sciatic nerve, which is easily found in this location. It can be evaluated in the thigh in the transverse section using the "elevator technique" which shows its course from its exit from the pelvis at the level of the piriformis down to its bifurcation into the tibial and common fibular nerves in the area closer to the popliteal fossa.

Scanning Technique in Thigh US

The soft tissues of the thigh are mainly examined in the transverse plane by sliding the transducer from the proximal to distal region; the manner of examination resembles the "elevator technique" used for peripheral nerve assessment. This enables initial scanning of the area. One must

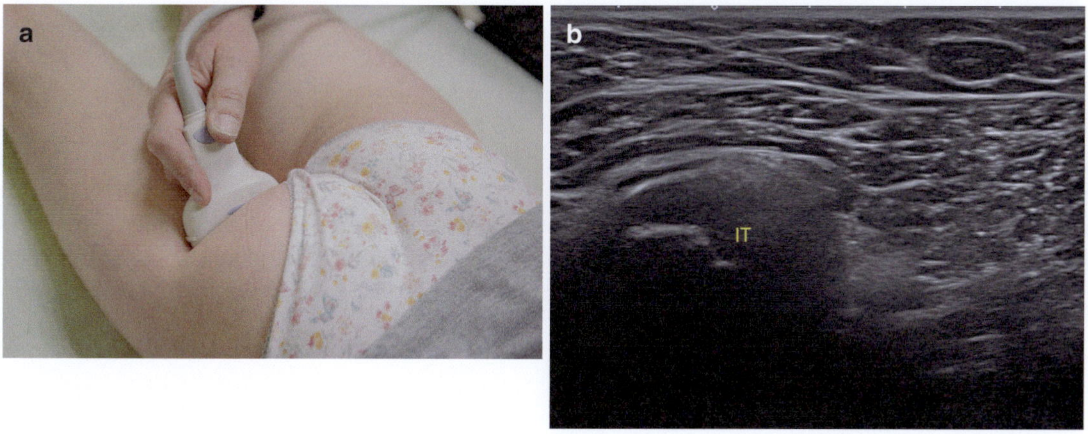

Fig. 9.8 (**a** and **b**) Transverse position of the probe in the area of the ischial tuberosity. Position of the transducer (**a**). Corresponding US image (**b**). IT the ischial tuberosity

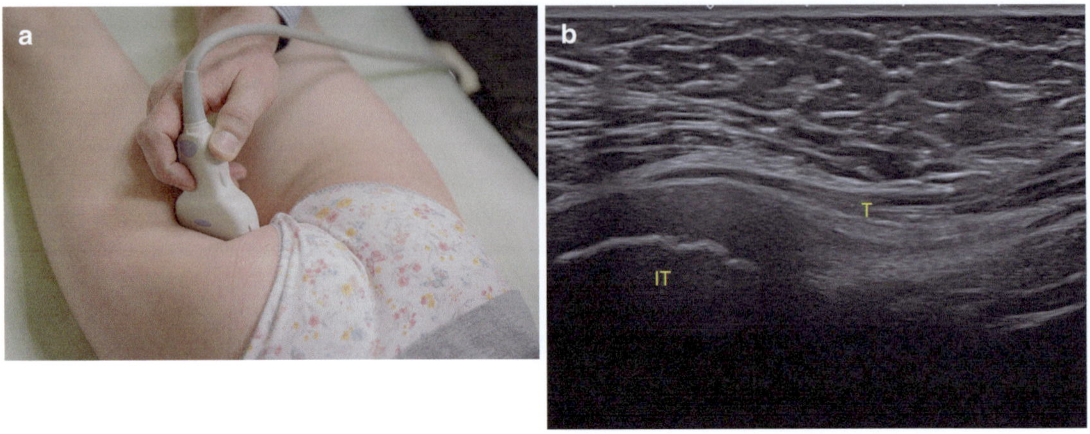

Fig. 9.9 (**a** and **b**) Longitudinal position of the probe in the area of the ischial tuberosity. Position of the transducer (**a**). Corresponding US image (**b**). IT the ischial tuberosity, T tendons of the posterior compartment of thigh

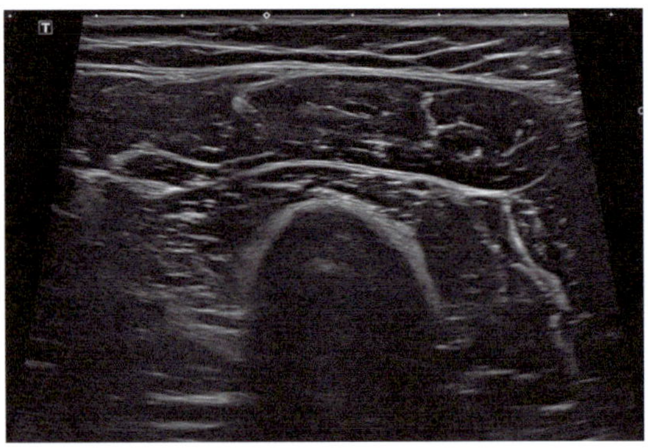

Fig. 9.10 Ultrasonographic cross-sectional image of the thigh in the anterior compartment; muscles of normal architecture. Deeper in the image, one may note a typical arch-like hyperechogenic reflection from the femoral cortical bone

remember that the examination should cover full soft tissue thickness with necessary visualisation of the cortical layer of the femur (Fig. 9.10).

Should any lesions be found in the US image, they must be assessed also in other planes, mainly in the longitudinal one.

The thigh is divided into three compartments: anterior, encompassing the quadriceps femoris; medial, encompassing the adductor longus, brevis and magnus; and posterior, encompassing the hamstrings. The proximal insertion of the adductor muscles and hamstrings as well as the rectus femoris muscle, which is one of the heads of the quadriceps femoris, has been described above.

As for local abnormalities, such as resistance on palpation, local thickening or localised pain, the examination should start from this very region as such abnormalities may have focal nature and local range.

Should any abnormalities be found in thigh US, their location must be determined. First of all, one should assess whether they are located epifascially (within the subcutaneous tissue and skin) or subfascially. In the case of the latter lesions, their location relative to the surrounding tissues should be evaluated: between muscle bellies or intramuscularly. A method that facilitates muscle identification is their tracing over a longer fragment, particularly to their insertions.

Normal and Pathological Hip and Thigh US Images

US Images of the Hip Joint

The primary goal of hip US in children is to assess the hip joint. Subsequently, periarticular structures undergo evaluation, with a focus mainly on clinically suspicious regions.

Sonographic assessment of the hip joint should involve:

- The articular capsule and potential abnormalities within it, such as thickening or decreased echogenicity

- Signs of inflammation in the articular capsule in the form of fluid and/or hypertrophic synovium
- Articular capsule vascularisation and possible intra-articular inflammatory changes using Doppler imaging (power and colour Doppler)
- The femoral head outline, echogenicity of the cartilage of the proximal femoral epiphyses as well as the shape of the ossification nucleus of the proximal femoral epiphysis
- The shape of the acetabulum as well as the anterosuperior and superior facets of the labrum

Hip joint assessment in ultrasonography plays a significant role in cases with suspected inflammation as US sensitivity reaches nearly 100% for its detection. The lack of inflammatory changes in the hip joints, as seen in the ultrasound, is a confirmation of their actual absence. If present, these changes can be seen as increased amount of fluid, synovial hypertrophy, thickening and lower echogenicity of the articular capsule.

Joint Capsule

The joint capsule is evaluated at the level of the anterior recess with the hyperechogenic outline of the cortical layer of the femoral neck. At this level, two adjacent layers of the capsule, anterior and posterior, can be observed [13]. Within the anterior recess, it is frequently possible to notice the "stripe sign", i.e. hyperechogenic reflection located in the interface between two layers of the capsule, which indicates non-distended joint cavity. For this sign to be spotted, the transducer should be placed parallel to the neck, which can be facilitated by the manoeuvre with asymmetrical probe compression mentioned in section "Hip Joint Scanning Technique". The anterior layer of the capsule is strengthened with the iliofemoral ligament, which makes it slightly thicker than the posterior part (Fig. 9.11).

In the healthy hip joint, the capsule is echogenic and of concave outline with the hip in external rotation [14]. In neutral hip position, the outline of the recess may be convex [15] (Fig. 9.12). In the paediatric population, the average thickness of both layers of the capsule at the level of the anterior recess is 5 mm. The thickness of the anterior recess is a good and reproducible parameter to be used in routine hip joint assessment. The thickness of the anterior recess is measured at its greatest thickness, which usually is found in its central segment, taking the distance from the cortical surface of the neck to the outer demarcation of the anterior articular capsule; the measurement is taken in the transverse plane relative to the long axis of the recess [16]. This parameter is dependent on and changes with age and height of a child; capsule thickness varies across age groups from 3.7 mm in the first year of life to 6.7 mm at the age of 16 years [17]. Furthermore, one must remember about the possibility to compare the thickness of the anterior

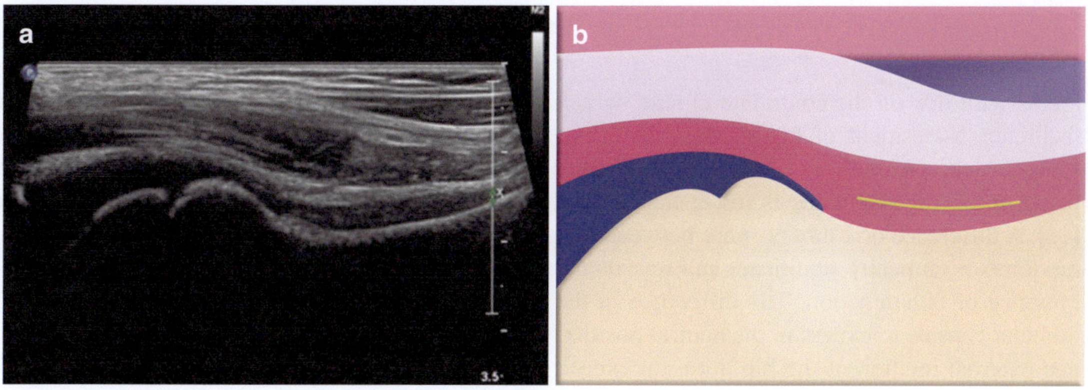

Fig. 9.11 (**a** and **b**) US, longitudinal section at the level of the femoral neck and the anterior recess of the hip joint – a "stripe sign" (**a**). A schematic of the image (**b**)

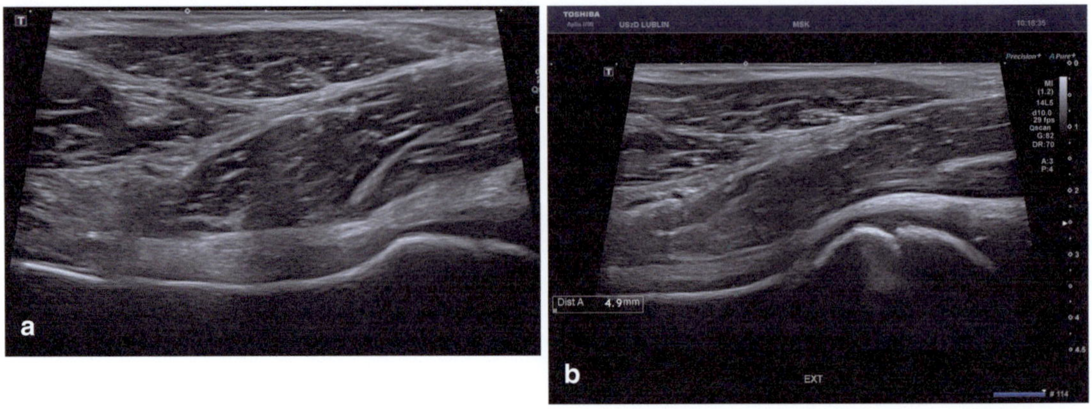

Fig. 9.12 (**a** and **b**) The longitudinal section of the anterior recess of the hip in the neutral position; convex articular capsule (**a**). Concave capsule with normal thickness in the transverse section at the external rotation (**b**)

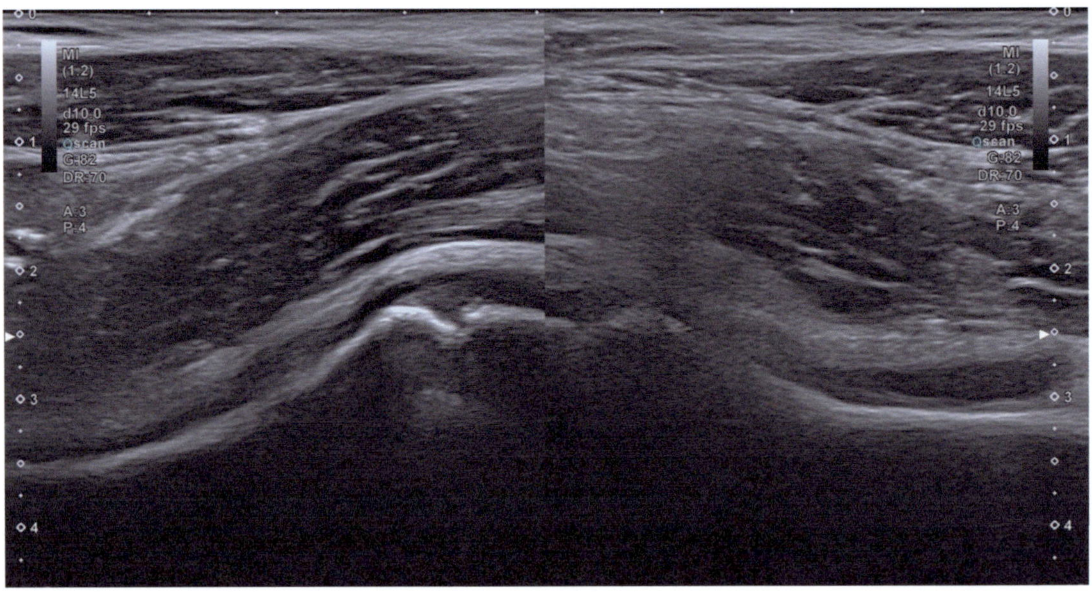

Fig. 9.13 Comparison of the right and left hip; fluid causes anterior recess distension in the left hip – inflammation

recess with that on the contralateral side, which facilitates assessment of hip joints with minor inflammatory changes (Fig. 9.13). A difference between healthy hip joints is lower than 1 mm [15]. A difference of 2 mm or more between two hip joints is clinically significant and reveals the presence of inflammation. The difference in the articular capsule thickness in the neutral position and external rotation of the hip does not exceed 1 mm. Additionally, one may assess the thickness of articular cartilage; it reflects differences in the joint image depending on age [15].

The first signs of hip joint involvement are a change of the articular capsule contour to a convex one and a decrease in its echogenicity as well as capsule thickening; the "stripe sign" is also absent (Fig. 9.14).

Synovial Membrane and Fluid

In more severe inflammation, the joint may present an increased amount of fluid or synovial hypertrophy, or both these signs [3]. The severity of inflammation should be evaluated in a semi-quantitative scale, specifying the degree of

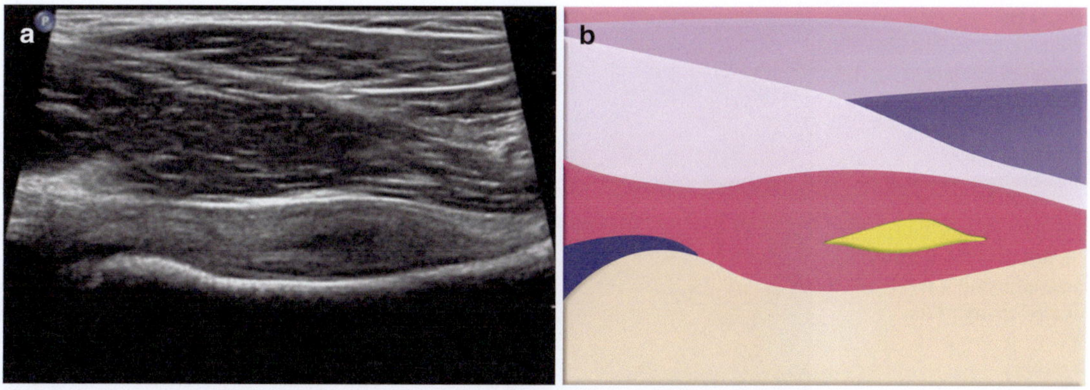

Fig. 9.14 (**a** and **b**) Slight inflammatory changes in the hip joint in the course of juvenile idiopathic arthritis. US appearance (**a**). Illustration of changes (**b**)

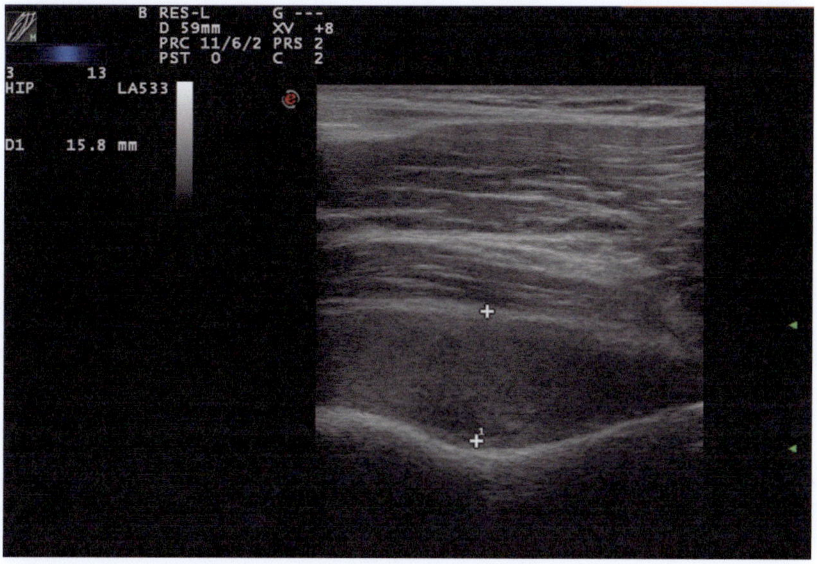

Fig. 9.15 Measurement of the thickness of the hip joint capsule in a patient with mucopolysaccharidosis type I (MPS I). The articular capsule is considerably thickened and hyperechogenic; thickness, 16 mm. Capsular thickness is measured to monitor the course of the disease. (Courtesy of Dr. Zbigniew ŻUBER)

involvement as minor, moderate or significant. Also, consecutive measurements of the anterior recess of the involved joint are helpful in the process of monitoring (Fig. 9.15). One may measure the total thickness of the anterior recess, encompassing both layers of the articular capsule and the dilated joint space between them, or, if possible, analyse the height of the dilated space in the anterior recess. The manner in which measurements are taken should be documented (Fig. 9.16).

The synovium and articular capsule may show enhanced vascularisation in power/colour Doppler imaging, which is correlated with the activity of inflammation [18]. The presence of vascularisation and its grade should be noted in an examination report. The normal articular capsule shows no signs of vascularisation (Fig. 9.17).

US imaging is of limited value in determining the aetiology of hip inflammation as it is characterised by low specificity. In these cases, differential diagnosis draws on clinical data and laboratory tests, e.g. based on the Kocher criteria [19]. Fluid echogenicity does not unambiguously indicate its nature even though hyperechogenic fluid in young children does suggest septic arthritis. In these cases, ultrasonography can be used for fluid aspiration for microbiological assess-

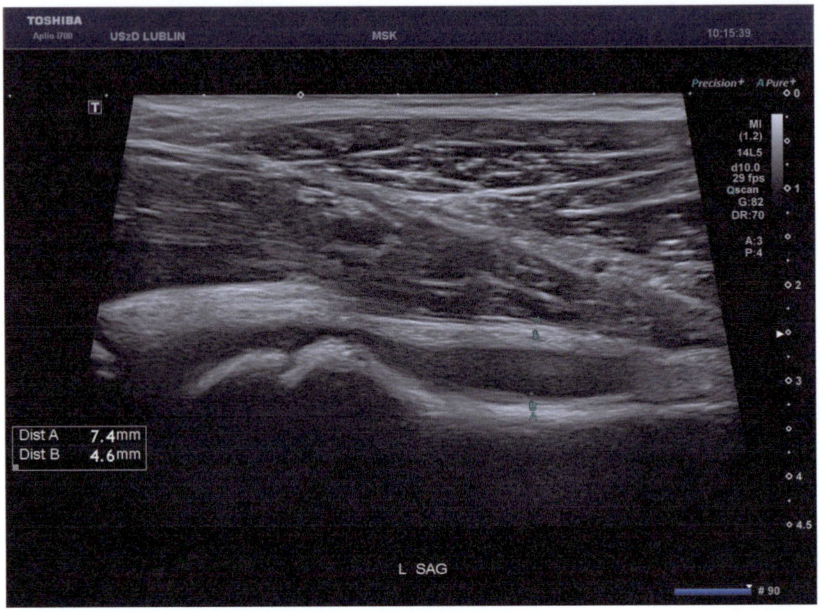

Fig. 9.16 Transient synovitis of the left hip. Increased amount of fluid in the joint cavity. Two ways to measure the recess: A, measurement of the anterior recess with the articular capsule layers (in this case 7 mm); or measurement of the dilated cavity of the recess (in this case 5 mm)

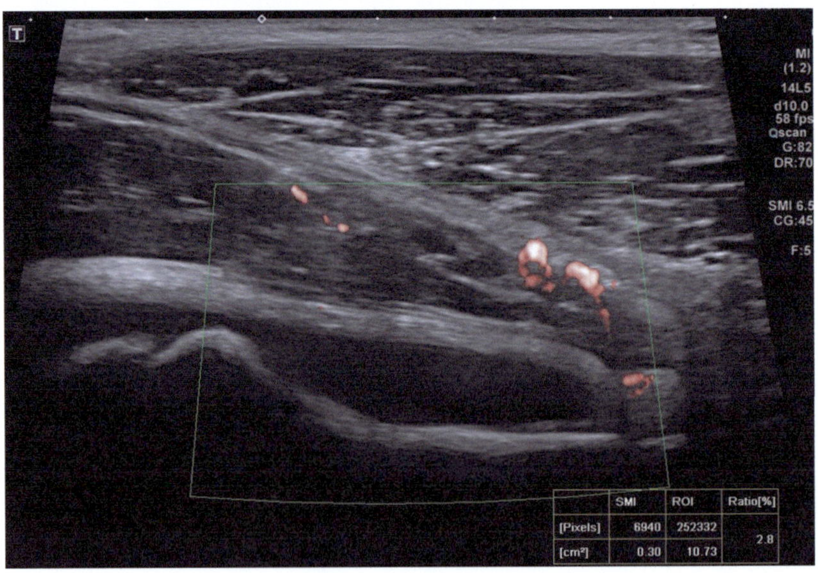

Fig. 9.17 Transient synovitis of the hip; power Doppler imaging to assess capsular vasculature. No vessels in the articular capsule. Single vascular segments in the periarticular soft tissues

ment. Also, markedly increased capsule and periarticular soft tissue vascularisation suggest an infectious nature of arthritis.

Femoral Head

Femoral head assessment is a permanent element of sonographic evaluation of the hip joint in children. The sonographic image of the femoral head changes significantly with the child's development. Even though slight ossification centres may appear in certain individuals as early as in the first weeks of life, the femoral head is usually completely cartilaginous up to month 4–5 of life [20]. Around month 5–6 of life, most children do have an ossification centre, initially of an irregular shape, within the cartilaginous femoral head. The ossification centre grows eccentrically towards the periphery, presenting a typical arch-like hyperechogenic reflection at the age of 2–3 years. In early childhood, considerable thickness of the hyaline cartilage is an important sign. It is a sum of epiphyseal hyaline cartilage, where one may observe echogenic reflections from the borders of vascular channels and single vascular segments in the cartilage, and articular hyaline cartilage, which is not vascularised. With age, the thickness of the hyaline cartilage in the femoral head decreases. In older children, the sonographic image of the femoral head resembles that of an adult. The difference is the interrupted continuity of the hyperechogenic outline of the head at the site of the growth place which is located between the epiphysis and metaphysis of the proximal part of the femur.

The assessment of the femoral head basically involves the shape, echogenicity of hyaline cartilage and outline of the ossification nucleus. These parameters combined and a comparison with the healthy side (bearing in mind pathologies that may affect both hip joints) make it possible to detect femoral head deformity that might develop in the course of hip diseases. Legg-Calvé-Perthes disease may serve as an example. It might cause flattening and distention of the head outline, increased echogenicity of hyaline cartilage and profoundly uneven contour of the ossification nucleus along with its fragmentation (Fig. 9.18). Pathological conditions that might lead to hip osteoarthritis, such as idiopathic juvenile arthritis or congenital hip dysplasia, may present with an abnormal image of the femoral head in US (Fig. 9.19).

A sonographic sign suggestive of slipped capital femoral epiphysis (SCFE) may be slight flattening of the upper femoral head outline and the lack of a visible space between the proximal epiphysis and metaphysis of the femur [21]. This sign is, however, difficult to find. That is why the identification and diagnosis of SCFE-type pathologies require other diagnostic tools.

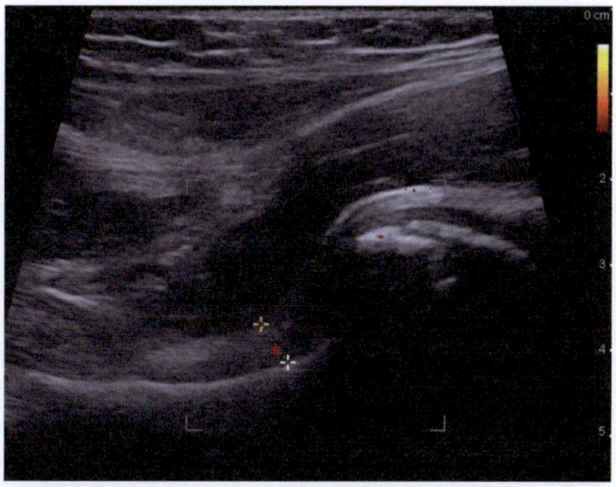

Fig. 9.18 Femoral head deformity in the course of Legg-Calvé-Perthes disease with flattened proximal epiphysis and marked distension of the proximal metaphysis of the femur. Inactive changes – no detectable inflammation in the joint cavity or signs of capsular vascularisation in power Doppler imaging

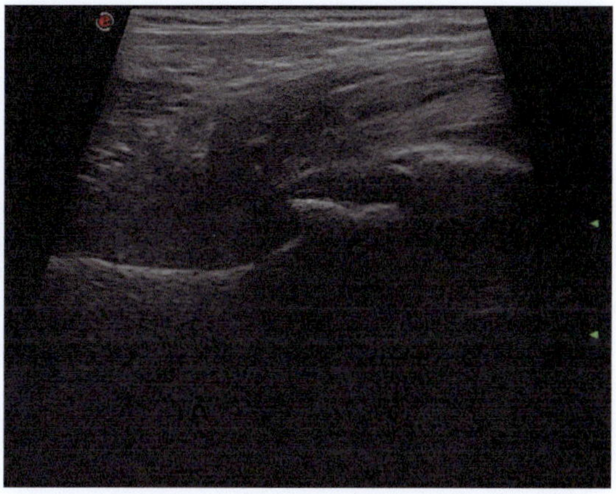

Fig. 9.19 Significant femoral head deformity in the course of untreated juvenile idiopathic arthritis (JIA). (Courtesy of Dr. Zbigniew ŻUBER)

Acetabulum and Labrum

The assessment of the shape of the acetabulum is correlated with the evaluation of the femoral head, and the combined analysis of both these structures may arouse a suspicion of a destructive or degenerative pathology.

The assessment of the acetabular margin is related to the evaluation of the anterosuperior part of the labrum, which is well accessible to US in this region. The labrum presents as a triangular hyperechogenic structure that closely adheres to the acetabular margin. A US scan may arouse a suspicion of labrum tear if the labrum is separated from the acetabular margin with a fluid space at the labral base, a linear or irregular area of low echogenicity located within the labrum or a fluid space located in the region of the labrum and communicating with it (i.e. a paralabral cyst) (Fig. 9.20). Labrum tears are rather uncommon in

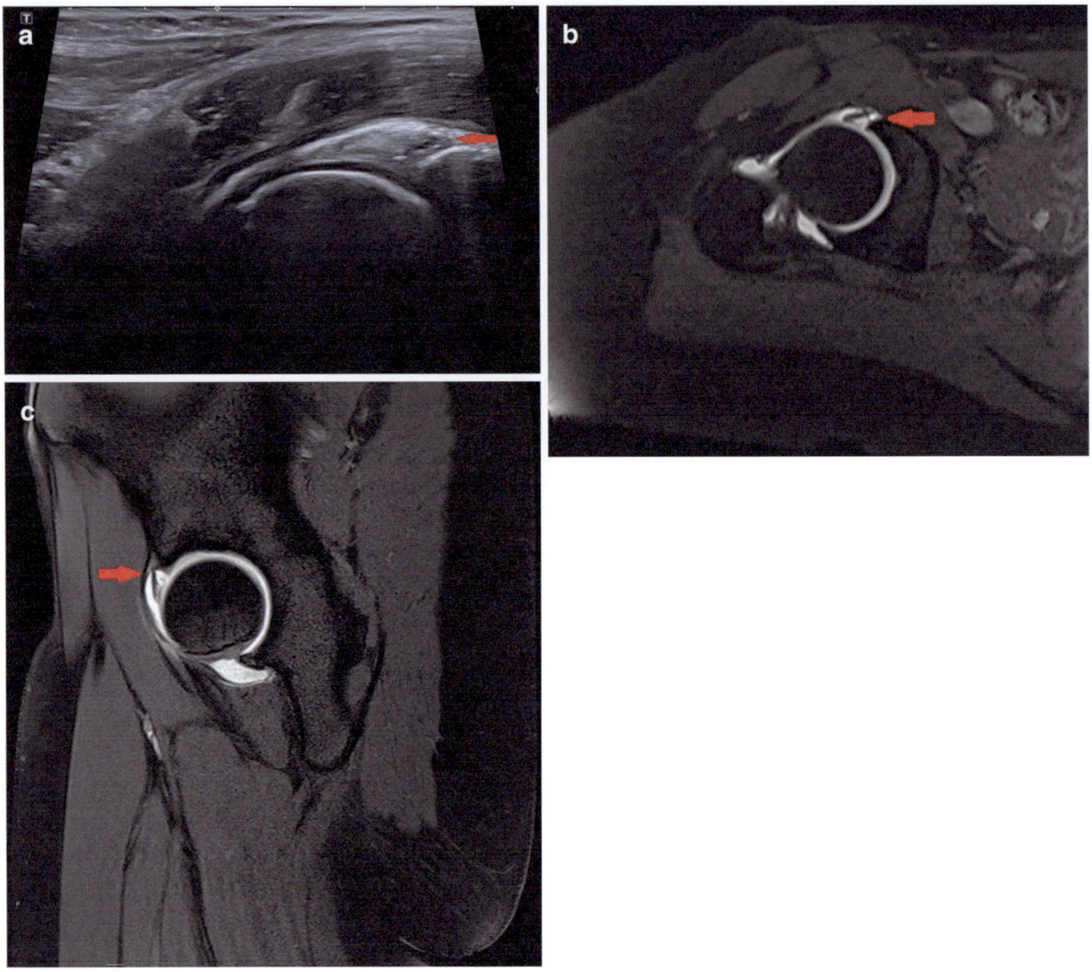

Fig. 9.20 (**a–c**) Injury to the anterosuperior part of the labrum in US (**a**), confirmed in subsequent MR arthrography in the transverse section (**b**) and sagittal section (**c**). Red arrow – a labral tear

the paediatric population. However, they may occur in older children, particularly when their joint structure predisposes to femoroacetabular impingement (FAI). Abnormalities detected on US are an indication to expand imaging diagnosis and perform MRI or MR arthrography [22].

Periarticular Structures in the Hip US

In the second part of the examination, one should visualise extra-articular structures that might be a source of pain within the hip. In the paediatric population, the focus is primarily on the region that might be the source of complaints and pain, and this is where abnormalities are sought for in the first place. In justified cases, such as an urgent scan or non-cooperative patient with a limited possibility to perform a full examination, the scan can be reduced to the evaluation of a suspicious region only.

The hip region is divided into four compartments: anterior, medial, lateral and posterior.

In the anterior region, the structures to be focussed on include the anterior inferior iliac spine and the anterior superior iliac spine. The common insertion of the adductor tendons and the inguinal region are the main focus in the medial compartment [23, 24]. In the lateral region, assessment involves the outlines of the greater trochanter and tendons that insert on it, such as gluteus minimus and medius tendons. Finally, in the posterior region, the ischial tuberosity and proximal insertion of the hamstring tendons should be analysed.

In the case of pain located in a non-standard region, sonographic evaluation may also be useful. The site of maximum pain frequently ideally correlates with abnormalities seen on US [25]. The examples of abnormalities of this type can be enthesopathies relating to the iliopsoas tendon insertion to the lesser trochanter (Fig. 9.21) or the proximal gluteus medius tendon to the iliac crest.

When evaluating soft tissues of the hip, one must remember about numerous muscle attachments in this area. Apophyses, which are numerous in the hip region, are sites of weaker resistance in the musculoskeletal structures and may undergo injury that might be of acute or chronic nature. Pathologies of soft tissues in the hip region can be generally divided into inflammatory, traumatic and focal. It must be remembered, however, that data from a paediatric patient's medical history and clinical examination may suggest a completely different pathology from the one found in US.

The basic images of the major soft tissue pathologies found in the hip region are presented in Clinical Applications and Typical Pathologies in Hip and Thigh US.

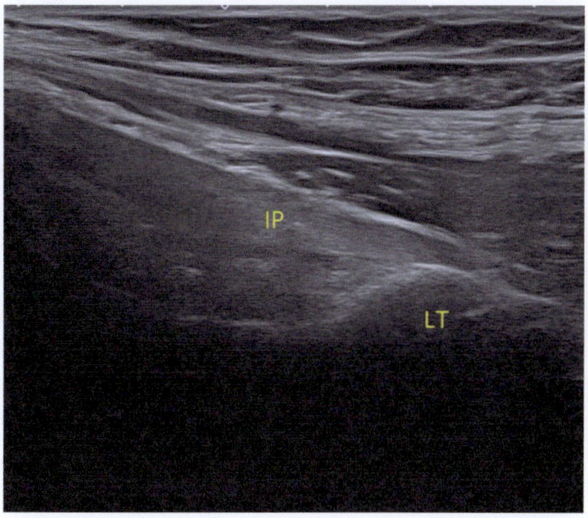

Fig. 9.21 US. Normal insertion of the iliopsoas tendon on the lesser trochanter; longitudinal position of the probe. LT the lesser trochanter, IP the iliopsoas tendon

Ultrasound Images of the Thigh

The thigh is made up mainly of muscles. That is why, proper knowledge of the sonographic muscle structure is important when interpreting US images. One should pay attention mainly to the ordering of the echotexture of visible tissues. In ultrasonography, muscle presents lower echogenicity with hyperechogenic fibroadipose septa that produce linear hyperechogenic reflections. Thicker hyperechogenic bands correspond with core tendons, usually of the typical distribution (Fig. 9.22). The knowledge about muscle division into compartments – anterior, medial and posterior – and the ability to distinguish between the individual muscles are useful to assess the extent and specify the exact location of a focal lesion, if detected, in given compartments, muscles or between normal thigh structures. In the case of superficial focal lesions, one should determine their location in relation to the fascia lata in order to distinguish between lesions located in the subcutaneous tissue from those located deeper, i.e. subfascially.

The examiner should pay attention to blurred muscle structures, including blurring of the fibromuscular septa and core tendons, as well as to areas of altered muscle echogenicity or the presence of fluid spaces. These abnormalities (apart from fluid collections) are usually more difficult to find than focal lesions and require more careful assessment; they can be either post-traumatic or

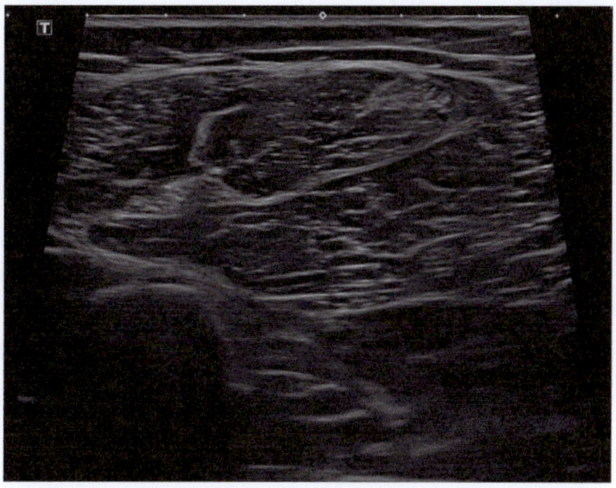

Fig. 9.22 US. Posterior thigh muscles in the transverse section. Normal echogenicity and muscle architecture. The sciatic nerve is visible in the centre

inflammatory. When a pathology is suspected in the examined region, Doppler evaluation is useful as both inflammatory and post-traumatic abnormalities tend to be accompanied by increased blood flow.

It is also significant to visualise the hyperechogenic bone cortical layer since a pathology which is the reason for conducting the scan might be located at the bone or cause bone tissue changes.

Clinical Applications and Typical Pathologies in Hip and Thigh US

This chapter discusses the most common pathologies that one may encounter in the hip joint ultrasound in children. The group of these pathologies is heterogeneous and characterised by a diversified sonographic appearance, which largely depends on the child's age. Ultrasonography is particularly useful in the assessment of inflammatory pathologies of the hip joints; inflammatory conditions are presented in the first part of the chapter. The second part discusses other pathological states in which ultrasonography may be of use. These abnormalities are mainly found in the periarticular soft tissues. Ultrasonography is highly useful in the differential diagnosis of articular and periarticular causes of pain in the hip. The third part of the chapter shows examples of pathological changes within the soft tissues of the thigh encountered in children.

Inflammatory Conditions

Transient Synovitis of the Hip

Transient synovitis of the hip joint is one of the most common causes of hip pain and limping in children. It has several synonyms including irritable hip, toxic synovitis, acute transient epiphysitis, coxitis fugax and others. It is a self-limited acute inflammation of the joint synovium and it is not specific to the hip [26].

The exact aetiology of the disease is unknown, and several theories were suggested pointing to its relation to viral infections, while other research showed that it is usually preceded by an upper respiratory tract infection. Trauma, vaccination and allergy were also proposed as common associations with this condition [27].

Transient synovitis has been reported to occur in children between the ages of 2 and 12; however, its most reported peak is around 3–8 years of age, and it is almost as twice as more common in boys than in girls. The disease has a benign course with no serious long-term complications; despite this, it is a disease diagnosed by exclusion due to the overlap of the clinical symptoms and signs with other serious hip pathologies in this age group. Septic arthritis, juvenile Rheumatoid arthritis and Legg-Calvé -Perthes disease should be ruled out first as the cause of hip pain and limping due to the complications related to these conditions [28, 29].

Clinically, patients present with an acute onset pain in the groin or the thigh associated with limping or refusal to bear weight on the affected side. Pain relief is achieved by flexion, abduction and external rotation of the hip to a degree where the patient feels comfortable, as this manoeuvre lowers the intracapsular pressure of the joint. Limited range of passive hip movement is seen as well during examination of the patients. Transient synovitis has no specific laboratory markers that help in achieving the diagnosis [26].

Plain radiography role in the diagnosis of transient synovitis is limited, as effusion is not seen on radiographs, and the joint will appear normal or mild joint space widening will be seen. The high sensitivity of ultrasound in detecting joint fluid renders it a valuable tool in these cases. Radiography, however, is of great value in excluding other causes of acute hip pain that have a more significant morbidity on the joint including fractures, Legg-Calvé-Perthes disease and slipped femoral capital epiphysis (SCFE) [27].

The aim of ultrasound examination of the hip in cases of transient synovitis is detection of effusion in the anterior recess of the joint.

The joint approached from its anterior aspect, the probe is placed to obtain a parasagittal plane along the long axis of the femoral neck as previously described in the scanning technique section (Fig. 9.1). The patient is examined in a supine position with the hip extended with slight external rotation, i.e. neutral position of the joint. Both joints should be examined and their appearances compared, even if the other is asymptomatic [30]. This technique of examination has been described by Seltzer et al. [31] and it is still in use till now.

Joint effusion is seen as a hypoechoic area anterior to the femoral neck and associated with anterior bulging of the anterior layer of the joint capsule. Effusion may not always be clear, and in some cases, turbidity of the fluid may be seen; thus turbid fluid does not always mean septic arthritis. It was found that anterior and posterior layers of the joint capsule are not thickened in transient synovitis. Bulging of anterior capsule is also found; however, it was found that concavity of the anterior joint capsule is a more reliable indicator of absent fluid within the joint. Cystic protrusion of the joint fluid through the anterior layer of the anterior joint capsule has also been reported forming a diverticulum-shaped lesion, and this is thought be secondary to a fluid leak through a defect in the fibrous capsule of the joint creating a pseudodiverticulum [13] (Fig. 9.16).

Some useful points to know to avoid misinterpretation of normal appearances of structures as pathology include recognition of the site where the anterior layer of the joint capsule joins the labrum as it could be seen on ultrasound showing fluid within as a hypoechoic triangular-shaped area resembling a tear. Another normal finding is the site of insertion of the joint capsule into the femoral neck. It is sometimes seen as a hump and was previously misinterpreted as turbid fluid [13, 30] (Fig. 9.23).

Since ultrasound is highly sensitive for the detection of hip joint effusion, it is not specific for transient synovitis or septic arthritis, and eventually a hip aspiration will be required. Ultrasound-guided aspiration has several advantages including the lack of radiation exposure, avoidance of vascular structures, availability, safety as well as being rapid. The technique can be performed easily in the emergency department. After taking an informed consent from the patient's parents or guardians, the patient is prepared and the choice of sedation or using local anaesthesia with proper patient retraining is determined. The procedure should be performed

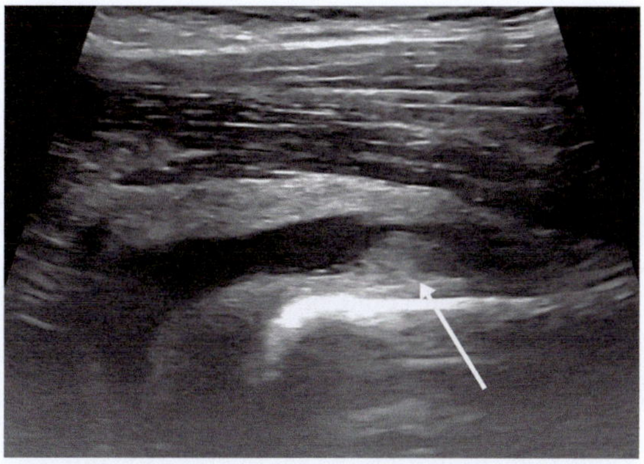

Fig. 9.23 Hip ultrasound of a patient with transient synovitis of the left hip joint showing fluid within the joint and bulging of the capsule as an echogenic hump is seen within the fluid (arrow) which is a frequent finding in transient synovitis; however, non-specific for this condition, it should not be misinterpreted as turbid fluid

under complete aseptic conditions including sterilisation of the skin and using a sterile probe sheath. A 19- or 22-G needle may be used, and it is aimed at the junction between the femoral head and neck, using a distal-to-proximal approach along the long axis of the femoral neck. The needle insertion site is marked on the skin by a surgical marker, and the needle is guided by the probe using an in-plane technique allowing its visualisation during its entry and advancement. Once the needle is in site, aspiration of the fluid could be performed. The absolute contraindication for this procedure is skin infection over the groin region [27, 29].

Septic Arthritis

Septic arthritis is commonly seen in infancy and early childhood, and this is related to rich blood supply of the joints as they are actively growing. Common causative organisms include *Staphylococcus aureus* and *Haemophilus influenzae*. Infection reaches the joint through the blood stream which may have originated in the upper respiratory tract, skin, adjacent osteomyelitis or any infected focus in the body. In infancy, capillaries from the richly blood supplied metaphysis traverse to the adjacent epiphysis facilitating a direct pathway for infectious pathogens spread if present; that is why septic arthritis is commonly associated with osteomyelitis. Septic arthritis in infants is easily diagnosed clinically as patients usually show an acute onset of pain, limping and fever. It is important however to early diagnose this condition to avoid its complications such as joint destruction and degenerative arthritis.

In neonates septic arthritis has a different presentation and could be diagnosed late unless there is high clinical suspicion. The earliest sign is the baby not moving his affected joint or limb; other signs of inflammation appear later. Ultrasound as in transient synovitis of the hip is an excellent tool in showing joint fluid which may be clear or turbid with debris as well as guide joint aspiration procedure. Doppler ultrasound may also show signs of increased vascularity of the joint capsule secondary to infection and inflammation [27, 28, 32] (Figs. 9.24, 9.25 and 9.26).

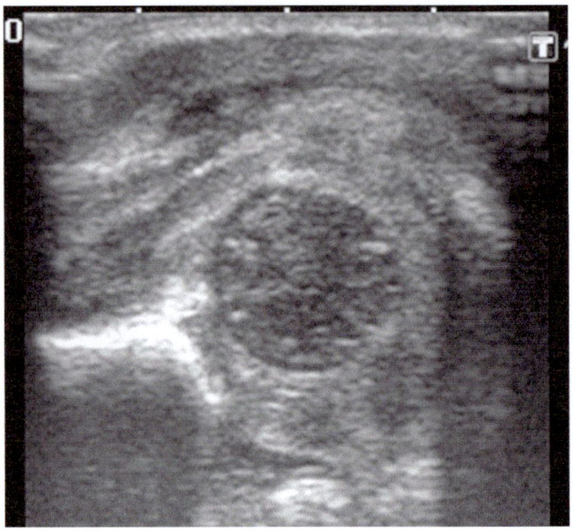

Fig. 9.25 Septic arthritis of the right hip in a neonate, known to have septicaemia, and presenting clinically with persistent right hip flexion and tenderness during passive movement of the joint. Image in the standard coronal plane shows the turbid fluid within the joint causing outward displacement of the femoral head simulating a dislocation. Acetabular measurements and morphology were normal however

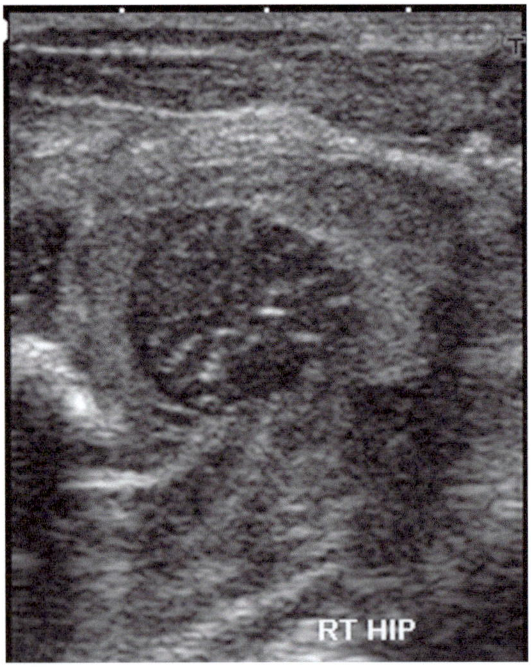

Fig. 9.24 Septic arthritis of the right hip in a neonate, known to have septicaemia, and presenting clinically with persistent right hip flexion and tenderness during passive movement of the joint. The ultrasound image shows a marked amount of turbid fluid within the joint circumferentially surrounding the femoral head

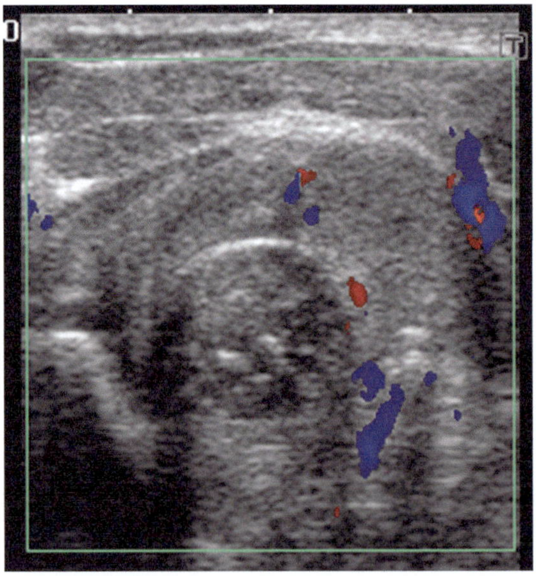

Fig. 9.26 Septic arthritis of the hip in a neonate; the ultrasound image shows a marked amount of turbid fluid within the joint circumferentially surrounding the femoral head; colour Doppler scanning shows increased vascularity in the joint capsule

Other Medical Conditions

Legg-Calvé-Perthes Disease (Kayser)

Legg-Calvé-Perthes (LCP) disease, also known as Perthes disease, is avascular necrosis of the femoral head, most commonly found between the ages of 4 and 9 and much more frequently in boys (4:1) [33, 34]. The disease can occur from the age of 2 years until puberty. In 10–20% of cases, both hips are affected. The disorder is caused by transient disruption of blood flow to the proximal femoral epiphysis, originating from the lateral epiphyseal vessels. It leads to ischaemia and bone infarctions [35, 36]. The natural course of the disease may vary; some patients develop irreversible changes and deformities (coxa magna, coxa vara and coxa breva) followed by secondary coxarthrosis [37].

Clinical signs and symptoms include pain, frequently radiating to the knee, and limping. Younger children present with reluctance to walk and load the affected extremity.

The basic imaging examination used to detect and assess abnormalities as well as to monitor the course of the disease is conventional radiography. It displays fragmentation and sclerosis of the femoral head as well as dilation and uneven outline of the proximal femoral metaphysis, frequently with cystic lesions in its vicinity. In later stages, one may observe a typical femoral head deformity [35].

In early stages, when there are no observable radiographic changes, magnetic resonance imaging (MRI) may prove useful. It may show alterations in the proximal femoral epiphysis signal and signs of impaired blood flow within the femoral head in contrast-enhanced sequences [35].

US is not the basic method in the assessment of Legg-Calvé-Perthes disease. However, it must be remembered that, in early stages, the disease may manifest as hip joint effusion, which can be easily identified in a US scan, and that a US examination is frequently ordered in patients with clinically suspected, so-called, irritable hip syndrome for the detection of joint effusion. If the joint effusion persists for more than 3–6 weeks, the differential diagnosis should always include LCP disease [38]. The contour of the femoral head, its sphericity and epiphyseal homogeneity are worth evaluating as well. If epiphyseal cartilage is found thickened or its echogenicity altered, the US image suggests a diagnosis other than transient synovitis of the hip.

In more advanced cases, signs typical of LCP disease, such as irregularity of the proximal epiphysis, rolled and markedly heterogeneous epiphyseal ossification centre, altered femoral head dimensions with its flattening as well as excessive lateralisation and ventralisation, are also detectable [39, 40] (Fig. 9.27). In order to gain more certainty in the hip joint assessment, it may be considered to evaluate the contralateral hip, bearing in mind the possibility of a bilateral pathology.

The course of the disease should be monitored in conventional radiography [35].

Traumatic Changes in Hip Ultrasonography

Conventional imaging tools used for the assessment of post-traumatic abnormalities within the hip, depending on injured structures, are radiography, CT and MRI. When bone changes are suspected, radiography is ordered, while CT is preferred for a more complicated picture due to the complex pelvic anatomy. CT is useful particularly with high-energy or multiple traumata; hip joint/pelvis examination is an element of the protocol in polytrauma [41].

The presence of chronic changes and suspicion of damage to the soft tissues are indications for MRI [42].

In post-traumatic changes in the hip, ultrasonography is useful mainly in selected cases, concerning mostly periarticular soft tissues. These tissues are located more superficially and hence are more accessible in the examination. In certain cases, an ultrasound scan can be the first diagnostic examination that may lead to the ultimate determination of the cause and end the diagnostic process, which is of particular significance in the paediatric population as radiation exposure or sedation needed for MRI can be avoided.

Of the most significant applications of ultrasonography in hip injuries typical of paediatric patients, assessment of tendon insertions on various apophyses found in the hip region and pelvis must be mentioned [35].

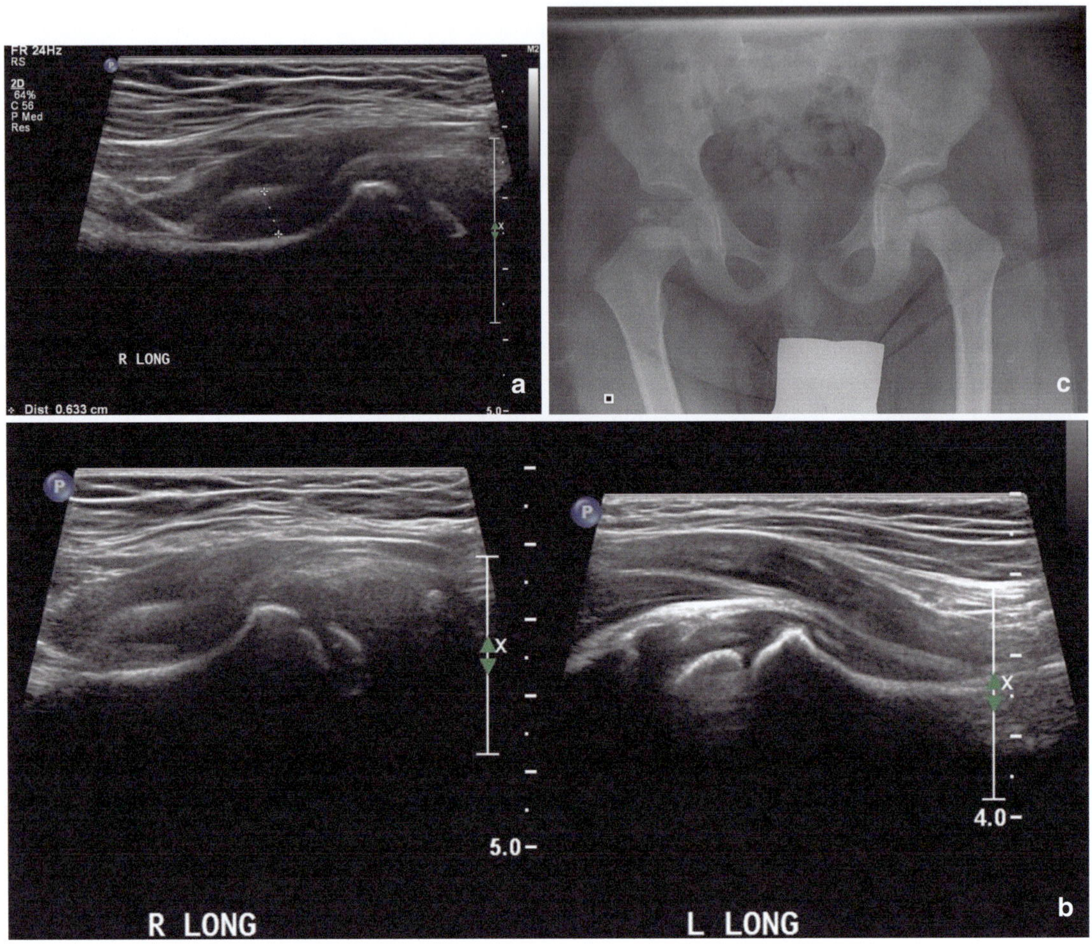

Fig. 9.27 (**a–c**) A 3-year-old boy with Legg-Calvé-Perthes disease suspected in US and confirmed in radiography. US of the right hip joint (**a**), a comparative US image of both hips with the normal left hip joint (**b**) and radiography (**c**)

Avulsion Fractures/Apophyseal Injuries

Ultrasonography is particularly valuable in the assessment of local abnormalities where it can be used for local evaluation and confirmation or exclusion of a pathology. When used in emergency settings, ultrasound imaging may help establish the correct diagnosis in a short period of time using a single probe application.

A typical example of this type of pathology is apophyseal injury [6, 43].

Tendon insertions to pelvic bones usually possess separate ossification centres and are areas of weaker resistance in children; the same trauma that may cause tendon and myotendinous junction injury in adults results in an avulsion fracture in children.

Apophyseal injury and avulsion fracture are mainly found in children older than 10 years of age and particularly in those older than 14 years of age. Trauma may be acute or chronic [44].

Acute apophyseal avulsion is of a fracture nature and is manifested by typical clinical signs and symptoms in the form of pain and oedema. Repeated injuries and chronic apophyseal overloading result in microfractures and overlapping secondary inflammatory changes. This type of injury affects physically active children, e.g. young athletes, engaged in sports involving kicking, jumping or running, i.e. sports which involve numerous acceleration and deceleration movements, for instance, soccer, hockey and gymnastics [45, 46].

Typical sites of avulsion fractures within the hip are (1) the anterior inferior iliac spine, the insertion of the straight tendon of the rectus femoris muscle; (2) the anterior superior iliac spine, the sartorius muscle insertion; (3) the lesser trochanter, the iliopsoas insertion; and (4) the ischial tuberosity, the hamstring insertion [47].

Routine imaging techniques involve radiography. When small bone fragments are separated and there are only low-grade apophyseal irregularities, the interpretation may be doubtful as pathological changes may be poorly visible or even undetectable in the picture [48].

In acute avulsion fracture, US may display a detached bone fragment and facilitate assessment of its dislocation as well as of the continuity and oedema of the tendon inserting on the detached fragment. Moreover, it can also present concomitant soft tissue oedema surrounding the insertion and show enhanced perfusion of soft tissues adjacent to the site of injury in power/colour Doppler imaging. A detached bone fragment presents as a hyperechogenic linear reflection, often with a marked acoustic shadow, which is joined to a tendon of a typical US appearance with preserved fibrillar structure and frequently with lower echogenicity secondary to oedema. At the bone separation site, the injured cortical bone outline is uneven (Figs. 9.28 and 9.29). In patients younger than 10 years of age, ultraso-

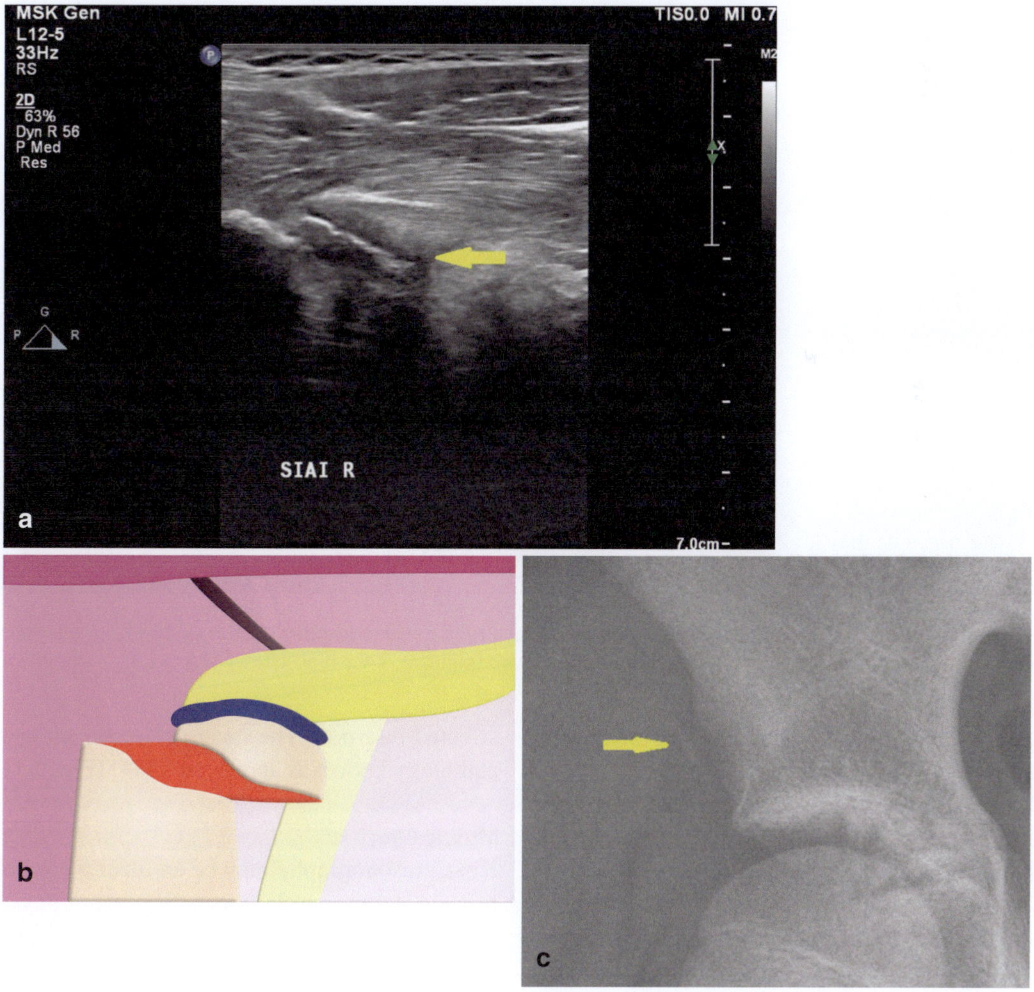

Fig. 9.28 (**a–c**) Avulsion fracture of the anterior inferior iliac spine: US appearance (**a**), a schematic (**b**) and correlation with radiography (**c**); the detached bone fragment is poorly visible in radiography. Yellow arrow – the detached bone fragment

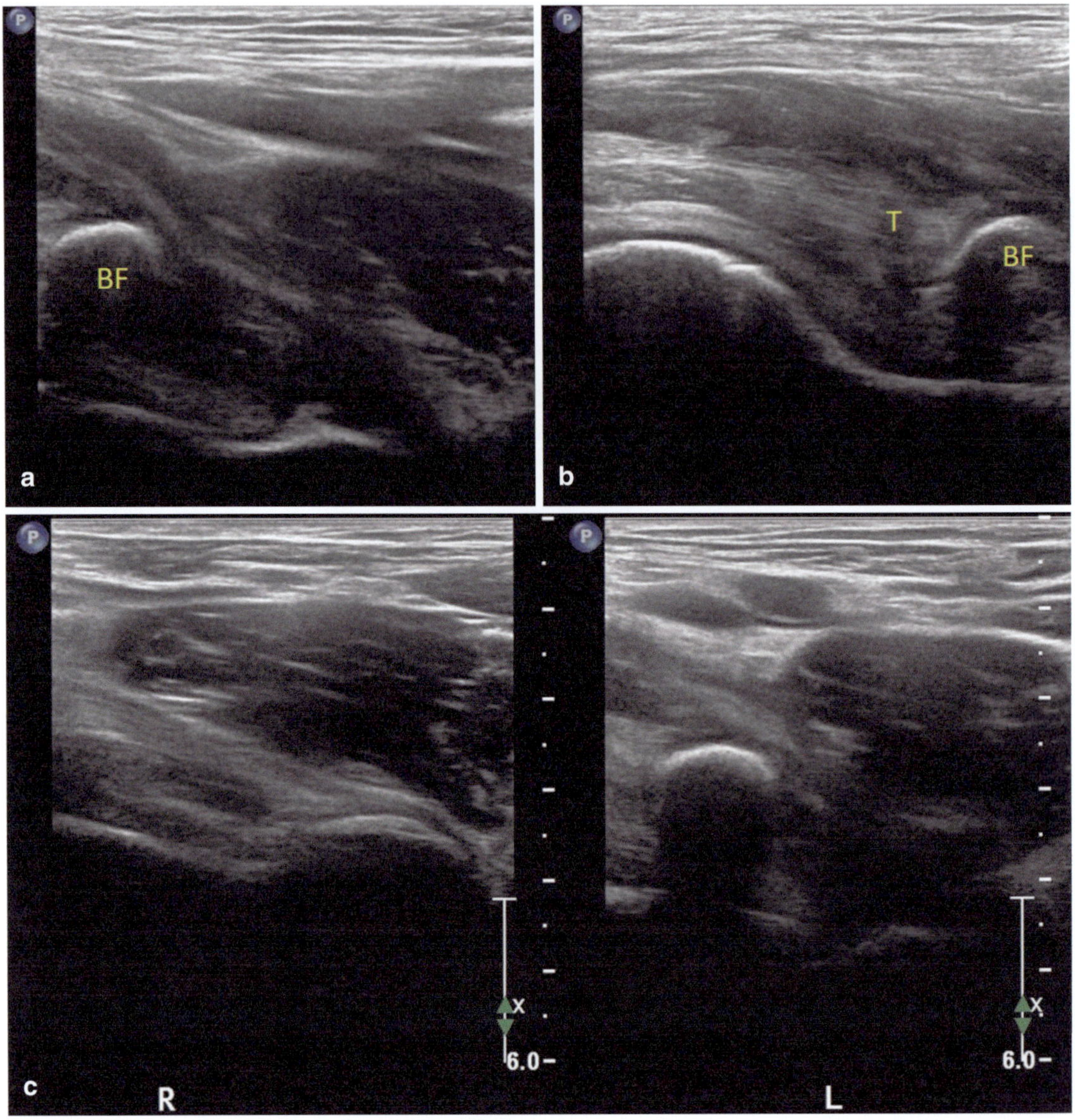

Fig. 9.29 (**a**–**c**) US. Avulsion fracture of the lesser trochanter: a separated and displaced bone fragment attaches the iliopsoas tendon (**a**, **b**). A comparative image (**c**). BF the bone fragment, T the iliopsoas tendon

nography may reveal a detached fragment composed solely of cartilage [38].

In the case of chronic changes, the bone insertion region is markedly irregular with possible additional small reflections corresponding with calcifications/periosteal reactions and changes in the structure of the inserting tendon with its decreased echogenicity and blurred structure (Fig. 9.30). Power/colour Doppler reveals markedly enhanced perfusion at the site of the affected insertion. The image corresponds with a pathology known as apophysitis [44] (Fig. 9.31).

Muscle Injury

Hip ultrasonography may be an ideal first-choice method in hip muscle injury. Increasing physical activity, particularly in older children and adolescents, is the reason for frequent pathologies of this type. The search for and the assessment of the site of muscle injury must be correlated with

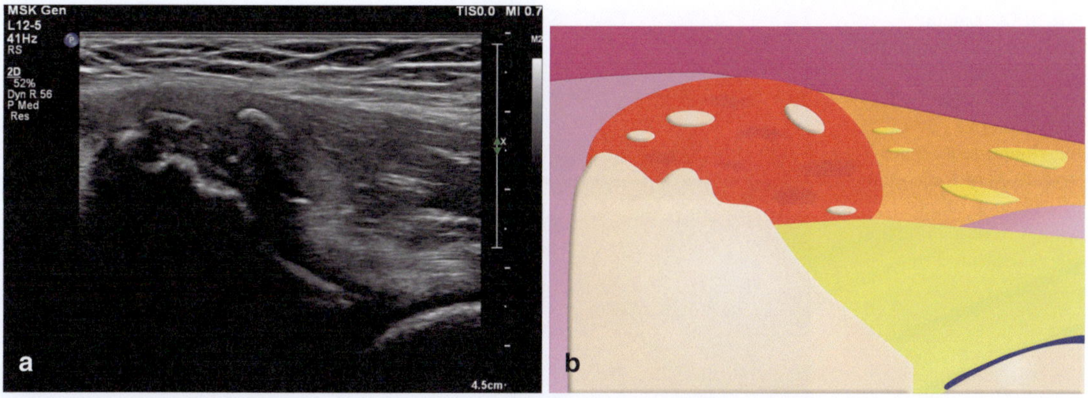

Fig. 9.30 (**a** and **b**) Chronic injury/avulsion of the enthesis on the anterior inferior iliac spine (SIAI). US appearance of the SIAI (**a**). A schematic (**b**)

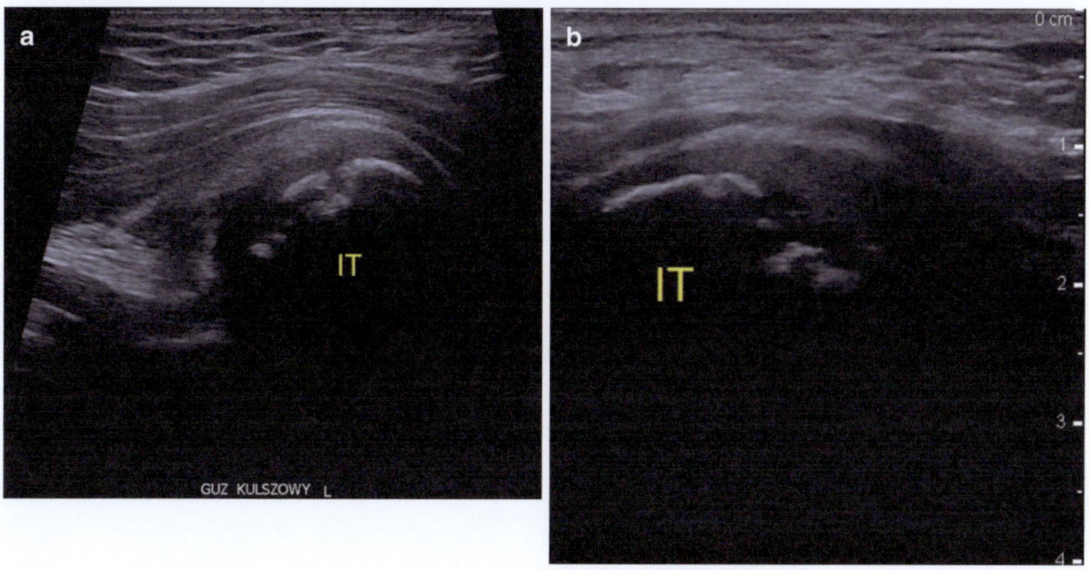

Fig. 9.31 (**a** and **b**) Apophysitis of the ischial tuberosity in a 15-year-old girl. Markedly uneven cortical outline of the ischial tuberosity with clinical signs and MRI abnormalities. Normal outline of the other tuberosity. Transverse section (**a**) and longitudinal section (**b**). IT the ischial tuberosity

the site of maximum clinical signs and symptoms (Fig. 9.32). In the hip area, particular attention must be paid to complaints within the inguinal/medial hip region [49, 50]. In this case, post-traumatic pain may be caused by injury to the proximal insertion of the adductor muscles, particularly the anterior-most adductor longus and gracilis muscle [51]. Ultrasonography enables assessment of the grade of injury and facilitates differentiation between low-grade injuries with muscle strain from complete muscle tear with retraction of its belly and a haematoma at the insertion. However, MRI may be needed for a more detailed assessment of the involvement of individual adductor muscles at their common insertion [52].

Muscle injuries within the hip occur more rarely than in adults, but their sonographic appearance and principles of their assessment are identical. More information about muscle

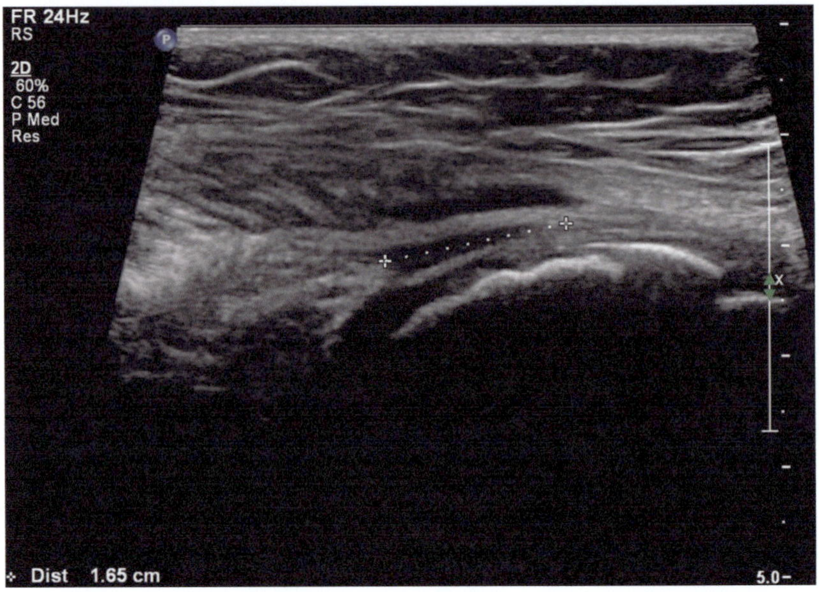

Fig. 9.32 Lateral hip – a site of maximum pain. Longitudinal section. Complete injury of the anterior part of the gluteus tendon in a 9-year-old girl; the grade of retraction of the tendon from its insertion site is measured

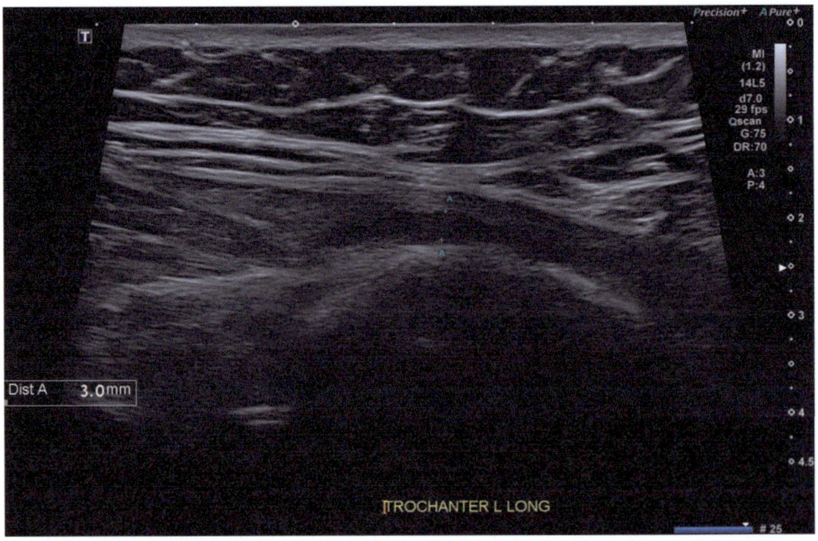

Fig. 9.33 Trochanteric bursitis. Slight bursa distension with a hypoechogenic area corresponding to the thickened synovium

injury, their appearance, assessment and grading in US is discussed in the chapter on thigh muscle injuries.

Greater Trochanteric Pain Syndrome

Ultrasonography may be used for the differential diagnosis of lateral hip pain [53]. The most common cause of pain in this area is a pathology in the greater trochanteric region: adjacent bursitis, enthesopathy, lateral snapping hip and, occurring more seldom in children, injury to tendons inserting on the greater trochanter.

However, one of the most common causes of lateral hip pain may be bursitis in the greater trochanteric region, mainly trochanteric bursitis [54]. The inflamed trochanteric bursa appears as an additional flat space between the iliotibial band and the greater trochanter. It is characterised by variable echogenicity: hypoechogenic with thickened and hypertrophied synovium or anechogenic with fluid in the bursa (Fig. 9.33). Depending on the inflammation activity, the bursa may show varied vascular patterns in Doppler imaging. Dilation of the bursa can be confirmed in a dynamic US scan. In this case, the bursa does not move together with the iliotibial band and greater trochanter and can be distinguished as a separate structure during movement.

Enthesopathies within the greater trochanter can be another cause of pain. These abnormalities may be local, associated with long-term overload or numerous microinjuries, or may result from the manifestation of a systemic disease, for example, JIA. In the case of enthesopathy, attention is typically drawn to evidently uneven outlines and blurred cortical structure with enhanced perfusion of the adjacent soft tissues as displayed in the power/colour Doppler imaging. Tendons inserting on the greater trochanter present oedematous changes with thickening and decreased echogenicity, but with preserved fibrillar structure.

Moreover, US also facilitates assessment of the gluteus muscle tendons in terms of their pathology. In the case of tendon degeneration, its echogenicity is decreased, fibrillar structure blurred and the tendon frequently thickened [55] (Fig. 9.34). In partial tendon injuries, depending on their grade, one may encounter a lower or greater tendon defect in the form of hypoechogenic/anechogenic area with focally invisible tendon structure. With complete tears, the tendon cannot be identified in the region of the proximal insertion and the cortical trochanteric layer is exposed.

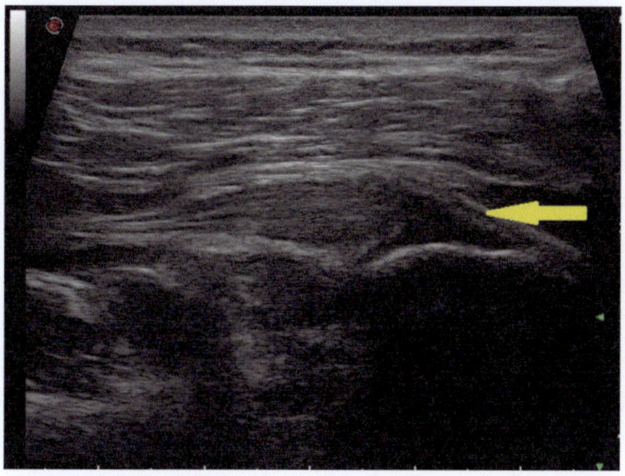

Fig. 9.34 Tendinopathy of the posterior part of the gluteus medius tendon in a 16-year-old boy with observable thickening and reduced echogenicity of the tendon. Yellow arrow – the posterior part of the gluteus medius tendon. (Courtesy of Dr. Zbigniew ŻUBER)

Lateral (external) snapping hip is discussed in the following subsection.

Snapping Hip

Ultrasonography is applied in the diagnostic process of pathological conditions that cause a snapping sensation felt in the hip region [56]. The usefulness of ultrasonography mainly results from the possibility to conduct a dynamic assessment of the cause of snapping and to directly visualise the conflict between structures. Snapping hip is typically divided into two groups, extra-articular and intra-articular, based on its causes. Ultrasonography is of more use in the former group due to the more superficial location of pathology and better accessibility to impinged structures. The two most common types of extra-articular snapping hip are lateral (external) snapping hip and anterior (internal) snapping hip [57–59].

As for lateral (external) snapping hip, the dynamic investigation in US helps reveal the impingement of the iliotibial band/gluteus maximus on the femoral greater trochanter by displaying the moment of a sudden dislocation/snap of the iliotibial band/gluteus maximus belly against the trochanter, frequently with an audible popping noise and pain. The pathology is assessed with the transducer placed transversely over the greater trochanter at hip rotation or flexion and extension. Sometimes, snapping of the structures above the trochanter occurs during more complex movement sequences; in these cases, patients should be asked to recreate this sequence during the examination. The iliotibial band can be thickened and have decreased echogenicity (Fig. 9.35). Between the band and the greater trochanter, there can be the dilated and reactively altered trochanteric bursa [60].

Anterior (internal) snapping hip occurs due to the impingement of the iliopsoas muscle on the surrounding tissues/structures [61]. The most frequent cause of internal snapping hip is snapping of the tendon against its own belly or impingement of the tendon on the iliopectineal eminence, which can also be documented in a dynamic scan

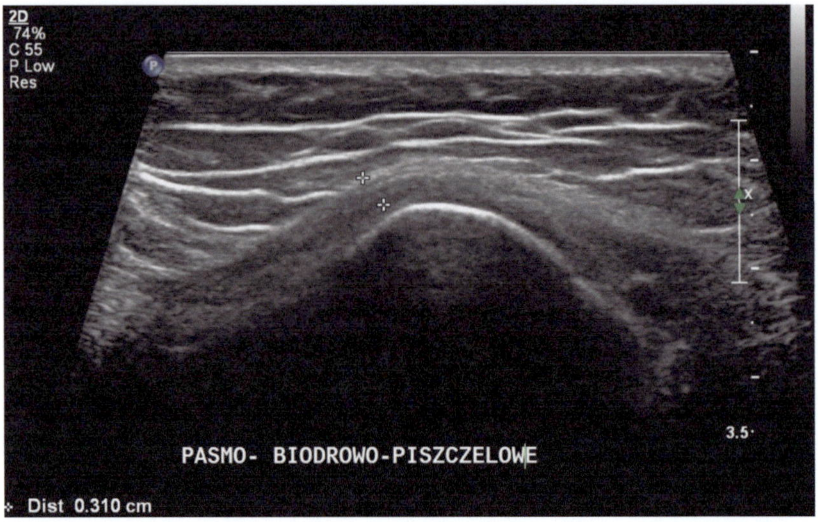

Fig. 9.35 The region of the greater trochanter in a patient with lateral snapping hip syndrome; changes confirmed in a dynamic US scan. Slight thickening and oedema of the iliotibial band

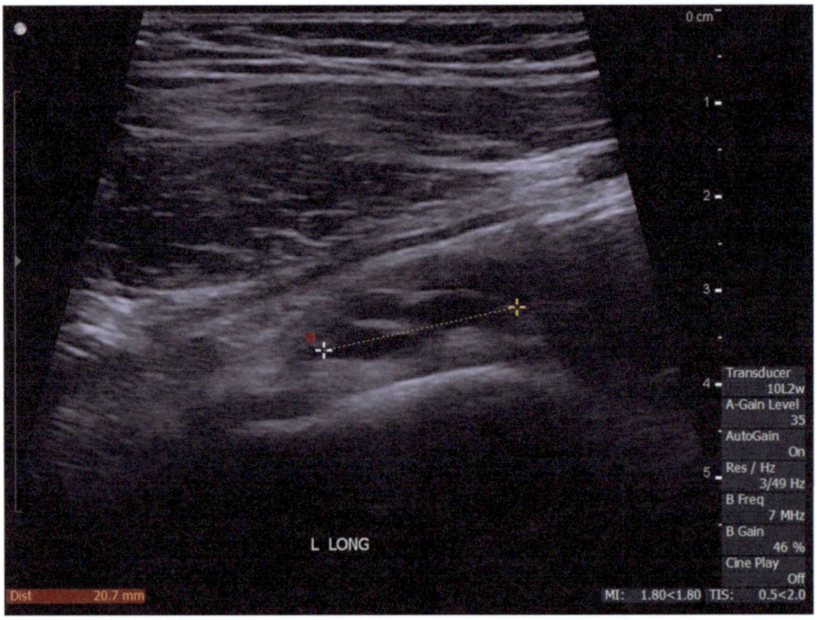

Fig. 9.36 A ganglion cyst originating from the anterior capsule of the hip joint

with the patient performing a sequence of movements that elicits the conflict or by abduction, flexion and external rotation of the hip followed by a return to the neutral position [62, 63].

In selected situations, US may contribute to the detection of intra-articular causes of snapping hip, which include labral tear. US is of use particularly in the assessment of the anterosuperior aspect of the labrum, i.e. one of the most common injury sites. Abnormalities appear as hypoechogenic or anechogenic spaces within the labrum or at its base. In some cases, at the labrum or at the anterior joint capsule, one may observe a cystic lesion corresponding with a paralabral cyst. The lesion should be differentiated from a ganglion cyst that may develop in the anterior part of the joint capsule; ultrasonography plays a significant role in the detection of a ganglion cyst latter as well (Fig. 9.36).

Labral tear may be secondary to hip deformation predisposing to femoroacetabular impingement and indicating the need for MR arthrography to precisely assess the morphology of the hip joint and its inner structures [64, 65].

Other causes of inter-articular snapping hip may include intra-articular foreign bodies or osteoarthritis secondary to pathological processes in the hip joint. These conditions are assessed with magnetic resonance imaging [66, 67].

Clinical Application and Typical Thigh Pathologies

Clinical indications for thigh ultrasonography in children mainly result from local signs and symptoms, such as pain, oedema, redness, tenderness upon compression, palpable local resistance or suspicion of a tumorous focal lesion. These signs and symptoms may be consequences of various pathologies, which can be generally classified into one of three large groups of causes: inflammation, trauma/overload and focal lesions. Ultrasonography is particularly helpful in establishing a correct diagnosis in children as clinical pictures are similar irrespective of the cause in this group of patients and there are no meaningful data from the interview and physical examination, while collected information frequently suggest a different pathology (Fig. 9.37). When evaluating a suspicious region in ultrasonography, the first thing to do is to detect potential discrepancies from the normal image. Next, these changes must be correlated with available data from the medical history, physical examination and possibly with laboratory and imaging findings, if available. However, in routine situations, US is the first imaging examination performed in children, especially in the case of soft tissue abnormalities, owing to all the advantages of ultrasonography in this group of patients.

Trauma

Ultrasonography is useful in the assessment of post-traumatic abnormalities within the soft tissues of the thigh in children and frequently ordered as the first examination. In many cases, it enables the final diagnosis to be established. However, basic limitations of this method must be borne in mind:

1. Abnormalities of low intensity may be undetected in US, and their proper assessment may require MRI.
2. Early post-traumatic abnormalities may be underestimated in US and suggest a lower grade of intensity. That is why their monitoring by repeated scanning in appropriately short time intervals is necessary as post-traumatic abnormalities are characterised by a significant variability of morphological images and evolution with time. US is an ideal tool for the monitoring of this evolution and of the healing

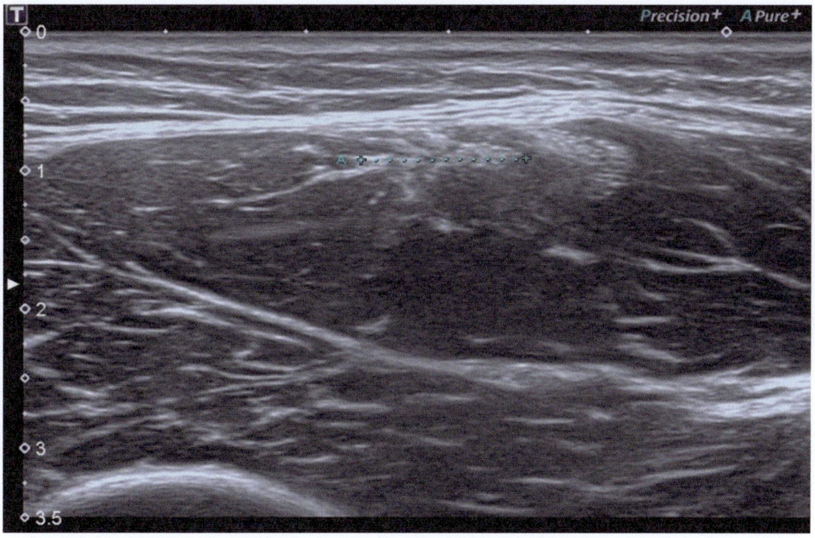

Fig. 9.37 US of the anterior thigh presents a scar at the site of the rectus femoris central core tendon after previous tendon injury. A 14-year-old patient with no recollection of injury. Suspicion of a pseudotumour in a clinical examination

process with the possibility to detect changes that are significant in treatment.

Post-traumatic changes in the soft tissues of the thigh may appear in a direct or indirect mechanism. Direct impact of forces causes local changes correlated with their extent and is restricted to the area upon which these forces act. In changes that have occurred indirectly, the soft tissue injury area lies beyond the site upon which the forces act and its extent is frequently considerable. In the case of trauma in children, it must be remembered that there is frequently no information pertaining to how the injury occurred, especially in terms of indirect or repeated minor injuries where children are unaware of the trauma or forget about it.

Muscle Injury

The severity of muscle injury is assessed on a three-grade scale, where:

- Grade 1 denotes slight changes with no visible damage to the muscle, in the form of muscle stretch.
- Grade 2 denotes partial changes with preserved muscle continuity, but with partial impairment of its structure and function.
- Grade 3 denotes complete injuries with complete loss of muscle continuity and function.

As for direct muscle injury, the following may appear on US depending on the injury grade: muscle oedema in the form of local area of lower muscle echogenicity with preserved tissue architecture, muscle belly contusion with its increased echogenicity and blurred structure of the muscle and fibromuscular septa, which corresponds with bleeding into the muscle tissue, and, in higher injury grades, macroscopic disruption of the muscle continuity with accompanying fluid collections corresponding with haematomas [68, 69] (Fig. 9.38). These haematomas may have various sizes, ranging from small lesions limited to the muscle belly to large intermuscular lesions separating the muscle bellies and/or disrupting their continuity. An important and constant feature of a haematoma is its temporal evolution; initially, haematomas present as hyperechogenic fluid collections that are not sharply delineated from the surrounding tissues, while, with time, fluid echogenicity decreases to practically anechoic lesions, haematoma demarcation improves as their outlines become smooth with a narrow transitory zone and abnormalities in the surrounding soft tissues regress [69].

One must remember that haematomas may appear even if they have not been spotted in US before, e.g. in areas of contusion. Haematomas may be subject to puncture under US guidance. Haematomas that persist despite applied therapy may indicate a predisposing pathology, e.g. a coagulation disorder.

Another significant role of US is the monitoring of the healing process and the ability to detect potential healing complications. Examples of abnormalities developing in the course of healing include post-traumatic calcifications and heterotopic ossification, i.e. myositis ossificans or muscle atrophy [69, 70]. Of these conditions, diagnostic difficulties may be associated particularly with cases of post-traumatic heterotopic ossification, especially when there is no information about a trauma-related nature of the examined abnormality. Careful observation of abnormalities with evidence of non-complete blurring of the muscle fibroadipose septa, rapid growth of the abnormality in consecutive scans and sudden appearance of numerous peripheral calcifications may be suggestive of the nature of the lesion. In many cases, the final diagnosis can be established only after correlation with other diagnostic methods, in particular CT that may show a typical distribution of calcifications (zonal phenomenon) [71, 72].

As for indirect injuries, muscle bellies located adjacent to bone structures, e.g. vastus intermedius in the anterior compartment of the thigh, are more susceptible to trauma.

Indirect muscle injuries tend to be characterised by greater range and extent of damage with more severe functional impairment and concomitant rupture and dislocation of the muscle bellies. Accompanying skin lesions in the form of petechiae and bruising frequently do not correlate with the site of actual muscle injury. Extensive oedema and diffuse pain result in the fact that

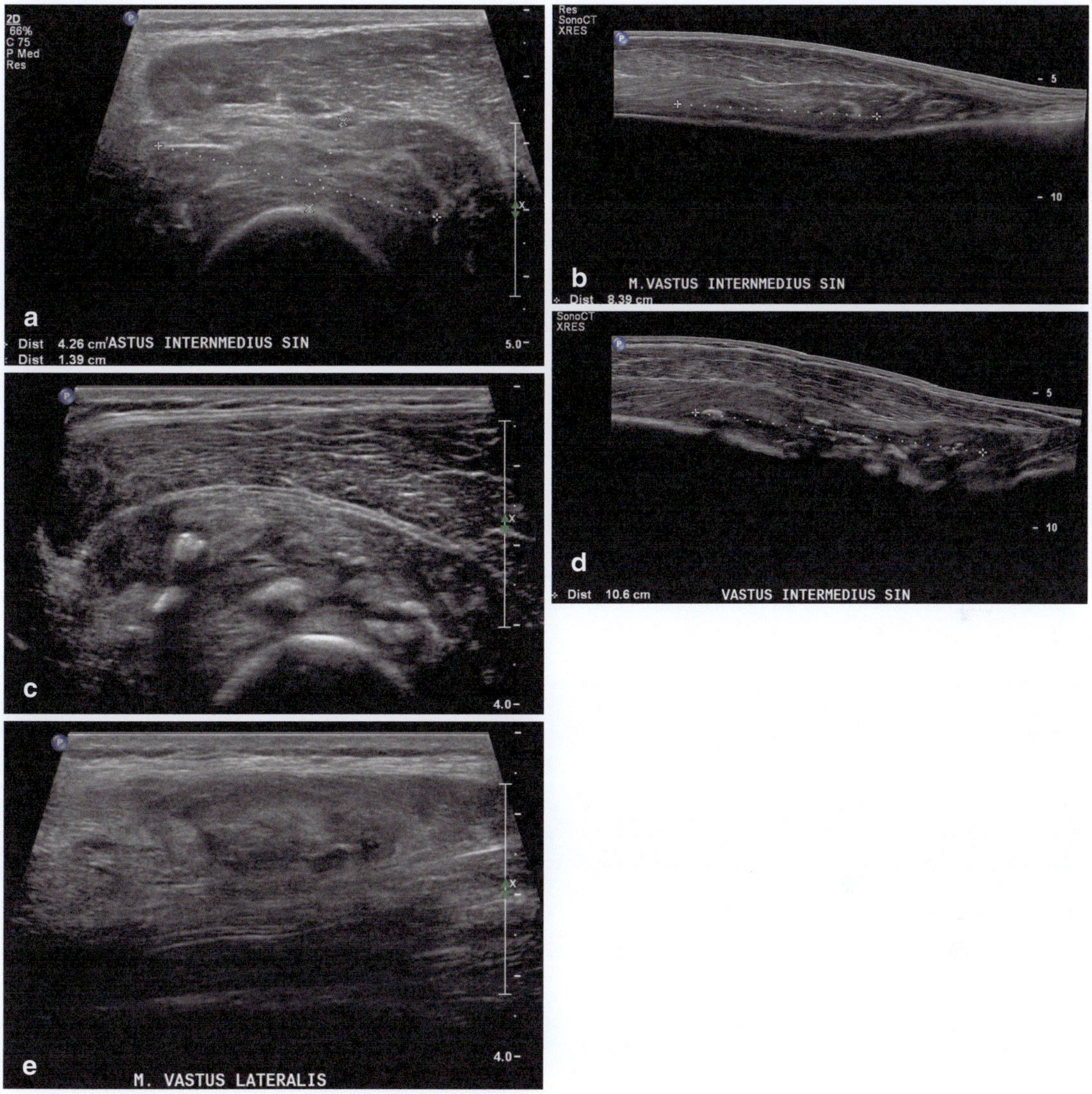

Fig. 9.38 Direct injury to the quadriceps femoris (medial and lateral heads) in a 15-year-old boy. Medial head US conducted several days after injury; transverse section and panoramic imaging show changes in the echotexture corresponding with muscle contusion (grade 2 injury) and enable assessment of the extensiveness of injury (**a** and **b**). A follow-up scan performed 2 weeks later displays numerous post-traumatic calcifications (**c** and **d**), which disappeared in subsequent scans. Lateral head contusion in the first examination (**e**)

greater areas of the thigh must be examined to locate and properly assess tissue injury. It is very important in indirect injury to assess the continuity of the muscle bellies, and if it is disrupted, to determine the location of the belly stumps, assess their retraction and evaluate the distance between them [73]. Panoramic ultrasound imaging may be of use as it enables visualisation of long fragments of the region of interest (Fig. 9.39).

One of the most frequently injured muscle bellies in the thigh is the rectus femoris muscle, usually in the direct mechanism. The structure of the belly of a "muscle-in-muscle" nature predisposes to injury, typically within the central core tendon located in the proximal and medial one-third of the muscle belly [74]. The central core tendon is oriented sagittally. Blurred outlines of the core tendon with slight oedema of the adja-

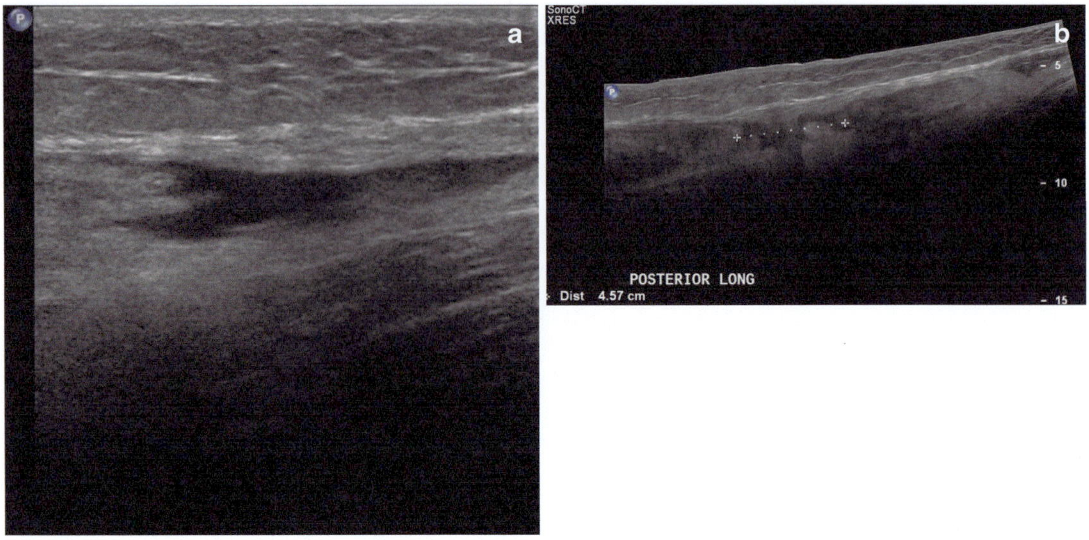

Fig. 9.39 Isolated injury to the gracilis muscle in a 16-year-old girl sustained while doing the splits. The proximal muscle stump is surrounded by a slight haematoma (**a**). Panoramic imaging shows the distance between the stumps (**b**)

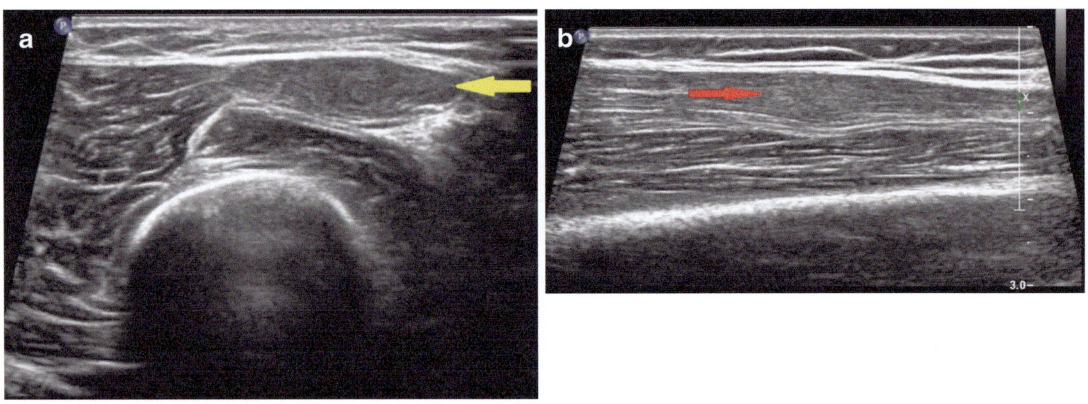

Fig. 9.40 Low-grade injury to the rectus femoris with visible blurring of the central core tendon and focal oedematous changes in the belly with local reduction of its echogenicity. Transverse section (**a**) and longitudinal section (**b**). Yellow arrow, the rectus femoris; red arrow, the lesion of the rectus femoris muscle

cent muscle is an early sign of injury (Fig. 9.40). More severe changes result in the loss of core tendon continuity with a defect in its structure. Similar images can be encountered in smaller secondary core tendons of the rectus femoris. Injuries of this type are common in young physically active boys, e.g. soccer players. Scars may be a remainder of core tendon injury, while retracted parts of the belly may mimic focal lesions in the clinical examination (a cause of so-called pseudotumours).

Moreover, injury may also induce changes in the subcutaneous tissue. Post-traumatic changes include: subcutaneous tissue oedema and haemorrhagic imbibition manifested as areas of markedly increased echogenicity compared with the surrounding subcutaneous tissue with blurred typical tissue architecture. Post-traumatic changes also include subcutaneous haematomas and serous fluid collections, called Morel-Lavallée lesions, which are located between the subcutaneous tissue and fascia, and develop in

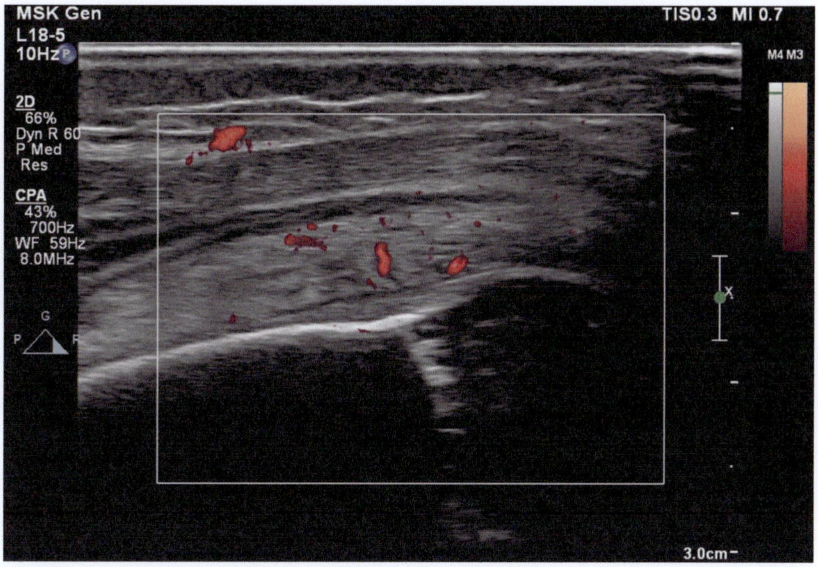

Fig. 9.41 Oedema and marked hyperaemia of the soft tissues in the region of the femoral cortical bone at its distal metaphysis; a US image suggests changes typical of osteomyelitis

the mechanism of separation and "rolling" of these structures [75, 76]. The location of these changes in the thigh is one of the most typical.

Thigh Tissue Inflammation

Ultrasonography is an acknowledged tool for the detection of inflammatory abnormalities within the thigh tissue. The assessment of the thigh tissues is easier in children than in adults owing to smaller area to be investigated and thinner subcutaneous tissue, which often facilitates the use of high-frequency transducers and enables evaluation of the entire region of interest, including deep tissues at the cortical layer of the femur. A significant reason for this considerable usefulness of ultrasonography in the detection of musculoskeletal system inflammation is short examination time, no need for sedation and growing availability, which, when combined with high sensitivity of this method, makes it often the only tool available in urgent settings that enables correct diagnosis.

Ultrasonography is a particularly important tool in emergency settings in patients with suspected osteomyelitis. An ultrasound scan is capable of displaying changes indicative of this pathology even 2–3 days after the onset, which is much earlier than radiography (minimum 10 days after the onset) [77].

The earliest signs in US are soft tissue oedema at the bone cortical layer with evidence of enhanced blood flow in power Doppler imaging (Fig. 9.41). The appearance of a subperiosteal fluid collection or a fluid space in the soft tissues near bones is practically a confirmation of osteomyelitis [77, 78]. These changes develop earlier in children due to the loose connection of the periosteum with the bone cortex and its easier separation by fluid with increased intraosseous pressure. The periosteum may be swollen, or thickened, with the thickness exceeding 2 mm, and with decreased echogenicity and signs of increased blood flow. In the later stage, this is followed by changes typical of bone destruction and markedly uneven cortical outline resulting from periosteal reactions (Figs. 9.42 and 9.43). Moreover, widespread soft tissue changes with their structural disorders, extensive infiltration and forming abscesses may appear (Fig. 9.44). Pathogen spread is usually of the haematogenous character [79]. In neonates and infants, inflammatory changes tend to originate from the adjacent joint or bone epiphysis. At this age, the growth plate does not constitute a barrier for the spread of the inflammatory process, and inflammation in the femur or soft tissues of the thigh is associated with arthritis, usually in the knee joint [80]. In

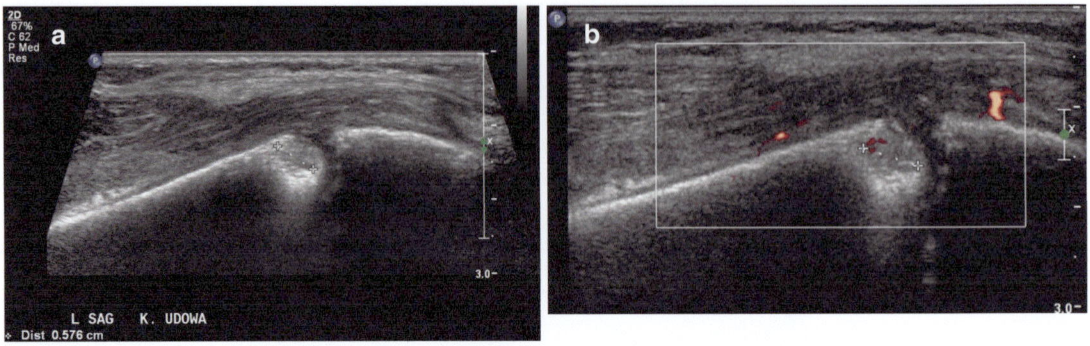

Fig. 9.42 A bone defect within the femoral distal metaphysis (**a**) and enhanced vascular flow in this region (**b**) the image of osteomyelitis

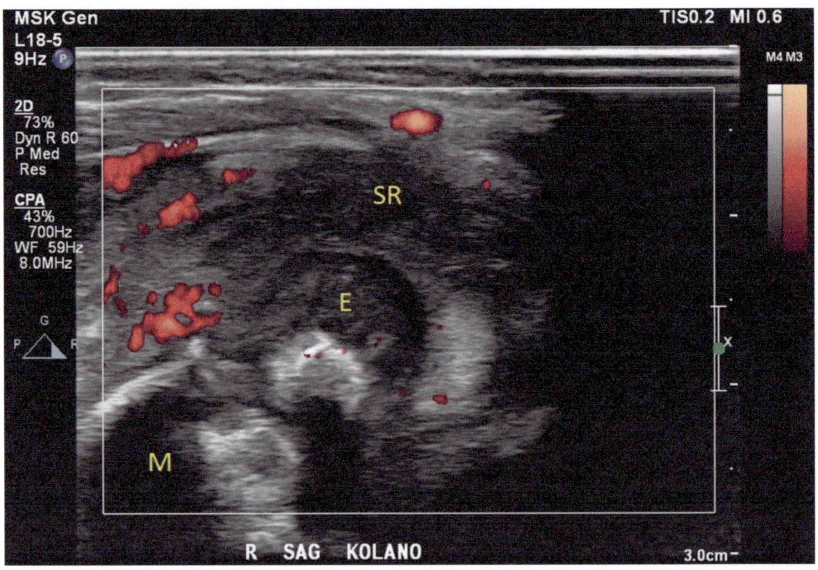

Fig. 9.43 A different patient. A 6-month-old girl. Considerable bone destruction within the distal femoral metaphysis with inflammatory infiltration in the adjacent soft tissues with high-grade inflammation. E the distal femoral epiphysis, M the distal femoral metaphysis, SR the suprapattelar recess with inflammatory changes

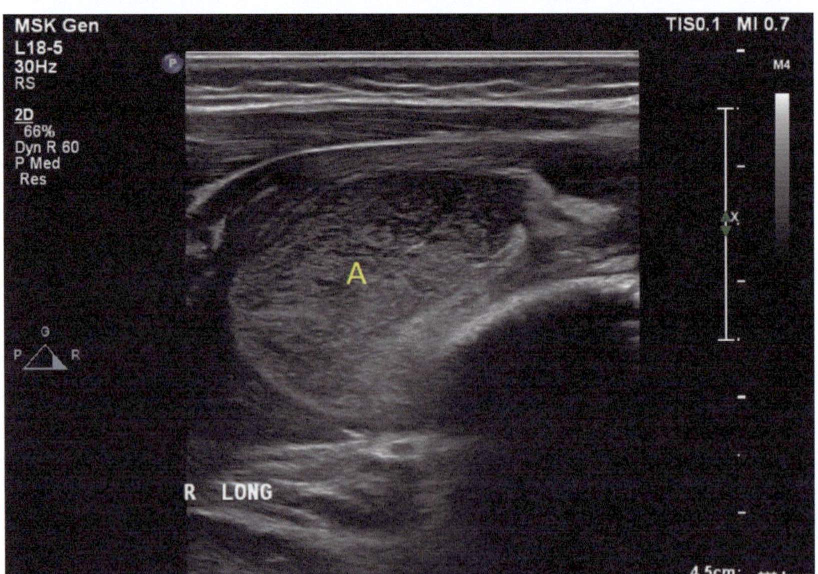

Fig. 9.44 The same patient. A large abscess in the soft tissues of the thigh (A)

older children, metaphyses are the primary location of these abnormalities.

Another cause of inflammation in the thigh in children is cellulitis [81, 82]. It typically manifests as local oedema, redness and pain, frequently accompanied by fever. Pathogens commonly responsible for infection are *Staphylococcus aureus* and *Streptococcus pyogenes*. Ultrasonography may reveal significant subcutaneous tissue oedema with marked elevation of its echogenicity and blurred tissue architecture with invisible fibrous septa. Also, hypoechogenic fluid spaces may appear within the affected area. Doppler scanning shows increased perfusion of the involved soft tissues. This examination can also be used for the monitoring of the disease and confirmation or exclusion of abscess formation.

A rare pathology of a fulminant course, induced by the same pathogens, is necrotising fascitis. In early stages, the sonographic image is similar to that in cellulitis, with extensive soft tissue oedema. The appearance of thickened fascial structures and fluid collections within the fascial region, around it and in deep tissues, suggests the correct diagnosis. Necrotising fascitis may also progress with the presence of soft tissue gas [79].

Another rare pathology is pyomyositis [79, 81]. Ultrasonography proves useful in determining local progression of the disease. In initial stages, US reveals not sharply delineated inflammatory infiltration of the muscle with disrupted tissue architecture, blurred fibroadipose septa and the presence of irregular fluid spaces. Later, an intramuscular abscess develops with variable echogenicity relative to adjacent tissues; echogenicity can be lower, similar or higher. In the case of anaerobic bacterial infection, one may notice hyperechogenic gas reflections within the abscess.

Muscle inflammatory diseases with generalised oedematous changes without distortion of the muscle structure may be very difficult to display in an ultrasound scan; in this case, MRI becomes the basis for diagnosis. An example of this type of pathology is dermatomyositis, frequently involving muscles of the proximal parts of the extremities, including thigh muscles. In this case, the lack of changes in ultrasonography does not preclude the pathology.

Focal Lesions Within the Thigh

The application of ultrasonography for the diagnosis of thigh focal lesions in children is one of the most common indications for thigh ultrasonography irrespective of the child's age. When a focal lesion in the soft tissues is suspected, the diagnostic algorithm may begin with US. The role of US is to confirm or rule out the presence of a focal lesion. If a focal lesion is excluded, ultrasonography may help find a cause of a so-called pseudotumour, e.g. asymmetrical subcutaneous fat distribution or history of muscle injury with abnormal retraction of its parts [83, 84].

If the presence of a focal lesion in the thigh tissues is confirmed, the most important steps are to differentiate its nature (either solid or cystic, while solid-cystic and cystic-solid lesions are treated as solid) and determine its location, particularly in relation to the fascia lata, as a subcutaneous or subfascial lesion.

When a lesion is identified as solid or comprises a solid component, or is suspicious of being solid, the analysis of its perfusion in colour and power Doppler imaging is an integral element of the examination (Fig. 9.45). The evidence of vessels in the lesion confirms its tissue nature, whereas their quantity and distribution deliver additional information useful in the differential diagnosis [85]. Elastography of focal lesions is still lacking an acknowledged place in imaging diagnosis, though "soft" lesions tend to be benign more often than "stiff" ones.

The most common benign focal lesions in children are vascular lesions, such as haemangiomas and vascular malformations, as well as lesions originating from the adipose tissue, such as lipoma and lipoblastoma [86] (Fig. 9.46). Vascular changes are characterised by a high number and density of vessels; they are usually hypoechogenic and may contain phleboliths. By contrast with vascular malformations, haemangiomas are of a tissue mass nature [87].

Lipomas originate from the adipose tissue and are usually well-circumscribed encapsulated and homogeneous tissue masses of an oval shape.

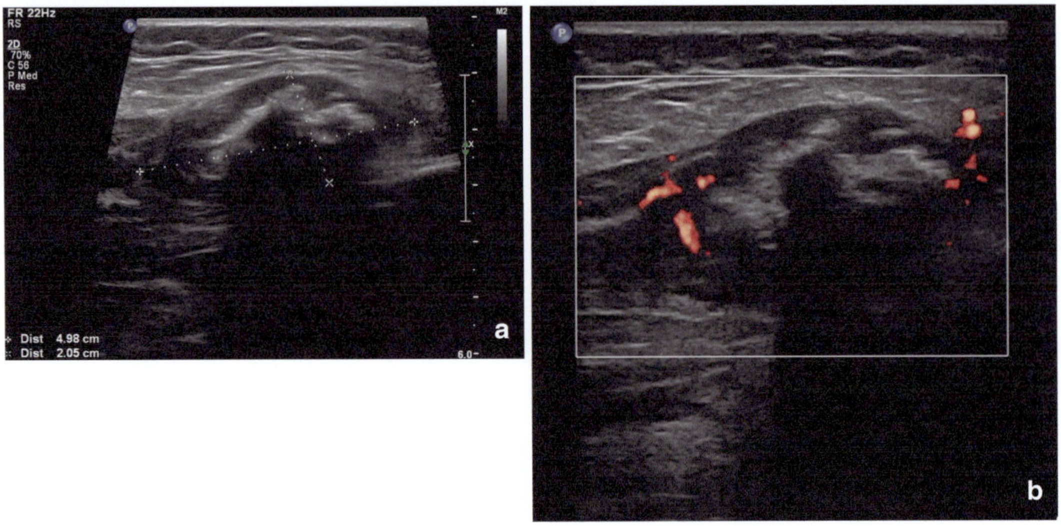

Fig. 9.45 (**a** and **b**) A focal lesion in the inferior part of the gluteus maximus in a 7-year-old boy. The lesion is hypoechogenic and solid with a central calcification and markedly enhanced vasculature in power Doppler imaging. A histopathological examination of the resected specimen revealed a focus of heterotopic ossification

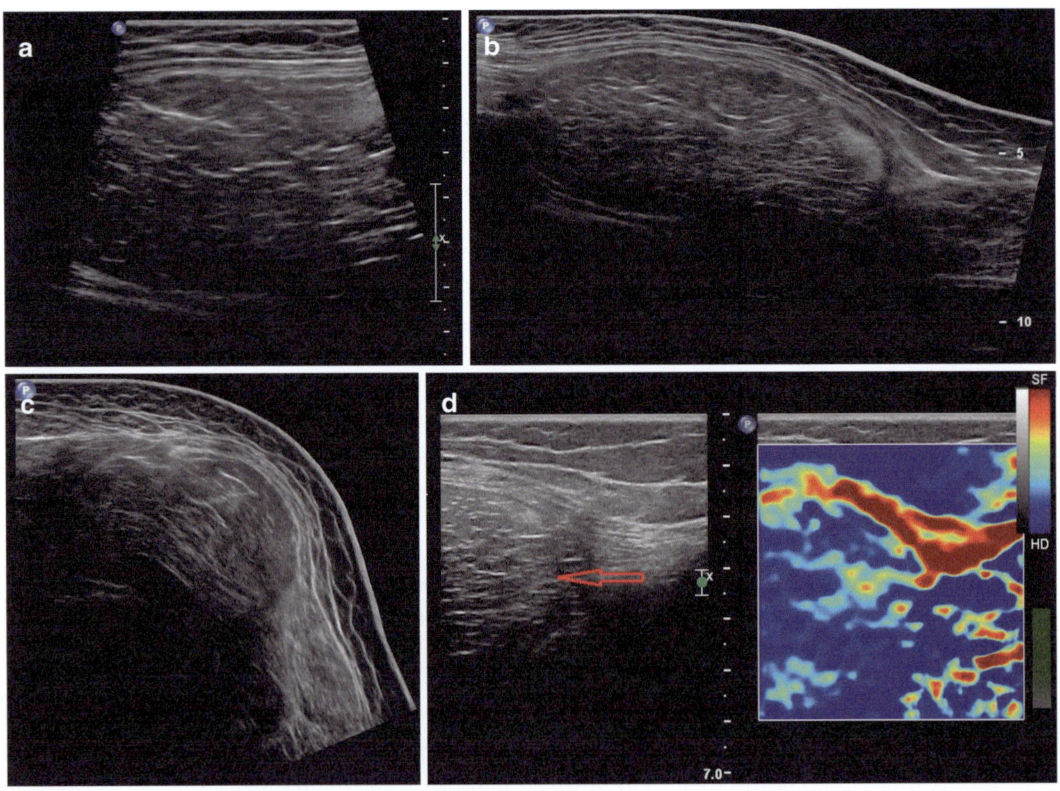

Fig. 9.46 (**a**–**d**) A 7-year-old boy with an intramuscular lipoma in the anterior compartment of the thigh. A large (over 6 cm) well-circumscribed tumour of hypoechogenic nature and structure resembling adipose tissue. US: the length of the tumour is greater than the length of the transducer's head, which may result in overlooking the lesion (**a**). A panoramic scan displays the size and shape of the tumour; longitudinal section (**b**) and transverse section (**c**). In elastography, the stiffness of the tumour is greater than that of the surrounding tissues (**d**). Red arrow, tumour of the thigh: an intramuscular lipoma

They tend to be hyper- or isoechogenic in relation to the surrounding tissues. Their location in the thigh may vary (subcutaneous, intramuscular, intermuscular). Lipomas are characterised by poor vasculature. However, lipoblastoma, which is a rarer lesion typical of the developmental age, can display greater structural heterogeneity and may not be sharply demarcated from the adjacent structures [83, 88, 89].

As for masses located along nerves, e.g. the sciatic nerve, neurogenic tumours can be encountered. Numerous neurofibromas of various sizes, located along the sciatic nerve, and presenting the "bag of worms" appearance can be seen in neurofibromatosis type 1 [90].

Another cause of tumorous lesions in the thigh is trauma, e.g. the above-mentioned haematomas, Morel-Lavallée lesions or post-traumatic subcutaneous tissue lesions. This group of lesions also includes muscle hernias associated with fascia lata injury and muscle protrusion to the subcutaneous tissue [91].

Malignancies within the thigh are rare in the paediatric population, with the most common being rhabdomyosarcoma-type tumours (RMS). After detection and suspicion of a malignant nature, MRI and histological verification are necessary. Thigh US is also capable of detecting primary malignancies originating from the bones as these lesions tend to be large (usually reaching over 5 cm in the longitudinal axis), cause bone destruction and protrude into/infiltrate the soft tissues. An example of a lesion of this type may be Ewing sarcoma, a malignant bone tumour localised in the femoral shaft [92] (Fig. 9.47).

Furthermore, ultrasonography is a very helpful method in cases of suspected foreign bodies within the soft tissues of the thigh. It enables their detection, localisation and monitoring for possible complications, e.g. suppurative conditions, or vascular or nerve damage [93].

Developmental Dysplasia of the Hip (DDH)

Developmental dysplasia of the hip (DDH) is a very common disorder in infancy. It has an estimated prevalence of 0.5–4% according to age, ethnicity and method of detection [94].

DDH include a spectrum of hip joint abnormalities, where there is an abnormal relation between the femoral head and the acetabulum. It may range between a subtle degree of femoral head uncovering by the acetabulum up to complete dislocation of the femoral head [95, 96].

DDH is more common in females, and other risk factors for it include breech position of the baby, positive family history and incorrect positioning of the lower limb when swaddling the babies [97].

Signs of DDH include leg length discrepancy, asymmetrical thigh or gluteal folds and limitation of movement in the affected hip. Ortolani and Barlow tests are used to assess the hip stability. Ortolani test is performed with the patient supine and the hips flexed 90°, the examiner holds the thighs with the thumb placed along the inner thigh and the index and middle finger placed above the greater trochanter. Gentle abduction of the hip while lifting the leg is then performed. This manoeuvre reduces a dislocated hip with palpable "clunk". The Barlow manoeuvre is performed with the patient supine and the hips flexed 90°; the examiner then adducts the hip and applies a gentle push-and-pull movement on the joint. It is considered positive if the femoral head has excessive mobility or a "clunk" is felt when it exits the acetabulum in lax hip joints (Fig. 9.48a, b) [98].

Sonoanatomy of the Hip Joint

The hip joint is a ball-and-socket articular joint providing stability and mobility in multiple planes. It is formed of multiple elements including bony, fibrocartilaginous, ligamentous and synovial structures. Muscles, tendons, synovial bursa and neurovascular structures are also involved in the joint structure and function [99].

The acetabulum has a cup-shaped cavity that accommodates the rounded femoral head. The acetabular labrum provides an attachment to capsular and ligamentous structures in addition to increasing the acetabular concavity and contact area with the femoral head [99].

Proper positioning of the femoral head within the acetabulum influences the normal development of both structures [100].

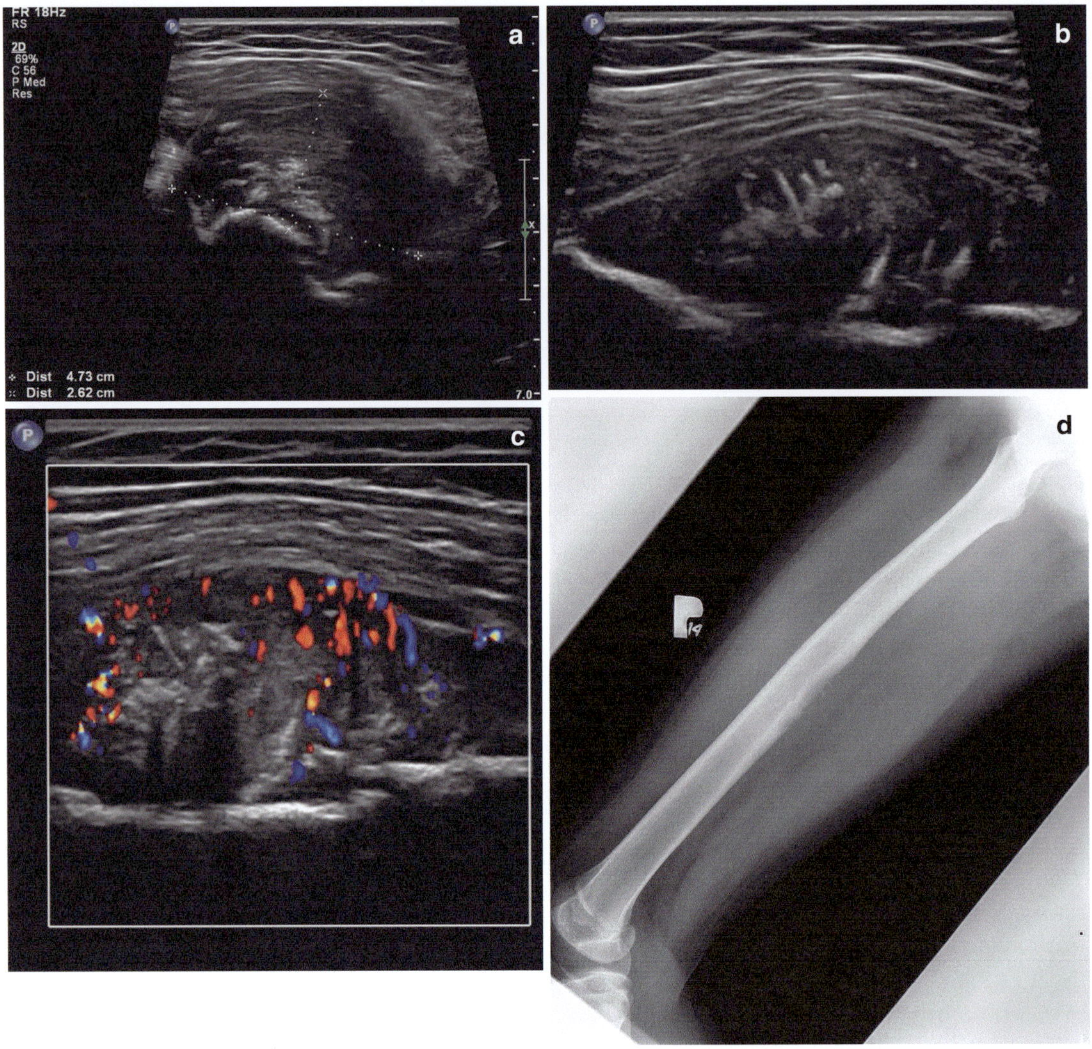

Fig. 9.47 (**a–d**) Ewing's sarcoma of the femoral shaft. US in the transverse (**a**) and longitudinal (**b**) planes displays the relationship of the lesion with the bone, its unclear delineation from the bone and pathological calcifications. Visibly enhanced vasculature of the tumour with chaotic arrangement of vessels (**c**). Radiography (**d**); attention is drawn to linear calcifications perpendicular to the bone at the level of the lesion: the image of "malignant" periosteal reactions

In infants the femoral head is mainly cartilaginous which allows it to be identified and assessed by ultrasonography together with the other fibrocartilaginous structures in the hip joint. Several ultrasound techniques are available for the assessment of the hip joint in cases of DDH. The joint is usually assessed both statically and dynamically. The most widely used techniques are the Graf and Harcke methods [101].

The standard coronal ultrasound view is the key view of assessment of the hip in both methods. The appearance of structures in this view could be related to viewing a plain anteroposterior radiograph of the hip joint, keeping in mind that the structures on the ultrasound image are horizontally projected rather than vertically [102] (Fig. 9.49).

The standard coronal plane should show the iliac bone as a straight line, the echogenic tip of

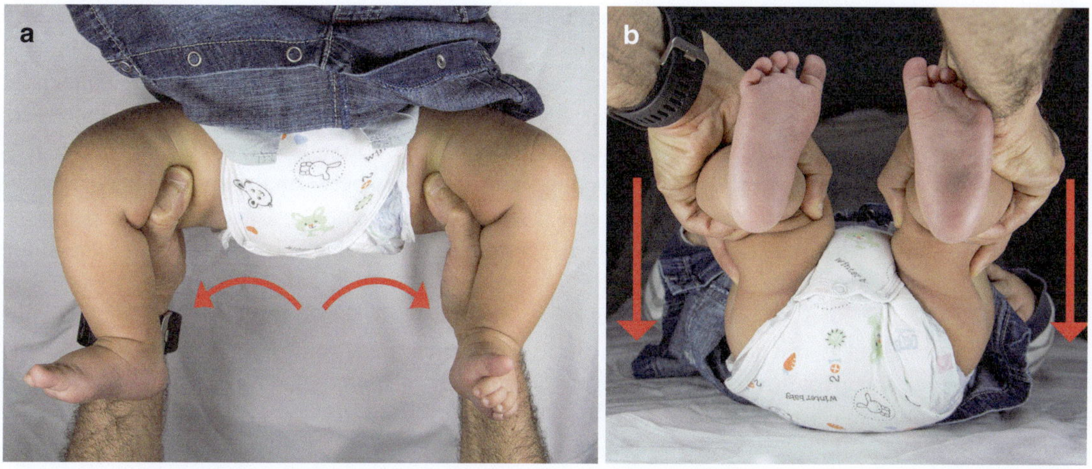

Fig. 9.48 (**a**) Showing Ortolani test. (**b**) Barlow's test

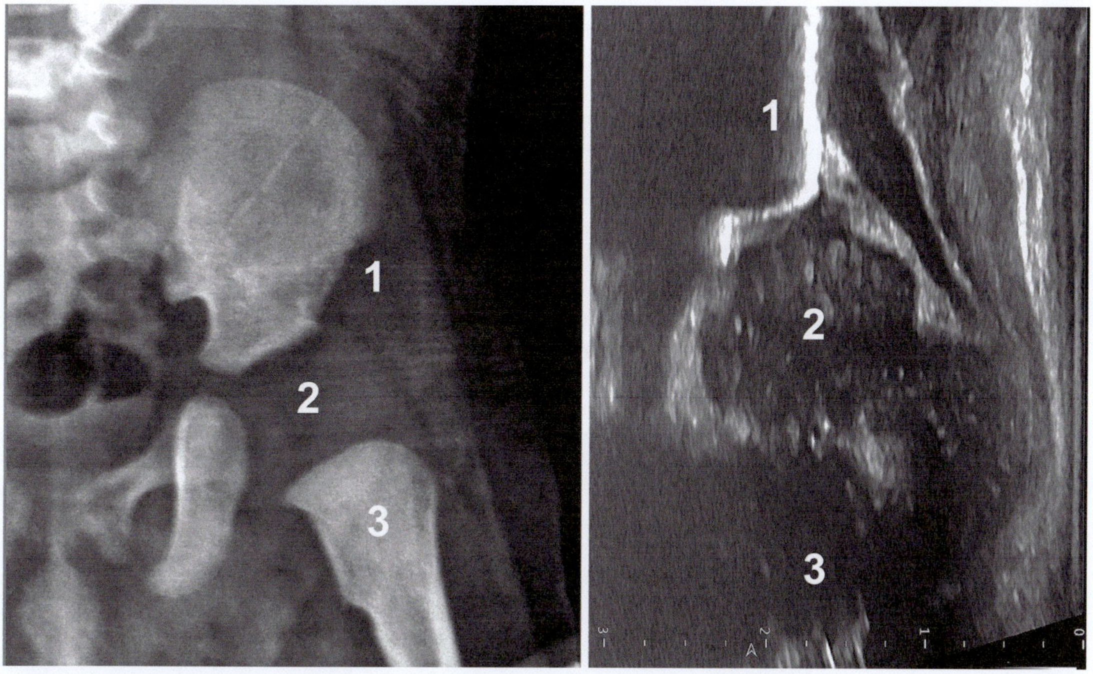

Fig. 9.49 Understanding how the hip ultrasound image is projected in the standard coronal view by comparing it to an antroposterior view of a hip joint X-ray. 1. Iliac bone, 2. femoral head, 3. femoral neck

the acetabular labrum and the tri-radiate cartilage. The chondro-osseous junction is also seen in this plane and appears as a highly echogenic line because of total ultrasound beam reflection by the bony structures of the femur through the epiphysial plate. It serves as an important hip ultrasound landmark to identify the femoral neck and surrounding anatomical structures. It also guides proper technique performance as its shape will change if improper placement of the transducer was done [103].

The femoral head in the newborn is cartilaginous, and it appears as a slightly oval structure of low echogenicity. The femoral head ossific centre may be present at birth or at 5–7 weeks of age. It has a variable shape, often oval, and variable in location rendering it of no value in assessing the position of the femoral head within the acetabulum. A large ossific centre may cause a shadow that obscures what is known as the lower limb of the iliac bone in the acetabular fossa which is a landmark for ultrasound ensuring that the imaging plane is passing through the centre of the acetabulum [103].

The joint capsule covers the lateral aspect of the femoral head and it is continuous with the perichondrium of the greater trochanter. It covers the femoral neck being firmly applied to it. The point where the capsule reflects off the femoral neck to become the perichondrium is known as the synovial fold. It appears as an ill-defined echogenic structure or as two parallel echogenic lines. Knowldge of this anatomical structure is important to avoid erronus identification of it as the actebuluar labrum [103].

The acetabulum is formed of a bony and cartilaginous portion. The labrum is the most peripheral part of the acetabulum and it is formed of fibrocartilage. It is seen in hip ultrasound as a triangular-shaped echogenic structure in contrast to the hyaline cartilage of the acetabular roof seen as a hypoechoic area between the femoral head and bony acetabular roof. Several structures are present in the acetabular fossa, the most significant of them from the ultrasound point of view is the lower limb of the os ileum which is an important landmark that should be clearly seen in the standard coronal view of the hip joint. It is almost centred between the anterior and posterior rims of the acetabulum just superior to the tri-radiate cartilage. The bony rim of the acetabulum is the most lateral point of the bony socket concavity, and it is identified on ultrasound as the zone where the concavity of the bony acetabular roof changes into the convexity of the ilium [103] (Figs. 9.50 and 9.51).

Scanning Technique

According to the recommendations of the American College of Radiology, the hip joint should be scanned in at least two orthogonal planes using a linear probe with a frequency between 7 and 10 Mhz. The coronal plane at rest and the transverse plane with the latter during hip flexion with and without stress [102]. It is best used in the first 4–5 months of life as the femoral head is mainly cartilaginous and its ossific centre is small or absent [104].

The scan could be performed with the patient in the supine or lateral decubitus positions; both are accepted. Immobilisation of the patient in the

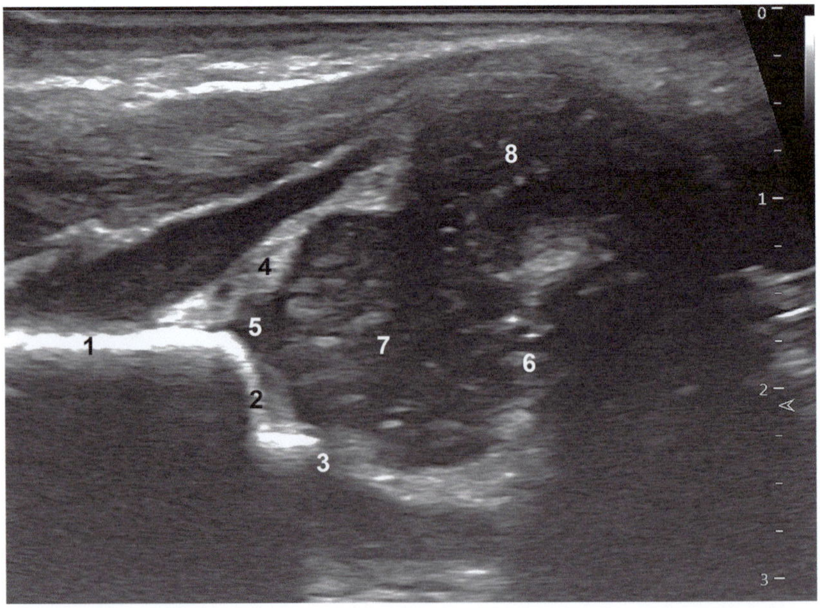

Fig. 9.50 Coronal ultrasound image of a normal hip joint in the standard plane. 1. Iliac bone. 2. Bony acetabular roof. 3. Tri-radiate cartilage. 4. Acetabular labrum. 5. Cartilagenous acetabular roof. 6. Chondro-osseous junction. 7. Femoral head. 8. Greater trochanter

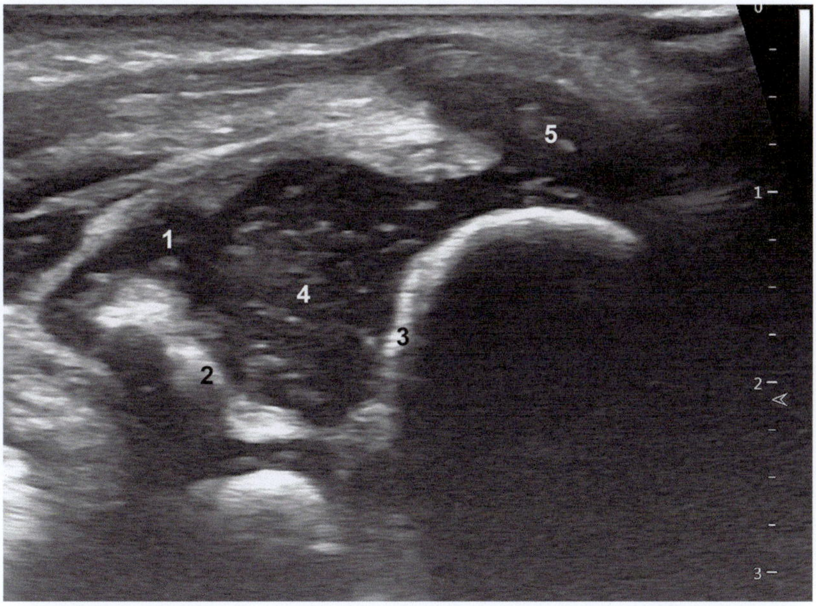

Fig. 9.51 Axial ultrasound image of a normal hip joint during adduction. 1. Posterior acetabular labrum. 2. Bony acetabulum (the tri-radiate cartilage is seen as a small hypoechoic disconsolation). 3. Chondro-osseous junction. 4. Femoral head. 5. Greater trochanter. Note the normal V-shaped relation between the bony acetabulum and chondro-osseous junction

lateral decubitus position can be achieved using a special cradle or foam pads. Feeding the babies during the examination may help in calming them down and reducing their movements [102].

The hip joint is assessed for its position, morphology and stability, all of which should be reported unless one or more of these items could not be fulfilled; then, the report should mention the cause of this limitation [102].

After the patient is placed in a supine or lateral decubitus position, the hip joint may be imaged in the neutral position, i.e. with 15–20° flexion or in the flexed position. The transducer is placed over the lateral aspect of the hip joint parallel to the patient's back, and fine adjustment of the position of the transducer by minimal rotation is performed in order to obtain the standard coronal view of the hip that is essential for proper evaluation [102] (Fig. 9.52a).

The transverse or axial view is performed with a 90° hip flexion. In this view the structures of the hip joint are projected resembling an anatomic axial plane like that of an axial computed tomographic image (Fig. 9.52b). The femoral shaft is seen ending in the femoral head which rests on the ischium. In both the coronal and transverse images, the chondro-osseous serves as an important landmark in the identification of femoral head. The transverse view is used to assess the position of the hip joint at rest and during passive abduction and adduction, gentle stress is then applied to check for hip stability [102]. In the transverse view of the hip, the relation of the echogenic chondro-osseous junction of the femoral metaphysis and the bony acetabulum form a U shape during abduction and a V shape during adduction [105] (Fig. 9.51).

Normal Findings

Graf's classification is a quantitative (morphological) method of assessing the acetabular roof, its bony part through α angle and the cartilaginous part through β angle. The age of the patient, changes in the cartilaginous roof structure, course of the cartilaginous acetabular roof perichondrium and β angle under stress are factors taken in consideration in order to describe and differentiate the different hip morphology types [101].

The α angle is that between the acetabular roof and vertical part of the iliac bone. This angle is mainly responsible for determining the hip type. A normal α angle is more than 60°. The β angle is between the cartilaginous acetabular labrum and the vertical part of the iliac bone. A β angle of more than 55° is abnormal; this can be explained

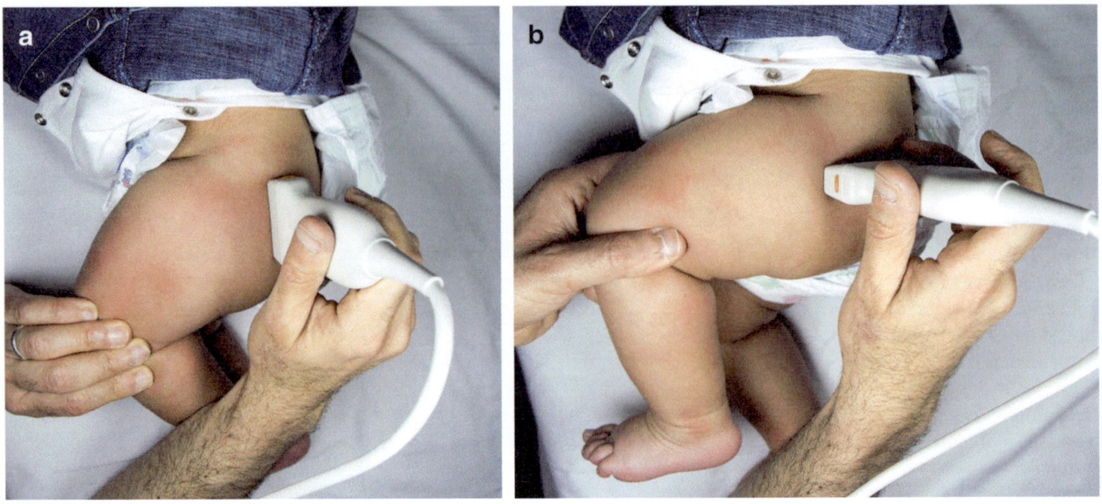

Fig. 9.52 Showing scanning technique and probe placement (**a**). Approach for standard coronal plane. (**b**) Approach for axial view

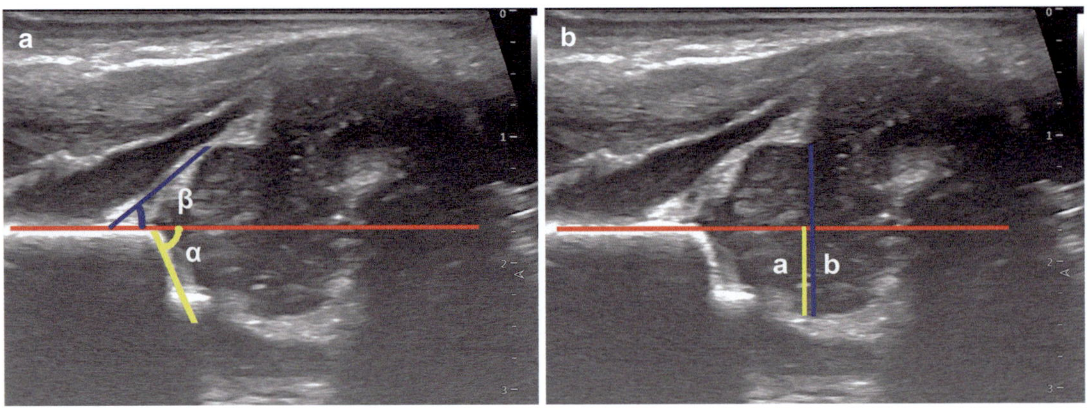

Fig. 9.53 (**a**) α angle and β angle measurements. The baseline is drawn along the iliac bone, α angle is between the acetabular roof and vertical part of the iliac bone, and β angle is between the cartilaginous acetabular labrum and the vertical part of the iliac bone. (**b**) Acetabular coverage calculation is performed by the following formula (a/b) × 100, where a is the length of the femoral head radius below the baseline and b is the radius of the femoral head in the coronal view at its widest part

by the fact that the femoral head when dislocated causes upward displacement of the labrum (Fig. 9.53a).

The other most accepted method of assessing DDH is the Harcke's method, which depends on acquiring several transverse and frontal (i.e. coronal) views of the hip during rest and application of stress. The views defined by Harcke include frontal views in neutral and 90° flexion and transverse views in neutral and 90° flexion. The imaging standard suggested by the American Institute of Ultrasound in Medicine (AIUM), and the American College of Radiology (ACR), includes the coronal view at rest and the 90° flexion transverse view with and without stress.

These views are used to assess and check the femoral head relation to the posterior acetabulum; any change that occurs in this relation means an unstable hip [102, 106].

In the standard coronal view, the acetabulum should cover at least 50% of the femoral head. A baseline is drawn passing along the straight part of the iliac bone. In normal children, this line passes through the femoral head dividing it into a part within the acetabulum and a part outside it. A perpendicular line is then drawn between the baseline and the furthest point of the femoral head within the acetabular fossa, and another line parallel to the latter is drawn across the furthest points of femoral head, i.e. its entire width. The first distance is then divided on the second and multiplied by 100 [32]. Acetabular coverage assessment is performed in both Graf's and Harcke's methods. Most paediatric radiologists usually assess the hip joint for DDH using the combination of both methods, and this was incorporated in the imaging standard by the American Institute of Ultrasound in Medicine (AIUM) and the ACR [102] (Fig. 9.53b).

Pathological Findings

Abnormal acetabular development can be judged by the degree of femoral head coverage by the bony acetabulum. A coverage of less than 50% is considered abnormal. The acetabulum in dysplastic hips is shallow and its roof is irregular and steep. The cartilaginous acetabular roof is usually thickened, more echogenic and shows upward displacement by the displaced femoral head. In severe cases of dislocation, it becomes deformed with inversion of the labrum into the acetabulum. The lateral osseous edge of the acetabulum is normally angular and sharp, while in dysplastic hips, it becomes blunt, rounded or flattened [105].

Another method of visual assessment of the femoral head displacement is by scanning the posterior aspect of the acetabulum in the coronal view; normally a small cartilage mound is seen, and no part of the femoral head should be visualised in this region. The femoral head may be seen adjacent to the ileum, posterior, lateral or superior to the acetabulum in advanced cases of hip dislocation [105] (Fig. 9.54).

In the Graf method, the hip is categorised into four types based on their α and β angle measurements. As mentioned earlier, a femoral head coverage of more than 50% and α angle of more than 60° are considered as normal (Type I) hip, and no treatment is required. Type II hip, according to Graf, is considered as an immature hip and further subdivided into four categories according to α and β angle measurements as well as the patient age if it is less than or more than 3 months. Patients falling into this type will need clinical follow-up to check if their hips mature or will proceed into subluxation and dislocation. Types III and IV have dislocated hips needing treatment with Type IV being more severe and showing interposition of the labrum between the femoral head and acetabulum [103] (Table 9.1) (Figs. 9.55, 9.56, 9.57 and 9.58).

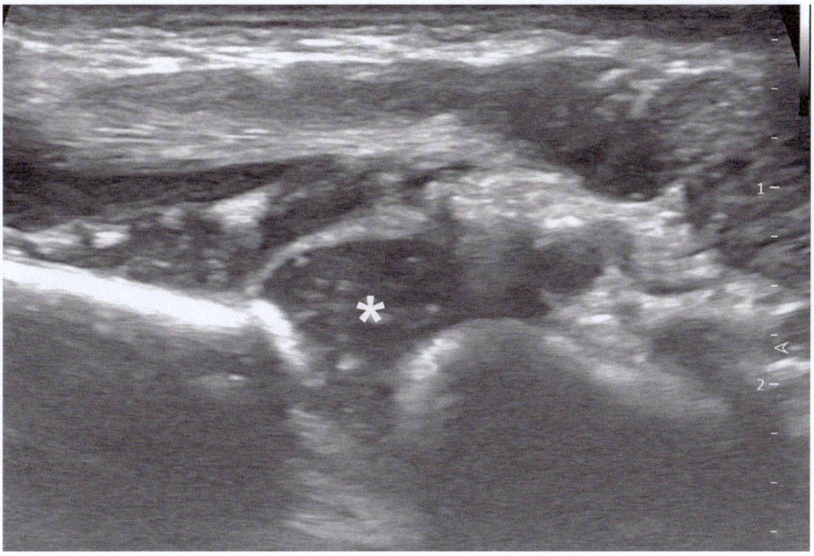

Fig. 9.54 Coronal view of the acetabulum, in a normal subject, posterior to the standard coronal plane showing the posterior aspect of the cartilaginous labrum (asterisk); no femoral head should be seen in this plane

Table 9.1 Graf classification of sonographic types of the hip joint [103]

Graf type	Age	Joint description	α Angle	β Angle	Comments
I	Any	Normal	≥60°		Mature hip with angular acetabulum and good coverage of the femoral head
II					
II a	Less than 3 months	Physiological immature hip	50–59°		Rounded bony acetabular rim
II b	More than 3 months	Delayed ossification	50–59°	<77°	
II c	Any	Critical zone	43–49°	<77°	Rounded or flattened acetabulum with deficient bony roof, cartilaginous roof still covers the femoral head
II d	Any	Sublaxed	43–49°	>77°	Displaced cartilaginous roof upwards
III	Any	Dislocated	<43°	>77°	Dislocated with shallow acetabulum
IV	Any	Dislocated	<43°	>77°	Dislocated with shallow acetabulum and interposition of the labrum between the femoral head and acetabulum

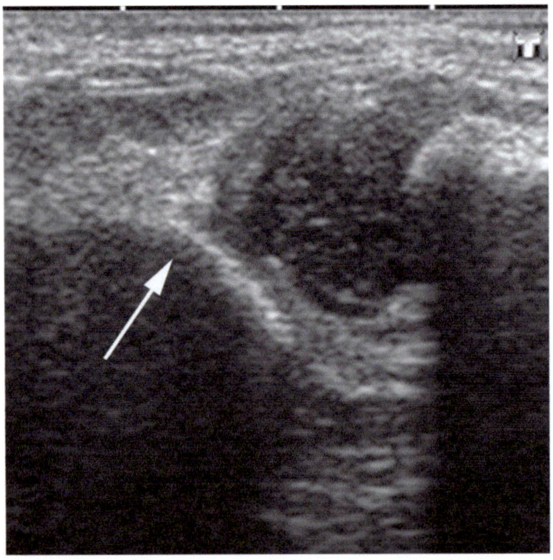

Fig. 9.55 Patient aged 1 month showing rounding of the bony acetabulum "arrow" and α angle of 55° conforming to Graf 2a hip (physiological immaturity)

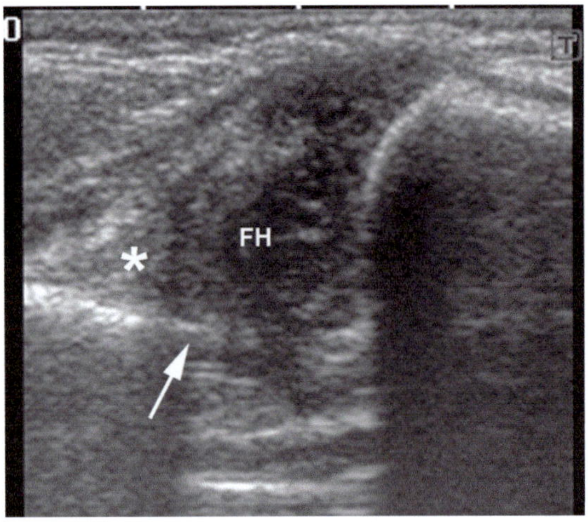

Fig. 9.56 Patient aged 2 months showing shallow, almost flattened acetabulum "arrow", and dislocation of the femoral head "FH"; the acetabular labrum "asterisk" is seen displaced upwards conforming to Graf 3 hip (dislocated without labrum inversion)

According to the Harcke's method, the hip joint could be classified into several categories. A normal hip is that showing a normal position of the femoral head within the acetabulum during rest, motion and during stress. A dislocated hip is that showing no acetabular coverage. If the femoral head coverage changes during motion and stress application, it could be further described as Lax, subluxated and dislocatable. A Lax hip shows normal position of the hip during rest and abnormal motion during stress, yet the femoral head stays within the acetabulum. A sublaxated hip would show lateral displacement of the femoral head during rest, but no dislocation occurs during stress application. A dislocatable hip is that showing sublaxation during rest and dislocation during stress. The acetabulum is reported as normal, immature or dysplastic as mentioned earlier based on its concavity and shape of its roof [105].

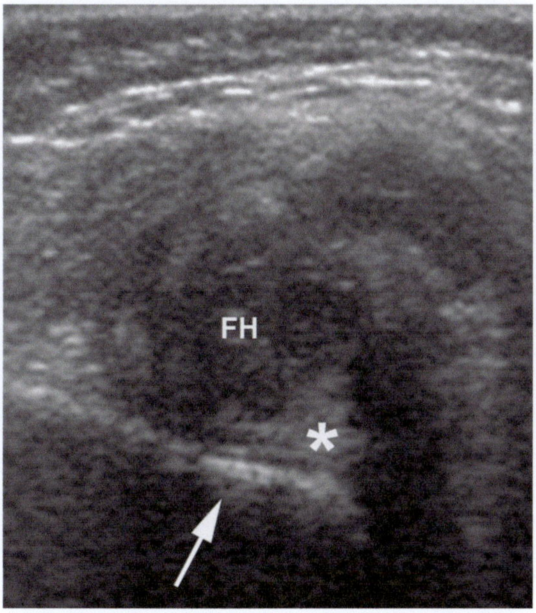

Fig. 9.57 Patient aged 1.5 months showing shallow, almost flattened acetabulum "arrow", and dislocation of the femoral head "FH" overriding the iliac bone; the acetabular labrum "asterisk" is seen everted below the femoral head conforming to Graf 4 hip (dislocated with inversion of the labrum)

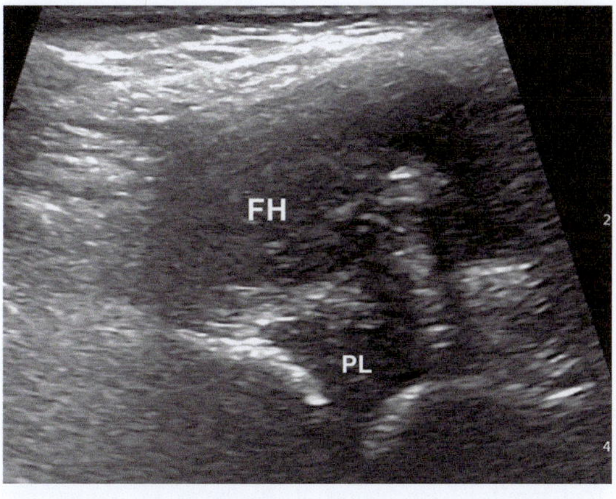

Fig. 9.58 Patient aged 9 months with complete hip dislocation. The femoral head (FH) is seen upwardly and posteriorly displaced; the latter is recognised by visualisation of the posterior cartilaginous labrum (PL), compared with Fig. 9.6

Pitfalls

As with any ultrasound examination, the examiner's experience is an important factor. The most common pitfall is scanning outside the standard coronal plane which can make a normal acetabulum look shallow.

In the transverse view of the hip, the transducer should be placed postrolaterally to the hip joint; lateral positioning of it may cause a normal joint to appear falsely abnormal.

The greater trochanter of the femur may be mistaken for a dislocated femoral head if the patient has a contracture or a varus deformity of the femoral neck.

Clinical Applications

Several clinical and imaging studies showed the patients with mild DDH and instability will show spontaneous resolution and improvement. On the contrary those on the extreme end of the disease will suffer from limping, leg length discrepancy and limited hip mobility if left untreated [97].

Ultrasound is an accurate tool in assessing DDH in early infancy. A controversy still exists about the methodology in neonatal hip screening programs, whether clinical alone is adequate and if ultrasound should be done for all newborns or for high-risk babies only [101].

There is lack of strong clinical evidence for the use of hip ultrasound as a screening tool in DDH; however, several programs are applied in different parts of the world. Universal ultrasound screening programs are applied in Austria and Germany since 1992 and 1996. In the UK and other parts of Europe, selective screening is performed. In the USA, the guidelines of the American Academy of Pediatrics advise against universal screening, and selective hip ultrasonography is considered at the age of 4–6 weeks in high-risk infants [98, 101, 107, 108].

Ultrasound of the hip joint is used to monitor DDH along its treatment course as it is more sensitive and specific than clinical and radiological assessment. Serial sonograms are usually performed to check for proper hip reduction after using splints such as the Pavlik harness. Osseous maturation of the acetabulum is also monitored. Scans performed during treatment may lack some of the information of the dynamic part of the study as they are performed with the harness in place, which causes limitation of hip movement. A full scan at the end of the treatment period may be performed after harness removal. Ultrasound of the hip during the treatment course are usually performed at a 2–3 weeks interval [105].

Conclusion

DDH is a common disorder seen in infancy with a wide spectrum of presentation ranging between mild laxity of the hip and complete dislocation. Neglected cases will suffer from complications leading to variable degrees of disability causing physical, psychological and financial burdens on the patient.

Early identification and diagnosis of this problem will lead to significant improvement in the outcome of the patient. DDH is assessed clinically, radiologically and by ultrasound. The latter is the most convenient and proper for the affected patient in several aspects including lack or radiation exposure, high sensitivity and specificity in the early stages of the disease and during treatment follow-up as well as its availability and reasonable cost.

The minimum standard hip ultrasound scan should include a morphological and dynamic assessment of the joint. The two most established methods are Graf's (morphological/static) and Harcke's (dynamic).

Graf's method classifies the hip joint into four types ranging from Type I (normal) to Type IV (dislocated with interposition of the labrum between the femoral head and acetabulum). Harcke's Method classifies the joint according to its behaviour during stress into normal, lax, subluxated, dislocatable and dislocated hip.

Both methods are easy to learn and apply and have a relatively short learning curve as long as the standard scan planes are followed and pitfalls are recognised and avoided.

References

1. Graf R, Tschauner C. Sonography of the infant hip. Sources of error, progress and current clinical relevance. Radiologe. 1994;34(1):30–8.
2. Tschauner C, Graf R. Ultrasound diagnosis of hip dysplasia – current status and future perspectives. Padiatr Padol. 1992;27(2):A19–22.
3. Backhaus M, Burmester G, Gerber T, Grassi W, Machold K, Swen W, et al. Guidelines for musculoskeletal ultrasound in rheumatology. Ann Rheum Dis. 2001;60(7):641–9.
4. Gill KG. Pediatric hip: pearls and pitfalls. Semin Musculoskelet Radiol. 2013;17(3):328–38.
5. Tagliafico A, Bignotti B, Rossi F, Sconfienza LM, Messina C, Martinoli C. Ultrasound of the hip joint, soft tissues, and nerves. Semin Musculoskelet Radiol. 2017;21(5):582–8.
6. Herregods N, Vanhoenacker FM, Jaremko JL, Jans L. Update on pediatric hip imaging. Semin Musculoskelet Radiol. 2017;21(5):561–81.
7. Czyrny Z. Standards for musculoskeletal ultrasound. J Ultrason. 2017;17(70):182–7.
8. Jacobson JA. Introduction to musculoskeletal ultrasound. Ultrasound Clin. 2007;2(4):569–76.
9. Serafin-Król M, Maliborski A. Diagnostic errors in musculoskeletal ultrasound imaging and how to avoid them. J Ultrason. 2017;17(70):188–96.
10. Fessell D, van Holsbeeck M. Ultrasound guided musculoskeletal procedures. Ultrasound Clin. 2007;2(4):737–57.
11. Pesquer L, Poussange N, Sonnery-Cottet B, Graveleau N, Meyer P, Dallaudiere B, et al. Imaging of rectus femoris proximal tendinopathies. Skelet Radiol. 2016;45(7):889–97.
12. Balius R, Pedret C, Blasi M, Miguel M, Vallejo B, Margalet E, et al. Sonographic evaluation of the distal iliopsoas tendon using a new approach. J Ultrasound Med. 2014;33(11):2021–30.
13. Robben SG, Lequin MH, Diepstraten AF, den Hollander JC, Entius CA, Meradji M. Anterior joint capsule of the normal hip and in children with transient synovitis: US study with anatomic and histologic correlation. Radiology. 1999;210(2):499–507.
14. Rohrschneider WK, Fuchs G, Troger J. Ultrasonographic evaluation of the anterior recess in the normal hip: a prospective study on 166 asymptomatic children. Pediatr Radiol. 1996;26(9):629–34.
15. Trauzeddel RF, Lehmann H, Windschall D, Ganser G, Berendes R, Haller M, et al. Age-dependent arthrosonographic reference values of the hip joint in healthy children and adolescents – a cross-sectional multicenter ultrasound study. Pediatr Radiol. 2017;47(10):1329–36.
16. Laurell L, Hochbergs P, Rydholm U, Wingstrand H. Capsular distance in the hip of the healthy child – normal values with sonography and MR imaging. Acta Radiol (Stockholm, Sweden: 1987). 2002;43(2):213–6.
17. Zuber Z, Owczarek A, Sobczyk M, Migas-Majoch A, Turowska-Heydel D, Sternal A, et al. Establishing percentile charts for hip joint capsule and synovial cavity thickness in apparently healthy children. Pediatr Rheumatol Online J. 2017;15(1):8.
18. Sudol-Szopinska I, Grochowska E, Gietka P, Plaza M, Pracon G, Saied F, et al. Imaging of juvenile idiopathic arthritis. Part II: ultrasonography and MRI. J Ultrason. 2016;16(66):237–51.

19. Kocher MS, Zurakowski D, Kasser JR. Differentiating between septic arthritis and transient synovitis of the hip in children: an evidence-based clinical prediction algorithm. J Bone Joint Surg Am. 1999;81(12):1662–70.
20. Paranjape M, Cziger A, Katz K. Ossification of femoral head: normal sonographic standards. J Pediatr Orthop. 2002;22(2):217–8.
21. Kallio PE, Lequesne GW, Paterson DC, Foster BK, Jones JR. Ultrasonography in slipped capital femoral epiphysis. Diagnosis and assessment of severity. J Bone Joint Surg. 1991;73(6):884–9.
22. Ziegert AJ, Blankenbaker DG, De Smet AA, Keene JS, Shinki K, Fine JP. Comparison of standard hip MR arthrographic imaging planes and sequences for detection of arthroscopically proven labral tear. AJR Am J Roentgenol. 2009;192(5):1397–400.
23. Goh LA, Chhem KR, Wang SC, Tho KS. Ultrasonographic features of an adductor longus tear: case report. Can Assoc Radiol J. 2001;52(4):252–4.
24. Sofka CM, Marx R, Adler RS. Utility of sonography for the diagnosis of adductor avulsion injury ("thigh splints"). J Ultrasound Med. 2006;25(7):913–6.
25. Deanehan JK. Point-of-care ultrasound identification of a psoas abscess in a child presenting with hip pain. Pediatr Emerg Care. 2017;33(6):437–9.
26. Nouri A, Walmsley D, Pruszczynski B, Synder M. Transient synovitis of the hip: a comprehensive review. J Pediatr Orthop B. 2014;23(1):32–6.
27. Teh J, Wilson D. Imaging of the irritable hip and hip infection. In: Davies AM, Johnson K, Whitehouse RW, editors. Imaging of the hip & bony pelvis: techniques and applications. Medical radiology diagnostic imaging. Berlin/New York: Springer; 2006. p. 141–57.
28. Ranson MDE, Babyn PS. The joints. In: Slovis TL, Caffey J, editors. Caffey's pediatric diagnostic imaging. 11th ed. Philadelphia: Mosby/Elsevier; 2008. p. 3013–48.
29. Plumb J, Mallin M, Bolte RG. The role of ultrasound in the emergency department evaluation of the acutely painful pediatric hip. Pediatr Emerg Care. 2015;31(1):54–8; quiz 9–61.
30. Pauroso S, Di Martino A, Tarantino CC, Capone F. Transient synovitis of the hip: ultrasound appearance. Mini-pictorial essay. J Ultrasound. 2011;14(2):92–4.
31. Seltzer SE, Finberg HJ, Weissman BN. Arthrosonography – technique, sonographic anatomy, and pathology. Investig Radiol. 1980;15(1):19–28.
32. Kang YR, Koo J. Ultrasonography of the pediatric hip and spine. Ultrasonography. 2017;36(3):239–51.
33. Guille JT, Lipton GE, Szoke G, Bowen JR, Harcke HT, Glutting JJ. Legg-Calve-Perthes disease in girls. A comparison of the results with those seen in boys. J Bone Joint Surg Am. 1998;80(9):1256–63.
34. Kayser R, Franke J, Mahlfeld K. Value of ultrasound diagnosis in Legg-Calve-Perthes disease. Praxis. 2003;92(24):1123–7.
35. Averill LW, Thacker MM. Avascular necrosis. In: Stein-Wexler R, Wootton-Gorges SL, Ozonoff MB, editors. Pediatric orthopedic imaging. Berlin/Heidelberg: Springer; 2015. p. 332–48.
36. Doria AS, Guarniero R, Cunha FG, Modena M, De Godoy RM Jr, Luzo C, et al. Contrast-enhanced power Doppler sonography: assessment of revascularization flow in Legg-Calve-Perthes' disease. Ultrasound Med Biol. 2002;28(2):171–82.
37. Erken EH, Katz K. Irritable hip and Perthes' disease. J Pediatr Orthop. 1990;10(3):322–6.
38. Martinoli C, Garello I, Marchetti A, Palmieri F, Altafini L, Valle M, et al. Hip ultrasound. Eur J Radiol. 2012;81(12):3824–31.
39. Robben SG, Meradji M, Diepstraten AF, Hop WC. US of the painful hip in childhood: diagnostic value of cartilage thickening and muscle atrophy in the detection of Perthes disease. Radiology. 1998;208(1):35–42.
40. Wirth T, LeQuesne GW, Paterson DC. Ultrasonography in Legg-Calvé-Perthes disease. Pediatr Radiol. 1992;22(7):498–504.
41. Leone A, Cassar-Pullicino VN, Perez MH, Guglielmi G. Emergency and trauma of the pelvic ring. Semin Musculoskelet Radiol. 2017;21(3):210–7.
42. Piccolo CL, Galluzzo M, Trinci M, Ianniello S, Tonerini M, Brunese L, et al. Lower limbs trauma in pediatrics. Semin Musculoskelet Radiol. 2017;21(03):175–83.
43. Pisacano RM, Miller TT. Comparing sonography with MR imaging of apophyseal injuries of the pelvis in four boys. Am J Roentgenol. 2003;181(1):223–30.
44. Vanhoenacker F, Jans L, Boutry N. The pediatric hip. In: Kramer J, Karantanas AH, editors. MRI of the hip. Horn: Breitenseher Publisher; 2016. p. 217–38.
45. Hogan KA, Gross RH. Overuse injuries in pediatric athletes. Orthop Clin North Am. 2003;34(3):405–15.
46. Sanders TG, Zlatkin MB. Avulsion injuries of the pelvis. Semin Musculoskelet Radiol. 2008;12(1):42–53.
47. Rossi F, Dragoni S. Acute avulsion fractures of the pelvis in adolescent competitive athletes: prevalence, location and sports distribution of 203 cases collected. Skelet Radiol. 2001;30(3):127–31.
48. Stevens MA, El-Khoury GY, Kathol MH, Brandser EA, Chow S. Imaging features of avulsion injuries. Radiographics. 1999;19(3):655–72.
49. Morley N, Grant T, Blount K, Omar I. Sonographic evaluation of athletic pubalgia. Skelet Radiol. 2016;45(5):689–99.
50. Pedret C, Balius R, Barcelo P, Miguel M, Lluis A, Valle X, et al. Isolated tears of the gracilis muscle. Am J Sports Med. 2011;39(5):1077–80.
51. Robinson P, Barron DA, Parsons W, Grainger AJ, Schilders EM, O'Connor PJ. Adductor-related groin pain in athletes: correlation of MR imaging with clinical findings. Skelet Radiol. 2004;33(8):451–7.
52. Hegazi TM, Belair JA, McCarthy EJ, Roedl JB, Morrison WB. Sports injuries about the hip: what the radiologist should know. Radiographics. 2016;36(6):1717–45.
53. Kong A, Van der Vliet A, Zadow S. MRI and US of gluteal tendinopathy in greater trochanteric pain syndrome. Eur Radiol. 2007;17(7):1772–83.

54. Hirschmann A, Falkowski AL, Kovacs B. Greater trochanteric pain syndrome: abductors, external rotators. Semin Musculoskelet Radiol. 2017;21(5):539–46.
55. Connell DA, Bass C, Sykes CA, Young D, Edwards E. Sonographic evaluation of gluteus medius and minimus tendinopathy. Eur Radiol. 2003;13(6):1339–47.
56. Khoury V, Cardinal É. Dynamic sonography of joints and soft tissues. Ultrasound Clin. 2007;2(4):699–709.
57. Pelsser V, Cardinal E, Hobden R, Aubin B, Lafortune M. Extraarticular snapping hip: sonographic findings. AJR Am J Roentgenol. 2001;176(1):67–73.
58. Choi YS, Lee SM, Song BY, Paik SH, Yoon YK. Dynamic sonography of external snapping hip syndrome. J Ultrasound Med. 2002;21(7):753–8.
59. Janzen DL, Partridge E, Logan PM, Connell DG, Duncan CP. The snapping hip: clinical and imaging findings in transient subluxation of the iliopsoas tendon. Can Assoc Radiol J. 1996;47(3):202–8.
60. Khoury V, Cardinal É, Bureau NJ. Musculoskeletal sonography: a dynamic tool for usual and unusual disorders. Am J Roentgenol. 2007;188(1):W63–73.
61. Kramer J, Karantanas AH. Snapping hip (Coxa Saltans). In: Kramer J, Karantanas AH, editors. MRI of the hip. Breitenseher Publisher; 2016. p. 217–38.
62. Flato R, Passanante GJ, Skalski MR, Patel DB, White EA, Matcuk GR Jr. The iliotibial tract: imaging, anatomy, injuries, and other pathology. Skelet Radiol. 2017;46(5):605–22.
63. Piechota M, Maczuch J, Skupiński J, Kukawska-Sysio K, Wawrzynek W. Internal snapping hip syndrome in dynamic ultrasonography. J Ultrason. 2016;16(66):296–303.
64. Schmaranzer F, Todorski IAS, Lerch TD, Schwab J, Cullmann-Bastian J, Tannast M. Intra-articular lesions: imaging and surgical correlation. Semin Musculoskelet Radiol. 2017;21(5):487–506.
65. Sutter R, Pfirrmann CWA. Update on femoroacetabular impingement: what is new, and how should we assess it? Semin Musculoskelet Radiol. 2017;21(5):518–28.
66. Schueller-Weidekamm C, Teh J. Inflammatory conditions of the hip. Semin Musculoskelet Radiol. 2017;21(05):589–603.
67. Kramer J, Karantanas AH. Hip osteoarthritis: what every radiologist wants to know. In: Kramer J, Karantanas AH, editors. MRI of the hip. Breitenseher Publisher; 2016. p. 217–38.
68. Miller TT. Common tendon and muscle injuries: lower extremity. Ultrasound Clin. 2007;2(4):595–615.
69. Peetrons P. Ultrasound of muscles. Eur Radiol. 2002;12(1):35–43.
70. Zamorani MP, Valle M. Muscles and tendons. In: Bianchi S, Martinoli C, editors. Ultrasound of the musculoskeletal system. Berlin/Heidelberg: Springer; 2007.
71. Kransdorf MJ, Meis JM, Jelinek JS. Myositis ossificans: MR appearance with radiologic-pathologic correlation. AJR Am J Roentgenol. 1991;157(6):1243–8.
72. McCarthy EF, Sundaram M. Heterotopic ossification: a review. Skelet Radiol. 2005;34(10):609–19.
73. Davis KW. Imaging of the hamstrings. Semin Musculoskelet Radiol. 2008;12(1):28–41.
74. Bianchi S, Martinoli C, Waser NP, Bianchi-Zamorani MP, Federici E, Fasel J. Central aponeurosis tears of the rectus femoris: sonographic findings. Skelet Radiol. 2002;31(10):581–6.
75. Mukherjee K, Perrin SM, Hughes PM. Morel-Lavallee lesion in an adolescent with ultrasound and MRI correlation. Skelet Radiol. 2007;36(Suppl 1):S43–5.
76. Chokshi FH, Jose J, Clifford PD. Morel-Lavallee lesion. Am J Orthop (Belle Mead NJ). 2010;39(5):252–3.
77. Zamorani MP, Valle M. Bones and joints. In: Bianchi S, Martinoli C, editors. Ultrasound of the musculoskeletal system. Berlin/Heidelberg: Springer; 2007.
78. Schmit P, Glorion C. Osteomyelitis in infants and children. Eur Radiol. 2004;14(Suppl 4):L44–54.
79. Mossa-Basha M, van Holsbeeck M. Musculoskeletal Infection. Ultrasound Clin. 2007;2(4):639–53.
80. Blickman JG, van Die CE, de Rooy JW. Current imaging concepts in pediatric osteomyelitis. Eur Radiol. 2004;14(Suppl 4):L55–64.
81. Robben SG. Ultrasonography of musculoskeletal infections in children. Eur Radiol. 2004;14(Suppl 4):L65–77.
82. Wilson DJ. Soft tissue and joint infection. Eur Radiol. 2004;14(Suppl 3):E64–71.
83. Fornage BD. Soft tissue masses: the underutilization of sonography. Semin Musculoskelet Radiol. 1999;3(02):115–33.
84. Beggs I. Ultrasound of soft tissue masses. Imaging. 2002;14(3):202–8.
85. Bodner G, Schocke MFH, Rachbauer F, Seppi K, Peer S, Fierlinger A, et al. Differentiation of malignant and benign musculoskeletal tumors: combined color and power Doppler US and spectral wave analysis. Radiology. 2002;223(2):410–6.
86. Adler RS, Hwang S. Sonographic evaluation of the musculoskeletal soft tissue masses. Ultrasound Clin. 2007;2(4):683–97.
87. Paltiel HJ, Burrows PE, Kozakewich HP, Zurakowski D, Mulliken JB. Soft-tissue vascular anomalies: utility of US for diagnosis. Radiology. 2000;214(3):747–54.
88. Wagner JM, Lee KS, Rosas H, Kliewer MA. Accuracy of sonographic diagnosis of superficial masses. J Ultrasound Med. 2013;32(8):1443–50.
89. Inampudi P, Jacobson JA, Fessell DP, Carlos RC, Patel SV, Delaney-Sathy LO, et al. Soft-tissue lipomas: accuracy of sonography in diagnosis with pathologic correlation. Radiology. 2004;233(3):763–7.
90. Fornage BD, Tassin GB. Sonographic appearances of superficial soft tissue lipomas. J Clin Ultrasound. 1991;19(4):215–20.
91. Reynolds DL, Jacobson JA, Inampudi P, Jamadar DA, Ebrahim FS, Hayes CW. Sonographic characteristics of peripheral nerve sheath tumors. Am J Roentgenol. 2004;182(3):741–4.
92. Craig JG. Ultrasound of ligaments and bone. Ultrasound Clin. 2007;2(4):617–37.
93. Shiels WE. Soft tissue foreign bodies: sonographic diagnosis and therapeutic management. Ultrasound Clin. 2007;2(4):669–81.

94. Olsen SF, Blom HC, Rosendahl K. Introducing universal ultrasound screening for developmental dysplasia of the hip doubled the treatment rate. Acta Paediatr. 2018;107(2):255–61. https://doi.org/10.1111/apa.14057. Epub 5 Oct 2017.
95. Gelfer P, Kennedy KA. Developmental dysplasia of the hip. J Pediatr Health Care. 2008;22(5):318–22.
96. Wright J, James K. Developmental dysplasia of the hip. In: Aresti NA, Ramachandran M, Paterson MJMH, Barry M, editors. Paediatric orthopaedics in clinical practice. 1st ed. London: Springer; 2016. p. 69–90.
97. Shaw BA, Segal LS, Section On Orthopaedics. Evaluation and referral for developmental dysplasia of the hip in infants. Pediatrics. 2016;138(6). pii: e20163107.
98. Clinical practice guideline: early detection of developmental dysplasia of the hip. Pediatrics. 2000;105(4):896–905.
99. Molini L, Precerutti M, Gervasio A, Draghi F, Bianchi S. Hip: anatomy and US technique. J Ultrasound. 2011;14(2):99–108.
100. Ponseti IV. Growth and development of the acetabulum in the normal child. Anatomical, histological, and roentgenographic studies. J Bone Joint Surg Am. 1978;60(5):575–85.
101. Ömeroğlu H. Use of ultrasonography in developmental dysplasia of the hip. J Child Orthop. 2014;8(2):105–13.
102. American Institute of Ultrasound in Medicine. AIUM practice guideline for the performance of an ultrasound examination for detection and assessment of developmental dysplasia of the hip. J Ultrasound Med. 2013;32(7):1307–17.
103. Graf R. Hip sonography. Diagnosis and management of infant hip dysplasia. 2nd ed. Berlin: Springer; 2006.
104. Zucker EJ, Lee EY, Restrepo R, Eisenberg RL. Hip disorders in children. Am J Roentgenol. 2013;201(6):W776–W96.
105. Dipietro MA, Harcke T. Developmental dysplasia of the hip. In: Slovis TL, Caffey J, editors. Caffey's pediatric diagnostic imaging. 11th ed. Philadelphia: Mosby/Elsevier; 2008. p. 3049–66.
106. Harcke HT. Imaging methods used for children with hip dysplasia. Clin Orthop Relat Res (1976–2007). 2005;434:71–7.
107. Sewell MD, Rosendahl K, Eastwood DM. Developmental dysplasia of the hip. BMJ. 2009;339:b4454.
108. Shorter D, Hong T, Osborn DA. Cochrane review: screening programmes for developmental dysplasia of the hip in newborn infants. Evid Based Child Health. 2013;8(1):11–54.

Knee and Leg

10

Adham Aboul Fotouh Khalil and
C. Hernández-Díaz

Introduction

Ultrasound is now a very useful tool to assess different joints and soft tissue areas. The knee joint and the surrounding soft tissue are no exception. Ultrasound provides very practically important plethora of information about this joint and region and is very practical to use especially in soft tissue examination with much less hazards and negative aspects compared to the other imaging modalities.

This chapter will discuss the importance of ultrasound in the knee and leg, together with description of the normal sonoanatomy and the most commonly encountered pathological findings.

The knee is a clinically accessible joint to review, and the use of imaging techniques to assess it depends on a more specific diagnostic indication as previously reported [1].

Knee anatomy is complex in the early stages of development because it contains a lot of cartilage and support structures that are still developing.

Ultrasonography (US) of the knee is simple and provides sufficient elements for the evaluation to determine damage of joint structures or soft tissues.

Normal Anatomy and Variants

Knee

Children knee is characterized by strong structures that provide stability and specialized movement to the thigh and the leg.

Extensor mechanism of the knee is provided by the quadriceps muscle group; these are formed by the rectus femoris muscle superficially, followed by the three vasti (medial, lateral, and intermedialis) muscles, which lie deeper to the rectus femoris, and are attached at the end to the medial or lateral margins of the rectus femoris to the patella, contributing to patellar stability. Also, the rectus femoris muscle contributes with anterior fibers to the attachment in the main body of the patellar tendon [2]. This contribution requires the presence of the largest sesamoid bone of the body, the patella, which is a cartilaginous structure in the early years of life, that ossifies between the age of 4–7 years; its ossification is fragmented in three facets that are not clearly seen; the medial one drives a change of patellar fibers orientation that eventually lead its way until the insertion in the tibial tuberosity. The patellar tendon is flat

A. A. F. Khalil (✉)
Egyptian School for Musculoskeletal Ultrasonography, Cairo, Egypt

C. Hernández-Díaz
Musculoskeletal ultrasound Laboratory, Instituto Nacional de Rehabilitación "luis Guillermo Ibarra Ibarra", Mexico city, Mexico
e-mail: cristy_hernandez@prodigy.net.mx

Y. El Miedany (ed.), *Pediatric Musculoskeletal Ultrasonography*,
https://doi.org/10.1007/978-3-030-17824-6_10

during the childhood, and its ossification in the adolescence can have more than one ossification centers [2], which may lead to different lesions.

At birth then shortly after vascularization of the meniscus takes place, but it decreases with growing until it almost disappears at the age of 10, maintaining blood vessels and nerves only in the peripheries [3].

There is scarce information related to other anatomical structures in the knee that have been studied or could change its aspect from childhood to adult; however, it is important to remember that there are some variants or incomplete forms especially in stabilizing structures such as the menisci [4], collateral ligaments, and popliteal ligaments.

Leg and Calf

There is no difference between the children and the adult anatomy; large bones are still developing, and ossification centers will be found at the margins, disappearing by the adolescence.

The importance in this region lies in the complex anatomy that could lead to vascular and nerve problems. In the muscular aspect, the distribution of the muscle structures determines the pathology in the area due to its distribution and biomechanical function, especially for fractures displacement and compartment syndrome [5].

Tibia ossifies from three centers, the proximal one is already present at birth, the second one appears around 12 years and soon fuses with the epiphysis; the distal appears around the first year of life and both proximal and distal epiphysis fuses at around 15 or 16 years [5]. Tibia is poorly covered by soft tissue, and it's predisposed to injuries easily.

On the other side, the fibula is not that complicated as the tibia, but each of its borders is associated with a particular group of muscles.

There are three main compartments in the leg: the anterior (extensor), the lateral (peroneal), and the posterior (flexor); each is enclosed by the deep fascia and separated by the bones and the interosseous membrane. These compartments can be also studied as two space compartments (anterolateral and posteromedial) according to its location with respect to the fascia and/or to its function.

Muscles in the leg consist of a group of extensors muscles that causes dorsiflexion of the ankle, a flexor muscle group that causes plantar flexion, and a lateral group that contributes to the walking mechanism.

The extensor mechanism is given by the extensor hallucis and common extensor tendons which continue to the foot and help during walking; with the contribution of the tibialis anterior and peroneus tertius, both also contribute to inversion and eversion mechanism, respectively.

The lateral compartment contains the peroneus brevis and peroneus longus muscles. Both evert the foot and do a plantar flexion of the ankle. Both muscles make a gap in which the peroneal nerve passes.

Finally, the posterior compartment is larger than the anterolateral, and its muscles are more powerful than the others. Due to its location, it is composed by deep and superficial muscles, separated by the transverse fascia. The superficial group is the gastrocnemius (medial and lateral), soleus, and the plantaris muscles. All of them contribute to plantar flexion of the foot, and the soleus is the only muscle related solely to the ankle because the others contribute to both ankle and knee movements.

The deep flexor group is formed by the popliteus in the proximal tibia acting as a knee rotator helping to stabilize the knee; and the flexor digitorum longus, flexor hallucis longus, and tibialis posterior muscles all of them act as plantar flexors of the ankle [5].

Ultrasound

The US of an infant's knee is relatively easy and can show musculoskeletal structures with great clarity. It is a good method to evaluate cartilaginous structures in the immature bone. Epiphysis appearance depends on the stage of ossification and is seen as a homogeneous hypoechoic or anechoic linear structure. Epiphyseal cartilage has a separate blood supply and vessels that can be evaluated with Doppler. The growth plate is clearly seen as an interruption of the bony cortex [6] and cannot be confused with fractures or erosions.

A short, thin, and densely hyperechoic reflection is noted consistently at the medial aspect of the distal femur representing the perichondral ring, a dense band of ossified connective tissue which helps support the cartilaginous epiphysis. The osseous/cartilaginous interface appears as a relatively sharp, thin, and hyperechoic line. The speckled, hypoechoic cartilage comprising the femoral condyles and tibial plateau is similar in its sonographic pattern to cartilage seen at other large joints in infants, like the femoral head [7].

Tendons are seen like in the adult, with a fibrillar hyperechoic structure; paratenon is seen as an undefined hypoechoic tissue surrounding the tendon margin [8]. Patellar tendon can readily be followed from the cartilaginous, hypoechoic tibial tuberosity to the patellae, the end of the quadriceps muscle [7, 9]. As cartilaginous content is abundant until adolescence, structures can be seen better than in adults.

Equipment, Technique, and Sonoanatomy

Knee

US equipment with musculoskeletal software is needed, linear transducers with 12–18 MHz are enough to evaluate the joint, but if hockey stick probe is available, it can be used.

The scanning technique does not differ from that suggested for adults [10, 11], but special considerations should be considered.

To begin, the child should be placed in a lying in a supine position with the knee flexed at 30°. The probe is placed midline sagittal on the thigh, with the distal end of the probe on the superior pole of the patella [12]. This position makes it easy to visualize the quadriceps tendon with a fibrillar pattern. A little amount of fluid can normally be seen in the suprapatellar recess as well as the bursa; both will be visualized as anechoic and be compressible. The patella in younger children is completely anechoic as an oval structure; sometimes, it will show tiny echoes according to child's age (Fig. 10.1).

Continuing with the examination, the knee is now flexed at 45° to scan the patellar tendon, and the probe is placed over the inferior pole of the patella and perpendicular to the tendon to visualize the enthesis [11]. The patellar tendon as in the adult will visualize fibrillar, but in the distal patella, this pattern could extend further according to the age of the child and ossification grade of the tibial plateau.

Then, the child is asked to fully extend the knee, to explore the medial and lateral recesses. The probe is placed in transverse view to look at the recess, one end of the probe is placed on the patella and the other on the femur condyle (medial or lateral); an anechoic image is seen particularly in the lateral recess, representing a little amount of fluid; normally in the medial aspect, a compact laminar band is seen representing the patellar retinaculum. The lateral retinaculum is not as compact and sometimes is difficult to differentiate from the adjacent soft tissues. In children, there are no data concerning imaging or anatomic descriptions of these structures [12, 13] (Fig. 10.2).

Then, a rational scanning of the medial and lateral regions should be performed, scanning and position are the same as in adults, but probably visual differentiation of the structures will be difficult due to the femoral and tibia cartilaginous structures especially in young children (Figs. 10.3 and 10.4).

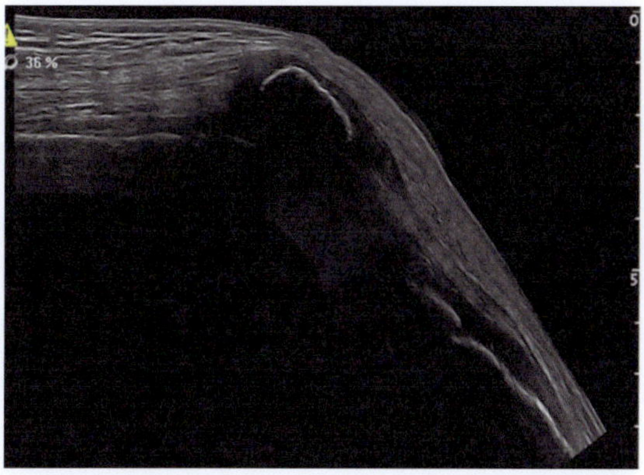

Fig. 10.1 Panoramic view of the anterior scanning in a normal knee of a 7-year-old child. Patella is ossified. Cortical in the tibial bone is in an ossified process

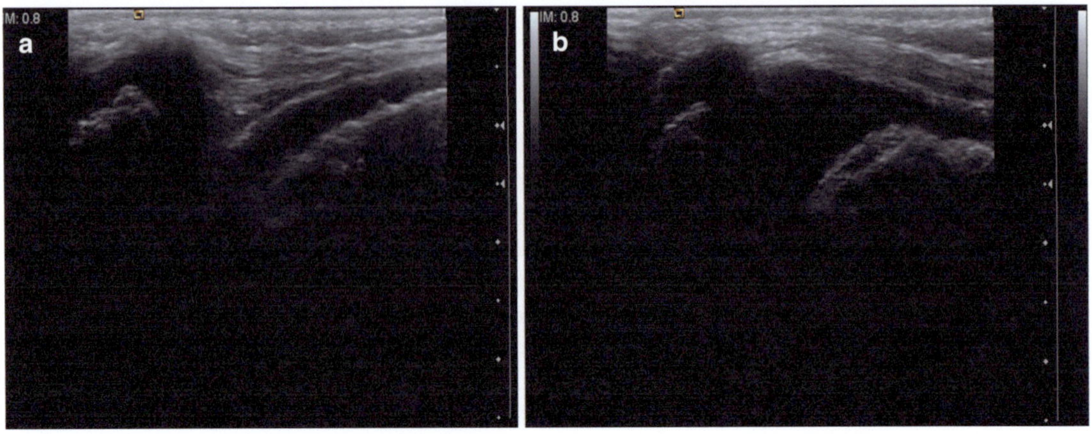

Fig. 10.2 (**a**) Medial recess in the knee, the patellar ligament is visible in its trilaminar aspect without fluid. (**b**) Lateral recess with a little amount of normal fluid. Both femoral cartilages are in ossifying process, and cartilage is seen hypoechoic and heterogeneous

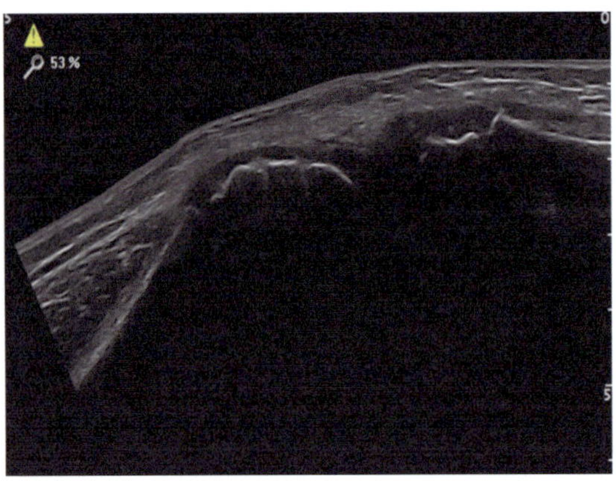

Fig. 10.3 Panoramic view of the medial region

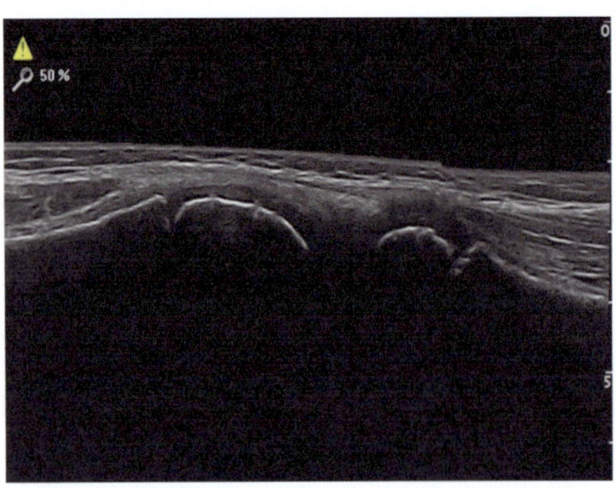

Fig. 10.4 Panoramic view of the lateral region

The posterior aspect is evaluated ideally with the child lying in a prone position with the foot out of the bed. The main structures to evaluate include the vascular and nerve bundle in the popliteal region, and there is a little possibility to find a bursa since the gastrocnemius-semimembranosus bursa develops in the adulthood [14], but sometimes, we can see a little amount of fluid in a newly developed bursa.

Leg and Calf

US scanning of the anterior leg muscles needs the patient to be in supine position, with the leg in a slight internal rotation. The US could begin in transverse view in order to easily locate muscle belly and tibial cortical bone [8]. Muscle is seen as in adults, with a relatively hypoechoic background reflecting the muscle fascicles and linear hyperechoic bands which clearly delimitated the perimysium; in transverse view, the typical image of small dot-like reflectors in a hypoechoic basis is the normal image [8].

US scanning must take into consideration the pennate organization and orientation of each muscle, in order to perform a clear and organized scanning. Most of the muscles have an oblique plane, and in the anterior compartment, the fascia is an important structure to evaluate. Intramuscular vessels are often seen and can be evaluated by color and power Doppler. Fascia is hyperechoic and better organized compared to the muscle belly. Dynamic scanning is preferable. During contraction, it can show changes in size and fascicle structure, transversely the muscle appearance is thicker and more hypoechoic; dynamic scanning is especially useful when a muscle hernia is suspected.

Tibialis posterior muscle is deep with a clear circumpennate appearance and lies between the flexor digitorum longus and the flexor hallucis longus, while the peroneus longus is rounded proximally and flat distally.

The peroneal nerve is easily observed in the lateral aspect of the leg, distally, it is more superficial and easier to locate between the peroneus longus and brevis and the extensor digitorum longus belly.

The triceps surae (gastrocnemius and soleus) has a particular anatomy; the gastrocnemius can be seen flat in the distal end of its margins just before the myotendinous junction with the Achilles tendon; the medial gastrocnemius is rounded and thicker and extends more distally than the lateral. The plantaris is thicker and small compared to the gastrocnemius. To evaluate the posterior aspect, patient should lie prone with the foot hanging out of the bed [8].

Pathology

Knee

The US added value is the accessibility to scan all structures in real time during daily practice. Beside inflammation disorders, the US of the knee is capable to detect masses, fractures, infectious diseases, and ligament lesions [15].

Several points must be considered during the scanning, especially that there are more cartilaginous structures than in the adult.

The main indications beside JIA to perform US on the knee and leg are:

- Noninflammatory entheseal pathology (apophysitis)
- Patellar dislocation or sleeve avulsion fracture
- Tendon tears
- Synovial impingement syndrome
- Soft tissue infections and abscesses
- Other tumors or masses in the leg
- Foreign bodies

Noninflammatory Entheseal Pathology

In children and adolescents, it is related to sports in which excessive force is applied to the knee such as Taekwondo, tennis, football, or similar. Pain is characteristic, and development of Osgood-Schlatter disease (OSD) could happen frequently.

OSD develops by a traction apophysitis caused by a repetitive strain of the patellar tendon and an avulsion of the tibial tubercle. Diagnosis is usually clinical. However, radiographic or ultrasound examination is helpful, and the latter can detect the condition early. Maturation stage can be observed together with an abnormal secondary ossification center of the tibial tubercle, which could lead to irregularities in the apophysis up to fragmentation of the tibial tuberosity later. It is important to evaluate the patellar tendon distal enthesis, as well as the cartilage and the apophyseal surface, in which depending on the stage of the disease, maturation and fiber attachment visualization are abnormal [16, 17]. OSD has been classified into three types or stages, in which type I is related to an igloo-like deformation of the internal ossification of the tibial tuberosity, deep infrapatellar bursitis, and changes of the patellar tendon. Type II refers to the fracture of the tibial tuberosity, with deep infrapatellar bursitis and inflammatory changes of the patellar tendon. And type III refers to fracture of the ossification center and an irregular deformation of the tuberosity, deep infrapatellar bursitis, and inflammatory changes in the patellar tendon with or without calcified lesions [18] (Figs. 10.5, 10.6, and 10.7).

Another disease related to sports, frequent in children between 10 and 14 years, is the Sinding-Larsen-Johansson syndrome where a pure osseous lesion in the inferior pole of the patella takes place without major cartilage involvement due to forceful contraction of the patellar tendon against resistance. Differential diagnosis includes the patellar sleeve avulsion in which extensive sleeve cartilage avulsion occurs. Magnetic resonance is the imaging diagnostic technique of choice, but US is also used to distinguish between both lesions. It can also differentiate from OSD by depicting calcified lesions and the deep infrapatellar bursa involvement [19, 20].

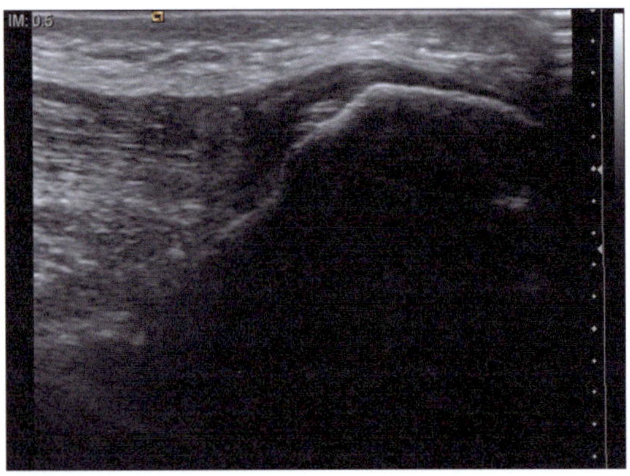

Fig. 10.5 Distal patellar tendon with mild tendon changes and hyperechoic dots in the enthesis in an adolescent practicing Tae Kwon Do

Patellar Instability

Patellar instability is the most common pathology in the knee during growth, the mean peak of incidence is around 15 years and girls are more affected than boys. The medial displacement is the most common, but there are four types of instability depending on the affected structures [21]. The imaging technique used to determine the type and severity of the disease is the plain radiography, then the magnetic resonance, but the US has been used to assess soft tissue-associated lesions and specially to determine the cartilaginous and osseous anatomy, with focus on the morphology of the trochlear groove. US is useful at the beginning to search for acute injury [22].

Patellar Sleeve Avulsion Injuries

This type of fracture is unique because of its pattern in plain radiograph in the immature children. It is different from the patella fractures caused by direct fall.

Patellar fracture occurs in the inferior pole related to an intense mechanism that involves a

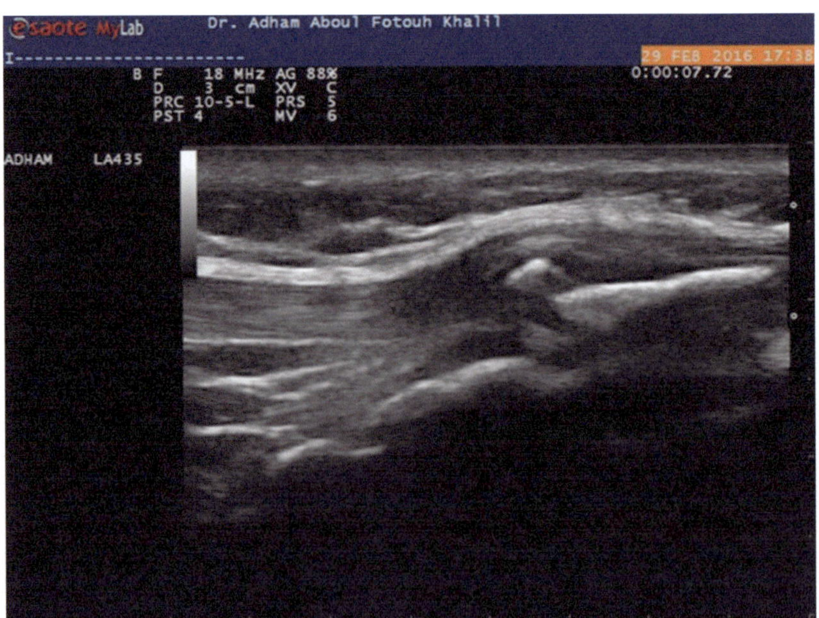

Fig. 10.6 Distal patellar tendon with marked changes at the level of the enthesis in a 13-year-old boy

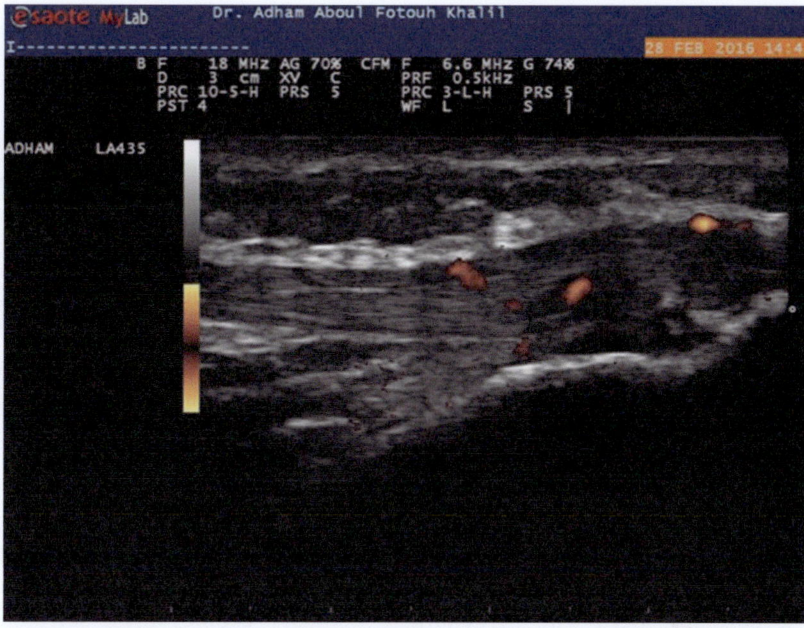

Fig. 10.7 Distal patellar tendon with marked tendon changes and Doppler signal in an adolescent practicing Tae Kwon Do

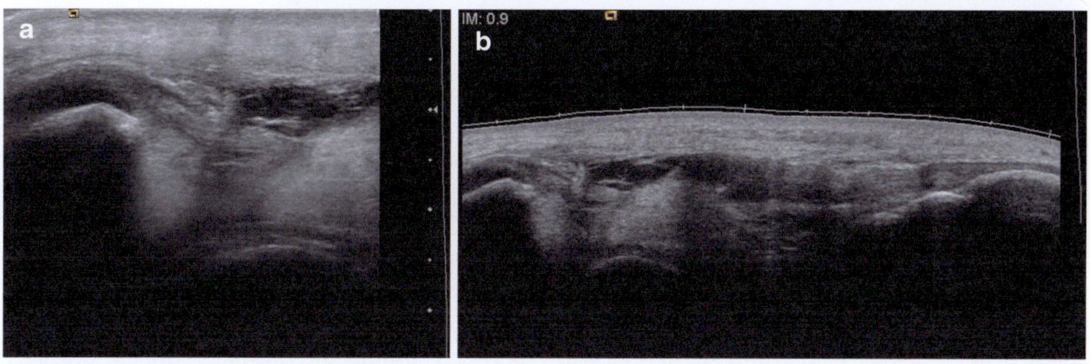

Fig. 10.8 (**a**) Total proximal patellar tendon disruption. (**b**) Panoramic view

high energy that causes a sleeve injury in the periosteum and patellar retinaculum medial or laterally, with a rapid contraction of the quadriceps tendon on a flexed knee, often related to a sport as skateboarding. The sleeve avulsion of the patella bone-forming tissue is from the full circumference of the patella and differentiates from osteochondral fragments because the avulsed tissue may continue to ossify independently. The disruption occurs over the body of the patella and slides distally causing an elongation of the quadriceps mechanism. Thus, rapid diagnosis and imaging are mandatory; radiographic findings are unspecific, and the US is used to demonstrate cartilage or osseous changes in the patella sleeve avulsion injury, as well as quantify the amount of osseous or cartilaginous fragments displacement [22, 23].

Tendon/Ligament Tear

Medial patellofemoral ligament is one of the most affected ligaments in the knee and in children; its lesion is associated in up to 78% with partial or total tear in the insertion site at the proximal pole of the patella in an isolated location. It is frequently related to an avulsion mechanism and, discordant to sleeve avulsion injuries, can be proximal or distal rather than central tear, and it predispose to a high-grade patellar chon-

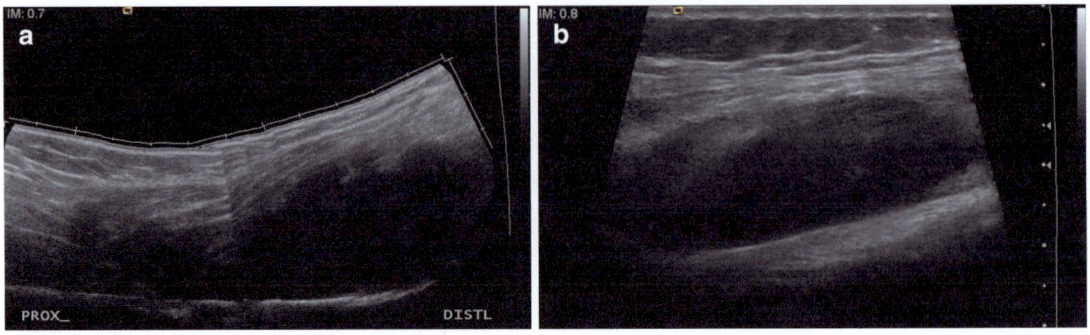

Fig. 10.9 A compose figure of an abscess caused by *S. aureus* in the lateral recess of the knee in an adolescent after a traumatic injury. (**a**) A panoramic view. (**b**) A view of the abscess with hypoechoic hardly compressible content in between the cortical femoral bone and the vastus lateralis muscle

dral lesion [24, 25]. Partial tears are seen as thickening and irregular contour with discontinuity of the fibrillar pattern with peritendinous edema; when the tear is complete, fibrillar pattern is absent, with extensive edema, and more than 5 mm between torn ends at dynamic examination can be observed [26]. Also, US can detect muscle lesions, particularly disruption of the vastus medialis muscle [27] (Fig. 10.8).

Synovial Impingement Syndrome

It is associated again with sports and is a frequent cause of anterior knee pain in athletes; it is caused by Hoffa's fad pad inflammation and patellar tendinosis related to edema and lateral patellar subluxation [28]. There is no much information about image by US because the diagnosis is clinical and by magnetic resonance; but some US studies had reported increases in the Hoffa's fat pad vascularity, especially in the superior lobe and focal inflammatory changes in the patellar tendon structure [29].

Soft Tissue Infections and Abscess

Soft tissue infection usually starts in children due to trauma, and the main organism is *Staphylococcus aureus*. It begins as cellulitis causing a pus collection. By US, it is variable but can be seen with or without a mass effect with a variable echogenic pattern (hypo- to hyperechoic) in the surrounding tissues, with a sharp margin and an echogenic rim accompanied by soft tissue edema with or without Doppler signal; sonographic fluctuation should be sought by a gentle pressure from the transducer or the examiner's hand. Doppler signal is very useful to discriminate between inflammatory and infectious diseases because in the second there is no signal in the content but there is in the surroundings, unfortunately, Doppler is not capable to discriminate from noninfectious collections. Additionally, US can detect fluid collections and abscesses between orthopedic artifacts (metal artifacts) [30] (Fig. 10.9).

Osteomyelitis is the infection of the bone marrow; again, *Staphylococcus aureus* is the common etiology, and then *Streptococcus pyogenes, E. coli*, *Pseudomonas aeruginosa* and *H. influenzae*. Symptoms are age-dependent, and hematogenous route is the most commonly implicated; in infants, the location of the diaphyseal vessels facilitates the pathogen spreading into the growth plate to reach the epiphysis. US can evaluate deep edema and detect subperiostic involvement and thickening, subperiosteal abscess formation and soft tissue inflammation, even several days before radiographs. During the course of the disease, US can evaluate cortical defects; Doppler is useful but just after a few days in which it is able to detect peripheral

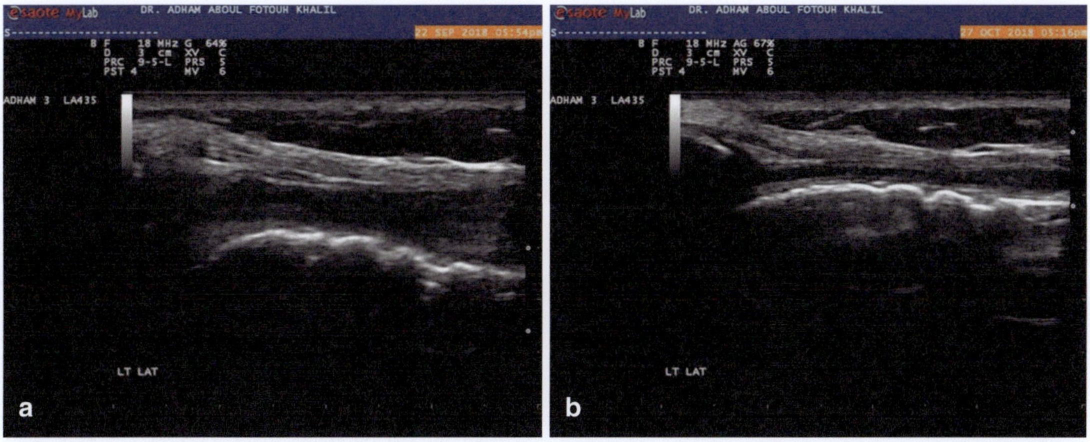

Fig. 10.10 JIA by Grayscale. (**a**) Active disease with synovial effusion and hypertrophy. (**b**) After treatment

hyperemia; in chronic cases, it can also depict cortical defects and fistulas [30–32].

Tumor and Other Masses

Not frequent in the knee, some of the most important tumors as osteochondromas and tenosynovial giant cell tumor begin in young adults or late adolescence, but US is not the gold standard imaging technique to evaluate them.

Foreign Bodies

They are usually associated to puncture wounds, the most frequent location is the plantar aspect of the foot, but sometimes they are related to sports or playing time and can affect the lateral aspect of the leg. In children association with limping is common, and soft tissue infection can be present.

Although US is not sensitive to detect them, it can be specific in determining its nature, especially wooden, plastic, and metal; it can detect the surrounding soft tissue reaction showing a hyperreflective focus with acoustic shadow or reverberation in case of metal; chronically, it can depict a granulomatous reaction with an anechoic halo surrounding the foreign body. Doppler signal can be used to detect metal [30, 32].

Juvenile Idiopathic Arthritis (JIA)

It is reported that juvenile idiopathic arthritis is the most common chronic arthritis affecting pediatric population [33].

Ultrasonography is a practical tool that is useful when combined with the clinical examination.

Some histologically active disease is found in asymptomatic joints [34]. In addition, musculoskeletal ultrasonography can be used in JIA to detect synovitis in clinically normal subjects (subclinical synovitis) [35].

All these points emphasize the particular importance of using musculoskeletal ultrasonography in JIA.

In addition, enthesitis is another phenomenon that can be detected using ultrasonography. Enthesitis was detected in enthesitis-related arthritis, in other categories of JIA, as well as in clinically silent enthesis [36].

OMERACT (Outcome Measures in Rheumatology) gave preliminary definitions in children [37] that included:

- Synovial effusion: abnormal intraarticular hypoechoic displaceable material
- Synovial hypertrophy: abnormal intraarticular hypoechoic nondisplaceable material, and that Doppler signal must be exhibited for the hypertrophy to be considered a sign of synovitis (Fig. 10.10)

Conclusions

Musculoskeletal ultrasound adds to clinical examination. It's handy and can aid in quickly diagnosing pediatric patients without major troubles. In some diseases, it is very sensitive to detect changes in asymptomatic patients and proves useful in classification and treatment decisions, together with follow-up. Remission criteria can be modified to include ultrasound in diseases where it proves useful.

References

1. Magni-Manzoni S, Collado P, Jousse-Jouline S, Naredo E, D'Agostino MA, Muratore V, et al. Current state of musculoskeletal ultrasound in pediatric rheumatology. Results of an international survey. Rheumatology. 2014;53(3):491–6.
2. Dwek JR, Chung CB. The patellar extensor apparatus of the knee. Pediatr Radiol. 2008;38:925–35.
3. Makris EA, Pasha Hadidi BS, Athanasiou KA. The knee meniscus: structure-function, pathophysiology, current repair techniques, and prospects for regeneration. Biomaterials. 2011;32(30):7411–31.
4. Constantine JL. Observations on discoid menisci. J Bone Joint Surg Am. 1950;32(3):649–52.
5. Nevell RLM. Leg. In: Standring S, editor. Gray's anatomy. The anatomical basis of clinical practice. 39th ed. Baltimore: Elsevier Churchill Livingstone; 2006. p. 1489–506.
6. Karmazyn B. Ultrasound of pediatric musculoskeletal disease: from head to toe. Semin Ultrasound CT MRI. 2011;32:142–50.
7. Keller MS. Musculoskeletal sonography in the neonate and infant. Pediatr Radiol. 2005;35:1167–73.
8. Bianchi S, Martinoli C. General: muscle and tendon and, Pediatric applications: pediatric musculoskeletal ultrasound. In: Ultrasound of the musculoskeletal system. Berlin: Springer; 2007. p. 45–96, 921–959.
9. Markowitz RI, Hubbard AM, Harty MP, Bellah RD, Kessler A, Meyer JS. Sonography of the knee in normal and abused infants. Pediatr Radiol. 1993;23(4):264–7.
10. Möller I, Janta J, Backhaus M, Ohrdorf S, Bong DA, Martinoli C. The 2017 EULAR standardized procedures for ultrasound imaging in rheumatology. Ann Rheum Dis. 2017;76:1974–9.
11. Bakchaus M, Burmester GR, Gerber G, Grassi W, Machold KP, Swen WA. Guidelines for musculoskeletal ultrasound in rheumatology. Ann Rheum Dis. 2001;60:641–9.
12. Paz CR, Esperanza, NS. Exploración de la rodilla. En: Médicos SA, Editores. Ecografía de la anatomía infantil. Primer Edición. Madrid: EDIMSA; 2007. p. 26–33.
13. Kim JS, Jong Yun S, Jin W, Young GK, Young Park S, Nam Ryu K. A focal defect at the lateral patellar retinaculum on clinical knee MRI and cadaveric study: a normal variant or pathologic lesion? AJR Am J Roentgenol. 2017;208(5):1103–9.
14. Herman AM, Marzo JM. Popliteal cysts: a current review. Orthopedics. 2014;37(8):e678–84.
15. Collado, Ramos P. Use of ultrasonography in the pediatric patient. In: Wakefield RJ, D'Agostino MA, editors. Essentials applications of musculoskeletal ultrasound in rheumatology. 1st ed. Saunders Elsevier; 2010. p. 207–10.
16. Kaneuchi Y, Otoshi K, Hakozaki M, Sekiguchi M, Watanabe K, Igari T, Konno S. Bony maturity of the tibial tuberosity regard to age and sex and its relationship to pathogenesis of Osgood-Schlatter disease. An ultrasonographic study. Orthop J Sports Med. 2018;6(1):2325967117749184.
17. Ducher G, Cook J, Spurrier D, Coombs P, Ptasznik R, Black J, Bass S. Ultrasound imaging of the patellar tendon attachment to the tibia during puberty: a 12-month follow-up in tennis players. Scand J Med Sci Sports. 2010;20:e35–40.
18. Zbigniew C. Osgood-Schlatter disease in ultrasound diagnostics – a pictorial essay. Med Ultrason. 2010;12(4):323–35.
19. Kuehnast M, Mahomed N, Mistry B. Sinding-Larsen-Johansson syndrome. SAJCH. 2012;6(3):90–2.
20. Patel DR, Villalobos A. Evaluation and management of knee pain in young athletes: overuse injuries of the knee. Transl Pediatr. 2017;6(3):190–8.
21. Hasler CC, Studer D. Patella instability in children and adolescent. EFORT Open Rev. 2016;1. https://doi.org/10.1302/2058-5241.1.000018.
22. Maloney E, Stanescu AL, Ngo AV, Parisi MT, Iyer RS. The pediatric patella: normal development, anatomical variants and malformations, stability, imaging, and injury patterns. Semin Musculoskelet Radiol. 2018;22:81–94.
23. Hunt DM, Somashekar N. A review of sleeve fractures of the patella in children. Knee. 2005;12(1):3–7.
24. Leschied JR, Gaetke Udager K. Imaging of the pediatric knee. Semin Musculoskelet Radiol. 2017;21:137–46.
25. Zhang G, Zheng L, Shi H, Ji B, Feng Y, Ding H. Injury patterns of medial patellofemoral ligament after acute lateral patellar dislocation in children: correlation analysis with anatomical variants and articular cartilage lesion of the patella. Eur Radiol. 2017;27(3):1322–30.
26. Zhang G, Zheng L, Ding H, Li E, Sun B, Shi H. Evaluation of medial patellofemoral ligament tears after acute lateral patella dislocation: comparison of high-frequency ultrasound and MR. Eur Radiol. 2015;25(1):274–81.
27. Trihka SP, Acton D, O'Reilly M, Curtis MJ, Bell J. Acute lateral dislocation of the patella: correlation of ultrasound scanning with operative findings. Injury. 2003;34(8):568–71.

28. O'Dell C, Jaramillo D, Bancroft L, Varich L, Longsdon G, Servaes S. Imaging of sports related injuries of the lower extremity in pediatric patients. Radiographics. 2016;36:1807–27.
29. Mikkilineni H, Delzel BP, Andrish J, Bullen J, Obuchowski NA, Subhas N, et al. Ultrasound evaluation of infrapatellar fat pad impingement: an exploratory prospective study. Knee. 2018;25(2):279–85.
30. Robben SGF. Ultrasonography of musculoskeletal infections in children. Eur Radiol. 2004;14:L65–77.
31. Garcés-Iñigo EF, Guasp Vizcaino M, Gomez Fernandez-Montes J. Musculoskeletal imaging in pediatrics emergencies: the basics through three clinical scenarios. Radiologia. 2016;58(Suppl 2):104–18.
32. Chaturvedi A, Cain U, Rupasov A. The acutely limping school and school-age child: an imaging perspective. Semin Musculoskelet Radiol. 2018;22: 46–56.
33. Ravelli A, Martini A. Juvenile idiopathic arthritis. Lancet. 2007;369:767–78.
34. Wakefield RJ, Green MJ, Marzo-Ortega H, Conaghan PG, Gibbon WW, McGonagle D, et al. Should oligoarthritis be reclassified? Ultrasound reveals a high prevalence of subclinical disease. Ann Rheum Dis. 2004;63:382–5.
35. Magni-Manzoni S, Epis O, Ravelli A, Klersy C, Veisconti C, Lanni S, Muratore V, Sciré CA, Rossi S, Montecucco C. Comparison of clinical versus ultrasound-determined synovitis in juvenile idiopathic arthritis. Arthritis Rheum. 2009;61:1497–504. https://doi.org/10.1002/art.24823.
36. Jousse-Joulin S, Breton S, Cangemi C, Fenoll B, Bressolette L, de Parscau L, Saraux A, Devauchelle-Pensec V. Ultrasonography for detecting enthesitis in juvenile idiopathic arthritis. Arthritis Care Res. 2011;63:849–55. https://doi.org/10.1002/acr.20444.
37. Roth J, Ravagnani V, Backhaus M, Balint P, Bruns A, Bruyn GA et al., Omeract Ultrasound Group. Preliminary definitions for the sonographic features of synovitis in children. Arthritis Care Res (Hoboken). 2016;16. https://doi.org/10.1002/acr.23130.

Ankle and Foot

11

Johannes Roth

Introduction

If there was one joint for which ultrasonography was made, it would be the foot and ankle region. It represents a complex anatomic area consisting of multiple joints as well as many tendons and entheses all of which can be affected by inflammatory changes as part of Juvenile Idiopathic Arthritis (JIA) [1, 2]. The ankle is the second most commonly affected joint in JIA further underlining the relevance of this area [3]. In addition, there are many other pathologies that can cause similar symptoms as inflammatory changes and need to be differentiated from findings related to JIA. Ultrasonography is uniquely positioned to provide crucial information – if desired at the point of care – in order to enhance the clinical assessment and provide a detailed diagnosis in real time.

Inflammatory lesions of the tibiotalar, subtalar, midfoot, and toe joints as well as tenosynovial changes can be demonstrated reliably with ultrasonography when technical standards are applied carefully. For the entheses ultrasonography due to its spatial resolution and detailed depiction can be superior to other imaging techniques including MRI [4]. The involvement of the various structures in JIA is highly variable, and patients may present with different combinations of synovitis and tenosynovitis. In one study a majority of JIA patients with swollen ankles in the oligoarticular group did not have any synovitis but tenosynovitis instead [1]. It is tempting to speculate that this variable pattern of structures affected by inflammation might explain why patients undergoing ankle injections are twice as likely to have an insufficient response or relapse early compared to patients receiving intraarticular knee injections [3].

Some areas of the ankle, due to the complexity with several bones as reference points and various structures potentially affected by inflammation can be relatively challenging to scan especially in younger children with incomplete ossification. It is therefore essential to understand the process of ossification but also the anatomy of the ankle overall in order to obtain the desired information reliably. I would very much encourage the sonographer to not separate the anatomic knowledge, physical exam, and ultrasonography but instead have a visual perception of the anatomic structures while examining this region clinically and then let the ultrasonographic assessment be guided by the clinical exam in turn. It is important to pay particular attention to the palpation of crucial anatomic landmarks before putting the probe on the patient and to ensure that the patient/the anatomic area in

J. Roth (✉)
University of Ottawa, Ottawa, ON, Canada

Division of Pediatric Dermatology and Rheumatology, Children's Hospital of Eastern Ontario, Ottawa, ON, Canada
e-mail: jroth@cheo.on.ca

Y. El Miedany (ed.), *Pediatric Musculoskeletal Ultrasonography*,
https://doi.org/10.1007/978-3-030-17824-6_11

question as well as the examiner are positioned in an optimal way to assess it. In the following I will start with a short review of the ossification process of the ankle and foot and then continue with the sonoanatomy followed by a review of relevant pathologic findings.

Ossification of the Ankle and Foot

From an imaging point of view, it is important to remember that depending on the age of the child, a significant part of what later becomes the bone or the bony portion of an enthesis is still composed of hyaline cartilage as well as fibrocartilage (in the case of the enthesis) and will therefore appear hypo- or anechoic on US [5]. The details of the enthesis, which is really considered an entheseal organ including bone, hyaline cartilage, fibrocartilage, fat, bursae, as well as the tendon, cannot be covered in detail in this chapter [6]. It is nevertheless fascinating to see how the development of these various tissues changes the imaging properties of a given anatomical region throughout childhood and adolescence. This is especially true for apophyseal regions and for the ankle region can be especially well observed at the Achilles tendon insertion [7] further detailed below. The progress of ossification is also dependent on gender and within the same gender on the degree of maturation, i.e., the pubertal stages. It has to be noted though, that especially inflammatory diseases like JIA can lead to a significant alteration of these time points, often in fact an acceleration of maturation of an affected skeletal area [8].

Ossification of the distal tibia and fibula starts early with the secondary ossification centers in both epiphyses appearing in the second year of life (Fig. 11.1). From an imaging point of view, it is important to know when scanning the medial and lateral ankle that the medial and lateral malleolus remain cartilaginous much longer. Ossification will be almost complete in these two areas by the age of 12 years only.

Ossification of the bones of the ankle and foot occurs and progresses at variable rates. It starts very early in the talus, calcaneus and cuboid bone

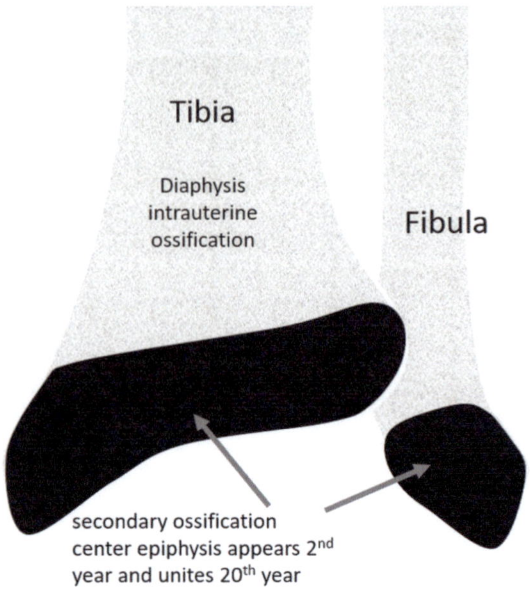

Fig. 11.1 Ossification of the distal tibia and fibula. Secondary epiphyseal ossifications centers are shown in black

during intrauterine life (Fig. 11.2), but parts of these bones will ossify later.

The clinically relevant areas are the posterior talus where a secondary ossification center can be present and sometimes show non-union with the main bone which is called an os trigonum. It also affects portions of the lateral talus which serve as reference points for the subtalar joint. For the calcaneus the sustentaculum tali may show significant amounts of cartilage until fairly late which needs to be differentiated from an effusion originating from the subtalar joint [5, 7, 9]. A significant portion of the lateral calcaneus will be unossified in younger children, making the assessment of the posterior subtalar joint more challenging. At the posterior calcaneus, a variable amount of hyaline cartilage is present, and the main ossification center will show significant changes of shape during maturation. In addition, fibrocartilage will be present at the posterior calcaneus as well as a secondary ossification center at the insertion of the Achilles tendon. This secondary ossification center can be fragmented physiologically. The ossification of the posterior calcaneus is as follows: (A) from 2 months to 3 years, no ossification of the secondary center of

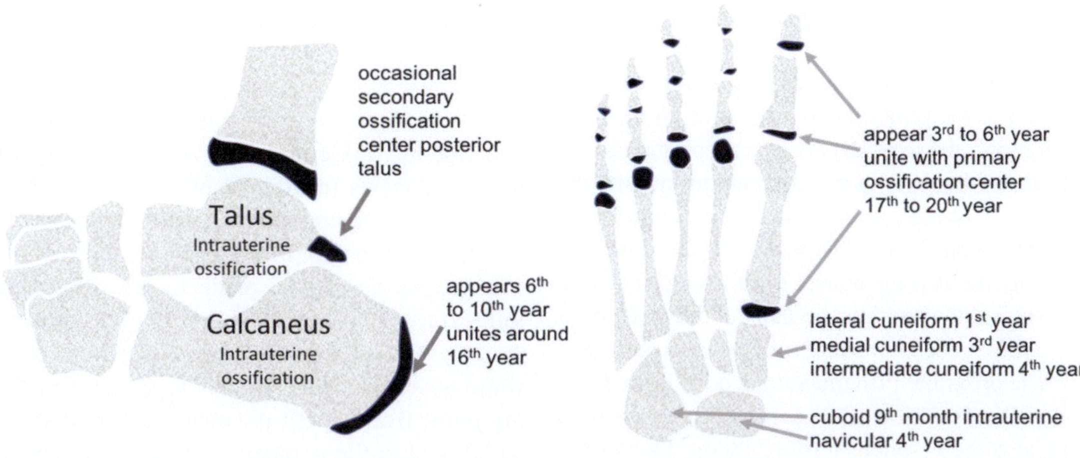

Fig. 11.2 Ossification of the bones of the ankle and foot. Secondary epiphyseal ossifications centers are shown in black

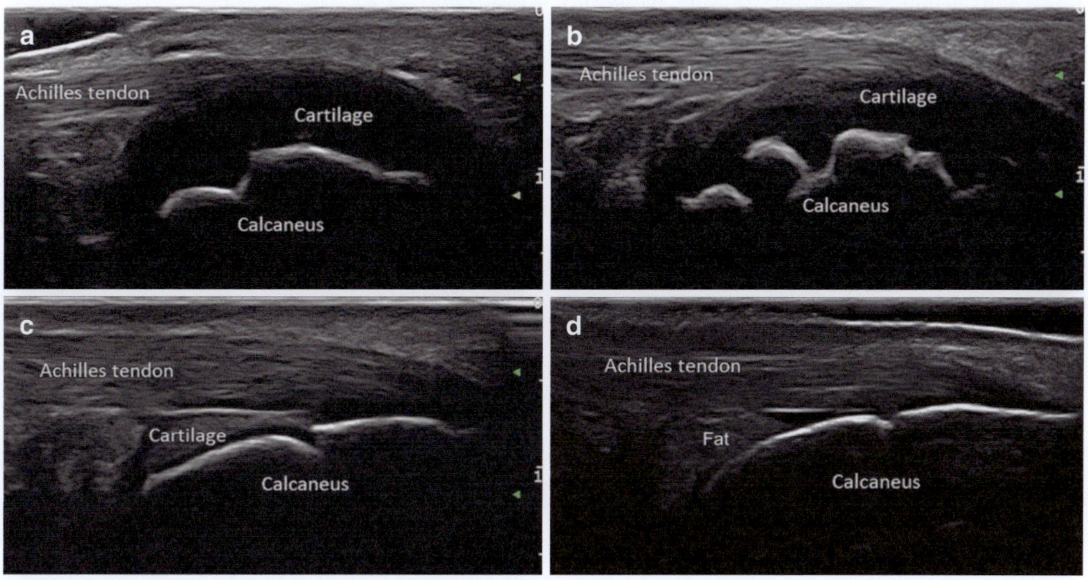

Fig. 11.3 Ossification of the posterior Calcaneus

calcaneus is visible; (B) from 4 to 6 years, early signs of the secondary ossification center appear; (C) from 7 to 11 years, the posterior bony contour of the primary ossification center of the calcaneus has got a wavy appearance; (D) from 12 to 18 years, the secondary ossification center then appears and full ossification of the apophyseal cartilage occurs [5, 7] (Fig. 11.3a–d).

In contrast to these three bones, the ossification of the navicular bone starts later, around the fourth year of life, and the cuneiform bones will start to ossify between the first to fourth year of life [5].

The navicular bone has the enthesis of the tibialis posterior tendon and a secondary ossification center in this area can show non-union with the main ossification center presenting as an accessory os naviculare (discussed in more detail in the pathology section).

The toes show an ossification pattern that is very similar to the fingers which is illustrated in Fig. 11.2. The diaphysis is fully ossified at birth with the metaphysis and epiphysis consisting of hyaline cartilage. Secondary ossification centers will develop within the epiphysis, and they are located in the proximal epiphysis for all the toes. In contrast, the secondary ossification center of the metatarsal bones is in the distal epiphysis with the exception of the first toe where it is found in the proximal epiphysis. This raises the question whether the first metatarsal bone should rather be considered the proximal phalanx of the first toe. At least the ossification pattern seems to suggest this.

The proximal fifth metatarsal bone is the location of the insertion of the peroneus brevis tendon and also the peroneus tertius tendon. Its secondary ossification center at the enthesis can show fragmentation physiologically. This needs to be taken into account when interpreting pathology in this area (Fig. 11.4).

An interesting feature is the fact that sesamoid bones also ossify at a later age and this can potentially cause confusion when scanning for example the volar aspect of MTP 1. An example is shown for a 10-year-old boy in Fig. 11.5.

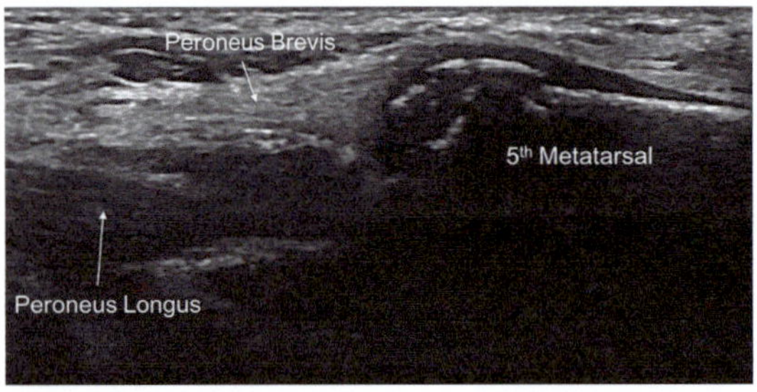

Fig. 11.4 Enthesis of the peroneus brevis into the proximal fifth metatarsal bone with physiologic fragmentation of ossification center

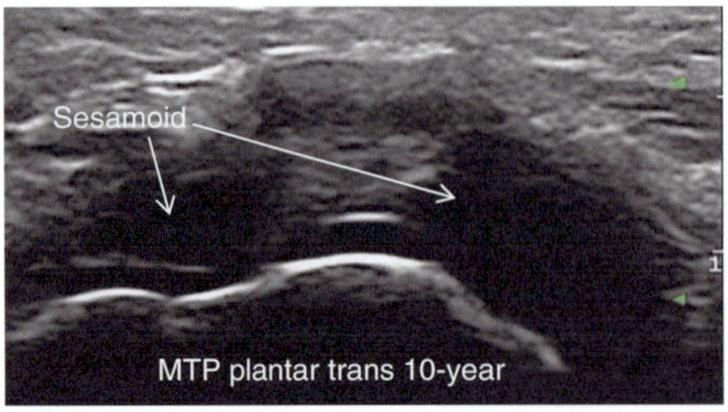

Fig. 11.5 Sesamoid bones on the plantar aspect of MTP 1 in a 10-year-old boy

Normal Sonoanatomy of the Ankle and Foot

In this section the assessment of the various areas of the ankle and foot will be described. Standard views to do so have been published for adults [10], but the pediatric standardization has only begun more recently, and recommendations have been made for the tibiotalar joint, for example [11]. It is important to note that these standard views are not meant to be static positions. Instead, they represent a starting point from which the evaluation will start, and it is essential to move both the probe across the joint area of the respective joint as well as the joint itself during the sonographic evaluation (Fig. 11.6).

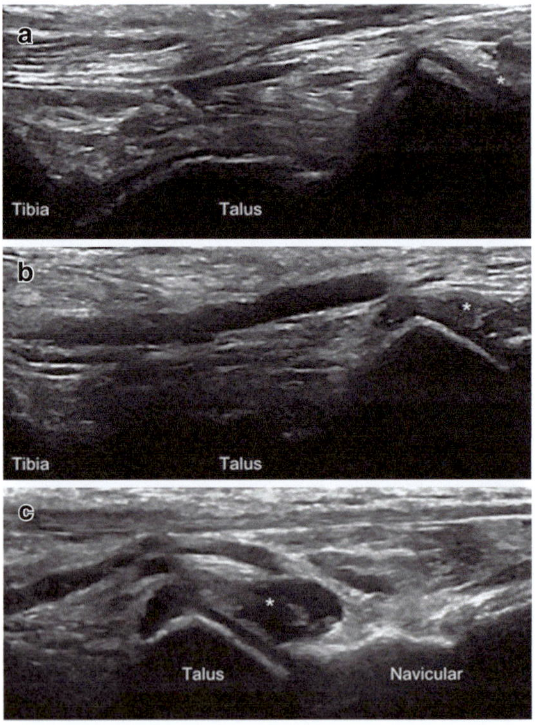

Fig. 11.6 Identification of talonavicular synovitis by moving across the joint area. A longitudinal view of the tibiotalar joint is shown including the talonavicular joint at the right side of the image (**a**). As the probe is moving across a synovial distension originating from the talonavicular joint becomes visible (asterix in **b**) that is not appreciated in image (**a**). Image (**c**) shows a detailed view of the synovitis with hypo- and anechoic components within the distended synovial recess (asterix)

Ankle anterior	Anterior tibiotalar and talonvavicular joint recess
	Tibialis anterior, Extensor hallucis longus, Extensor digitorum tendons
Ankle medial	Subtalar joint recess
	Tibialis posterior, Flexor digitorum, Flexor hallucis longus tendons
	Deltoid ligament
Ankle lateral	Subtalar joint recess
	Peroneus longus and brevis tendons
	Anterior tibiofibular, anterior talofibular, calcaneofibular ligaments
Ankle posterior	Achilles tendon
	Posterior bursae
	Tibiotalar and Subtalar joint
Foot plantar	Plantar fascia
Midfoot dorsal	Midfoot joints
	Extensor tendons
Forefoot	Dorsal joint recesses toes

Fig. 11.7 Checklist of the ultrasonographic exam of the ankle and foot

This will ensure the identification of focal pathologies and also facilitate the distinction between cartilage and soft tissue changes especially in younger children. Through the movement of the probe, the sonographer will essentially achieve a tomography of the joint by the addition of multiple slices even though the technology per se is a two-dimensional method. In addition, the respective joints can be moved as well during the assessment which will help clarifying findings. Care should also be taken to position the foot in an optimal way for each of the scans in order to give optimal access for the probe while at the same time ensuring a comfortable position for the patient and the examiner. Any scanning position might have to be modified in younger, possibly non-cooperative patients, who might also feel much more comfortable on a parents lap.

Finally, the settings including depth, frequency and focus might have to be adjusted during the assessment as the various structures of the ankle lie at very different levels.

Figure 11.7 provides a checklist of the structures that would commonly be assessed through ultrasonography of the ankle. It is important to note though, that depending on the clinical scenario, a more focused exam may be completely appropriate and save significant time.

Tibiotalar Joint

The sonographic assessment of the ankle and foot region typically starts with the tibiotalar joint in longitudinal view (Fig. 11.8). The foot can be placed flat on the exam bed with the knee in flexion. This is inline with recent recommendations on the standardization of ultrasonography [11], although reference [11] suggests the foot to be dorsally extended, whereas in fact the opposite should be done (plantar flexion). Further standardization of the ultrasonographic assessment of the ankle and other joints is ongoing and may help to optimize scanning further in the future.

Alternatively, the leg can be straight, and the examiner can plantar flex the foot with his other hand. This has the advantage that the tibiotalar joint can be moved during the assessment which may help to clarify pathology.

For the joint itself, it is easier to start in longitudinal view putting the probe along the distal

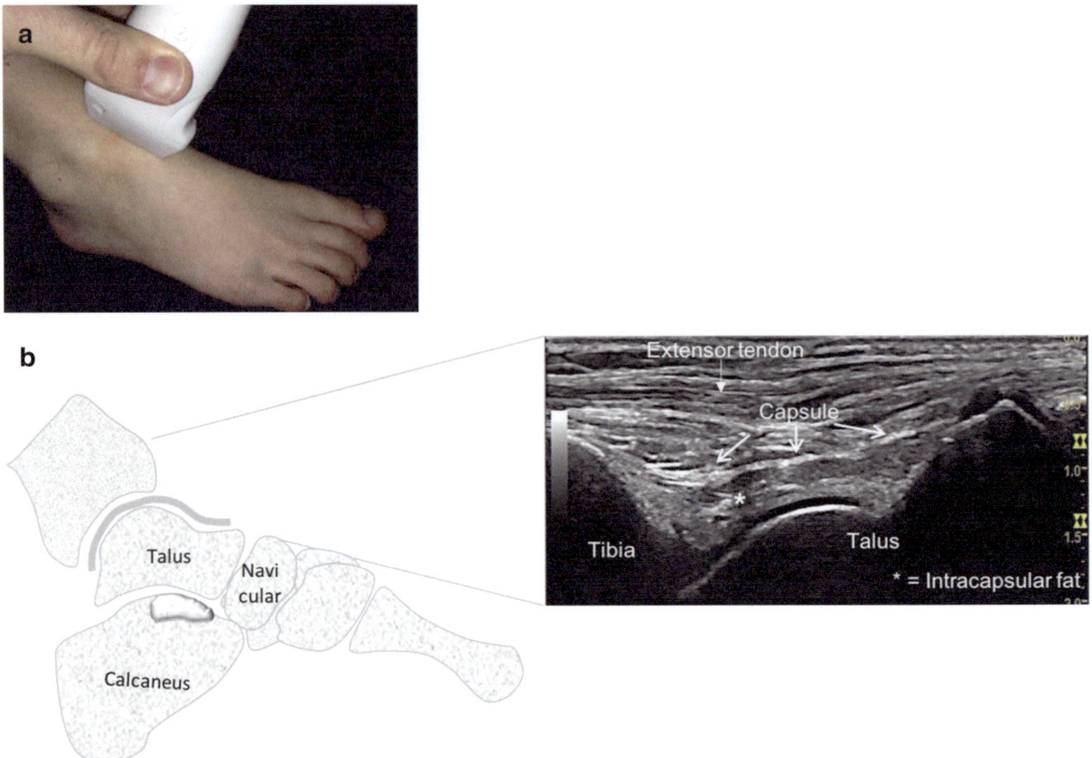

Fig. 11.8 Tibiotalar joint longitudinal view. (**a**) Probe position. (**b**) Schematic anatomic structures and ultrasound image

tibia and the talus. Depending on the footprint of the probe and the size of the child, it is important to visualize the entire talar dome with the cartilage on top and also the distal talus with the talonavicular joint. Only the very distal part of the tibia needs to be visualized. In addition to the bony landmarks, the joint capsule is important to identify. It is usually well visible as a fibrillar structure running from the tibia to the distal talus. Below the joint capsule and already in an intraarticular location is fat. This intraarticular fat is nevertheless extrasynovial and Doppler signals that are seen within this area can be physiologic. In a healthy joint, only a small amount of fluid is usually seen in the deep corner between the tibia and the talus. A localized accumulation of fluid can nevertheless be seen on top of the talar dome distal to the cartilage and just before the neck. This physiologic fluid accumulation is usually very focal and does not cover the entire width of the joint which can be shown in transverse view. Superficial to the joint capsule and depending on the exact location of the probe the anterior tendons of the ankle can be seen in longitudinal view. Once the bony landmarks and especially the cartilage are well visualized, the probe should be moved medially and laterally covering the entire width of the tibiotalar joint.

Normative data on the cartilage thickness of the talar cartilage have been published [12]. The thickness was assessed in the anterior longitudinal scan between the first and second metatarsal bone. The anterior demarcation of the cartilage on the medial part of the dome of the talus was identified. From this point, a distance of 5 mm in the proximal direction was measured and the cartilage thickness was measured perpendicularly to the bone surface [12]. Based on these data, the 95% confidence interval would indicate a range in boys of 0.8–1.6 mm at the age of 8 decreasing to 0.4 to 1.4 mm at the age of 16. In girls the respective

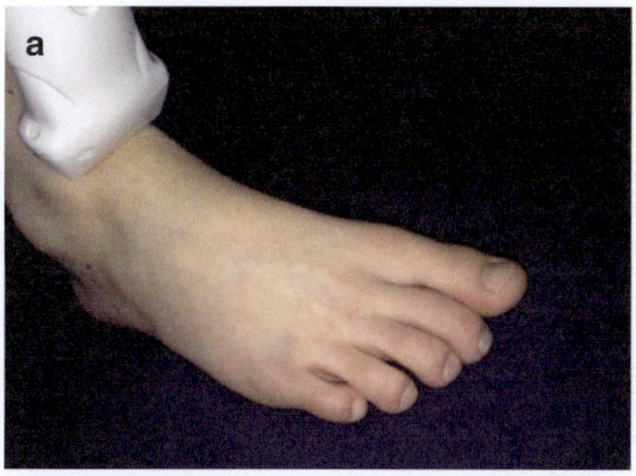

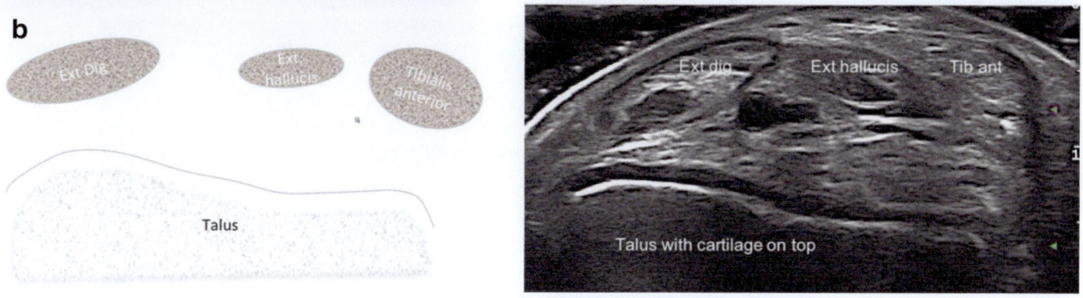

Fig. 11.9 (**a**) Probe position anterior ankle trans. (**b**) Schematic Anatomic structures and ultrasound image

numbers would be 0.7–1.4 mm at the age of 8 decreasing to 0.4 to 1.2 mm at the age of 16.

Following the longitudinal assessment, the probe will be positioned in transverse visualizing the talus with the cartilage on top and then moving it proximally and distally (Fig. 11.9).

The transverse view is also an important view for the assessment of the anterior tendons which are from medial to lateral the tibialis anterior, extensor hallucis longus, extensor digitorum tendons as well as the peroneus tertius tendon, the latter is absent in 10–20% of humans. A mnemonic to remember the tendons (except for the peroneus tertius) is: Tom (Tibialis Anterior) hates (Extensor Hallucis Longus) Dick (Extensor Digitorum). Again, the probe has to be moved proximally and distally to assess the entire extent of the tendons. The tibialis anterior tendon inserts into the medial cuneiform bone and the first metatarsal bone. Its distal fibers twist and there can be a bifid variant. It is also important to avoid anisotropy and to note that the myotendinous junction can be quite variable. In some people it is fairly distal especially for the extensor hallucis longus tendon, and the muscle surrounding the tendon should not be mistaken for hypertrophic synovium. It is easy to clarify this my moving the probe proximally. In the case of muscle, the tissue seen around the tendon will enlarge further and show the typical echotexture of muscle.

Medial Ankle

The assessment of the medial ankle has the following objectives: the visualization of tendons and their entheses, the neurovascular bundle as well as the assessment of the medial aspect of the subtalar joint (discussed in detail in the section on the subtalar joint). In addition, the various components of the deltoid ligament as well as the spring ligament can be demonstrated.

The tendons, blood vessels, and tibial nerve pass through the tarsal tunnel which lies posterior and inferior to the medial malleolus and is roofed by the flexor retinaculum, which extends from the medial malleolus to the calcaneus. The floor consists of the medial surfaces of the tibia, talus, and calcaneus [13].

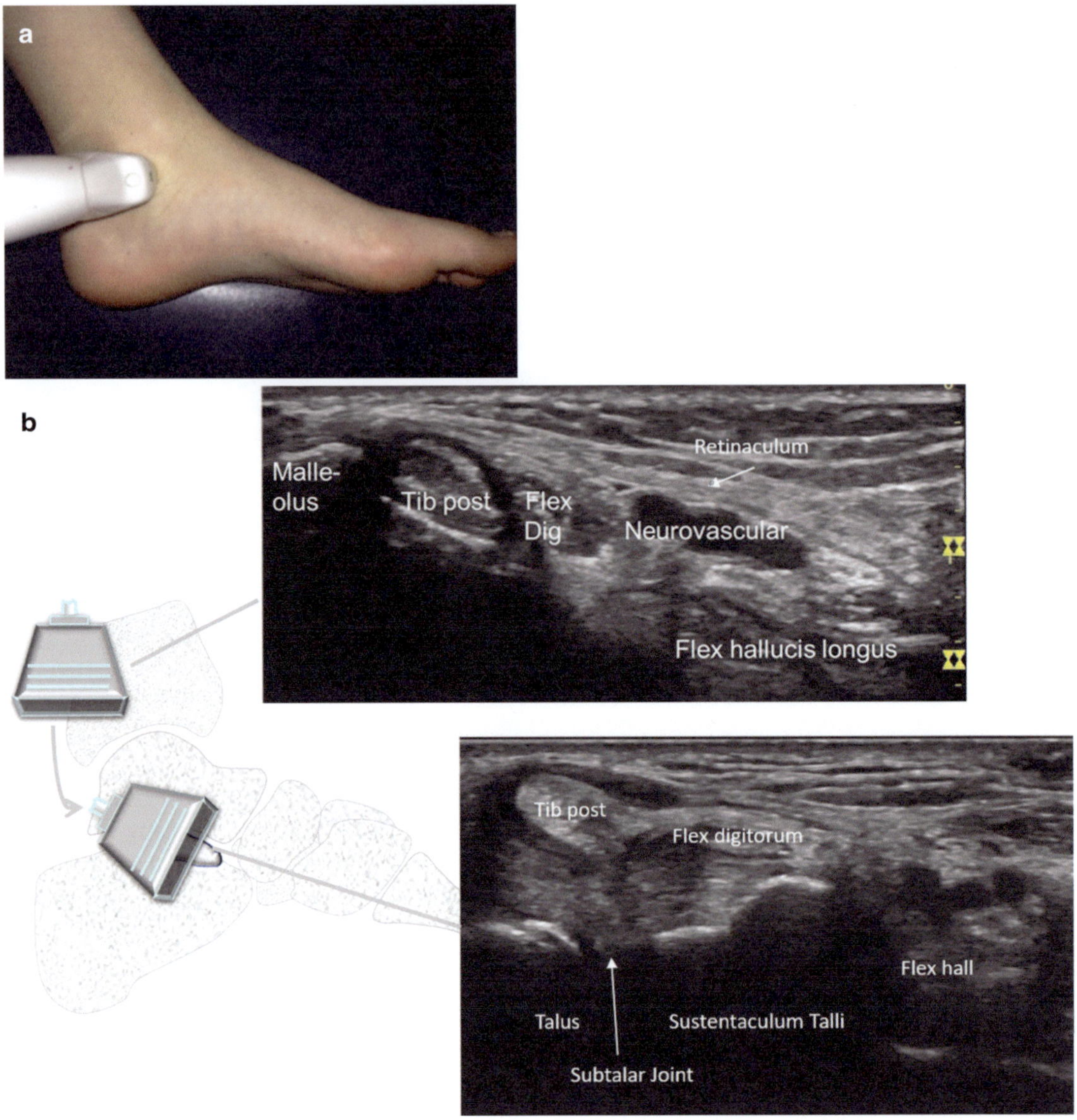

Fig. 11.10 (**a**) Probe position. (**b**) Schematic anatomic structures and ultrasound image

It can be assessed initially either in longitudinal or transverse view, but pathology will need to be confirmed in a second plane. The following tendons need to be identified from anterior to posterior (Fig. 11.10): Tibialis posterior tendon, flexor digitorum and flexor hallucis longus tendons. Between the flexor digitorum and flexor hallucis longus tendon, the neurovascular bundle is located consisting of the posterior tibial artery, the tibial nerve, and multiple veins. The tibial nerve divides into the medial and lateral plantar nerves and also sends the medial calcaneal nerve to the heel providing sensory fibers for the posteromedial aspect of the heel and heel fat pad. The separation of the tibial nerve into these branches can vary and especially the medial calcaneal nerve can branch off proximal to the tarsal tunnel or within the tunnel [13].

A mnemonic to remember the tendons, vessels and nerve is: Tom (Tib post), Dick (Flexor Digitorum) and (Artery) the very (Vein) nervous (Nerve) Harry (Flexor Hallucis Longus).

If one takes the longitudinal approach to scan this region, the probe will be positioned just posterior to the medial malleolus and after the tibialis posterior tendon has been identified moved slowly posterior in order to identify the other structures. It can be difficult to know exactly which tendon is being assessed at any given moment and this is why a lot of sonographers prefer a transverse approach that will allow to visualize all three tendons as well as the neurovascular bundle at the same time. The probe is being positioned at the level of the medial malleolus in transverse and tilted slightly backward. *It is very helpful to rotate the leg/foot externally if possible to place it almost flat on the exam bed with the medial ankle upward, and further pronation of the ankle/foot may be helpful to expose the tendons better when scanning.* Careful technique has to be applied to get rid of anisotropy that may be present by angulating the probe. It has to be noted though that not all tendons may always run at the same angle and therefore anisotropy of one or two tendons may be present while the other one is well visible. Similar to what has been discussed for the anterior tendons, the myotendinous junction especially of the flexor hallucis tendon may be located quite distally, and in a proximal position of the probe, a significant amount of muscle may be seen with tendon fibers centrally. This should not be mistaken for proliferative tenosynovitis. The tibialis posterior tendon has a much larger diameter than the flexor digitorum tendon with which it runs closely together proximally. As the examiner follows the tendons more distally, the probe will turn clockwise by 90 degrees, and as it gets more distal, the flexor hallucis longus tendon will dive deep and pass below the sustentaculum tali. The insertion of the tibialis posterior tendon is clinically most relevant and will need to be assessed in transverse as well as longitudinal view. This tendon has multiple insertions on the medial, plantar, and lateral aspect of the foot, and only some of its fibers will insert into the navicular bone. As the other fiber bundles turn in different directions to reach their respective entheses, this tendon will lack the regular fibrillar pattern as it gets closer to its insertion. Additional ossification centers can be present at the insertion into the navicular bone and give rise to pathology that will be discussed below. At various points, especially when the tibialis posterior tendon gets close to bone, a triangular fluid collection can be observed between tendon and bone that is not circumferential but located within the tendon sheath. It is typically completely anechoic and does not show synovial hypertrophy. This should not be confused with tenosynovitis as it represents merely a little fluid cushion to offset the mechanical strain on the tendon.

The Deltoid ligament is a stronger and more extensive band than the lateral ligaments. It consists of a combination of superficial and deep layers of fibers with the tibiotalar ligament (posterior, superficial and deep layer), tibiocalcanear ligament (intermediate, superficial) and tibionavicular ligament (anterior, superficial) that blend into each other.

In order to visualize these various components, it is important to position the ankle to stretch out the respective parts. For the posterior tibiotalar and tibiocalcaneal portion, the foot is best brought into a dorsiflexion and for the tibionavicular portion into a plantar flexion (Fig. 11.11).

When the probe is positioned along the distal tibia, calcaneus, and sustentaculum tali, it can be turned counterclockwise by 90 degrees to visualize the spring ligament that inserts on the sustentaculum tali proximally and the undersurface of the navicular bone distally.

Lateral Ankle

The assessment of the lateral ankle has the objectives of assessing the peroneus tendons and their entheses, the lateral aspect of the subtalar joint (discussed in detail in the section on the subtalar joint), as well as the anterior tibiofibular, the talofibular, and the calcaneofibular ligament.

Similar to the assessment of the medial ankle, the tendons can be assessed initially either in longitudinal or transverse view, but pathology will need to be confirmed in a second plane. The

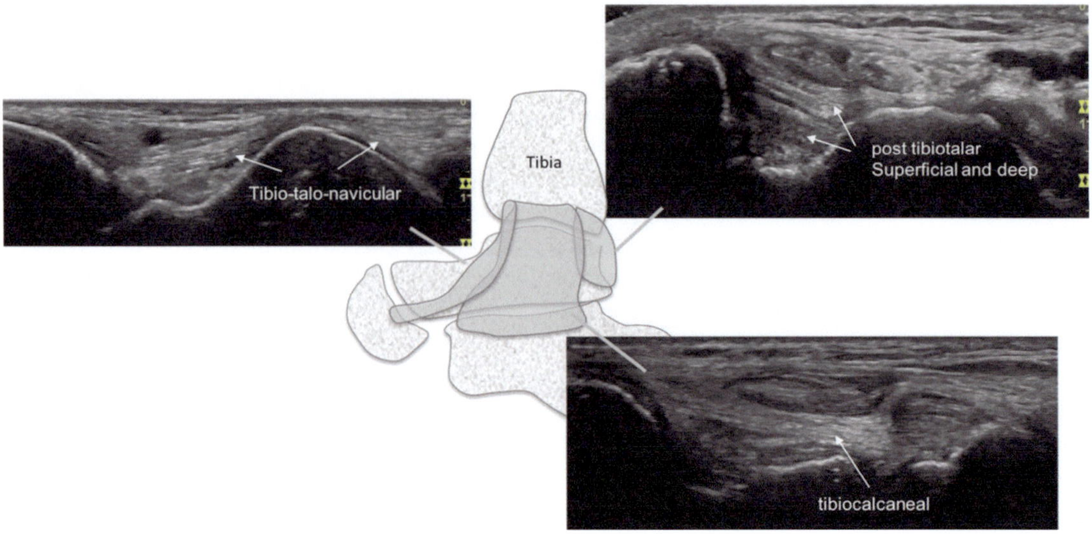

Fig. 11.11 Deltoid ligament

tendons of the peroneus brevis and peroneus longus muscles have a common tendon sheath and pass posterior to the lateral malleolus and deep to the superior and inferior retinaculum. They will then diverge on the lateral surface of the foot. The peroneus longus and brevis tendons need to be identified, and the peroneus brevis tendon will typically be closer to the bone, but this can vary, and another reliable way is to move the probe proximally – the peroneus brevis tendon will transition into muscle more distally than the peroneus longus tendon which remains a pure tendon until more proximally. An additional muscle and tendon, the peroneus quartus can be identified in 10–20% of humans.

With the transverse approach, the probe is being positioned at the level of the lateral malleolus in transverse and tilted slightly backward (Fig. 11.12).

It is very helpful to rotate the leg/foot internally if possible to place it flat on the exam bed with the lateral ankle upward, and further supination of the ankle/foot may be helpful to expose the tendons better when scanning. The examiner will follow the tendons distally turning counterclockwise around the malleolus. Copious amounts of gel may be necessary to ensure good coupling and visualization of the tendons and toggling of the probe will be necessary to avoid anisotropy. Following the peroneus tendons distally, a bony prominence of variable size, the peroneal tubercle, will come into view on the lateral aspect of the calcaneus. At this point the two tendons will diverge, and it is often impossible to show both of them without anisotropy in a single image due to their different directions. The peroneus brevis tendon can be followed distally to its insertion on the fifth metatarsal bone, and the peroneus longus tendon can be followed crossing on the plantar aspect of the midfoot and inserting on the medial cuneiform and first metatarsal base.

For the ligaments it might be best to position the probe along the distal fibula and tibia to visualize the tibiofibular ligament. The probe can then be turned clockwise until the talofibular ligament is found. This is best achieved by plantarflexion of the foot which will put tension on the ligament. It runs from the anterior border of the lateral malleolus to the lateral surface of the talar neck and blends with the joint capsule. It is the weakest, most frequently injured and restrains the anterior talar motion. Finally, the probe will be positioned at a 45 degree angle pointing to the heel from the fibula to visualize the calcaneofibular ligament which lies underneath the peroneus tendons. With a dorsiflexion and inversion of the foot tension will be put on this ligament pushing up the peroneus tendons like a hammock if the ligament is intact.

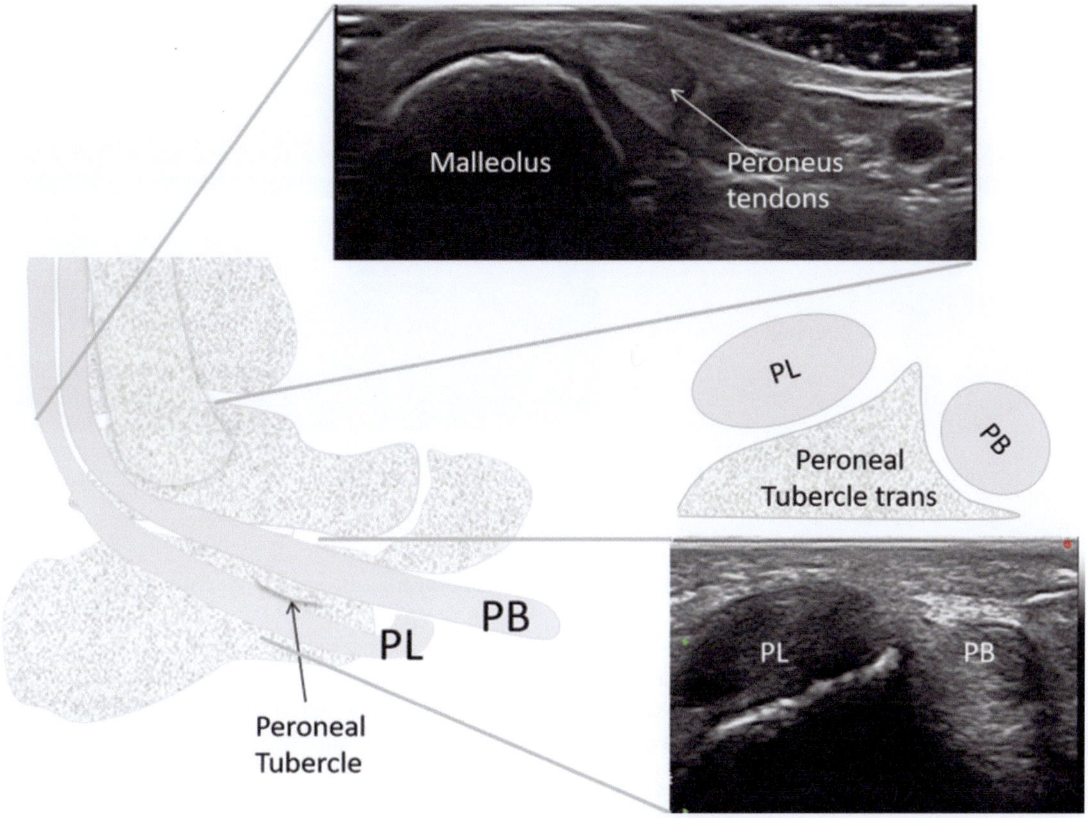

Fig. 11.12 Schematic anatomic structures and ultrasound image of the peroneus brevis and longjus tendons

Posterior Ankle

At the posterior ankle tendon, the main structure to assess is the Achilles tendon (running together with the plantaris tendon) including its enthesis into the posterior calcaneus and the retrocalcaneal bursa. In addition, the tibiotalar and subtalar joint can be visualized from posterior (Figs. 11.3 and 11.13). The Achilles tendon and its insertion will best be visualized with relatively high frequencies and reduced depth. It is formed by the fusion of the aponeurosis of the two heads of the gastrocnemius muscle superficially and the soleus muscle as the deep layer. These two layers of it can usually be distinguished on ultrasonography.

The accompanying plantaris tendon cannot be distinguished usually and may only become visible in the case of Achilles tendon rupture as a remaining fibrillar band. The Achilles tendon is not surrounded by a tenosynovium but by a paratenon instead. The paratenon represents an elastic sleeve made of collagen I and III fibers with synovial cells that allows gliding of the tendon [14]. At the level of the posterior calcaneus the tendon will run along the bone proximally and then, in the case of the fully mature bone, transition through an anechoic layer of fibrocartilage to insert into the cortex more distally ([14, 15], Fig. 11.3). This enthesis consists of a considerable length. In younger children, the posterior calcaneus looks quite different. Until the age of 6 years, a significant portion of the posterior calcaneus is anechoic representing hyaline cartilage but a more superficial layer will be hypoechoic, likely representing fibrocartilage (even though the layer of fibrocartilage in the fully mature bone appears anechoic). This superficial layer of hypoechoic cartilage will become even more prominent from 7 to 11 years when the posterior bony contour of the primary ossification center of the calcaneus has got a wavy appearance. From 12 to 18 years, the secondary ossification center then appears and

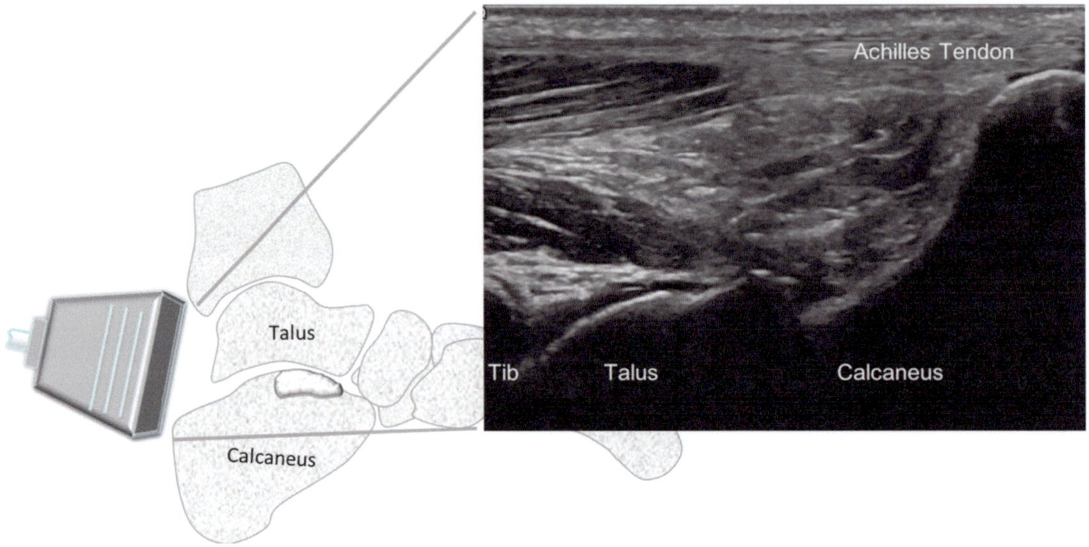

Fig. 11.13 Posterior longitudinal view showing the achilles tendons superficially and the posterior tibiotalar and subtalar joint deeper

full ossification of the apophyseal cartilage occurs (Fig. 11.3). During this process the proximal part of the posterior calcaneus still remains cartilaginous initially with a hypoechoic appearance again. This should not be confused with Karger's fat pad (Fig. 11.3). An easy way to tell the difference is to move the ankle and see this hypoechoic area move exactly with the rest of the calcaneus without changing shape.

The retrocalcaneal bursa is often not visible or detectable as a thin layer in the angle between Karger's fat pad, the bone and the tendon.

In order to assess the posterior aspect of the tibiotalar and subtalar joint, the depth will have to be increased significantly, the frequency lowered and the focus points moved for optimal visualization. It can also be helpful to move to do dorsi- and plantarflexion in order to clarify the structures (Fig. 11.13).

Subtalar Joint

The subtalar joint is functionally a single joint that, anatomically, is divided into an anterior part, the talocalcaneonavicular joint (ASTJ) and a posterior part, the (posterior) talocalcaneal joint (PSTJ) [15]. The ASTJ is formed by the navicular bone and the head of the talus anteriorly and the anterior and middle facets of the talus and the calcaneus (sustentaculum tali) inferiorly. The spring ligament supports the joint inferiorly. The ASTJ and the talonavicular joint therefore from a continuity [15]. The ASTJ is separated from the PSTJ by the sinus tarsi and tarsal canal with several strong ligaments within the sinus tarsi. The PSTJ consists of the posterior facets of the talus and the calcaneus [15]. It is difficult to assess clinically but the various components can well be assessed sonographically. Several approaches to do so have been suggested. In a recent publication focused on the anatomic and sonographic description of the subtalar joint in adults [15], a set of four scans for the subtalar joint has been proposed as follows:

Anterior Subtalar Joint

Medial scan 1 Starting with the proximal pole of the transducer placed on the medial malleolus and the distal pole placed on the sustentaculum tali, while the distal pole remains fixed on the sustentaculum tali, the proximal pole is rotated anteriorly toward the navicular bone until the spring ligament overlying the talar cartilage is visualized, along with the anterior subtalar joint.

Posterior Subtalar Joint

Medial scan 2 Starting with the proximal pole of the transducer placed on the medial malleolus and the distal pole placed on the sustentaculum tali, the transducer is then shifted behind the medial malleolus to visualize the flexor hallucis longus tendon in long axis and the posterior subtalar joint beneath the tendon.

Lateral scan: The proximal pole of the transducer is placed on the lateral malleolus with the distal pole pointing to the sole of the foot and shifted slightly anteriorly to visualize the posterior subtalar joint between the talus and the calcaneus.

Posterior scan: The transducer is placed on the calcaneus, aligned along the long axis of the Achilles tendon. By increasing the depth and lowering the focus, the posterior subtalar joint is visualized deep to Kager's fat pad, adjacent and distal to the bony contour of the talus.

The problem with this approach is that it suggests specific scan positions without movement of the probe to identify unusual extensions of the synovial recesses in the case of pathology. Some of the scans are also slightly complicated in terms of the probe positioning and landmarks may be more difficult to identify especially in young children where ossification of the bones is incomplete.

Essentially all components of the subtalar joint can be assessed during the anterior longitudinal scan of the ankle (talonavicular joint), the medial and lateral scans moving the probe along the tendons as well as the posterior longitudinal scan when increasing the depth to visualize the posterior subtalar joint. Sometimes it can nevertheless still be difficult to clearly identify the PSTJ from lateral as the gap between talus and calcaneus can be very narrow and it might equally be difficult to distinguish effusion/synovial hypertrophy from cartilage in young children. I would therefore like to suggest a very simple yet complete way to assess the various components of the subtalar joint including the dynamic assessment in order to better distinguish pathology from normal anatomic structures.

The ASTJ is first assessed through the scan of the talonavicular joint as part of the longitudinal assessment of the anterior ankle with the tibiotalar joint by simply moving the probe more distally to include the talonavicular joint (Fig. 11.14).

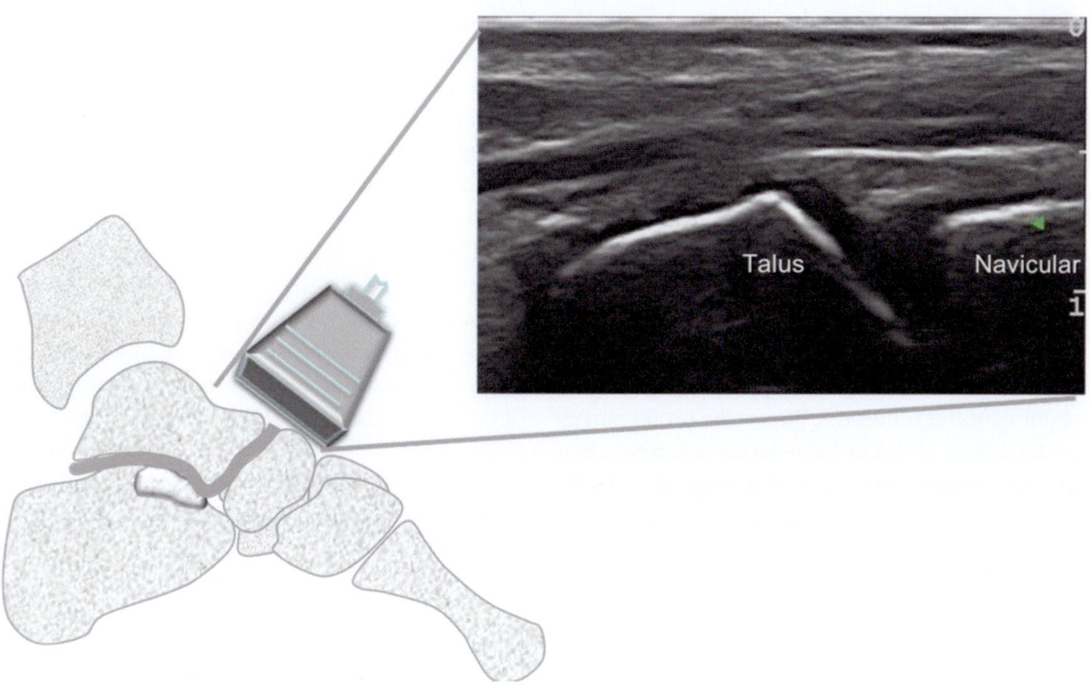

Fig. 11.14 Assessment of the talonavicular joint

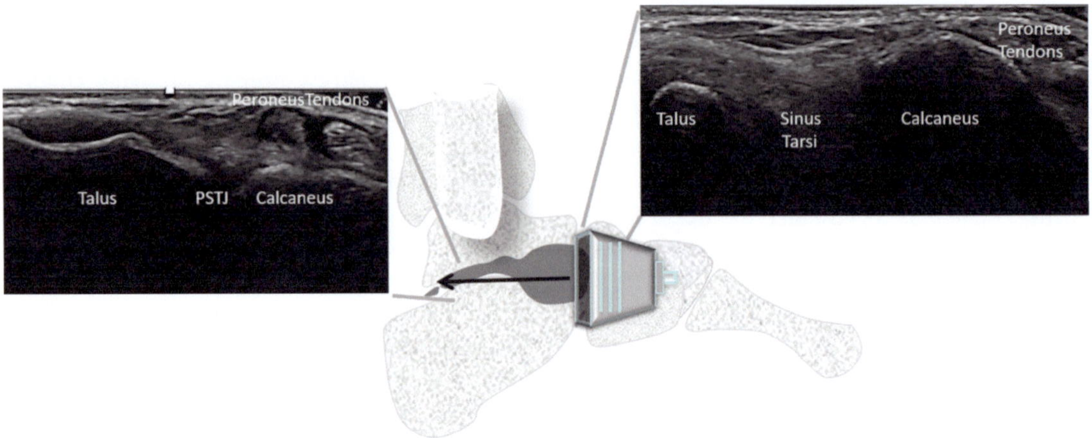

Fig. 11.15 Lateral subtalar joint

It is important though to move the probe medially and laterally in order to not miss pathology which can be focal (Fig. 11.6).

The probe can then be positioned medially in a 45-degree angle pointing at the heel identifying the sustentaculum tali and talus. In fact the examiner can also decide to palpate the sustentaculum tali and then put the probe directly on it. This will visualize part of the ASTJ from medially (Fig. 11.10b). The probe will need to be moved toward the midfoot/toes to ensure full assessment of the anterior subtalar joint and also toward the heel to capture pathology of the posterior subtalar joint.

The PSTJ will mainly be assessed from lateral and also posterior. For the lateral assessment a very simple and reliable approach is to position the probe on top of the sinus tarsi – which can be easily identified through palpation – at a 90 degree angle to the sole. The probe will then be moved posteriorly while remaining initially at 90 degrees and then just turning a little bit. The examiner will be able to appreciate the wide opening of the sinus tarsi, and as the probe moves posteriorly, it will narrow to the tight gap between the talus and calcaneus forming the PSTJ (Fig. 11.15). Through this maneuver it is very easy to document the subtalar joint from lateral and the examiner will not miss pathology as the entire extent of the articulation of the talus with the calcaneus will be assessed. It is important to recognize that for the assessment of the sinus tarsi, the examiner may have to decrease the frequency more than for some of the more superficial structures of the ankle.

The assessment of the posterior subtalar joint has already been described in the section on the posterior ankle.

Plantar Foot

The main structure that will be assessed at the plantar surface of the foot is the plantar fascia. It is important to note that the main bundle of the fascia is located rather medially. The patient can be in a prone position but may also be lying on the side or the examiner may simply hold the foot of a child even sitting on the lap of a parent and put the probe on the sole with the proximal end positioned on the calcaneus and the distal end pointing to the midfoot. Due to the relatively thick fat pad over the calcaneus, the frequency might have to be lowered in order to identify the fibrillar plantar fascia that – depending on the age of the child – might insert into fully ossified bone or cartilage. The normal thickness is up to 4 mm (Fig. 11.16).

Midfoot

The midfoot is being assessed from dorsal by putting the probe longitudinally in midline and then sliding medial and lateral. The navicular-cuneiform as well as the various cuneiform-

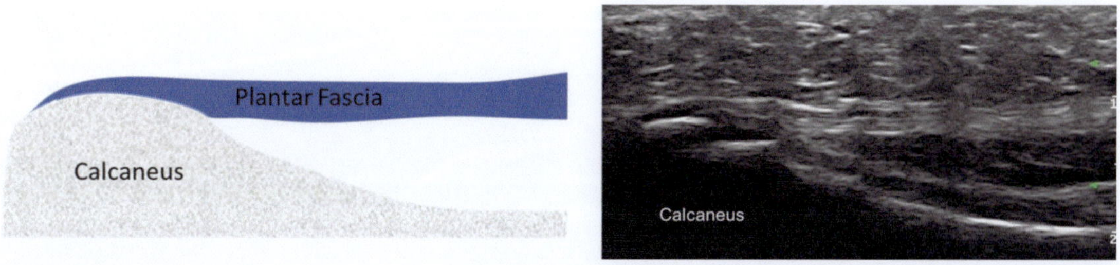

Fig. 11.16 Plantar Fascia

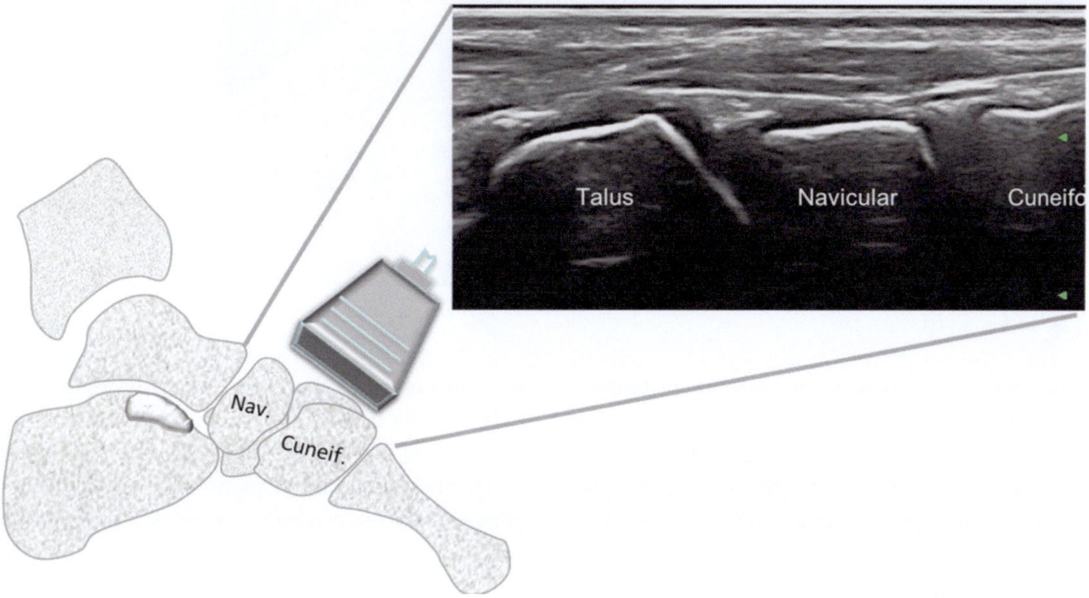

Fig. 11.17 Midfoot longitudinal scan

metatarsal joints will be assessed as well as the extensor tendons with their tendon sheaths more superficially (Fig. 11.17). More laterally the calcaneocuboid joint can also be assessed. The articulations between the three cuneiform bones can best be assessed in transverse view, and this view will also help to assess the tendons and confirm potential pathology in a second plane.

Forefoot

The forefoot is an interesting area with relevant pathology in relation to the nerves and also the bursae and vessels. In adults the differential diagnosis of forefoot pain includes bursitis, Morton Neuroma, and thrombosis of plantar veins. In children these pathologies nevertheless do not play a significant role and this area is not part of the standard ultrasonographic assessment.

Toes

The toes will be assessed in longitudinal and transverse view mainly from dorsal, in contrast to the fingers (Fig. 11.18). The plantar assessment might nevertheless be necessary in the case of more focal pathology. The MTP and IP joints will show the bone contour with variable amounts of cartilage depending on the age as well as the synovial recess. Especially in the case of MTP 1 and 2, a small amount of physiologic fluid and distension of the recess is often present. Please

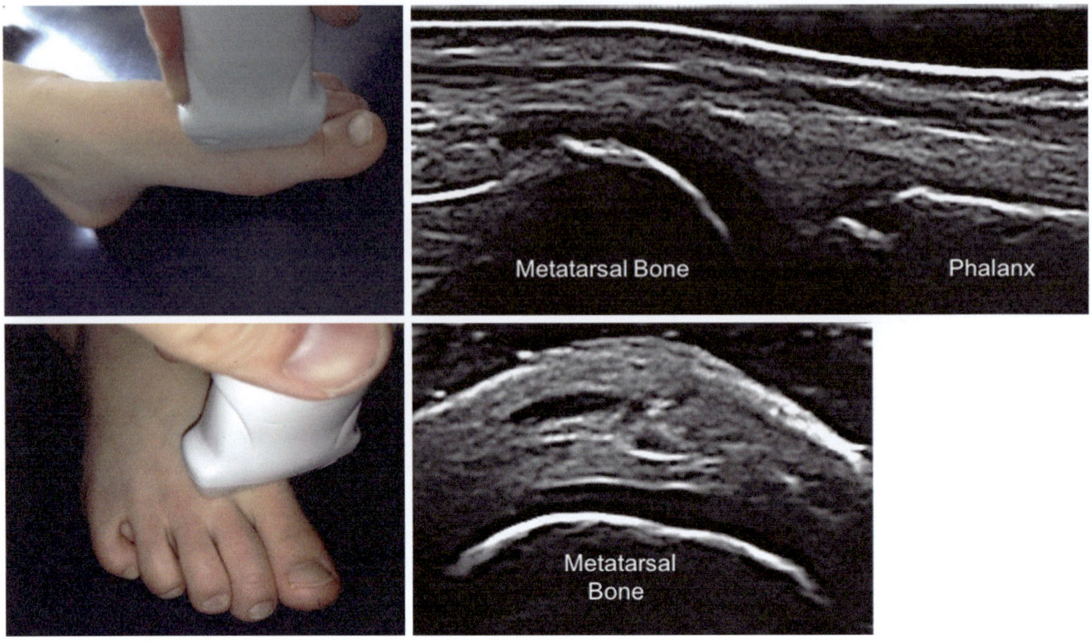

Fig. 11.18 MTP

note that the synovial recess extends proximally, and ensure that the probe is positioned accordingly, i.e., the image is divided approximately 2/3 proximally and 1/3 distally from the joint space. As mentioned in the chapter on ossification, the sesamoid bones found typically on the plantar surface of MTP 1 may be anechoic due to the fact that ossification may not yet have occurred (Fig. 11.5).

Pathology and Differential Diagnosis

The main pathologies that will be assessed in the context of pediatric rheumatology are synovitis, tenosynovitis, and enthesitis.

Synovitis

As per the Omeract pediatric definitions, the detection of synovitis in children should include both B-Mode as well as Doppler techniques but allows the diagnosis based on B-mode findings only [16]. This is especially important for deeper structures where sensitivity of Doppler may be less. In contrast, synovitis cannot be diagnosed based on the detection of Doppler signals only to ensure, that physiologic intraarticular blood flow is not misinterpreted as pathologic. In the pathogenesis of synovitis, synovial hyperplasia detected as thickening of the synovium is the primary process and increased blood flow detected as Doppler signals has to be shown within an area of thickened synovium. Despite the fact that the pathologic process in synovitis is synovial hyperplasia and not hypertrophy, the latter term is commonly used in the rheumatology literature. The Omeract group therefore decided to use the term synovial hypertrophy in their synovitis definitions but in this chapter the term synovial hyperplasia will be used. The Omeract consensus defines synovial effusion as an abnormal, intraarticular, anechoic or hypoechoic material that is displaceable. Synovial hypertrophy is defined as an abnormal, intraarticular, hypoechoic material that is non-displaceable [16].

Synovitis in the tibiotalar joint will often be detected in the anterior longitudinal view first and subsequently confirmed in the transverse view (Fig. 11.19).

It is important to ensure the complete assessment of the joint by moving the probe medially and

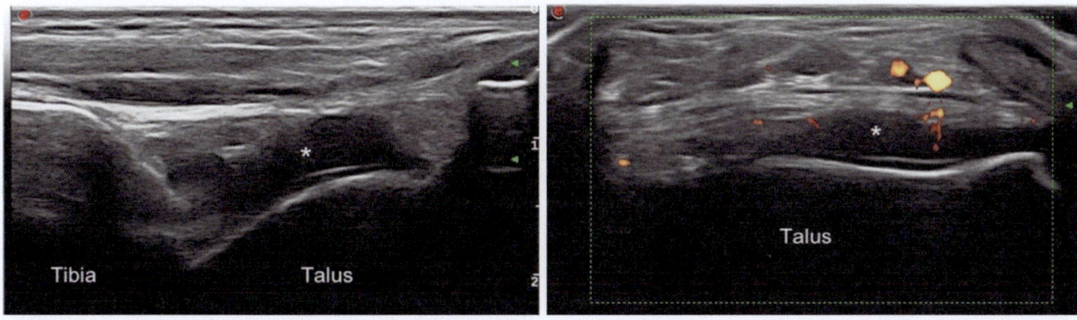

Fig. 11.19 Synovitis of the tibiotalar joint in longitudinal and transverse view, the asterix marks the area of synovial distension long and trans

laterally. Especially chronic synovial proliferation may be more focal and not extend across the entire joint. Synovial Fluid and proliferation will accumulate in the angle between the proximal talus and tibia first and then increasingly push up the intraarticular fat. It will extend along the talar dome and reach the area distal to the visible cartilage. It is important to recognize that small amounts of fluid may be normal in the angle between the tibia and talus and also in the distal area. Flexion and extension of the foot while scanning can help to visualize synovial changes and distinguish them from the cartilage. Great care should be taken to clearly demonstrate the cartilage surface interface sign by ensuring orthogonal insonnation through optimal positioning of the ultrasound probe. Sometimes synovitis will extend into unusual locations, and synovial cysts may be found in an anterior or anterolateral and anteromedial location especially in the case of chronic, long-standing synovitis [17]. Communication with the principal synovial recess cannot always be demonstrated.

No normative data exist for the pediatric ankle to suggest what amount of synovial distension should be considered pathologic. A recent publication on the standardization of pediatric ultrasonography and normal age-related findings does not provide data on the normal dimensions of the synovial recess. It focuses on the tibiotalar joint only and emphasizes that in none of the age groups, intrasynovial Doppler signals were demonstrated, whereas they were present in some healthy volunteers in the intraarticular but extrasynovial fat as well as in the epiphyseal cartilage of the distal end of tibia, mainly in younger children (2–4 and 5–8 years) [11].

Quantification of findings has not been standardized either. Measurements of the distension of the recess can be difficult due to the rapid change of the dimensions depending on the probe position and the positioning of the foot (flexion and extension). A scoring system that was previously proposed does in fact not apply to the tibiotalar joint as demonstrated by the illustration in this very same publication [18].

A not yet validated and published semiquantitative scoring of the tibiotalar joint may be done as follows:

Grade 0
No fluid, possibly some fluid in the distal part of the tibiotalar joint.

Grade 1
The anterior recess is minimally distended with a concave or flat shape.

Grade 2
The anterior recess is moderately distended with a convex shape of the synovium.

Grade 3
Synovium occupies >50% of the expected full volume of the recess.

Doppler Signals Will Be Scored As

Grade 0 None

Grade 1 Single signals (up to three) within the synovial recess

Grade 2 More than three signals within synovial recess or confluent signals in less than 50% of synovial recess

Grade 3 Confluent signals in more than 50% of the recess

Blood vessels crossing the synovial recess and entering the bone or growth plate are considered feeding vessels and should not be included in the scoring.

Subtalar Joint/ Talonavicularcalcaneal Joint

The detection of synovitis in the subtalar joint can best be achieved by assessing the talonavicular joint as well as the talocalcaneal joint from medial, lateral and posterior. The ultrasonographic detection of synovial abnormalities may vary among patients, i.e., some patients will demonstrate more significant changes on the medial aspect of the ankle, whereas in others, changes are most visible on the lateral aspect [19]. Whether the posterior approach will demonstrate synovitis that is otherwise not visible is not clear. Some authors have demonstrated variations in the sensitivity especially of Doppler ultrasonography to show intrasynovial blood flow [20], which may be most sensitive for the lateral scan of the PSTJ. This may not be surprising given the variable depth at which the synovial changes can be found. With increasing depth Doppler will become less sensitive to pick up signals of small vessels as they are present in synovitis. Instead of using standardized settings, the frequency of B-Mode as well as Doppler may have to be lowered especially when assessing the sinus tarsi and the subtalar joint on the posterior longitudinal view. The dynamic assessment from anterior (talonavicular joint), medial, lateral, and posterior will ensure capture of pathology in most cases.

Positioning the probe in longitudinal view over the talonavicular joint a distension of the joint recess originating from the gap between the two bones can be demonstrated (Fig. 11.6). It is important though, as mentioned previously, to move the probe across the joint medially and laterally to not miss pathology. On the medial aspect of the ankle, positioning the probe over the talus and the sustentaculum tali distensions of the synovial recess of the anterior subtalar joint will be shown (Fig. 11.20). Due to the insertion of the deltoid ligament on the sustentaculum tali, the recess will tend to expand proximally, unless the ligament has been damaged or is very loose. It has to be differentiated from the distension of the tibiotalar synovial recess which will extend from proximal to distal.

Physiologic communications between the two joints also exist physiologically in about 20% of humans. The communication and coalescence of synovial recesses/tissue may also happen in the case of chronic, significant synovitis, similar to what can be seen in the wrist with the radiocarpal, midcarpal and carpometacarpal recesses. Moving the probe posterior on the medial aspect of the ankle, the distensions of the synovial recess of the PSTJ may also be seen.

On the lateral aspect the PSTJ will be assessed mostly with a variable presence of B-Mode and Doppler findings within the sinus tarsi or more posterior extending from the relatively narrow

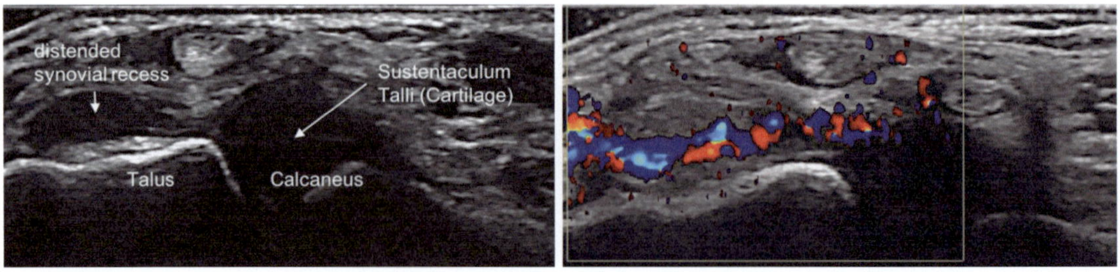

Fig. 11.20 Synovitis of the anterior subtalar joint from medial in B-mode (*left*) and Doppler (*right*)

space between the talus and calcaneus and – similarly to the medial ankle – extending proximally along the talus (Fig. 11.21).

Finally, on the posterior longitudinal view of the ankle, a distension of the synovial recess can be detected originating from the gap between talus and calcaneus when the depth is increased and the frequency lowered.

Calcaneocuboid Joint and Midfoot

Scanning across the calcaneocuboid, navicular-cuneiform and cuneiform-metatarsal joint extensions of the synovial recess can be detected (Fig. 11.22).

It is important to distinguish cartilage from synovial hypertrophy and fluid especially in younger children with incomplete ossification. This is best done by demonstrating the cartilage interface sign which will usually be even better visible when fluid is present as the change of impedance between fluid and cartilage is stronger than between soft tissue and cartilage and the reflection of the ultrasound therefore is stronger than in the absence of fluid making the white line on top of the cartilage better visible. In juvenile spondylarthropathies but also other subtypes of JIA, midfoot involvement is frequent and may be more prominent than expected from the clinical exam alone [21].

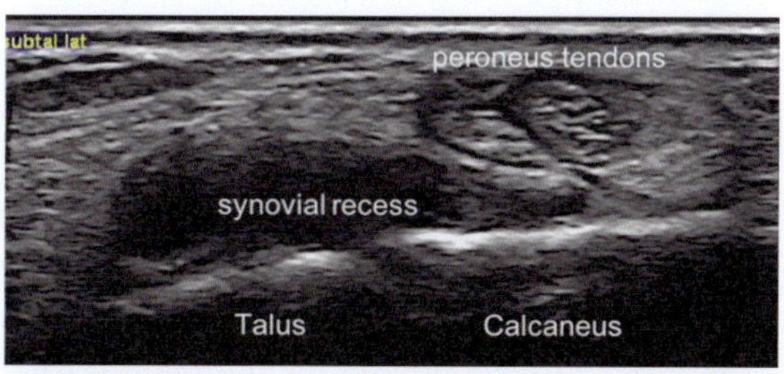

Fig. 11.21 Lateral scan of the posterior subtalar joint

MTP and IP Joints

Distensions of the synovial recess originating from the MTP and IP joints will tend to extend proximally (Fig. 11.23). As mentioned previously, small amounts of fluid may be normal especially in MTP 1 and 2, but no pediatric normative data are published at this point.

Involvement of Extrasynovial Tissues in Inflammatory Arthritis

Especially in psoriasis arthritis, other tissues than the synovial joint recesses and tendon sheaths may be involved [22]. This includes soft tissue edema, local enthesitis (extensor tendon insertions and collateral ligaments), involvement of the plantar & palmar plate and paratenonitis of the extensor tendons as well as osteoproliferation. Unfortunately no data exist at this point on extrasynovial findings in children with psoriasis arthritis or other subtypes of JIA.

Differential Diagnosis of Inflammatory Arthritis

Septic Arthritis and Hemarthros may present with increased echogenicity of the joint fluid but there are no sonographic criteria that would allow a specific diagnosis of the two conditions. Instead, the diagnosis of these conditions will

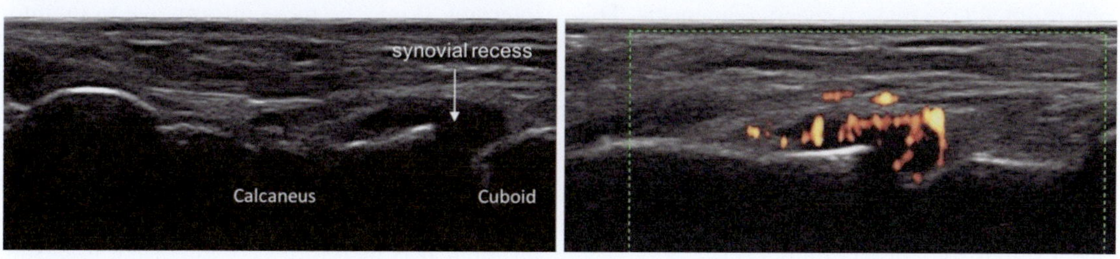

Fig. 11.22 Synovitis of the calcaneocuboid joint on B-mode (*left*) and Doppler (*right*)

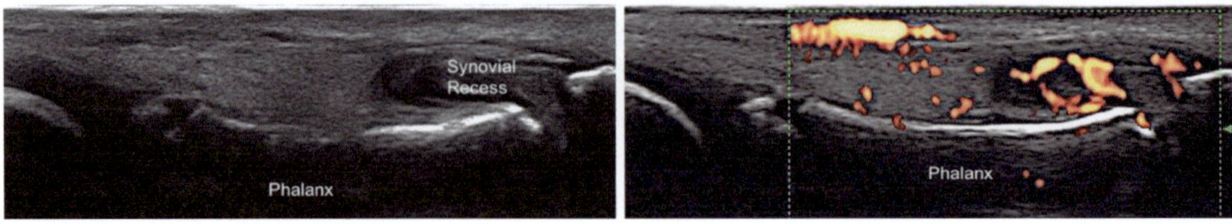

Fig. 11.23 Synovitis of the IP joint

have to be made on clinical grounds – taking into account the imaging findings – but will often also require joint aspiration, which in turn can be guided very well through ultrasonography [23–25].

In this context it is also important to differentiate echogenic fluid from synovial hypertrophy. This can be done by compression with the transducer, showing displaceability in case of fluid. For deeper joints this may nevertheless be difficult to achieve. Increased echogenicity, showing as hypoechoic material may also be present in inflammatory arthritis with a high cell count and protein content of the fluid.

Hemorrhage into a joint may initially appear an- or hypoechoic and echogenicity will increase over time with the organization and resolution of the intraarticular blood. With recurrent hemorrhages, for example in hemophilia, synovial proliferation and secondary damage to the cartilage and bone can be observed [25]. However, inflammatory changes are expected to be histologically milder in hemosideritic synovial tissue with less of a vascular response [23–25]. Less Doppler signals are therefore observed than in inflammatory arthritis [25] and this may be similar to what can be seen in Osteoarthritis or mechanical joint problems [26].

Villonodular synovitis can present with significant synovial proliferation but ultrasonography is not able to make a specific diagnosis. This may be different with MRI where Magnetic susceptibility artifact (blooming) within the affected joint space on GRE images is characteristic. This artifact is related to the local magnetic field that is created by iron present in hemoglobin, which causes spinning nuclei to dephase and a subsequent signal void, or blooming [27].

Ultrasonography is an excellent modality to detect loose bodies within the joint, some of them originating from within the joint/the adjacent bones as in Osteochondritis dissecans [28] and others having been introduced from extraarticular.

Finally, disease processes originating in the adjacent bones may present with joint effusions, with or without synovial proliferation, something that can be observed, for example, in osteonecrosis as well as chronic recurrent multifocal osteomyelitis. These conditions illustrate the value of the combination of imaging techniques, especially baseline radiographs in addition to the ultrasound assessment.

Cartilage Damage and Bone Erosions

No pediatric literature exists on characteristics of bone erosions as seen on ultrasonography for the ankle. Cartilage thickness in patients with JIA was compared to normative data in healthy children [29] and mean cartilage thickness measured in the total JIA cohort was significantly lower in the knee, wrist, and second PIP joints compared with the healthy control group but not the tibiotalar joint. Looking at the range of thickness described in the section on the normal tibiotalar joint [12], it is also conceivable that a single cross-sectional measurement might be difficult to interpret. It may be more informative to monitor cartilage thickness over time, but the problem in the pediatric age group is that it will decrease anyways due to the ongoing maturation of the bone. Finally, large parts of the cartilage are not very well accessible to the ultrasonographic assessment, for example, in the case of the subtalar joint. It is therefore very important to ensure monitoring of the cartilage and the overall structural integrity of the joint through other imaging methods, including radiographs and MRIs. With regard to the cartilage on the talar dome, which is very accessible to ultrasonography, it may be more important to demonstrate the integrity of the cartilage surface through the demonstration of the cartilage interface sign. In the case of cartilage damage, the first abnormality to detect, even before the reduction of cartilage thickness, is the inability to demonstrate the cartilage interface sign [30].

Tendon Pathology

The following tendon pathologies can be observed when scanning the ankle: Tenosynovitis, Paratenonitis, Tendinosis, Enthesopathy, Tendon tears and rupture as well as calcifications.

Tenosynovitis results from the proliferation of the parietal and visceral layer of the tendon sheath with increased fluid secretion and circumferential widening of the tendon sheath (Fig. 11.24). The fluid presents as hypoechoic or anechoic material that is displaceable and the synovial hyperplasia as thickened hypoechoic tissue which may exhibit Doppler signals [31]. Assessment will often be done in the transverse plane and pathology can then be confirmed longitudinally. It is important to follow the tendons along as pathology may occur at specific levels of the tendon. Especially the medial tendons can communicate with the tibiotalar but also the subtalar joint and fluid within the tendon sheath may originate from those joints rather than representing primary tendon pathology [13]. The demonstration of synovial proliferation within the tendon sheath nevertheless suggests the presence of true tenosynovitis.

Tenosynovitis is very prevalent in Juvenile Idiopathic Arthritis affecting the ankle. Studies have shown that in clinically swollen ankles 50% of JIA patients may have tenosynovitis only [1, 2]. The medial ankle and the tibialis posterior tendon may be very frequently involved but isolated tenosynovitis of the Flexor hallucis longus tendon, anterior ankle tendons or peroneus tendons will also be seen regularly [19]. While the ankle is the second most commonly affected joint in JIA, the relapse rate following joint injections is double than that of the knee [3]. It is tempting to speculate that incomplete or inappropriate identification of target structures may contribute to the reduced efficacy of joint injections in this anatomic area. Careful identification of target structures and imaging guided injection may improve outcomes [19]. The extensor tendons of the foot running along the midfoot do also have a tendon sheath and pathology will therefore present as tenosynovitis in this region as well (Fig. 11.25).

Other pathologies of the tendon sheath can mimic tenosynovitis clinically and to some extent also on ultrasonography. Especially when the clear architecture of the tendon with the surrounding tendon sheath cannot be demonstrated the differential diagnosis needs to be considered and additional imaging as well as tissue sampling may be necessary. This may also occur in children with an existing diagnosis of JIA. In Fig. 11.26 the transverse image of the peroneus tendons is shown in an 11-year-old girl with long-standing JIA presenting with lateral ankle swelling. The tendon architecture is not visible but has been replaced by an amorphous structure. The classic findings of tenosynovitis cannot be seen either. A subsequent MRI confirmed the

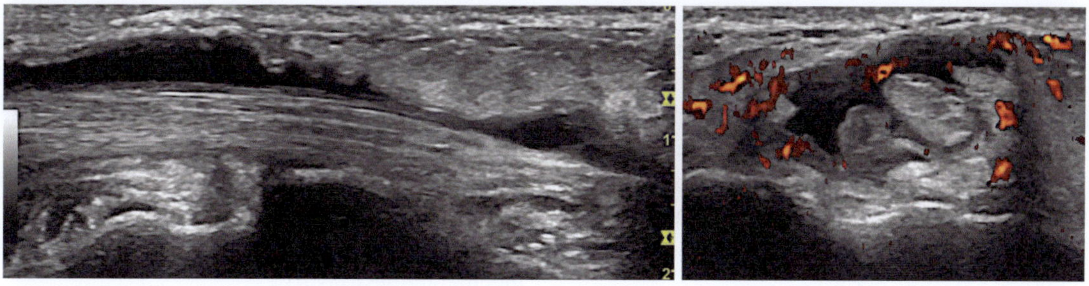

Fig. 11.24 Tenosynovitis peroneus tendons

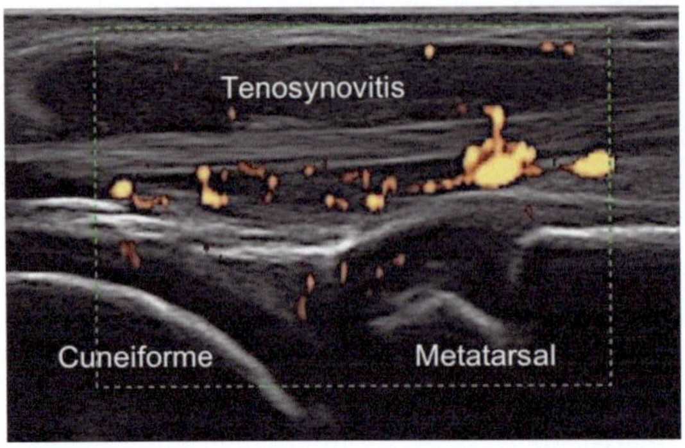

Fig. 11.25 Tenosynovitis of the extensor digitorum tendons in the midfoot area

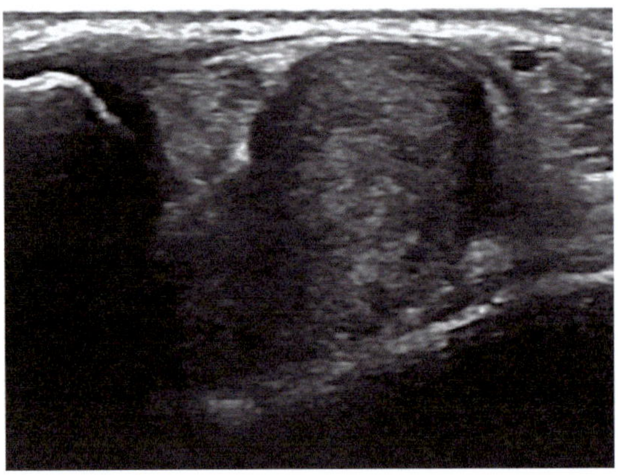

Fig. 11.26 Giant cell tumor of the tendon sheath of the peroneus tendons

suspicion of pathology other than tenosynovitis and biopsy confirmed the presence of a giant cell tumor of the tendon sheath.

Paratenonitis describes the inflammation of a tendon without a tendon sheath, in the case of the ankle region this applies to the Achilles Tendon. Tendons which do not have a tendon sheath have a paratenon instead, which is an elastic sleeve surrounding the tendon that consists of type 1 and 3 collagen and also synovial cells in a single layer. Paratenonitis presents as hypoechoic or anechoic thickened tissue with or without fluid around the tendon, which is seen in 2 perpendicular planes and which may exhibit Doppler signal. Paratenonitis is well described as a characteristic feature of Psoriatic Arthritis but can also be seen in Rheumatoid Arthritis. No data on findings in children exist currently.

Tendinosis describes changes of the tendon body and not the tendon sheath or paratenon prior to the insertion into bone (enthesis). The term tendinosis rather than tendonitis has been used to acknowledge the fact that these changes are often degenerative in nature and not necessarily primarily inflammatory. On ultrasonography it will appear as a hypoechoic, fusiform swelling especially of the Achilles tendon but without disruption of the tendon fibers. Increased blood flow on Doppler may be demonstrated due to neovascularization (Fig. 11.27).

Enthesitis

The Omeract group has developed a definition of enthesopathy. This definition is also used for enthesitis specifically but ultrasonography cannot distinguish between mechanical lesions and spondylarthropathies ultimately [6], no pediatric definition exists for enthesopathy or enthesitis currently. The Omeract definition states:

Enthesopathy is defined as an abnormally hypoechoic (loss of normal fibrillar architecture) and/or thickened tendon or ligament at its bony attachment (may occasionally contain hyperechoic foci consistent with calcification), seen in 2 perpendicular planes that may exhibit Doppler signal and/or bony changes including enthesophytes, erosions, or irregularity.

In the pediatric setting, it is especially challenging to differentiate physiologic blood flow around the enthesis from pathologic Doppler signals [6]. In addition, it is not clear whether structural changes like enthesophytes, erosions or bone irregularities would be very frequent. In order to make a cautious but reliable diagnosis, similar to the approach for synovitis where only Doppler signals within an area of synovial proliferation will be considered as pathologic, the presence of B-mode abnormalities (hypoechogenicities) should be an essential feature for the diagnosis of enthesitis as well (Fig. 11.28). The distinction between mechanical lesions and enthesitis has to be done on the clinical background and some entheses are more prone to mechanical lesions [6].

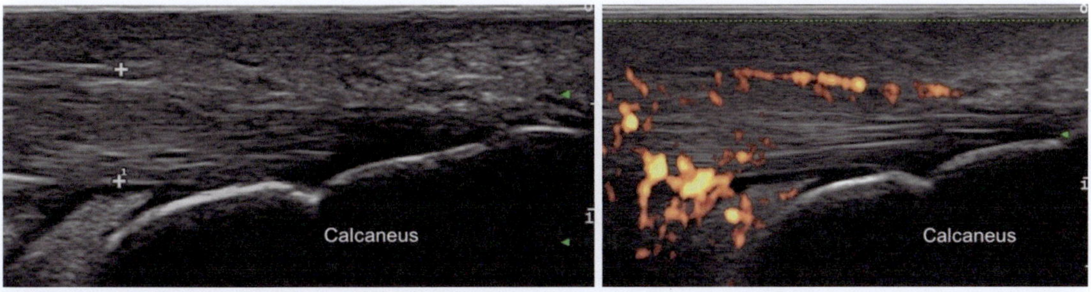

Fig. 11.27 Tendinosis of the Achilles tendon

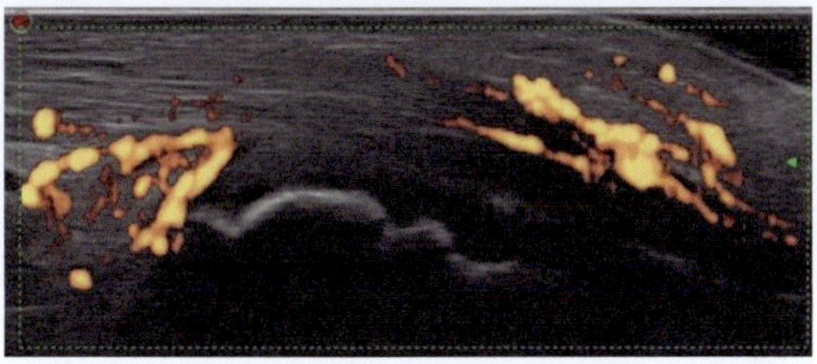

Fig. 11.28 Enthesitis of the Achilles tendon

Traction Apophysitis

During growth forces on entheses at bony protuberances (apophyses) increase. As a result inflammatory changes of the entheses may occur including thickening, hypo- and anechogenicity, and bursal distension but also fragmentation of the ossification center [6]. This condition is called apophysitis and may manifest at the tibial tuberosity (Osgood Schlatter), posterior calcaneus (Sever's), distal patella (Sindig Larssen Johannsen) and other locations. The clinical (symptoms) and imaging correlation is variable, and the examiner also needs to take into account that the presence of several ossification centers is physiologic at the posterior calcaneus, proximal fifth metatarsal bone, and other locations. Apophysitis is an important differential diagnosis of enthesitis as part of spondylarthropathy.

Accessory Navicular Bone

An accessory navicular bone, also referred to as the "os tibiale externum," can be found in about 10–15% of children [13]. It can present as a Type-I sesamoid bone that lies within the tibialis posterior tendon and is separate from the navicular (Fig. 11.29) or as a Type-II that is united to the navicular by a cartilaginous or fibrocartilaginous bridge (secondary ossification center connecting the tendon to the navicular during the first 10 years of life). Especially the Type-II represents an important differential diagnosis of medial ankle/foot pain.

Tendon Tears and Rupture

Tendon tears may occur as partial-thickness or full-thickness tears. Partial-thickness tears will appear as intrasubstance anechoic or hypoechoic areas or clefts that partially disrupt the tendon fibers. It needs to be demonstrated in two planes ideally. A longitudinal split of the tendon which may extend to one or two tendon surfaces is also called a transfixed tear. It will be best demonstrated on transverse view and needs to be differentiated from anatomic variants like the distal bifid tibialis anterior tendon or an accessory peroneus quartus tendon. In the case of the latter, distal imaging will help as the peroneus quartus will insert onto the retrocochlear eminence of the calcaneus. Full-thickness tears will result in tendon rupture, and this can be shown as a complete discontinuity of the tendon fibers especially in longitudinal view. Dynamic maneuvers may help to clarify this pathology. In the case of the Achilles tendon rupture, an intact plantaris muscle tendon may mimic an intact Achilles tendon through the continuity of the plantaris fibers, but the diameter and thickness will be significantly less than what would be expected with the Achilles tendon.

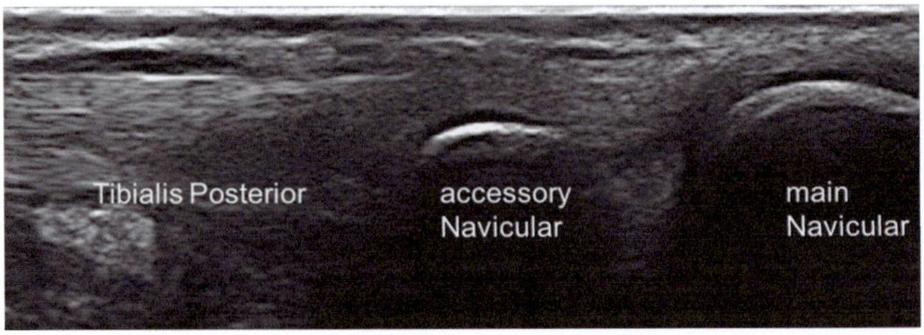

Fig. 11.29 Type-I accessory navicular bone

Contrary to adults, the weakest point of the tendon in children is at the insertion and not in the tendon body itself, likely due to the lower incidence of degenerative changes in the tendon body. Rather than tendon ruptures, avulsions of tendons at their insertion can be seen either acute or chronic, the latter usually presenting as apophysitis (see above). Acute avulsion will show discontinuity of the tendon prior to its insertion when the tendon only got avulsed. In other instances the fibrocartilage, cartilage, or parts of the bone may be avulsed as well, and the separation of the avulsed fragment attached to the tendon and separated from the main bone can be demonstrated, often enhanced by dynamic maneuvers.

Rupture of the ankle ligaments can be shown similarly than tendon ruptures and will best be seen when tension is put on the respective ligaments as described in the section on the normal sonoanatomy thus enhancing the separation of the torn ends. Associated soft tissue changes including subcutaneous edema, hemorrhage, synovial fluid, osseus lesions and in the more chronic phase calcifications can also be shown. In chronic active synovitis, there may be an increased incidence of ligament lesions due to damage to the ligaments secondary to the ongoing inflammation. It is therefore useful to include the common ligaments in the assessment of patients with inflammatory arthritis at certain time points or with symptomatology suggestive of ligament pathology.

Masses Around the Ankle and Foot

Masses around the ankle and foot include synovial cysts (including inflammation of bursae as well as atypical cysts), Ganglion cysts and other soft tissue masses. The most frequent synovial cyst is the bursitis of the retrocalcaneal bursa (Fig. 11.30) that is often seen in conjunction with inflammation of the enthesis. The retro-Achilles bursitis in turn is more frequently induced by mechanical causes.

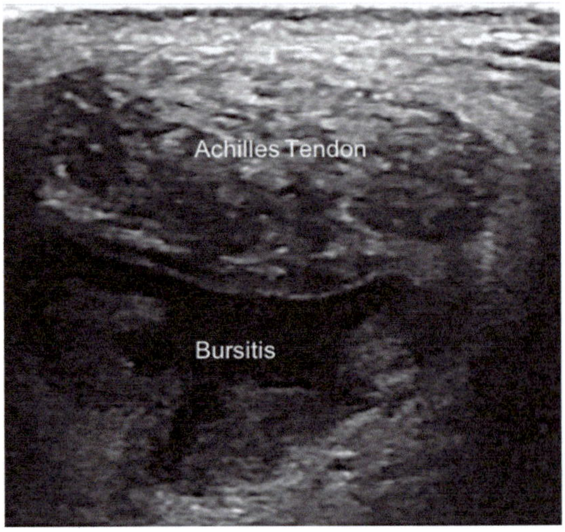

Fig. 11.30 Retrocalcaneal bursitis

In contrast to synovial cysts, ganglion cysts do not have an inner lining with synovium but with an epithelium instead. They can be found in the ankle and foot region as well and Fig. 11.31 shows an example of a ganglion cyst on the dorsal midfoot. It is important to differentiate the cyst from tenosynovitis or synovitis through longitudinal and transverse assessments. In this case it lies next to the tendons but clearly does not include the tendon sheath and also does not display Doppler signals as would be expected in the case of a synovial cyst.

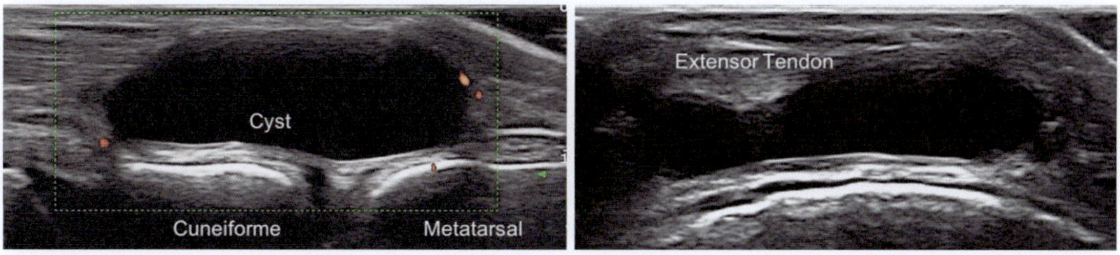

Fig. 11.31 Ganglion cyst of the midfoot

Talocalcaneal coalition

Talocalcaneal coalition (TCC) is a congenital fibrous, cartilaginous, or bony fusion of the subtalar joint predominantly involving the middle facet of the talus and the underlying sustentaculum tali of the calcaneus [32]. TCC is an important cause of medial ankle pain and typically becomes symptomatic in the second to fourth decades of life. These coalitions can be difficult to detect on standard radiographs. Owing to its tomographic capabilities ultrasound can detect TCC. Confirmation of the coalition by CT or MRI is required in the preoperative assessment to better assess the type and extent of the congenital anomaly as well as the adjacent joints [32]. The diagnostic ultrasound criteria for fibrous coalition are a reduced joint space of the medial aspect of the anterior talocalcaneal joint associated with an irregular, pointed appearance of its outline, while osseous coalition was diagnosed in patients with a smooth continuity of the hyperechoic bone surface between the medial talus and the sustentaculum tali.

Tarsal Tunnel Syndrome

Tarsal tunnel syndrome is a painful condition in which the tibial nerve and/or its divisional branches are impinged or compressed as they travel through the tarsal tunnel. It is a controversial entity, specific causes are identified in only 60%–80% of cases. Bone and joint disorders, space-occupying lesions, accessory muscles and congenital varus or valgus deformity of the foot may contribute to the clinical symptomatology.

Summary

Ultrasonography of the ankle and foot allows for a complete assessment of this complex anatomic area at the point of care. The exam can be tailored individually and be very focused or consider the wide range of differential diagnosis depending on the clinical situation. The dynamic assessment on ultrasonography and the high spatial resolution provide a specific advantage of this imaging technique over other methods. Different imaging methods might nevertheless be complementary and will ultimately ensure improved clinical outcomes in an anatomic area that can lead to severe functional impairment in case of damage [33–35].

Acknowledgment Illustrations in this chapter were designed based on illustrations by Carlo Martinoli, Genoa, Italy.

References

1. Rooney ME, McAllister C, Burns JF. Ankle disease in juvenile idiopathic arthritis: ultrasound findings in clinically swollen ankles. J Rheumatol. 2009;36(8):1725–9.
2. Pascoli L, Wright S, McAllister C, Rooney M. Prospective evaluation of clinical and ultrasound findings in ankle disease in juvenile idiopathic arthritis: importance of ankle ultrasound. J Rheumatol. 2010;37(11):2409–14.
3. Zulian F, Martini G, Gobber D, Agosto C, Gigante C, Zacchello FWH. Comparison of intra-articular triamcinolone hexacetonide and triamcinolone acetonide in oligoarticular juvenile idiopathic arthritis. Rheumatology. 2003;42:1254–9.
4. Malattia C, Rinaldi M, Martini A. The role of imaging in juvenile idiopathic arthritis. Expert Rev Clin Immunol. 2018;20:1–14.

5. Johnson, Kennedy JA. Radiographic anatomy of the human skeleton. Edinburgh/London: ES Livingstone; 1970. ISBN 044300268 1.
6. Weiss PF, Chauvin NA, Roth J. Imaging in juvenile Spondyloarthritis. Curr Rheumatol Rep. 2016;18:75.
7. Grechenig W, Mayr JM, Peicha G, Hammerl R, Schatz B, Grechenig S. Sonoanatomy of the Achilles tendon insertion in children. J Clin Ultrasound. 2004;32(7):338–43.
8. Roth J, Jousse-Joulin S, Magni-Manzoni S, Rodriguez A, Tzaribachev N, Iagnocco A, Naredo E, D'Agostino MA, Collado P. Outcome measures in rheumatology ultrasound group. Definitions for the sonographic features of joints in healthy children. Arthritis Care Res. 2015;67:136–42.
9. Ogden JA, McCarthy SM. Radiology of postnatal skeletal development. VIII. Distal tibia and fibula. Skelet Radiol. 1983;10(4):209–20.
10. Möller I, Janta I, Backhaus M, Ohrndorf S, Bong DA, Martinoli C, Filippucci E, Sconfienza LM, Terslev L, Damjanov N, Hammer HB, Sudol-Szopinska I, Grassi W, Balint P, Bruyn GAW, D'Agostino MA, Hollander D, Siddle HJ, Supp G, Schmidt WA, Iagnocco A, Koski J, Kane D, Fodor D, Bruns A, Mandl P, Kaeley GS, Micu M, Ho C, Vlad V, Chávez-López M, Filippou G, Cerón CE, Nestorova R, Quintero M, Wakefield R, Carmona L, Naredo E. The 2017 EULAR standardised procedures for ultrasound imaging in rheumatology. Ann Rheum Dis. 2017;76(12):1974–9.
11. Collado P, Vojinovic J, Nieto JC, Windschall D, Magni-Manzoni S, Bruyn GA, Iagnocco A, D'agostino MA, Naredo E. Omeract ultrasound pediatric group. Toward standardized musculoskeletal ultrasound in pediatric rheumatology: normal age-related ultrasound findings. Arthritis Care Res. 2016;68:348–56.
12. Spannow AH, Pfeiffer-Jensen M, Andersen NT, Herlin T, Stenbøg E. Ultrasonographic measurements of joint cartilage thickness in healthy children: age- and sex-related standard reference values. J Rheumatol. 2010;37(12):2595–601.
13. Bianchi S, Martinoli C. Ultrasound of the musculoskeletal system. Berlin Heidelberg: Springer; 2007.
14. Kannus P. Structure of the tendon connective tissue. Scand J Med Sci Sports. 2000;10(6):312–20.
15. Mandl P, Bong D, Balint PV, Hammer HB, Miguel M, Naredo E, Terslev L, Möller I. Anatomy for the image study group. Sonographic and anatomic description of the subtalar joint. Ultrasound Med Biol. 2018;44:119–23.
16. Roth J, Ravagnani V, Backhaus M, Balint P, Bruns A, Bruyn GA, Collado P, De la Cruz L, Guillaume-Czitrom S, Herlin T, Hernandez C, Iagnocco A, Jousse-Joulin S, Lanni S, Lilleby V, Malattia C, Magni-Manzoni S, Modesto C, Rodriguez A, Nieto JC, Ohrndorf S, Rossi-Semerano L, Selvaag AM, Swen N, Ting TV, Tzaribachev N, Vega-Fernandez P, Vojinovic J, Windschall D, D'Agostino MA, Naredo E, OMERACT Ultrasound Group. Preliminary definitions for the Sonographic features of synovitis in children. Arthritis Care Res. 2017;69:1217–23.
17. Roth J, Scheer I, Kraft S, Keitzer R, Riebel T. Uncommon synovial cysts in children. Eur J Pediatr. 2006;165:178–81.
18. Collado P, Naredo E, Calvo C, Gamir ML, Calvo I, García ML, Merino R, Graña J, Bustabab S, Garrido J, ECO-JIA Study Group. Reduced joint assessment vs comprehensive assessment for ultrasound detection of synovitis in juvenile idiopathic arthritis. Rheumatology. 2013;52:1477–84.
19. Laurell L, Court-Payen M, Nielsen S, Zak M, Boesen M, Fasth A. Ultrasonography and color Doppler in juvenile idiopathic arthritis: diagnosis and follow-up of ultrasound-guided steroid injection in the ankle region. A descriptive interventional study. Pediatr Rheumatol Online J. 2011;9(1):4.
20. Lanni S, Bovis F, Ravelli A, Viola S, Magnaguagno F, Pistorio A, Michele Magnano G, Martini A, Malattia C. Delineating the application of ultrasound in detecting synovial abnormalities of the subtalar joint in juvenile idiopathic arthritis. Arthritis Care Res (Hoboken). 2016;68(9):1346–53.
21. Phatak S, Mohindra N, Zanwar A, Aggarwal A. Prominent midfoot involvement in children with enthesitis-related arthritis category of juvenile idiopathic arthritis. Clin Rheumatol. 2017;36:1737–45.
22. Kaeley GS. Review of the use of ultrasound for the diagnosis and monitoring of enthesitis in psoriatic arthritis. Curr Rheumatol Rep. 2011;13(4):338–45.
23. Roosendaal G, Van Rinsum AC, Vianen ME. Haemophilic arthropathy resembles degenerative rather than inflammatory joint disease. Histopathology. 1999;34:144–53.
24. Valentino LA, Hakobyan N. Histological changes in murine haemophilic syn- ovitis: a quantitative grading system to assess blood-induced synovitis. Haemophilia. 2006;12:654–62.
25. Martinoli C, Della Casa Alberighi O, Di Minno G, Graziano E, Molinari AC, Pasta G, Russo G, Santagostino E, Tagliaferri A, Tagliafico A, Morfini M. Development and definition of a simplified scanning procedure and scoring method for haemophilia early arthropathy detection with ultrasound (HEAD-US). Thromb Haemost. 2013;109:1170–9.
26. Beitinger N, Ehrenstein B, Schreiner B, Fleck M, Grifka J, Lüring C, Hartung W. The value of colour Doppler sonography of the knee joint: a useful tool to discriminate inflammatory from non-inflammatory disease? Rheumatology. 2013;52:1425–8.
27. Bitar R, Leung G, Perng R, et al. MR pulse sequences: what every radiologist wants to know but is afraid to ask. Radio Graphics. 2006;26:513–37.
28. Kröger L, Piippo-Savolainen E, Tyrväinen E, Penttilä P, Kröger H. Osteochondral lesions in children with juvenile idiopathic arthritis. Pediatr Rheumatol Online J. 2013;11:18.
29. Pradsgaard DØ, Spannow AH, Heuck C, Herlin T. Decreased cartilage thickness in juvenile idiopathic

arthritis assessed by ultrasonography. J Rheumatol. 2013;40(9):1596–603.
30. Filippucci E, da Luz KR, Di Geso L, Salaffi F, Tardella M, Carotti M, Natour J, Grassi W. Interobserver reliability of ultrasonography in the assessment of cartilage damage in rheumatoid arthritis. Ann Rheum Dis. 2010;69:1845–8.
31. Bruyn GA, et al. Ann Rheum Dis. 2014;73(11): 1929–34.
32. Bianchi S, Hoffman D. Skelet Radiol. 2013;42: 1209–14.
33. Bugni Miotto eSilva V, de Freitas Tavares da Silva C, de Aguiar Vilela Mitraud S, Nely Vilar Furtado R, Esteves Hilário MO, Natour J, Terreri MT. Do patients with juvenile idiopathic arthritis in remission exhibit active synovitis on joint ultrasound? Rheumatol Int. 2014;34:937–45.
34. Janow GL, Panghaal V, Trinh A, Badger D, Levin TL, Ilowite NT. Detection of active disease in juvenile idiopathic arthritis: sensitivity and specificity of the physical examination vs ultrasound. J Rheumatol. 2011;38:2671–4.
35. Rebollo-Polo M, Koujok K, Weisser C, Jurencak R, Bruns A, Roth J. Ultrasound findings on patients with juvenile idiopathic arthritis in clinical remission. Arthritis Care Res. 2011;63:1013–9.

Spine: Neonatal and Infant Spine

12

Alka Karnik

Introduction

Spinal ultrasound (SUS) is a safe, non-invasive, highly sensitive imaging modality for evaluating intraspinal contents in neonates and infants younger than 4 months. Lack of ossification of the posterior elements of the spine allows excellent delineation of the terminal cord, conus and the cauda equina. The scan is best performed up to 4 months of age after which increasing ossification limits beam penetration. However if there is a defect in the posterior elements, imaging may be possible even after 6 months of age. Magnetic resonance imaging (MRI) till date has been considered the imaging gold standard, however new-generation ultrasound machines with high-frequency linear array transducers and extended field-of-view capability now permit diagnostic sensitivity equal to MRI in neonates [1, 2]. Comparative advantages of SUS over MRI are wide availability, no risks of sedation or general anaesthesia and absence of MRI-related cerebrospinal fluid (CSF) pulsation and vascular flow artefacts [3].

SUS is widely used as a first-line screening tool to look for spinal dysraphism (SD) in babies with lumbar cutaneous stigmata (like atypical dimples, skin tag or tail, haemangiomas, hairy patches) and skin-covered masses and in SD-associated syndromes (such as anorectal and urogenital malformations, including the VATER group). It helps image cord abnormalities in spina bifida, meningocoele, myelocoele, lipomeningomyelocoele, diastematomyelia, syringomyelia, tethered cord and intradural masses. It is suggested that SUS be used as the primary screening tool, reserving MRI for cases where SUS has equivocal findings or has revealed a definite abnormality [1]. Acquired intraspinal diseases following birth trauma, transient alterations after lumbar puncture and in meningitis can also be detected with SUS [4].

Embryology

To understand spinal anomalies, knowledge of embryonic development is necessary. In the third week of gestation the central nervous system starts to form, by a process of 'primary neurulation' during which the neural plate thickens bilaterally to form the neural folds, then folds upon itself and fuses dorsally to form the neural tube. The closure begins in the upper thoracic level and proceeds both cephalad and caudally [5]. The cephalic end closes before the caudal end. The proximal neural tube forms the brain and caudal one-third of the neural tube and neural crest form the spinal cord. When closure is complete, the neural tube separates

A. Karnik (✉)
Nanavati Super Speciality Hospital, Mumbai, India

Y. El Miedany (ed.), *Pediatric Musculoskeletal Ultrasonography*,
https://doi.org/10.1007/978-3-030-17824-6_12

from the ectoderm by the process of dysjunction. This is followed by 'secondary neurulation', a process of canalisation in the caudal cell mass at the distal end of the neural tube, resulting in an ependyma-lined tube that unites with the neural tube to form the primitive spinal cord. This is followed by 'retrogressive differentiation', a process whereby the caudal cell mass and neural tube regress in size to form the fetal conus medullaris, ventriculus and filum terminale.

Abnormal closure and dysjunction leads to various forms of spinal dysraphism (SD). Complete failure of dysjunction causes non-skin-covered defects such as myelocoele and meningomyelocoele. Focal incomplete dysjunction causes a dorsal dermal sinus. Premature dysjunction causes skin-covered lipomyelocoele, lipomyelomeningocoele, and terminal and intradural lipomas [6].

Abnormal canalisation and retrogressive differentiation leads to a spectrum of abnormalities ranging from tethered cord to filum terminale lipomas to severe anomalies like terminal myelocystocoele, sacral agenesis and caudal regression syndrome and sacrococcygeal teratomas [6].

Abnormal notochord splitting leads to diastematomyelia, neurenteric cysts, butterfly vertebrae and neurenteric fistulae [6].

Sonographic Examination

Preparation

Obtaining relevant history and explaining the procedure to the parents/accompanying guardian should precede the examination. Examination is carried out in a warm environment with all clothing removed. Ideally neonate should be fed prior to the ultrasound; however if pre-procedural feeding is not possible, a pacifier dipped in glucose can be helpful to keep the infant still.

An incontinence sheet should be spread on the examination couch. The neonate is placed in prone position preferably over a rolled pillow or bolster, to achieve adequate spinal flexion and increase spacing of spinous processes to provide an ideal acoustic window for examination. Elevation of the neonatal head allows CSF to distend the distal thecal sac improving visualisation of distal cord. If prone position is not possible, the neonate can be examined in lateral decubitus position. In the decubitus position, however one should remember that the spinal cord and nerve roots may gravitate to the dependent side [2].

Scanning Technique

A high-frequency linear 17–5 MHz transducer is used as it gives a larger image in the near-field and has a higher spatial resolution. In older infants, a lower- frequency may be necessary for better penetration. Panoramic function is used in imaging a long segment of the spine and thus aids in identifying the vertebral levels [2, 4]. A high-frequency, small footprint convex transducer is used to evaluate the craniovertebral junction.

The spinal cord is assessed in the sagittal and axial planes, with right and left labelled on axial images. Examination begins with an initial quick sweep of the transducer in axial plane from the thoracic region up to the sacrococcygeal region, to identify any posterior arch defects or gross anomalies [2].

Scanning in the sagittal plane starts at the level of sacrococcygeal junction. The level of termination of the conus, the filum terminale and termination of the thecal sac, should be documented. Normal oscillation of the cord and fibrillary movements of the cauda equina, synchronising with the cardiac-related pulsations of the spinal CSF, should be documented with cine-sequences, during crying and flexion of the spine or with M-mode [2].

Axial images are essential to assess integrity of the posterior neural arches and to identify diastematomyelia. Vertebral bodies are checked for alignment, shape and symmetry in both axial and sagittal planes. Off-centre scanning avoids refraction artefact that may resemble diastematomyelia [2].

In cases with sacral dimple or identified skin defect, a high-frequency hockey stick or small footprint transducer should be used to identify the fistulous communication. Minimal pressure should be applied to avoid compression and obscuration of the tract. Leakage of CSF from the dimple is an indication to perform MRI spine in these cases.

Areas of abnormal fluid accumulation in the central canal are documented and levels noted. Colour Doppler (CD) may be used as and when required in addition to the B-mode examination.

Documentation of the craniovertebral junction on sagittal suboccipital scanning completes the SUS evaluation and helps in detecting associated Chiari 2 malformation in cases of spinal dysraphism. This requires a small footprint convex transducer.

Normal Sonoanatomy

On sagittal scanning, (Fig. 12.1a) the spinal cord is seen as a hypoechoic, tubular structure surrounded by echo-free CSF and with an echogenic central canal [4, 7, 8]. The echogenic margins of the spinal canal are the ventral and dorsal dural surfaces. The cord tapers at the caudal end to form the conus medullaris which continues as the echogenic cord-like filum terminale, surrounded by echogenic nerve roots or the cauda equina which shows oscillatory movements. The normal filum measures less than 2 mm in thickness and passes through the subarachnoid space and through the dura mater to insert on first coccygeal vertebral body [7, 8]. In addition to the conus and filum terminale, the termination of the thecal sac, typically located at S2 should also be documented.

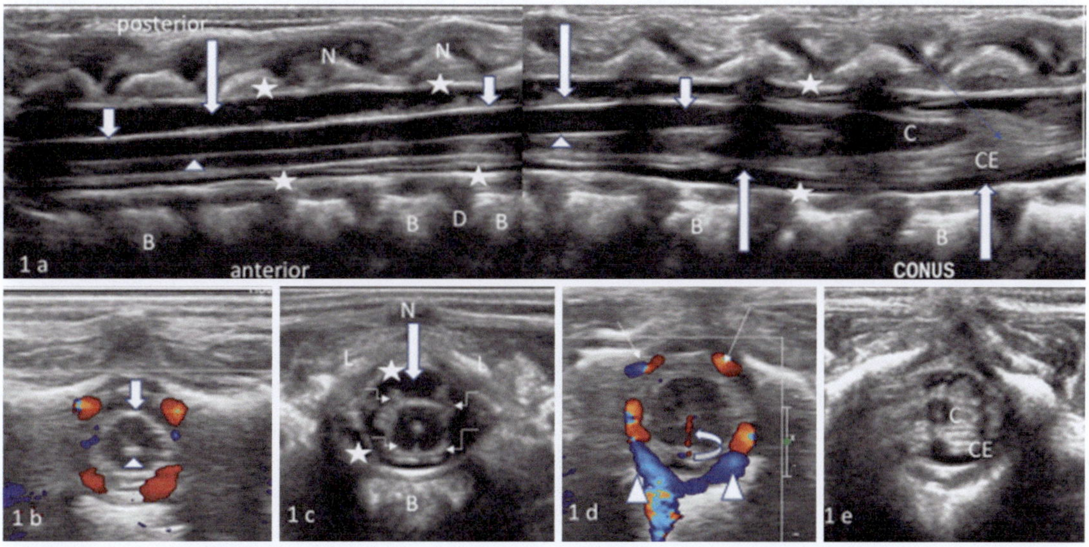

Fig. 12.1 Normal anatomy. (**a**) Sagittal scan shows the Spinal cord as a hypoechoic tubular structure (thick short arrow) with an echogenic central canal (arrow head). Lumbar enlargement of cord seen; distal to this the cord tapers to form the conus medullaris (C), which continues as the filum terminale surrounded by echogenic nerve roots (CE). Anteriorly is the anterior subarachnoid space (thick long arrow), anterior dura (star) and the vertebral bodies (B). Posteriorly is the posterior subarachnoid space (thick long arrow), posterior dura (star) and the neural arch (N). (**b** and **c**) Axial scan of thoracic cord. Spinal cord seen as a hypoechoic rounded structure (thick short arrow) with an echogenic central canal (arrow head). The cord is centrally placed in the spinal canal. The anterior and posterior nerve roots (angled arrows) are seen arising from the cord. Anteriorly is vertebral body (B), anterior dura (star) and the anterior subarachnoid space (thick long arrow). Posteriorly is the posterior subarachnoid space and posterior dura. Posteriorly is the neural arch comprising of the unossified spinous process (N) and ossified bilateral laminae (L), which appear echogenic. (**d**) Axial scan of lumbar cord. Colour Doppler showing the anterior spinal artery (curved arrow), paired posterior spinal arteries (thin arrows), anteromedial and anterolateral veins (arrowheads). (**e**) Axial scan at conus. Shows rounded hypoechoic tip of conus (C) surrounded by the echogenic cauda equina fibres (CE)

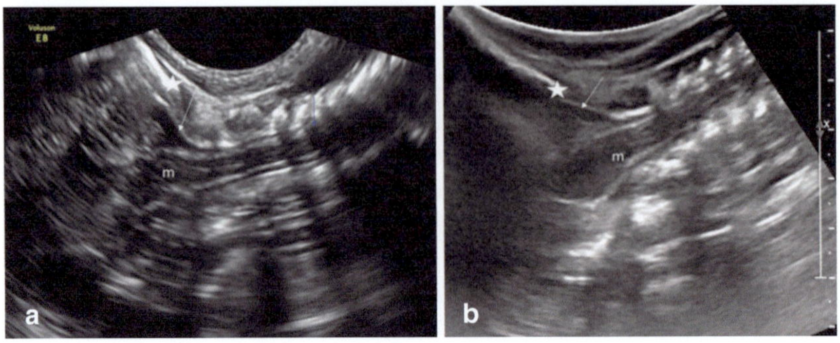

Fig. 12.2 Sagittal suboccipital scan at the craniovertebral junction. (**a**) Normal anatomy: The pons, medulla oblongata (m) and cervical cord are seen as hypoechoic structures with echogenic borders, surrounded by CSF in the subarachnoid space. The cisterna magna (arrow) with anechoic CSF noted caudal to the echogenic cerebellum (C). The echogenic border of the bony foramen magnum identified dorsally (star). (**b**) 5 day old neonate operated on day 2 for a lumbar meningomyelocoele. Scan shows attenuated cisterna magna (arrow) and a low placed medulla oblongata (m) as in a Chiari 2 malformation

In the axial section the spinal cord is hypoechoic, oval or round with an echogenic central echo-complex and is surrounded by the anechoic CSF-containing subarachnoid space. The cord is positioned centrally in the canal with the echogenic, paired nerve roots arising from it, which demonstrate oscillation with infant respiration (Fig. 12.1c). Anterior to the cord are the anterior subarachnoid space, dura, and vertebral bodies and posterior are the posterior subarachnoid space, dura, and neural arch. The spinal cord should remain round in the axial plane through the thoracolumbar region but may become more oval superiorly within the cervical region. The cord diameter is variable and is the largest at the cervical and lumbar levels, which are known as cervical and lumbar "enlargements". Axial scan at the conus shows rounded hypoechoic tip of conus surrounded by the echogenic cauda equina fibres.

The subarachnoid space is anechoic, interrupted by normal hyperechoic linear nerve roots and dentate ligaments (Fig. 12.1c).

Although colour Doppler (CD) imaging is not routinely used to evaluate the spinal vessels, with the advent of new-generation scanners, further insight into the vascular anatomy can be obtained. The midline anterior spinal artery, posterior paired spinal arteries, and anteromedial and anterolateral plexus of veins can be seen (Fig. 12.1b, d). Abnormal vascular channels can be seen in vascular malformations (Fig. 12.14).

On sagittal suboccipital evaluation of the normal craniovertebral junction with a small footprint convex transducer, the pons, medulla oblongata and cervical cord are seen as hypoechoic structures with echogenic borders, surrounded by CSF in the subarachnoid space. The cisterna magna with anechoic CSF is noted caudal to an echogenic cerebellum (Fig. 12.2a). The echogenic border of the bony foramen magnum is identified dorsal to the brain stem. Identifying the normal level of the medulla in relation to the foramen magnum helps in evaluating for Chiari 2 malformations in cases of SD.

Identifying the Level of the Conus

The conus normally lies at or above the L1–2 to L2–3 disk space in term neonates [9]. At 40 weeks gestational age, no conus was found below L2–3 and no conus was seen above T12-L1 [10]. In preterm infants, a conus located at mid L3 level may be identified [10]. A routine follow-up in such cases is recommended once the neonate attains a corrected age between 40 weeks gestation and 6 months of age [9, 10].

Accurate identification of the vertebral body level is required to comment on the level of conus termination. The first coccygeal segment has variable ossification at birth. If ossified, it can be distinguished by its rounder shape compared with the

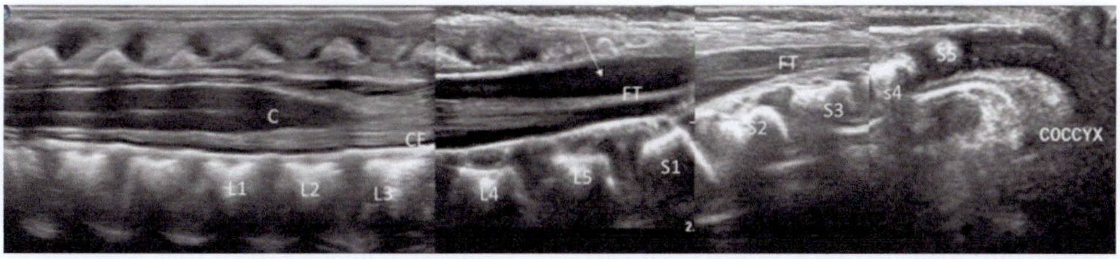

Fig. 12.3 Normal anatomy. Sagittal view of the distal spinal canal. The cord is seen as a hypoechoic tubular structure with an echogenic central canal tapering to form the Conus (C), which continues as the cord-like filum terminale (FT) surrounded by echogenic nerve roots of the cauda equina and anechoic CSF in the subarachnoid space (arrow). Coccyx is unossified cartilage and appears hypoechoic. The last sacral segment shows an echogenic ossification (S5). At the L5-S1 junction, the distinction between oblique orientation of the sacral vertebrae and horizontal orientation of the lumbar vertebrae is evident. Cranially, the vertebral bodies are numbered and conus is seen at L2–3 disc level

square or rectangular shape of the sacral bodies. Usually in term infants, the coccyx is identified as an unossified cartilage mass (Fig. 12.3). Counting cephalad to the coccyx identifies the 5 sacral vertebral bodies and the lumbosacral junction at L5-S1 [4, 5]. At the L5-S1 junction, the distinction between the oblique orientation of the sacral vertebrae and horizontal orientation of the lumbar vertebrae is evident (Fig. 12.3). Further cephalad counting of the vertebrae is done from the L5-S1 junction up to L1. The last rib-bearing vertebra can be presumed to be T12, and counting downward the lumbar level of the conus can then be determined.

In cases of transitional vertebra or when the level of the conus is indeterminate, a radiopaque marker is placed on the skin at the level of the conus determined by sonographic guidance, followed by a correlative AP spine radiograph [2].

Signs of Tethering of the Cord to Look for on SUS

A tethered spinal cord, with a fixation of the spinal cord in caudal location, is commonly associated with many spinal malformations. Incomplete separation of neural tube from the ectoderm may result in cord tethering [1]. Neurologic symptoms may not be present in newborns, but stretching with growth causes progressive neurological involvement. Because some paediatric neurosurgeons believe early surgical correction of SD may avoid these sequelae, early diagnosis of tethered cord is important [1]. Signs of tethered spinal cord to look for during SUS are as follows: (1) low conus, the level of termination of the cord below L2–L3; (2) abnormal conus configuration, a dorsal position of conus/filum in the spinal canal; (3) thickened echogenic filum terminale (>2 mm); (4) decreased or absent oscillation of conus/filum on real-time study; and (5) caudal tissue mass [6, 11].

Sometimes (in tight filum syndrome), the conus may be normally placed, but cord can still be tethered, and diagnosis is made on the basis of loss of pulsatility [6, 11].

Fluid Collections in the Spinal Cord

Fluid collections in the spinal cord are often seen in association with various spinal abnormalities. The lumen of the neural tube forms the central spinal canal. Accumulation of CSF in the ependyma-lined central canal of the spinal cord is hydromyelia and dissection of CSF through the ependyma with paracentral cavitation is termed syringomyelia. However, on imaging, distinguishing between the two entities is not always possible, and on SUS these are seen as an anechoic fluid-filled distension and widening of the echogenic central canal. They are often seen in association with anomalies like myelomeningocoele, diastematomyelia. Hydromyelia and syringomyelia always occur cranial to the placode and may be focal (Fig. 12.6a, Fig. 12.10a, Fig. 12.14a) or involve the entire spinal cord (Fig. 12.5 c,d). If untreated, these conditions may cause rapid development of scoliosis [4].

Identifying Normal Variants

1. **Ventriculus terminalis** – Seen as a transient fluid-filled anechoic fusiform widening of the central echo-complex (spinal canal), occasionally seen in normal neonates in the conus medullaris (Fig. 12.4b). This is a variant of no clinical significance and disappears within first few months of life [4, 12].
2. **Filar cyst** – Seen as a midline, anechoic, fusiform simple cystic mass within the filum terminale just below conus (Fig. 12.4c), as opposed to the conus medullaris location of the ventriculus terminalis. This finding is better seen on SUS than MRI and is of no clinical significance [4, 7, 8, 13].
3. **Prominent filum terminale** – A prominent filum terminale is echogenic in comparison with other nerve roots (Fig. 12.4d). It is distinguished as normal by its thickness and typical midline course [7, 8].
4. **Pseudomass of the cauda equina** – This entity is noted during SUS performed in decubitus position and is due to nerve root clumping (Fig. 12.4e). It disappears when scan is performed in prone position [7].
5. **Pseudosinus tract** – Seen as an echogenic, fibrous cord-like structure extending from the

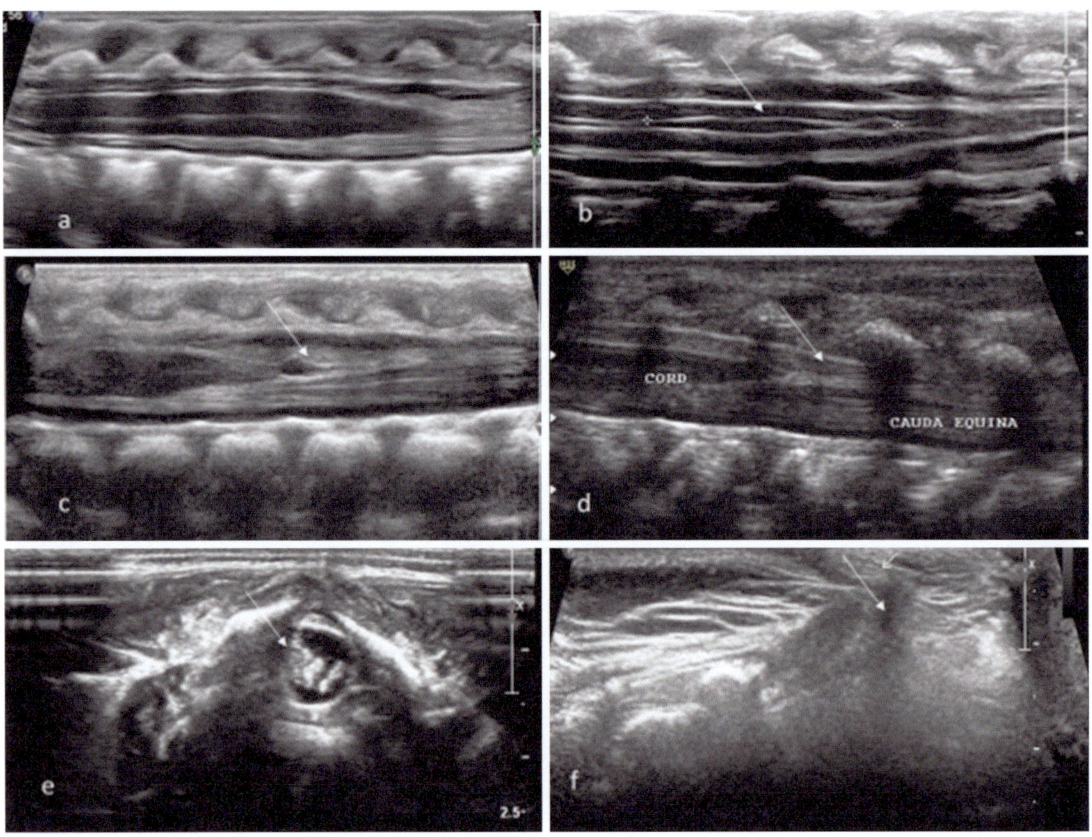

Fig. 12.4 Normal Variants. (**a**) Normal conus medullaris with echogenic central canal. (**b**) Ventriculus terminalis (arrow) seen as a transient fluid-filled anechoic widening of the central spinal canal in the conus medullaris. (**c**) Filar cyst (arrow) seen as an anechoic, fusiform simple cystic mass within the filum terminale just below the conus. (**d**) Prominent filum terminale (arrow) appears echogenic in comparison with surrounding nerve roots. (**e**) Pseudomass (arrow) of the cauda equina due to nerve root clumping. (**f**) Pseudosinus tract (arrow) seen as an echogenic, fibrous cord-like structure extending from the coccyx to an overlying sacral skin dimple

coccyx to an overlying sacral dimple (Fig. 12.4f). No fluid collections or masses should be identified along the tract. True dermal sinus tracts rarely occur at the tip of the coccyx and are typically found in a more cranial location [7].

6. **Dysmorphic coccyx** – Variations in the shape and ossification of the coccyx at birth can pose challenges in neonates with a palpable lump clinically [7].

Spinal Dysraphism

Incomplete or absent fusion of the posterior spinal tissues gives rise to a spectrum of anomalies labelled as "spinal dysraphism". These are broadly classified into two groups based on clinical findings: (a) Spina bifida aperta or open, non-skin-covered lesions and (b) Occult spinal dysraphism, or skin-covered lesions. The second group is further divided as skin-covered defects with a subcutaneous mass and occult spinal dysraphism without a mass [6, 9].

Open Spinal Dysraphism

Failure of fusion of the posterior spinal elements, causes spina bifida aperta or non-skin-covered or open defects such as myelocoele and myelomeningocoele. The neural tissue is exposed to the amniotic fluid *in utero*. Intracranial changes of Chiari 2 malformation are usually seen and help in early in utero diagnosis. Incidence is 2 per 1000 live births with a slight female preponderance [4]. Clinical diagnosis of open, non -skin-covered lesions (like myelocoele, meningomyelocoeles) is obvious at birth.

The lesion affects mostly the lower back with the following frequency distribution: thoracic, 2%; thoracolumbar, 32%; lumbar, 22%; and lumbosacral, 44% [4]. Lumbar or sacral myelocoele and myelomeningocoele are always associated with tethering of the spinal cord [1, 4]. Clinical symptoms like severe neurologic disturbances mainly of lower extremities and bladder bowel dysfunction are often seen.

In open SD, SUS is usually avoided owing to risk of injury and infection [4]. Examination may be performed with strict aseptic precautions after covering the probe with a sterile cover, covering the defect with a sterile plastic wrap, using sterile gel and non-latex-covered gloves [6]. On SUS there is widening of the bony posterior neural arch. The unfused neural plate called as neural placode is seen as a flat hypoechoic plaque of neural tissue with nerve roots arising from the ventral surface [5, 9]. Caudal displacement of the conus with tethering is seen [4, 5]. The neural placode is flush with the plane of the dorsal skin in patients with myelocoele. In patients with myelomeningocoele, there is an expansion of the ventral subarachnoid space which displaces the placode dorsally (Fig. 12.5a, b) leading to protrusion of the placode beyond the dorsal skin surface, into a CSF- filled sac [5, 9].

The imaging of the proximal skin-covered spine is usually after primary repair of the open defect, mainly to look for associated findings like syringomyelia (40–80% of patients) (Fig. 12.5 c, d), diastematomyelia (20–40% of patients) and arachnoid cyst (2% of patients). Chiari 2 malformation occurs in 99% of patients with open spinal defect [4]. Cranial sonography is done to assess degree of hydrocephalus (Fig. 12.5f). Associated abnormalities like hypoplasia or aplasia of corpus callosum and Dandy Walker malformation may be seen [4, 6].

The sagittal scanning of the craniovertebral junction to look for Chiari 2 malformation (Fig. 12.2b) shows a downward displacement of the pons, medulla oblongata and cranial part of cervical spinal cord [4]. The cerebellar vermis herniates through the foramen magnum into the cervical spinal cord [4] (Fig. 12.5e).

Post-operative complications like re-tethering of the cord, inclusion epidermoid, inclusion lipoma, hydromyelia, arachnoid cyst can be evaluated by sonography [4, 9].

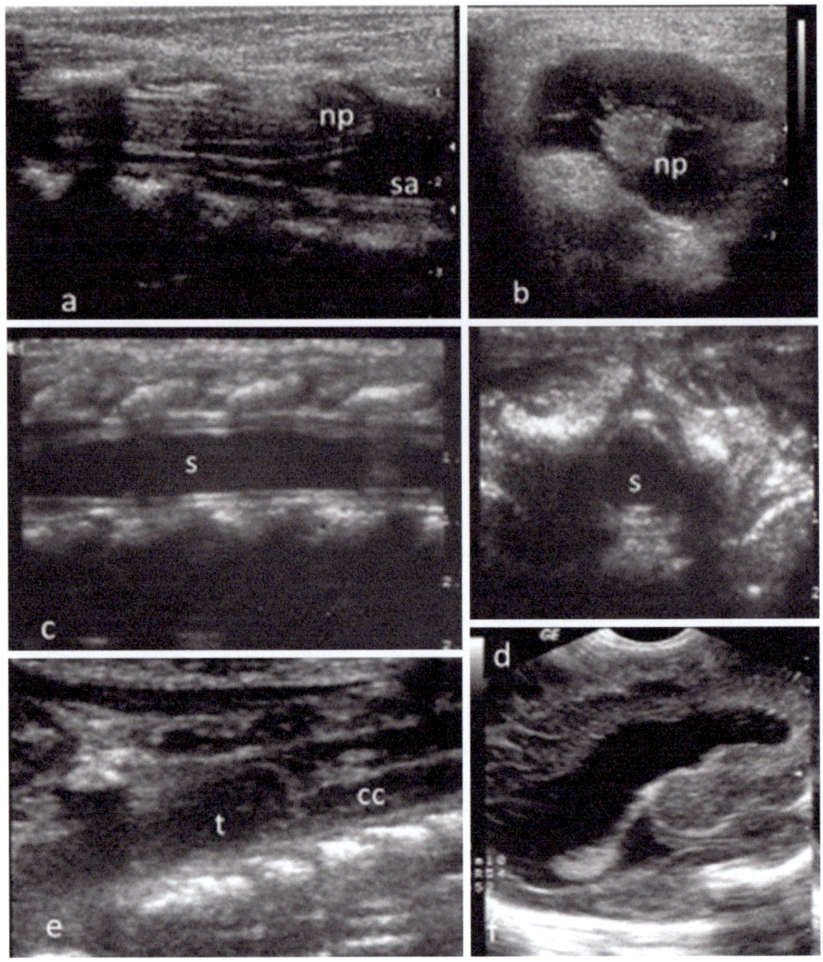

Fig. 12.5 Open spinal dysraphism – Meningomyelocoele and Chiari 2 malformation. (**a** and **b**) Sagittal and transverse sections of a lumbar meningomyelocoele with a thin partial membrane covering the soft tissue protrusion. Subcutaneous location of the neural placode (n) and widened anterior subarachnoid space (sa) noted. (**c** and **d**) Sagittal and transverse sections of the thoracic cord shows associated syringomyelia. (**e**) Sagittal scan at the craniovertebral junction shows brain stem and cerebellar vermis herniation (t) posterior to the cervical cord (cc). (**f**) Cranial USG reveals associated ventriculomegaly with dangling choroid plexus

Occult Spinal Dysraphism

Abnormal closure and dysjunction causes occult, skin-covered spinal dysraphism where, the neural tissue is deep to intact skin. This group is further divided as skin-covered defects with a subcutaneous mass and occult spinal dysraphism without a subcutaneous mass. Focal incomplete dysjunction causes a dorsal dermal sinus. Premature dysjunction causes skin-covered lipomyelocoele. Incidence is about 2 per 1000 births [6].

Occult spinal dysraphism may not be clinically evident, especially if not associated with a subcutaneous mass. Lumbar cutaneous stigmata like masses, skin tags, tuft of hair, dimples and haemangiomas are associated with a higher risk of having an occult spinal dysraphism and are seen in about 50% of cases.

Symptomatic manifestation becomes apparent as the vertebral column grows and there is increasing traction on the tethered spinal cord, leading to back pain, bladder-bowel dysfunction and lower limb abnormalities. Surgical intervention before onset of severe symptoms is associated with better results, hence early diagnosis by screening in patients with cutaneous stigmata is indicated [1, 6, 14].

Spinal Lipomas

Spinal lipomas are distinct collections of fat and connective tissue that are at least partially encapsulated and have a definite connection with the spinal cord [9]. These are caused by premature dysjunction, which allows mesenchyma to be trapped between the unfused neural folds and remain in contact with the neural placode [1, 3]. Spinal lipomas are composed of normal fat, may grow significantly during the first year of life, and may change in size with weight [11]. They may be intradural, extradural, or a combination of both. In addition to fat 84% of lipomas also contain neural tissue or meninges [3, 4]. Associations include tethered cord, dysraphism (4%), fatty filum or lipoma of filum (12%), and vertebral anomalies [1, 3, 4]. On SUS the fat is echogenic; intradural lipomas are sometimes better seen on MRI as the mass follows fat signal. The prognosis of these lesions is varied depending on their ability to be resected and the presence and type of various associated anomalies. Treatment consists of resection, when possible, or debulking [11].

Lipomas comprise 20–40% of occult SD and are classified as (a) lipomyelocoeles or lipomyelomeningocoele (84%); (b) fibrolipoma of the filum terminale (12%); (c) Intradural lipoma (4%) [1, 4]. The lipomyelomeningocoeles present as skin-covered masses; however the latter two may not show a subcutaneous mass.

Skin-Covered Defects with a Subcutaneous Mass

Lipomyelocoeles and Lipomyelomeningocoeles

These are a form of occult spinal dysraphism with a skin-covered osseous defect of the posterior spinal elements, through which various combinations of neural elements (neural placode), meninges, CSF, and adipose tissue protrude into subcutaneous tissues and merge with subcutaneous fat. Accounts for 20% of skin-covered lumbosacral masses and 50% of occult dysraphic spinal lesions [3–5]. The neural tissue is not exposed to the amniotic fluid *in utero* and intracranial changes of Chiari 2 malformation are not usually seen.

SUS shows an open neural arch with widely separated posterior osseous elements. There is a combination of neural placode, meninges, CSF and adipose tissue protruding out through the dorsal spinal defect, with a superimposed subcutaneous lipoma [6, 11].

There is a low-lying tethered spinal cord which distally shows an undulating deformed contour (Fig. 12.6b). The spinal cord is dorsally cleft forming a flattened hypoechoic neural placode, with the ventral and dorsal nerve roots arising ventrally owing to failure of dorsal fusion. An echogenic intraspinal lipoma may be seen adjacent to the deformed spinal cord (Fig. 12.6a) and merging with subcutaneous fat. In a lipomeningocoele the neural placode is in plane with the cutaneous surface (Fig. 12.6a). In a lipomyelomeningocoele there is a dilated subarachnoid space and a combination of deformed neural placode and adipose tissue protrude dorsally, with a superimposed subcutaneous lipoma (Fig. 12.6b).

It is the most common cause of tethered cord. Syringomyelia (Fig. 12.6a) is present in 25% of cases, diastematomyelia in 10% of cases and can be detected easily with SUS [4]. Vertebral segmentation abnormalities, partial sacral agenesis and genitourinary and anorectal abnormalities are also known associations.

Simple Meningocoeles

It presents with a skin-covered soft subcutaneous mass which may change in size, when the child cries [6]. Neurologic deficits are rare with simple meningocoeles. It is a protrusion of fluid and meninges through a dorsal spinal defect into the subcutaneous soft tissues. 80% are located in

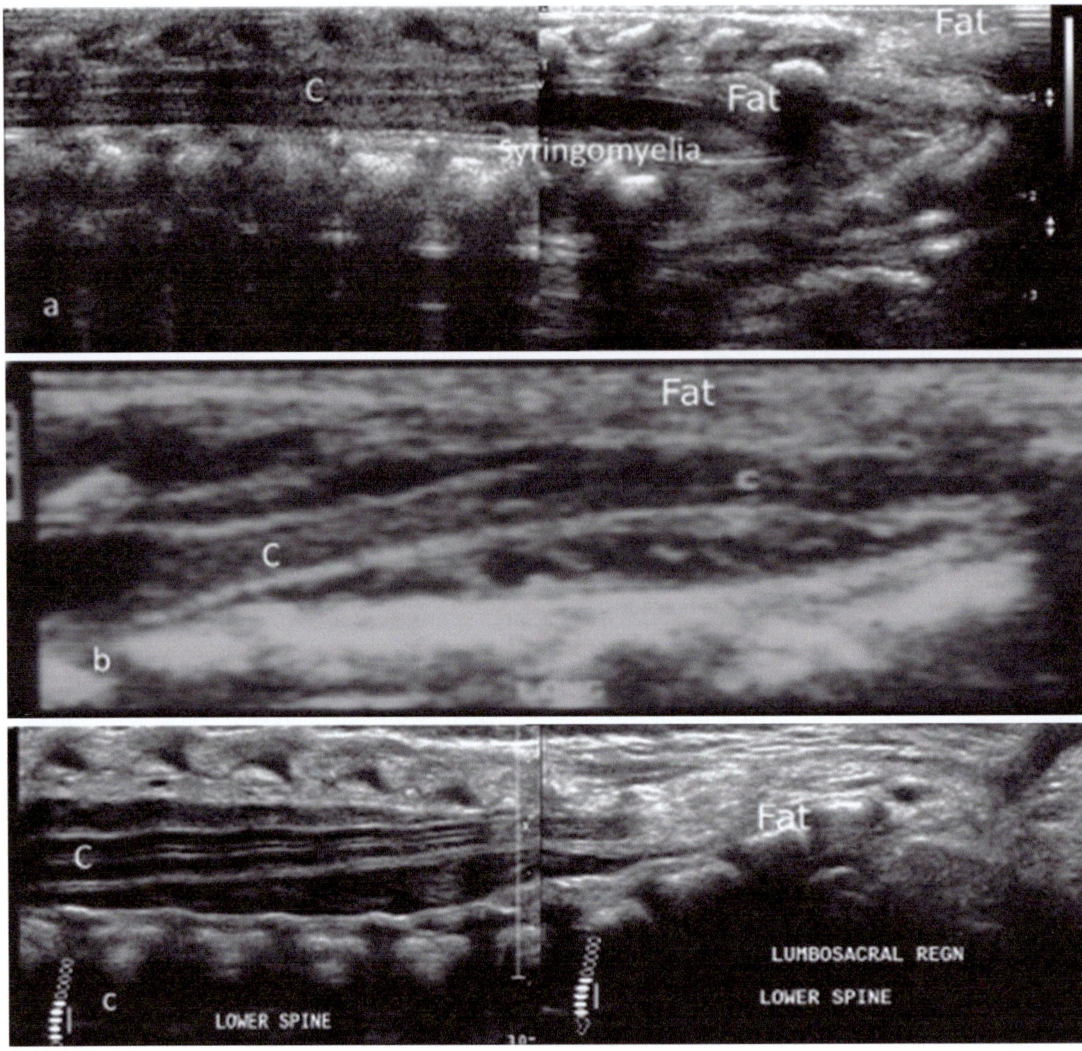

Fig. 12.6 Skin covered defects with a subcutaneous mass and spinal lipomas. (**a**) Lipomyelocoele. Sagittal scan shows a skin covered echogenic fatty mass continuous with spinal cord. Echogenic intradural fat seen adjacent to the cord with associated focal syringomyelia. The lipoma- neural placode interface is positioned within the spinal canal consistent with lipomyelocoele. (**b**) Lipomyelomeningocoele. Sagittal scan shows a skin covered echogenic fatty mass continuous with spinal cord. There is a widened anterior subarachnoid space with outward ballooning through dorsal osseous spinal defect. The lipoma-neural placode interface lies outside the spinal canal merging with subcutaneous fat consistent with a lipomyelomeningocoele. (**c**) Filum terminale lipoma. Sagittal scan shows a low placed conus at level of L5 and fusiform echogenic fatty tissue involving the filum consistent with a filum terminale lipoma

the lumbosacral region. Lateral meningocoeles are protrusions through the neural foramina. Congenital simple meningocoele is a relatively rare abnormality and occurs in 0.01% of all live births, and the embryology is unclear.

On SUS there is a focal spina bifida with a thin-walled anechoic cystic lesion, in continuity with the arachnoid space. No neural tissue is present (Fig. 12.7b). On sagittal scan posterior displacement of the cord may be seen at this level (Fig. 12.7a). It is rarely associated with other spinal cord anomalies.

Terminal Myelocystocoele

Terminal myelocystocoele is rare and comprises 1–5% of skin-covered lumbosacral masses. It is

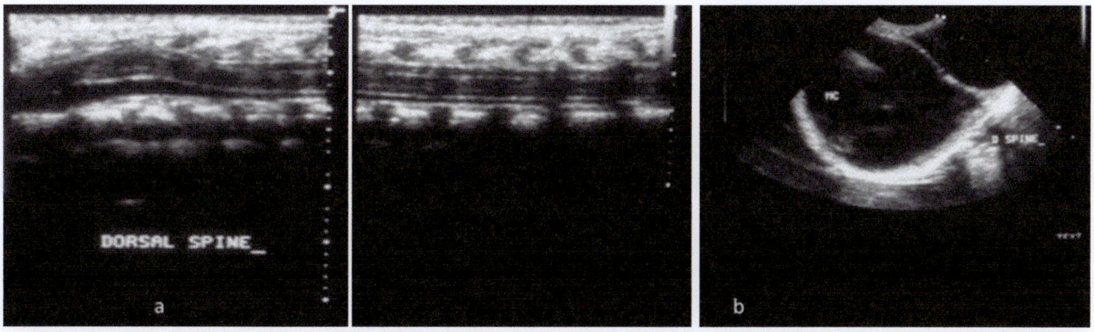

Fig. 12.7 Skin covered defects with a subcutaneous mass – Meningocoele in a 10 day neonate with a midline soft, smooth skin covered mid dorsal mass. (**a**) Sagittal scan shows a posteriorly pulled spinal cord at the level of meningocoele. (**b**) Axial scan over the mid dorsal mass shows a subcutaneous, fluid filled thin walled cystic anechoic mass, continuous with the spinal canal through the dorsal osseous spinal defect

often associated with epispadias, bladder extrophy, caudal regression syndrome and severe hindgut and genitourinary abnormalities [9]. Myelocystocoeles result from an error in formation of the caudal cell mass or failure of closure of the posterior neuropore [5, 6].

The lesion consists of a posterior spina bifida with an intact skin, hydromyelia with protrusion of the cord, meninges and the subarachnoid space into dorsal subcutaneous plane forming a meningocoele. Dilated distal cord bulging below the level of meningocoele prevents ascent of cord leading to a tethered cord [9].

SUS shows a dilated spinal cord surrounded by a dilated subarachnoid space (meningocoele) that is in direct continuity with the subarachnoid space of the spinal canal, a large cyst distal to the meningocoele, insertion of the cord on the posterior wall of the meningocoele, and the nerve roots exiting the spinal cord [6].

Skin-Covered Defects Without a Subcutaneous Mass

Filum Terminale Lipoma

Fatty filum and filar lipomas are due to a minor anomaly of canalisation and retrogressive differentiation with persistent or differentiated fatty tissue [3]. They are varying sized collections of fat within the filum terminale. Small lipomas occur in the filum itself, larger lipomas are usually found at lower dorsal dural attachment. Minimal fat in the filum is often asymptomatic and has been seen in 6% of normal spines at autopsy [1, 5, 11] and is considered a normal variant.

On SUS a thick echogenic filum terminale >1–2 mm in diameter is seen associated with a low-lying conus and restricted nerve root movements due to tethered cord [6]. When the fatty tissue forms a mass, a filar lipoma is diagnosed (Fig. 12.8e). The treatment and prognosis vary depending on the clinical symptoms and specific anomalies present.

Dorsal Dermal Sinus

A dorsal dermal sinus develops as a result of faulty neurulation with focal inadequate dysjunction between the superficial and neural ectoderm, resulting in an epithelial-lined tube connecting the skin to the spinal cord, cauda equina, or arachnoid. Commonly occurs in the lumbosacral region and very rarely seen in cervical and dorsal spine [6]. Clinically seen as a dimple or an opening with or without fluid discharge. A dorsal dermal sinus occurring in a paramedian location is often associated with an intraspinal dermoid or epidermoid [4]. A dimple which is high > 2.5 cm from the anus, > 5 mm in size and is eccentrically placed is associated with a higher risk of having an occult spinal dysraphism [6]. Infections and recurrent meningitis, epidural or subdural abscess, and intramedullary spinal cord abscess are known complications of a dorsal dermal sinus [4]. A dorsal dermal sinus should be differenti-

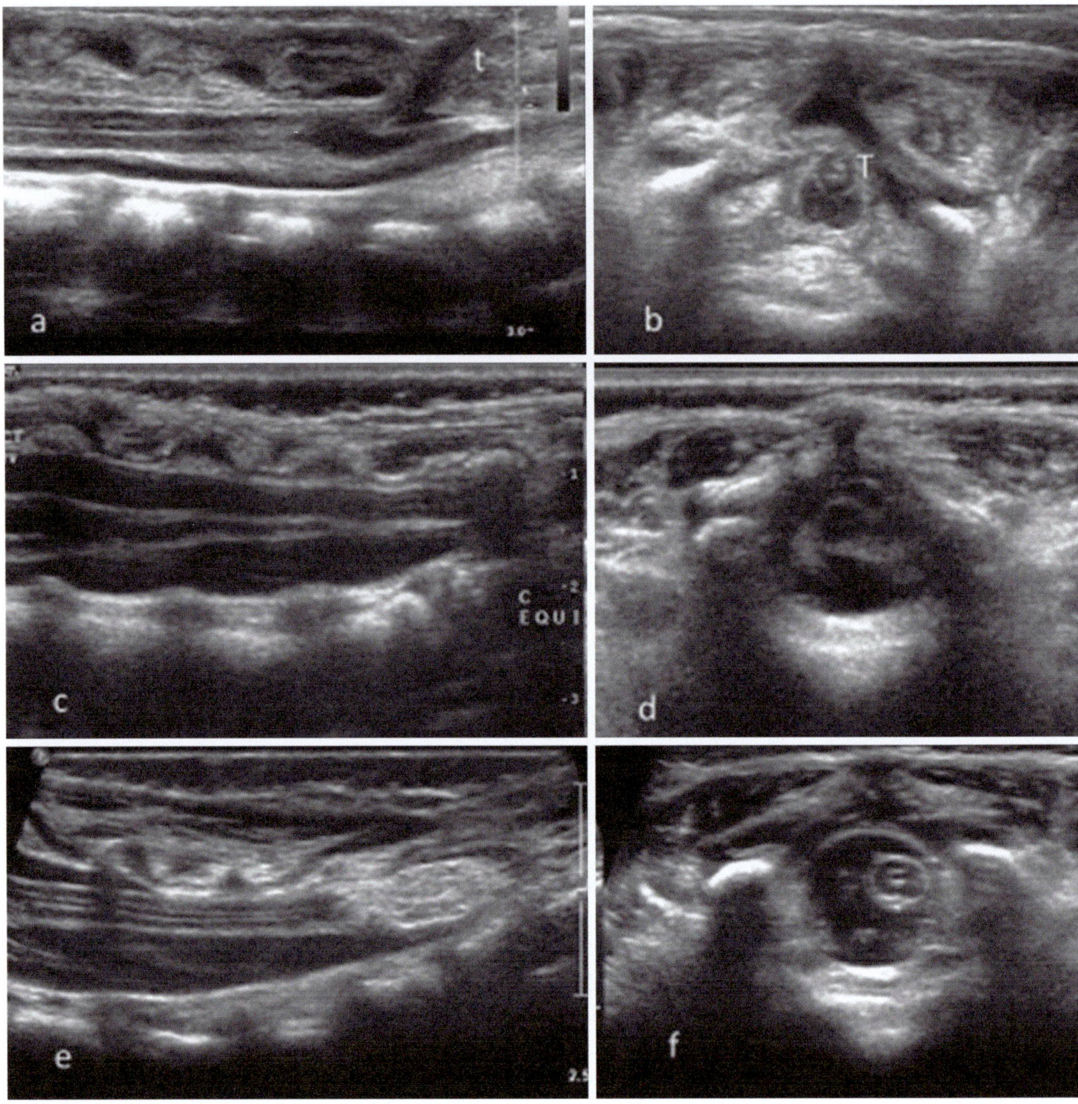

Fig. 12.8 Skin-covered defects without a subcutaneous mass. (**a** and **b**) Dorsal dermal sinus. (**a**) Sagittal scan in the lumbar region at level of the skin dimple shows an epithelial-lined tract extending from the skin to the spinal cord. The tract is hypoechoic in the subcutaneous tissues (t) with low-lying conus at L4–5 level. (**b**) Axial view shows the tract (T) close to the dorsal surface of the flattened and deformed neural placode. The tract appears echogenic surrounded by anechoic CSF in the subarachnoid space. Absent oscillatory movements noted on real time examination. (**c** and **d**) Thickened filum terminale. (**c**) Sagittal scan in the lumbar region shows a tethered cord with a low-lying conus at the level of L4. Thickened echogenic filum terminale seen surrounded by CSF. (**d**) Axial view shows a dorsally placed distal cord in the spinal canal. Absent oscillatory movements noted on real time examination. (**e** and **f**) Filum terminale lipoma. (**e**) Sagittal scan in the lumbar region shows a tethered cord and low-lying conus at L5 level, with an oval echogenic filum terminale lipoma. (**f**) Axial view shows dorsal and lateral displacement of the distal cord. Absent oscillatory movements noted on real time examination

ated from a simple sacral dimple or pilonidal sinus which does not extend to neural structures.

On SUS the tract is seen as a single line or double (railroad) lines corresponding to the lumen and walls of the tract [9] at level of skin dimple. This elongated tract is hypoechoic in the subcutaneous tissues (Fig. 12.8a). It may extend into the spinal canal where it appears hyperechoic surrounded by anechoic CSF [4] (Fig. 12.8b). If a low-placed conus is seen it suggests intraspinal extent with a tethered cord. It may be associated with intraspinal lipomas and deep dermoid, epidermoid tumours which cause compression of neural structures with neurologic symptoms.

Dermoid and Epidermoid Tumours

In absence of dermal sinus, the congenital epithelial rests may give rise to epidermoid tumours [9]. These comprise 1–2% of spinal cord tumours at all ages and 10% of all tumours below the age of 15 years [9]. 20% are formed in association with dermal sinuses.

Epidermoid tumours may also arise as a result of iatrogenic implantation of viable dermal elements during back surgeries or spinal taps performed with needles without a trochar [9]. Dermoid cysts are seen as unilocular or multilocular cystic masses, lined by epithelium containing stratified squamous epithelium, skin appendages like hair follicles, sweat glands and sebaceous glands. Epidermoid cysts are lined with membrane which contains only of the superficial elements of the skin [9].

Imaging findings of a spinal cystic mass which at surgery was a dermoid cyst are described in Fig. 12.9. The sagittal and axial SUS images of the lumbosacral spine (Fig. 12.9a and b) show a large unilocular hypoechoic cystic mass widening the spinal canal abutting and displacing and the filum terminale. The conus is low-lying with a tethered filum terminale. MRI images of the lumbosacral spine showed a large predominantly hypointense intraspinal mass on the T1 weighted images, with a thin crescentic hyperintense area within. The mass was displacing the filum and the conus which appeared stretched out and displaced. The lesion appears hyperintense on the T2-weighted image with septa within (Fig. 12.9d, e and f).

Diastematomyelia

Diastematomyelia or split cord malformation develops very early during embryogenesis and may be caused by an adhesion between the ectoderm and endoderm with splitting of the early notochord. A diastematomyelia is characterised by a sagittal cleft in the spinal cord dividing it into

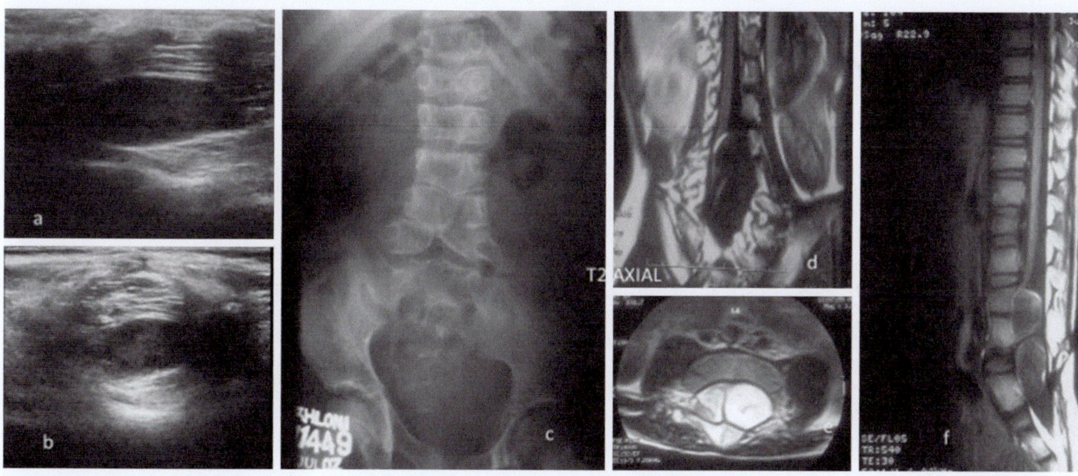

Fig. 12.9 Dermoid. (**a** and **b**) Sagittal and axial ultrasound images through the lumbosacral spine showing a large hypoechoic mass widening the spinal canal, displacing and abutting the filum terminale. The conus is low-lying with a tethered filum terminale. (**c**) AP radiograph of the lumbosacral spine showing segmentation anomalies of the lower lumbar vertebrae with widened interpedicular distance. (**d**, **e** and **f**) T1W coronal, T2W axial and T1W sagittal images of the lumbosacral spine showing a large predominantly hypointense intraspinal mass on the T1W images. This shows a thin crescentic hyperintense area within supero-laterally on the right in the coronal image (**d**) and postero-superiorly and inferiorly in the sagittal image (**f**). The mass displaces the filum and the conus which appear stretched out and displaced anteriorly and to the right. The lesion appears hyperintense on the T2W axial image with septa within. Images courtesy: Dr. Priscilla Joshi, Head, Dept of Radiodiagnosis, Bharati Vidyapeeth (DTU) Medical College Hospital, Pune

two hemicords. This vertical split may be by a fibrous septum, bony or a cartilaginous septum.

Split cord malformations are divided into two types [6] – Type 1 shows two hemicords within separate dural sacs separated by a rigid osseous-cartilaginous septum (Fig. 12.10a, d). Type 2 shows two hemicords which have no septum and lie in a single dural sac (Fig. 12.11d).

These split cord malformations involve the lower thoracic to lower sacral segments and are most commonly seen at the lumbar level. The spinal canal is most often widened. Often associated abnormalities of vertebral bodies like hemivertebra, butterfly vertebrae and kyphoscoliosis are also seen. An occult skin-covered SD, diastematomyelia is suspected clinically due to presence of cutaneous stigmata which are seen in 50–75% of patients. Club foot is seen in almost 50% of patients, and non-specific neurological symptoms are also commonly seen.

SUS performed in the axial plane shows a sagittal cleft in the spinal cord with two symmetric or asymmetric hemicords seen in cross-section, each with a central canal and ipsilateral nerve roots (Figs. 12.10, 12.11). In patients with a fibrous, cartilaginous, or osseous septum, each hemicord has a separate dural sheath, whereas a single sheath surrounds both hemicords when no rigid septum is present [1, 4]. Cranial to the split a fluid-filled focal dilatation of the central canal or cord cyst may be seen (Fig. 12.11a, c). In most cases, the hemicords reunite caudal to the cleft [4] (Fig. 12.10e, Fig. 12.11e). Occasionally, the cleft extends unusually low and the hemicords remain distinct, with two separate coni medullaris (Fig. 12.12). Abnormally low conus medullaris, thickening of the filum terminale and tethering may be seen.

Other anomalies like myelocoeles, meningocoeles, lipomas, hydromyelia and cord tethering are seen in 80% of cases. Most severe forms of split notochord syndrome have enteric fistulas characterised by communication between the gastrointestinal tract and dorsal skin in the midline [6].

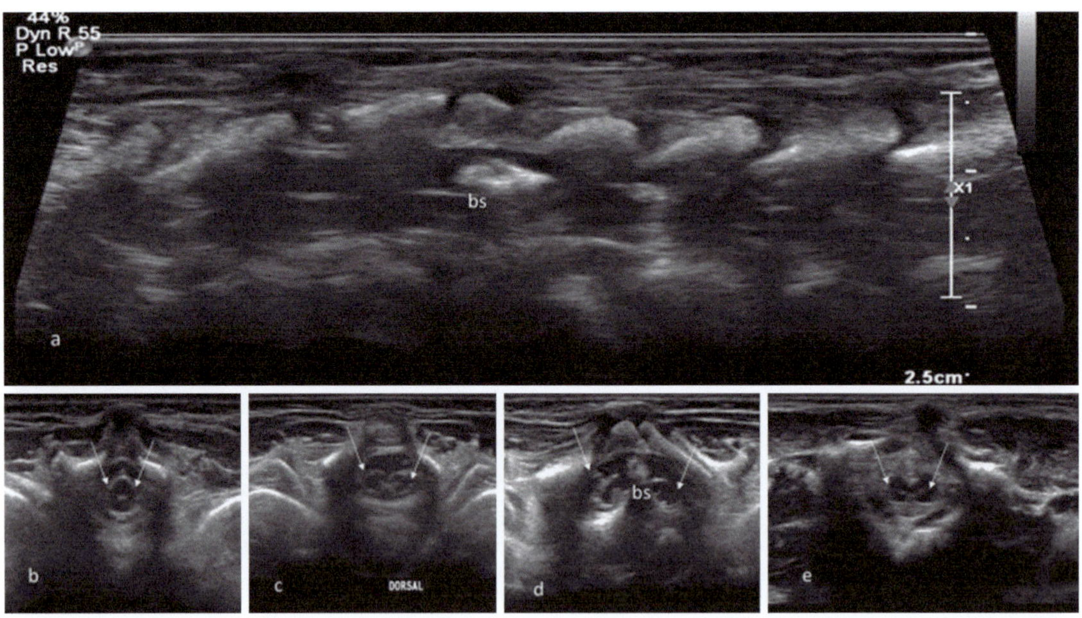

Fig. 12.10 Diastematomyelia with bony spur. (**a**) Sagittal scan of the thoracolumbar spine shows an echogenic bony spur (bs). (**b**) Axial scan of mid thoracic spine shows a single rounded hypoechoic cord (arrows) with single echogenic central canal. (**c**) Axial scan of lower thoracic spine shows two rounded hypoechoic cords (arrows) in a single dural sac.(**d**) Axial scan of upper lumbar spine shows a vertical bony spur (bs) with two rounded hypoechoic cords (arrows), each in a separate dural sac. (**e**) Axial transverse scan of distal lumbar spine shows two cords close together and partially fused in a single dural sac

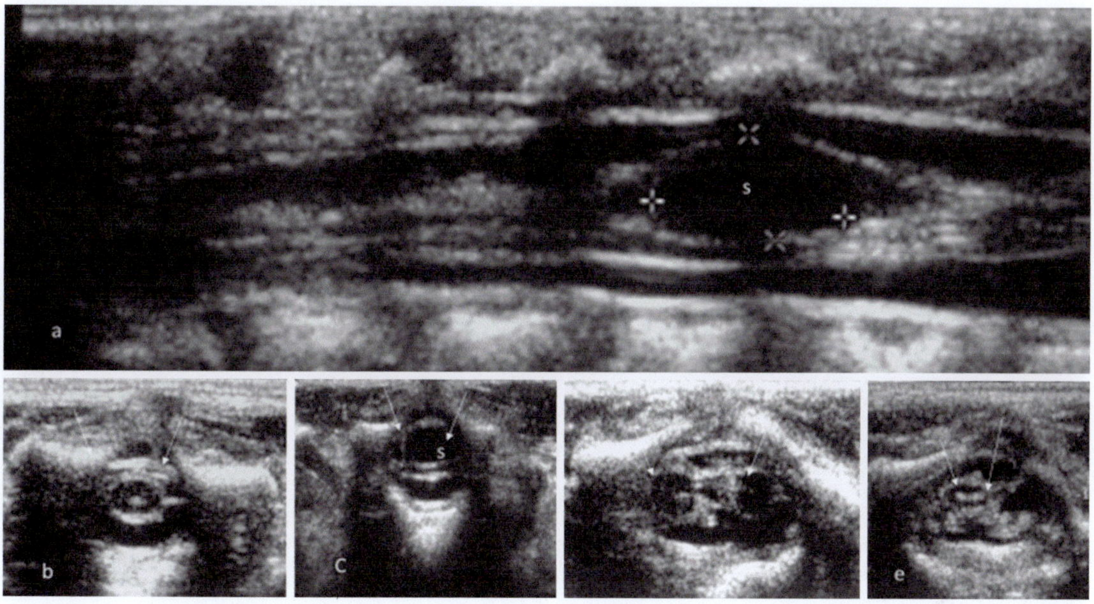

Fig. 12.11 Diastematomyelia with fibrous septum. (**a**) Sagittal scan of the thoracolumbar spine shows a localized focal fluid-filled dilatation of the central canal – cord cyst (s). (**b**) Axial scan of lower thoracic spine shows a single rounded hypoechoic cord (arrows) with single echogenic central canal. (**c**) Axial scan of upper lumbar spine shows a single rounded hypoechoic cord (arrows) with fluid filled dilatation of central canal – cord cyst (s). This is seen just above level of the split. (**d**) Axial scan of lumbar spine just distal to the level of cord cyst, shows two rounded hypoechoic cords (arrows) of equal size in a single dural cavity, split by a fibrous septum. (**e**) Axial scan of distal lumbar spine shows the two cords close together and partially fused

Caudal Spinal Anomalies

Caudal regression syndrome is due to dysembryogenesis of the caudal cell mass with failed development of the lumbar and sacral spine [7, 11]. This leads to a spectrum of anomalies of the caudal end of the trunk. Malformations vary from isolated partial agenesis of the sacrococcygeal spine to more severe deformities like sirenomelia [9], and associated malformations like imperforate anus, genitourinary anomalies, and renal dysplasia. The incidence of Caudal regression syndromes is about 1 in 7, 500 children. It occurs most often in children of diabetic mothers [9].

In group 1, SUS demonstrates a blunt, deformed conus medullaris that terminates above the normal level of L1 (Fig. 12.13). In group 2, the conus medullaris is elongated and tethered by a thickened filum terminale or intraspinal lipoma and ends below L1. Patients in group 1 have major sacral deformities, whereas neurological disturbances are more severe in group [3, 4].

Sacrococcygeal Teratoma

Incidence is 1 in 40, 000 births and forms approximately 1% of fetal and neonatal germ cell tumours [6, 9]. They arise from the caudal cell mass and are not associated with bony abnormalities of the sacrum. They are classified into 4 types according to location: Type 1 is almost entirely external; Type 2 is predominantly external with large intrapelvic component; Type 3 is predominantly intrapelvic with a small external component (Fig. 12.15); Type 4 is entirely presacral [9].

SUS shows the location and internal architecture of the mass and confirms whether solid or cystic components are present. Malignant tumours have larger solid components and the benign tumours are predominantly cystic. Colour Doppler shows flow in the solid components with arteriovenous shunting in the malignant masses.

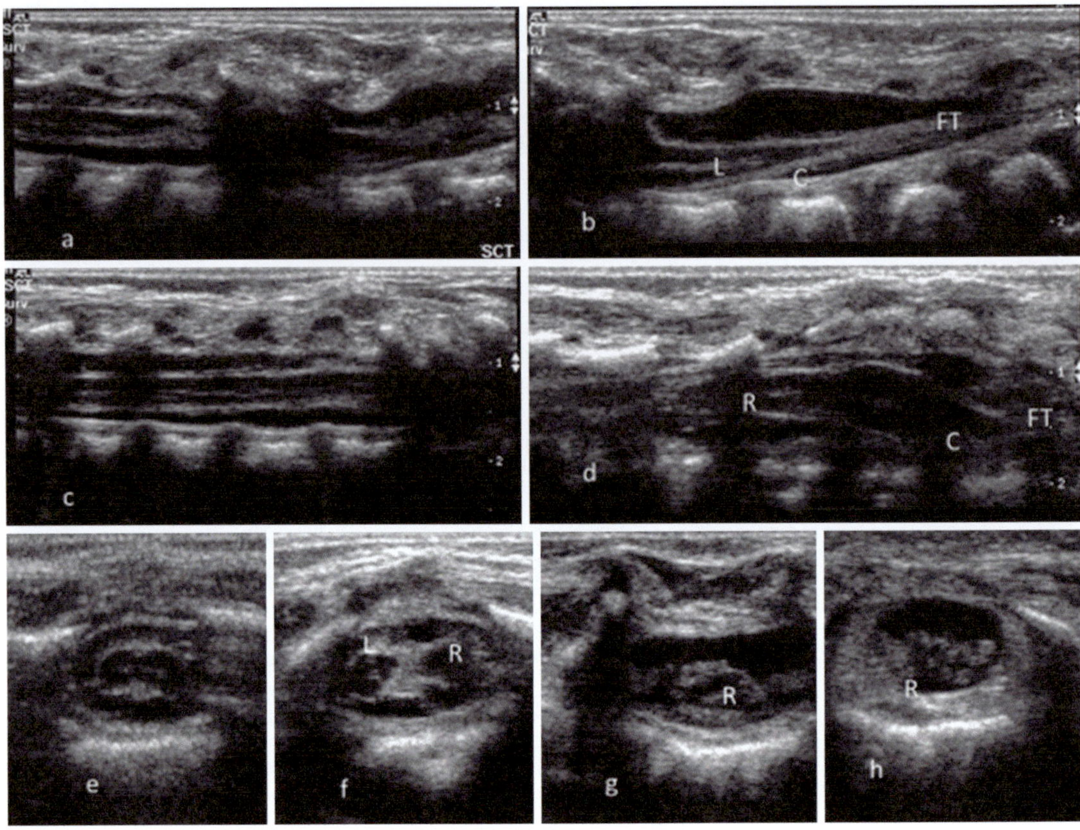

Fig. 12.12 Diastomatomyelia with fibrous septum. The cleft extends unusually low with two hemicords showing two separate coni medullaris. (**a**) Sagittal scan, Vertebral abnormality with echogenic fused posterior elements causing shadowing. (**b**) Sagittal scan of left hemicord (L) showing an abnormally low conus medullaris (C) with thickening of the filum terminale (FT) and tethering. (**c**, **d**). Sagittal scan of right hemicord (R) is thicker and bulbous and conus medullaris (C) is lower with tethering and a short filum terminale (FT). (**e**) Axial scan showing split. (**f**) Axial scan showing split and discordant sizes of the hemicords, Right (R) larger than the left (L). (**g**, **h**) Axial scan showing the Right (R) hemicord extends lower than the left

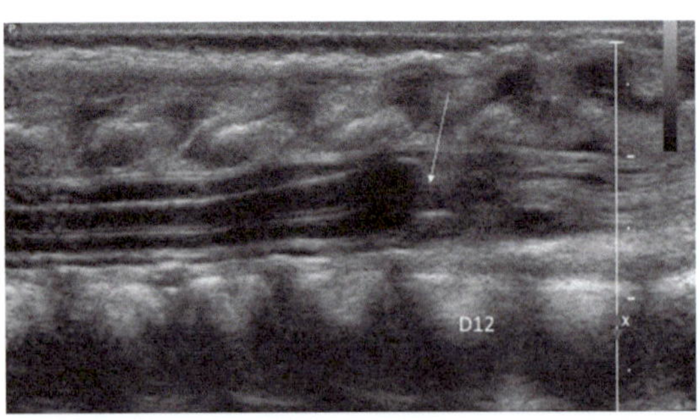

Fig. 12.13 Caudal regression syndrome: A 1-month-old neonate with arthrogryposis. Sagittal scan of the thoraco-lumbar spine shows a blunt-ending spinal cord at the level of D12 vertebra

Tumours

Intraspinal tumours seen in neonates are largely congenital and include teratomas, dermoids, epidermoids, hamartomas, lipomas, and enterogenous cysts. Intramedullary tumours cause cord enlargement and extramedullary tumours displace the cord (Fig. 12.14).

Haemangiomas

Vascular masses like haemangiomas and arteriovenous malformations can be seen in the spinal canal as echogenic masses with tiny cystic areas which show flow on colour Doppler (Fig. 12.14).

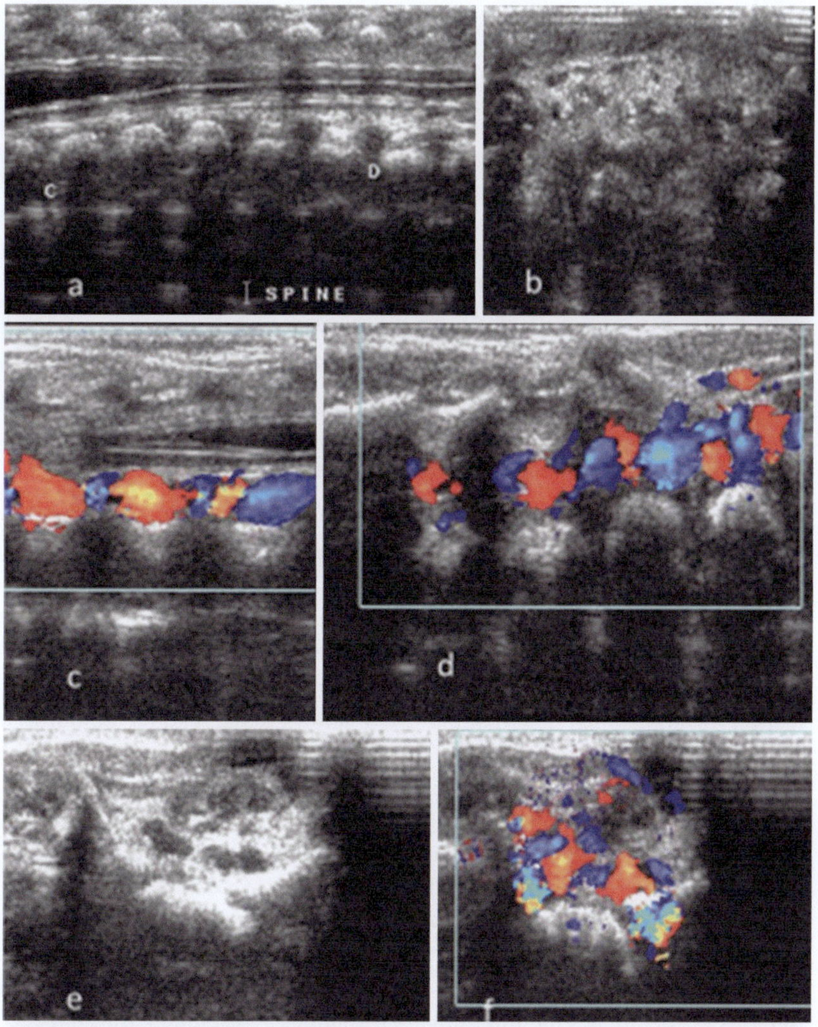

Fig. 12.14 Spinal vascular malformation in a 15 day neonate with a skin covered lumbar swelling. (**a**) Sagittal scan of cervical cord shows a syringomyelia. (**b**, **c** and **d**) Sagittal scan of thoracolumbar region shows the cord surrounded by echogenic tissue with tiny anechoic cystic areas. On colour Doppler (**c** and **d**), these cystic areas show presence of flow, consistent with a vascular malformation. (**e** and **f**) Axial scan showing dorsal osseous spinal defect in addition to the B-mode and colour Doppler findings of a vascular malformation surrounding the cord

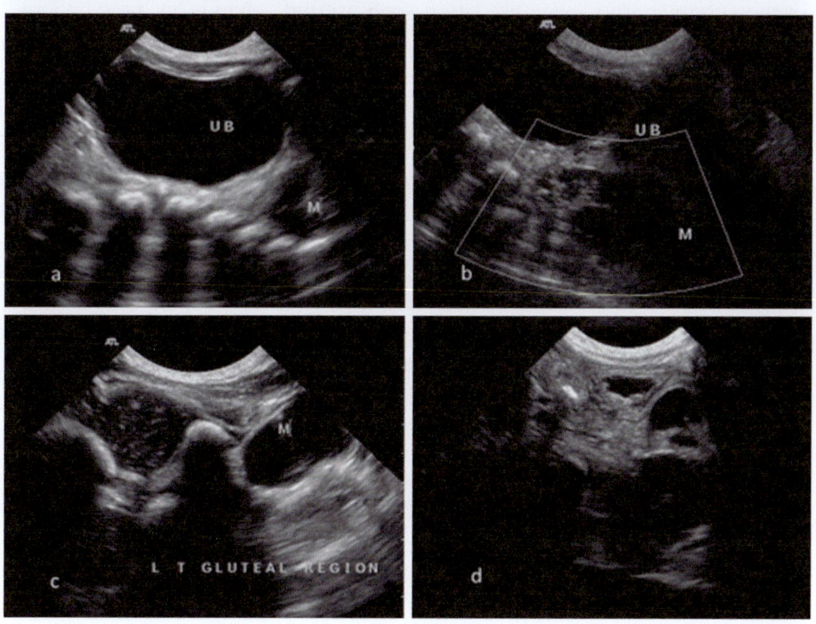

Fig. 12.15 Sacrococcygeal teratoma in a neonate with a sacrococcygeal and left gluteal swelling. (**a** and **b**) Axial and sagittal scan of the pelvis reveals a hypoechoic predominantly solid mass with small cystic areas (M) situated anterior to the lumbosacral spine. Colour Doppler shows no significant vascularity within. (**c** and **d**) show the mass extending into the left gluteal region (M) with large cystic components

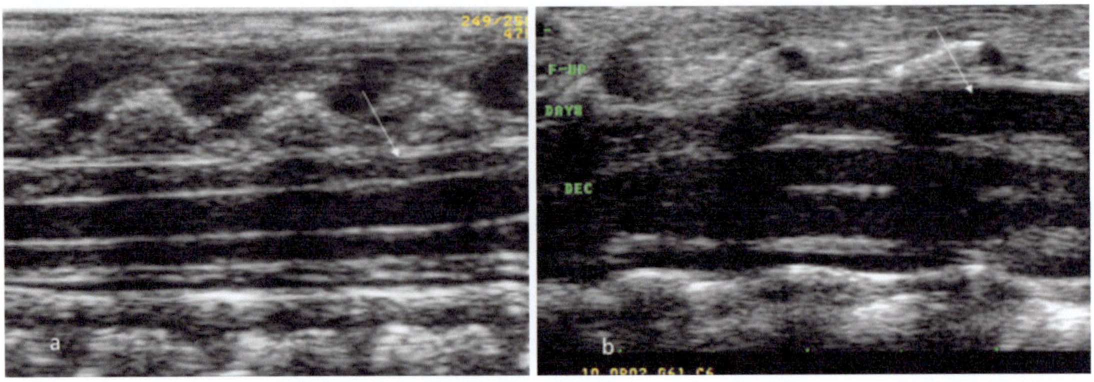

Fig. 12.16 Meningitis. (**a**) Sagittal scan shows internal echoes in the CSF within the posterior subarachnoid space (arrow). (**b**) Follow-up after 7 days of treatment shows clearing of the CSF within the posterior subarachnoid space (arrow)

Acquired and Miscellaneous Conditions

Trauma

Excessive traction on the spinal cord during delivery can lead to spinal cord injury, cord transection or intraspinal haematoma SUS shows increased cord echogenicity due to traumatic oedema or subdural/epidural haematoma with cord displacement. SUS can also help look for epidural and subdural haematomas following a traumatic lumbar puncture. Evolution/regression of haematoma can be seen in follow-up scans.

Infection: Meningitis

In cases of meningitis the inflammatory changes in the subarachnoid space are often seen around the spinal cord. SUS reveals increased echogenicity and septations in the CSF in the subarachnoid space (Fig. 12.16a). Real-time sonography may show decreased or absent pulsations of the spinal cord and nerve roots, and is an additional finding in meningitis [15–17]. Follow-up examination shows a clearing of the CSF after treatment (Fig. 12.16b).

Guided Procedures

Lumbar Puncture: The Conus ascends by 40 weeks to the level above L2–3 disc space. Hence level L3–4 is safe for lumbar puncture if entry into the lower spaces is difficult. In premature infants puncture at this level will generally avoid the spinal cord but a SUS can be used for guidance [10]. SUS can be used to evaluate the cause of failed lumbar puncture and to estimate the likelihood of success of further lumbar puncture attempts [18]. Therapeutic uses of SUS include guidance for paediatric caudal anaesthesia, caudal epidural blocks used for blocking lumbar and sacral nerve roots, where blind punctures might be difficult [18, 19].

Conclusions

MRI is no doubt the gold standard in spinal cord evaluation, however with the advent of newer high-resolution transducers, SUS especially in expert hands has now become a reliable and highly accurate method of examining the spinal cord and spinal canal in newborns and young infants up to 4–6 months of age. Babies, with lumbar cutaneous stigmata like atypical dimples, skin tags or tails, haemangiomas, hairy patches and skin-covered lumbar masses or having SD-associated syndromes such as anorectal and urogenital malformations, and the VATER group should undergo early SUS to screen for spinal dysraphism and associated cord abnormalities. Indications also include deformities of the spinal column neurological disturbances like paresis, bladder or bowel dysfunction and in suspected spinal cord injury due to traumatic birth to look for cord compression.

In neonates with cord abnormalities and tethering of the cord, early detection and timely intervention has shown better results. A systematic ultrasound examination of the spinal canal and its contents helps to rule out significant pathology of the cord with a sensitivity and specificity close to an MRI scan. In neonates with completely normal SUS further evaluation can be avoided. In patients with abnormal or equivocal findings on SUS, it helps in choosing the type and timing of therapeutic intervention and decide further MRI examination can be performed at the time of the elective surgical intervention. In addition, SUS also helps in evaluation and follow up of neonatal spinal cord trauma and infections. It is also useful as an image guidance modality for certain procedures and therapeutic applications.

Acknowledgements Figures 12.11, 12.13, 12.14 and 12.15 reproduced with permission from Ultrasound Examination of Paediatric Musculoskeletal Diseases and Neonatal Spine. Karnik AS, Karnik A, Joshi A. Indian J Pediatr. 2016 Jun; 83(6):565–77. doi: 10.1007/s12098-015-1957-2. Epub 2016 Feb 1.

References

1. Dick EA, Patel K, Owens CM, de Bruyn R. Spinal ultrasound in infants. Br J Radiol. 2002;75:384–92.
2. American Institute Of Ultrasound In Medicine (AIUM). Practice guideline for the performance of an ultrasound examination of the neonatal spine. 2007. (updated 2012).
3. Byrd SE, Darling CF, McLone DG. Developmental disorders of the pediatric spine. Radiol Clin N Am. 1991;29:711–52.
4. Unsinn KM, Geley T, Freund MC, Gassner I. US of the spinal cord in newborns: Spectrum of Normal findings, variants, congenital anomalies and acquired diseases. Radiographics. 2000;20:923–38.
5. Barkovich AJ. Congenital anomalies of the spine. Pediatric neuroimaging. 4th ed. Philadelphia: Lippincott Williams & Wilkins; 2005. p. 704–72.
6. Coley BD, Siegel MJ. Spinal sonography. Pediatric sonography. 4th ed. Philadelphia: Lippincott Williams & Wilkins; 2011. p. 647–74.
7. Lowe LH, Johanek AJ, Moore CW. Sonography of the neonatal spine: part 1, normal anatomy, imaging pitfalls, and variations that may simulate disorders. AJR. 2007;188:733–8.
8. Malas MA, Salbacak A, Buyukmumcu M, Seker M, Koyluoglu B, Karabulut AK. An investigation of the conus medullaris termination level during the period of fetal development to adulthood. Kaibogaku Zasshi. 2001;76:453–9.
9. Naidich TP, Raybaud C. Congenital anomalies of the spine and spinal cord. Riv Neuroradiol. 1992;5(suppl 2):113–30.
10. Beek FJ, de Vries LS, Gerards LJ, Mali WP. Sonographic determination of the position of the conus medullaris in premature and term infants. Neuroradiology. 1996;38(suppl 1):S174–7.
11. Lowe LH, Johanek AJ, Moore CW. Sonography of the neonatal spine: part 2. Spinal Disord 2AJR. 2007;188:739–44, 0361–803X/07/1883–739.
12. Kriss VM, Kriss TC, Babcock DS. The ventriculus terminalis of the spinal cord in the neonate: a normal variant on sonography. Am J Roentgenol. 1995;165:1491–3. https://doi.org/10.2214/ajr.165.6.7484594.
13. Coleman LT, Zimmerman RA, Rorke LB. Ventriculus terminalis of the conus medullaris: MR findings in children. Am J Neuroradiol. 1995;16:1421–6.
14. Zalel Y, Lehavi O, Aizenstein O, Achiron R. Development of the fetal spinal cord: time of ascendance of the normal conus medullaris as detected by sonography. J Ultrasound Med. 2006;25:1397–401.
15. Kinare A, Chaudhari S, Vaidya U, Kadam S, Khairnar B, Abnave A. Ultrasound imaging of neonatal spine in meningitis. Ultrasound Med Biol. 2009;35(8):S204.
16. Baruah D, Gogoi N, Gogoi RK. Ultrasound evaluation of acute bacterial meningitis and its sequale in infants. Indian J Radiol Imaging. 2006;16:553–819.
17. Nepal P, Sodhi KS, Saxena AK, Bhatia A, Singhi S, Khandelwal N. Role of spinal ultrasound in diagnosis of meningitis in infants younger than 6 months. Eur J Radiol. 2015;84(3):469–73.
18. Nair N, Sreenivas M, Gupta AK, Kandasamy D, Jana M. Neonatal and infantile spinal sonography: a useful investigation often underutilized. Indian J Radiol Imaging. 2016;26:493–501.
19. Senoglu N, Senoglu M, Oksuz H, Gumusalan Y, Yuksel KZ, Zencirci B, et al. Landmarks of the sacral hiatus for caudal epidural block: an anatomical study. Br J Anaesth. 2005;95:692–5. 2015;84:469–73

Nerves: Pediatric Neuromuscular Ultrasound

13

Eman A. Tawfik, Francis O. Walker, and Michael S. Cartwright

Introduction

Neuromuscular ultrasound refers to scanning of peripheral nerves and skeletal muscles using high-resolution ultrasound to diagnose, follow up, and guide interventions in primary neuromuscular disorders. The neuromuscular ultrasound field started in the early 1980s when Heckmatt and Dubowitz investigated the role of ultrasonography in the diagnosis of muscle diseases [1]. In the 1990s, the attention was directed toward the applications of ultrasound in focal neuropathies and remained so for decades [2–7]. Recently, the applications of neuromuscular ultrasound widely expanded to include traumatic nerve injuries, polyneuropathies, anterior horn cell diseases, and myopathies [8–16].

Although the first study in the neuromuscular ultrasound was performed on children, the pediatric neuromuscular ultrasound field is still not fully explored.

A neuromuscular disorder is defined as any disorder affecting the peripheral nervous system. Pediatric neuromuscular disorders are highly versatile and include disorders of motor neuron, nerve root, peripheral nerve, neuromuscular junction, and muscle. The diagnostic process of pediatric neuromuscular disorders is usually complex and requires a combination of electrophysiology, serology, genetic testing, and neuromuscular imaging in addition to muscle biopsy in myopathic diseases.

One of the essential and beneficial tools in the diagnostic workup of pediatric neuromuscular disorders is electrodiagnostic testing which includes motor and sensory nerve conduction studies, late responses, needle electromyography, evoked potentials, repetitive nerve stimulation, and single fiber electromyography. The electrodiagnostic studies can differentiate between neuropathic and myopathic disorders, determine the nature of pathology in neuropathic disorders, localize the lesion, predict prognosis, and in many cases lead to a definite diagnosis. However, there are several limitations of electrodiagnosis especially in children. First of all, electrodiagnostic testing represents a painful experience to the child as well as to the parents. Secondly, the nerve conduction and electromyography protocols are usually extensive and can be time-consuming. Moreover, the child may become intolerant to the test to the degree that obligates the physician to end the study. A major limitation of electrodiagnostic tests is that they give no clue about the anatomical/structural aspect of the neuromuscular system. Also, in many instances, electrodiagnosis fails to localize the

E. A. Tawfik (✉)
Department of Physical Medicine and Rehabilitation, Faculty of Medicine, Ain-Shams University, Cairo, Egypt
e-mail: eman_Tawfik@med.asu.edu.eg

F. O. Walker · M. S. Cartwright
Department of Neurology, Wake Forest School of Medicine, Winston-Salem, NC, USA
e-mail: fwalker@wakehealth.edu; mcartwri@wakehealth.edu

Y. El Miedany (ed.), *Pediatric Musculoskeletal Ultrasonography*, https://doi.org/10.1007/978-3-030-17824-6_13

lesion. Neuromuscular ultrasound is an attractive complementary tool to electrodiagnostic tests and can provide valuable information that cannot be obtained by the electrodiagnostic tests alone. Ultrasound can localize the lesion in traumatic nerve injuries and focal neuropathies, detect an underlying structural cause of neuropathies, identify nerve tumors, and be used as a rapid screening tool to differentiate between nerve and muscle disorders [9, 17–20]. Ultrasound is also an ideal modality to follow up children with neuromuscular disorders [21] given its advantages of being painless, portable, rapid, inexpensive, dynamic, and radiation-free tool. Unlike other neuroimaging modalities like CT scan and MRI for children, ultrasound does not require sedation or prescheduling.

The ideal setting of the ultrasound machine for neuromuscular ultrasound applications is the electromyography lab and the power of neuromuscular ultrasound as a diagnostic tool for adult or pediatric neuromuscular disorders depends on its integration in electromyography labs because clinical-electrodiagnostic-sonographic correlation is a prerequisite for accurate diagnosis and optimum patient care.

Approach for Pediatric Neuromuscular Ultrasound

When a child is referred to the electromyography lab for suspected neuromuscular disease, the first step is full history taking and meticulous neurological examination to reach a provisional diagnosis or a list of differential diagnosis and subsequently design the electrodiagnostic and sonographic protocols. In cases of suspected neuropathic disorders, electrodiagnosis is usually performed prior to ultrasound study, but there are situations where ultrasound is performed first. For example, it is better to start with the ultrasound study if the child is apprehensive or if the anatomical course of a nerve is altered to ensure accurate nerve conduction technique.

In suspected myopathic disorders, ultrasonography is commonly performed prior to needle electromyography to screen muscles and to choose the most appropriate ones for the needle examination.

Machine Setting and Image Optimization

Any ultrasound machine with a broadband linear array transducer is optimum for pediatric neuromuscular ultrasound. A hockey stick transducer is better in neonates and young children especially in curved or narrow areas like scanning the ulnar nerve at the elbow and scanning the brachial plexus in neonates with short neck. A curved array transducer is rarely needed in children unless the child has high body mass index.

Adjusting the frequency in children follows the same general rule of ultrasound; superficial structures need high frequency and deeper structures need lower frequency. To obtain best resolution and high-quality images of the peripheral nerves, a frequency of 16–20 MHZ is the optimum to scan the superficial nerves. In neonates, infants, and young children, it is usually unnecessary to use very low frequency even with scanning of deep nerves and muscles. Low frequency may be needed in obese adolescents.

To optimize the image, depth should be adjusted according to the depth of the target nerve and/or muscle. For superficial nerves and muscles, a depth of 2 cm is sufficient, while a depth of 4–5 cm can be suitable for deep nerves like the sciatic. The optimum depth is the depth at which the nerve and/or muscle under the study occupies the center of the ultrasound image with good visualization of the surrounding structures and bone profiles. The zoom function may allow detailed assessment of nerve echogenicity and its fascicular pattern. Adjusting the focus is highly important to improve the lateral resolution. The focus should be adjusted at the level of the target nerve or the muscle (Fig. 13.1). For peripheral nerve scanning, one focal point is recommended and for muscle scanning, 2–3 focal points may be used according to the thickness of the scanned muscle. However, it is important to put in mind that increasing the number of focal points decreases the frame rate which in turn affects the real-time imaging.

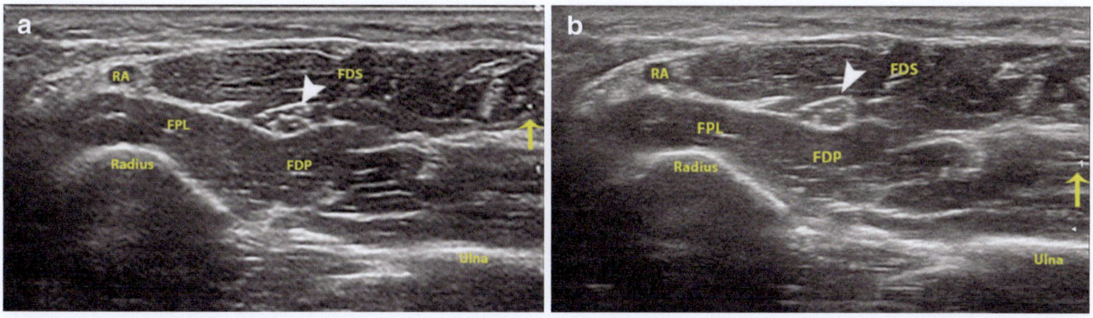

Fig. 13.1 Focus adjustment. (**a**) Proper focus position (yellow arrow) properly adjusted at the level of the nerve (white arrowhead) results in optimum lateral resolution. Also, note the clear distinction between the nerve and the surrounding muscle reflecting optimum gain adjustment. (**b**) Improper focus position (yellow arrow) below the level of the nerve (white arrowhead) results in poor lateral resolution. FDP Flexor digitorum profundus, FDS Flexor digitorum superficialis, FPL Flexor pollicis longus, RA radial artery

Gain in nerve and muscle ultrasonography should be adjusted so that the nerves can be clearly distinguished from surrounding blood vessels, tendons, and muscles, and the muscles can be differentiated from the surrounding fascia or aponeurosis with clear visualization of the intermuscular and peri-muscular connective tissue as hyperechoic septa (Fig. 13.1a).

Time gain compensation adjusts the gain in layers. During nerve scanning, knobs of the time gain compensation are usually kept at the middle to ensure uniform gain of the entire image. Gain of the deep layers can be minimized to reduce noise or can be maximized to compensate for the attenuation of ultrasound beam in deep tissues. For accurate quantitative assessment of muscle echogenicity, time gain compensation should not be adjusted to avoid over- or underestimation of muscle echo intensity.

Continuous adjustment of the frequency, depth, focus position, and gain according to the anatomical course of each nerve is an essential principle during nerve tracing.

To create a child-friendly environment, the study should be explained to the parents and to the child if old enough. Engaging the child in the study and allowing him/her to see the ultrasound images can be exciting to the child and ensure his/her cooperation if needed. No sedation should be used during dynamic muscle assessment to allow the child to actively contract the muscle. On the other hand, assessment of muscles for fasciculations/fibrillations may necessitate using a light sedative to achieve full child relaxation.

Peripheral Nerve Ultrasound

Nerve Structure and Sonographic Characteristics

Each peripheral nerve consists of parallel bundles of nerve fibers. The nerve fibers within the nerve collect in the form of bundles known as nerve fascicles. Three connective tissue sheaths wrap the nerve. The endoneurium is a delicate connective tissue that encases the individual nerve fibers and separates the axons from each other. The perineurium is a fine membrane that surrounds the fascicles and is made of connective tissue. The whole nerve is surrounded by an outer sheath known as the epineurium and is made of connective tissue composed of elastic fibers. From the epineurium, inner septa arise to separate the nerve fascicles [22].

When the ultrasound waves strike the nerve, the nerve fibers absorb most of the incident waves and thus appear hypoechoic. On the other hand, the connective tissue sheaths reflect most of the incident waves and thus appear hyperechoic. In the axial view, the nerve acquires a honeycomb or reticular appearance in which multiple rounded hypoechoic areas are embedded in a hyperechoic background and the outer nerve sheath appears as a hyperechoic border [23, 24] (Fig. 13.2). The hypoechoic areas represent the nerve fascicles, and the hyperechoic background represents the interfascicular connective tissue [23]. In the longitudinal view, the nerve appears tubular with internal hypoechoic thin bands separated by hyperechoic bands [23, 24]. The hypoechoic bands represent the nerve fascicles, and the hyperechoic thin bands represent the interfascicular connective tissue. The epineurium encases the nerve and appears as two echogenic bold lines in the longitudinal view (Fig. 13.3). The echogenicity may differ from one nerve to another depending on the fascicle diameter and the fascicular pattern [25].

The nerve exhibits other sonographic properties. It is relatively immobile compared to the tendons, preserves its echogenicity on probe inclination [24], and gives no signal on color or power Doppler.

The nerve sonographic appearance in children does not differ significantly from adults, and the typical honeycomb appearance of the nerve in the axial view is distinct even in infants younger than 1 year old (Fig. 13.4).

In children, the main nerves including the median, ulnar, radial, tibial, and fibular are easily visualized and traced along their full anatomical courses via ultrasound. Smaller nerves like musculocutaneous nerve can also be traced in children including neonates as young as 5 months old [26]. Tiny branches like the superficial radial, posterior interosseus, and deep peroneal nerves which can be challenging even in adults can be readily visualized in children (Figs. 13.5, 13.6 and 13.7).

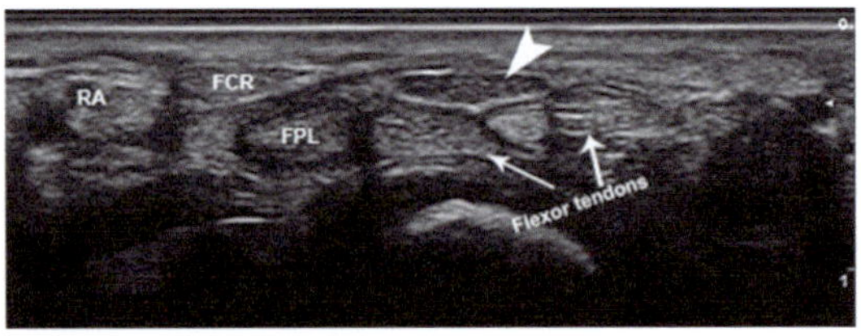

Fig. 13.2 B-mode ultrasound image of the median nerve (white arrowhead) at the wrist showing the normal sonographic appearance of a nerve in the axial view in which multiple hypoechoic round areas are embedded in a hyperechoic background (honeycomb appearance). FCR Flexor carpi radialis, FPL Flexor pollicis longus, RA Radial artery

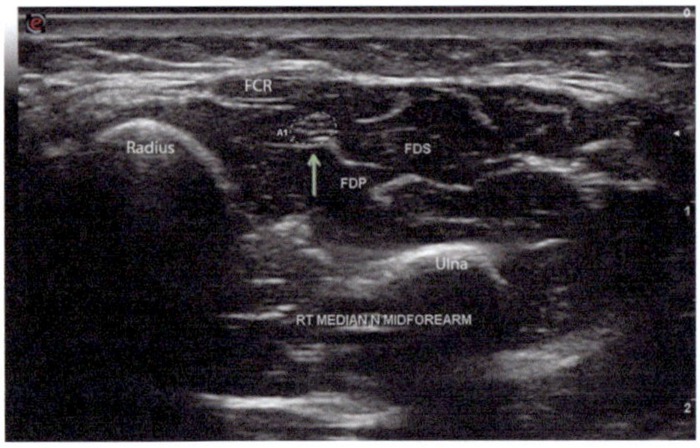

Fig. 13.4 Axial view of the median nerve (arrow) at the mid-forearm in an 8-month-old. The typical honeycomb appearance of the nerve is clear

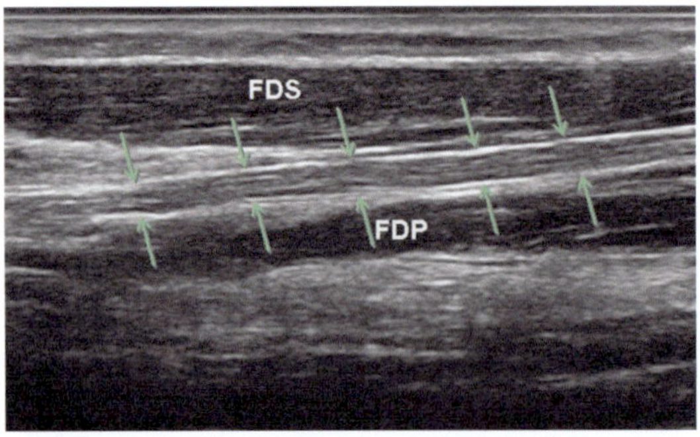

Fig. 13.3 B-mode ultrasound image of the median nerve (arrows) at the mid-forearm showing the normal sonographic appearance of the nerve in the longitudinal view. FDP Flexor digitorum profundus, FDS Flexor digitorum superficialis

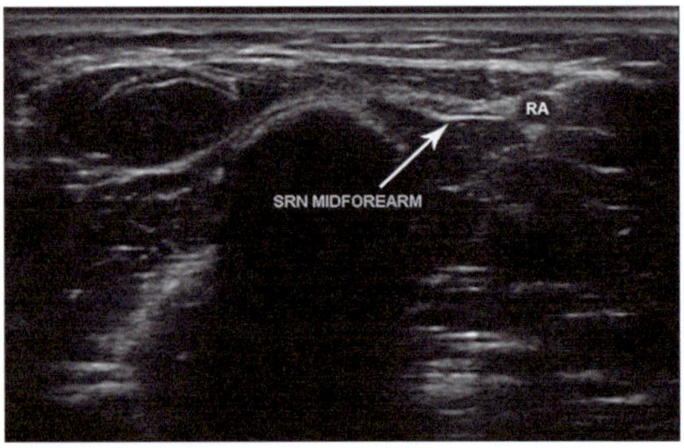

Fig. 13.5 B-mode ultrasound image showing axial view of the superficial radial nerve (arrow) at the mid-forearm. RA Radial artery

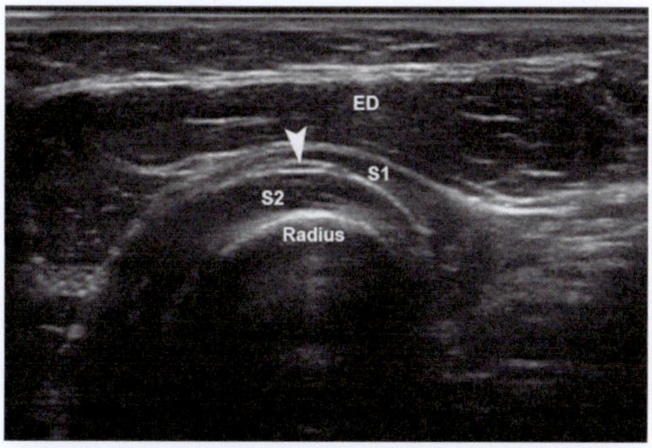

Fig. 13.6 B-mode ultrasound image showing axial view of the posterior interosseus nerve (arrowhead) between the superficial head (*S1*) and deep head (*S2*) of the supinator muscle. ED Extensor digitorum

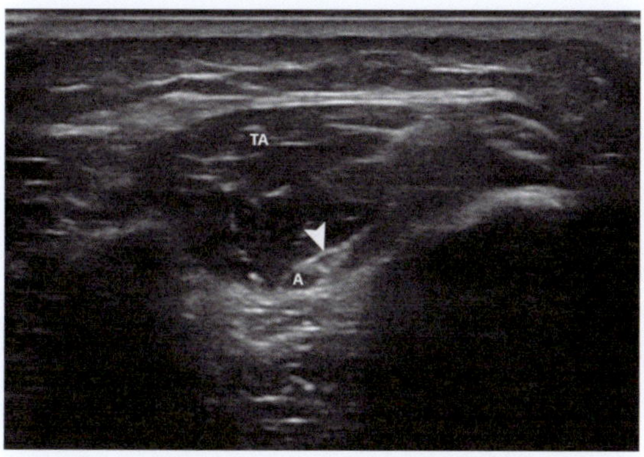

Fig. 13.7 B-mode ultrasound image showing axial view of the deep peroneal nerve (white arrowhead) adjacent to the deep peroneal artery (*A*) near the interosseus membrane and deep to the tibialis anterior (*TA*)

How to Identify the Nerve in the Ultrasound Image?

It is better to identify any nerve first in the axial view as it is easier to distinguish the characteristic honeycomb appearance of the nerve in the axial view, while in the longitudinal view, it can be difficult to distinguish a nerve from an adjacent tendon. In the axial view, the nerve typically appears as a honeycomb or cribriform structure composed of hypoechoic round areas on a hyperechoic background and surrounded by a hyperechoic outer sheath. This typical appearance however does not apply to all nerves at all anatomical levels. For example, the median nerve at the palm and the ulnar nerve at the ulnar groove normally appear hypoechoic (Figs. 13.8 and 13.9), and the median nerve at the forearm appears relatively hyperechoic compared to its appearance at the distal wrist crease. These normal variations of the echogenic properties of the nerves at different levels along their courses should be well known to the sonographer to avoid misinterpretation of such variations as pathological findings. To identify the nerve in the longitudinal view, the probe is rotated 90° from the axial view.

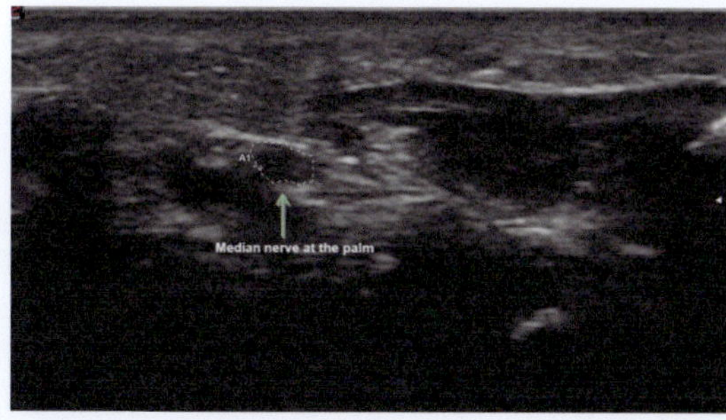

Fig. 13.8 Axial view of the median nerve (arrow) at the palm where the nerve normally appears hypoechoic

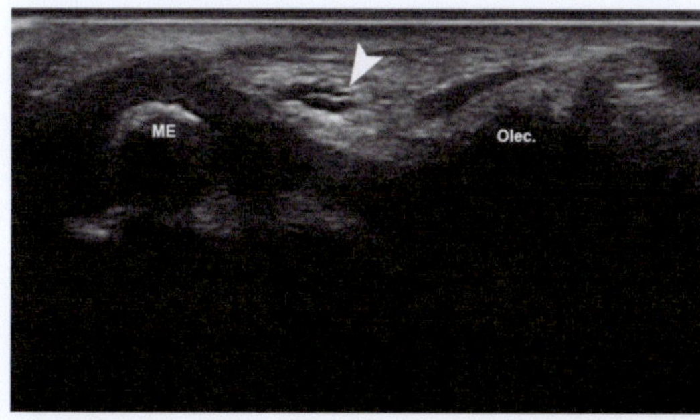

Fig. 13.9 Axial view of the ulnar nerve (arrowhead) at the ulnar groove, the nerve normally appears hypoechoic

The most accurate technique to identify nerves is by using specific anatomical landmarks along the anatomical course of the nerves. Most nerves lie in close proximity to a blood vessel, a bone, a tendon or lie between fascial planes of two muscles. The sonographer can utilize these nearby structures as anatomical sonographic landmarks to ensure accurate nerve identification. For example, the ulnar nerve at the Guyon's canal level lies medial to the ulnar artery and lateral to the pisiform bone (Fig. 13.10), the median nerve at the mid-forearm lies in the fascial plane between flexor digitorum superficialis and profundus (Fig. 13.1), and the tibial nerve at the popliteal fossa lies superior and lateral to the popliteal artery (Fig. 13.11). Tracking the nerve back and forth from one scanning level to another, active contraction of surrounding muscles or tilting the probe while in place can delineate an unclear nerve.

One can differentiate a nerve from a nearby tendon by inclining the probe and observing the change in the echotexture of the confusing structure. The tendon turns hypoechoic while the nerve relatively keeps its echotexture.

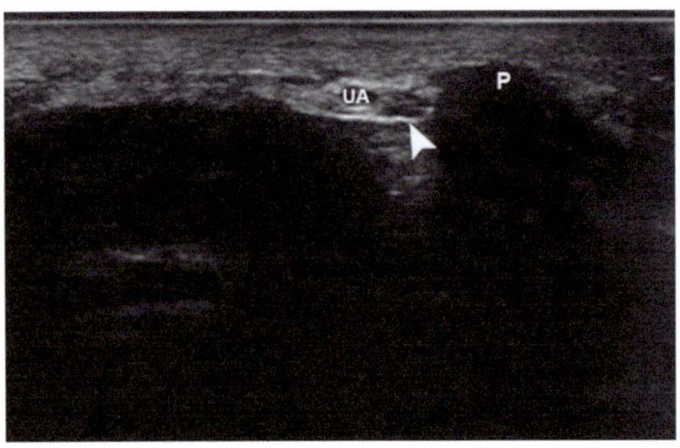

Fig. 13.10 Axial view of the ulnar nerve (arrowhead) at the Guyon's canal, the nerve lies lateral to the pisiform bone (*P*) and medial to the ulnar artery (*UA*)

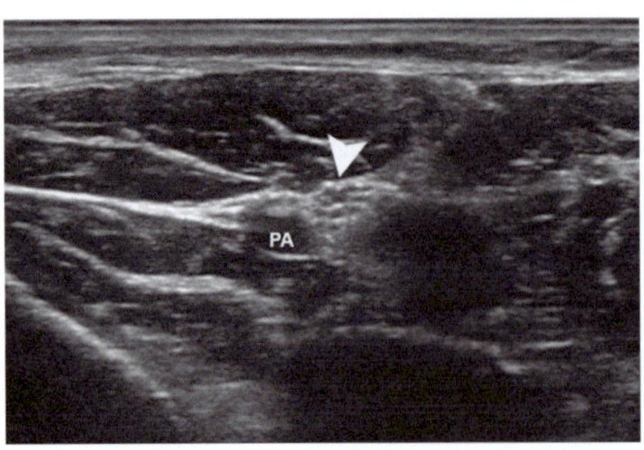

Fig. 13.11 Axial view of the tibial nerve (arrowhead) at the popliteal fossa, the nerve lies superior and lateral to the popliteal artery (*PA*)

Dynamic assessment by active or passive movement of the tendon in question can also discriminate between a nerve and a tendon. Moreover, tendons acquire a different echotexture from the nerves. In the axial view, the tendons appear as hyperechoic round or oval structures and acquire a fibrillar pattern with parallel hyperechoic lines in the longitudinal view [27–29].

The blood vessels possess distinctive features that distinguish them from a nerve. The blood vessels are anechoic and show Doppler signal. Additionally, the artery pulsates, and the vein collapses upon compression by the probe.

Technical Principles

Workplace Setup

The most important setup is to adjust the patient and the scanned limb in a proper position. For every nerve, there is a favored patient position, but child's comfort is a priority. Neonates and infants can be held by the parent. The limb should be properly positioned to allow smooth nerve tracing. For upper limb nerves, older children can lie in supine position for full tracing of brachial plexus, median, ulnar, and radial nerves. For limited scanning of median or ulnar nerve at the arm, forearm or wrist, the child can sit opposite to the sonographer with the arm and hand resting on the examination table. For lower limb nerves, the child can lie in prone position for tracing of sciatic, tibial, sural, and proximal portion of the fibular nerves, while supine position is preferred when tracing deep and superficial fibular nerves.

The sonographer's position is also important. The sonographer should adjust the work area so that he/she has easy access to the machine knobs during scanning. The sonographer's forearm and hand should gently rest on the patient to achieve optimum control and easy sliding of the probe during nerve tracing. The height of the sonographer's chair should be adjusted to match the bed height and the ultrasound screen should be at the eye level. Good posture of the spine, shoulder, and hand is encouraged at all times to avoid musculoskeletal injuries and postural malalignments.

Scanning Level

There is no fixed rule as at which level the sonographer should start tracing the nerve and it is a matter of personal preference. However, it is easier to visualize certain nerves at specific levels, and these levels can be used as the starting point for nerve tracing (Table 13.1).

Table 13.1 Starting point for tracing of common nerves

Nerve	Starting point
Median	Start scanning at the mid-forearm level where the nerve lies in the fascial plane between flexor digitorum superficialis and flexor digitorum profundus, and then trace the nerve distally to the palm and proximally to the axilla
Ulnar	Start scanning at the mid-forearm level where the nerve lies between flexor carpi ulnaris and flexor digitorum profundus, and then trace the nerve distally to the Guyon's canal and proximally to the axilla Or start scanning at the Guyon's canal where the nerve is easily identified medial to the ulnar artery and lateral to pisiform bone, and then trace the nerve proximally to the axilla
Radial	Start scanning at the elbow where the nerve lies between brachioradialis and brachialis, and then trace the nerve proximally to the axilla. Next, from the elbow level, trace the deep radial branch distally to the level where the posterior interosseus nerve passes between the two heads of supinator. The superficial radial nerve is traced from its origin from the radial nerve at the elbow to the wrist
Tibial	Start scanning at the ankle where the nerve can be easily identified posterior to tibial arteries and veins at the tarsal tunnel, and then trace the nerve proximally along the leg to the level of popliteal fossa
Fibular	Start scanning the nerve at the level of popliteal fossa where the nerve lies in its lateral aspect lateral to biceps femoris tendon, and then trace the nerve distally to fibular head
Sciatic	Start scanning at the popliteal fossa and follow the tibial and fibular nerve proximally to the point where they unite to form the sciatic nerve, and then trace the nerve proximally to the level of ischial tuberosity

To track a nerve along its entire course, the nerve is usually traced from distal to proximal in what is known as the teleferic technique. In focal pathological conditions such as focal neuropathies and traumatic nerve injuries, it is better to start scanning at a level distant from the expected lesion site and then trace the nerve to the lesion level.

Proper Probe Handling

A linear array transducer with medium-sized footprint (Fig. 13.12) or small-sized footprint is best suited for peripheral nerve and muscle scanning in the pediatric age group. The linear probe provides good image quality and adapts well to the surfaces of upper and lower limbs. The smaller hockey stick probe is helpful in scanning small and irregular areas, but it provides narrow field of view. The curvilinear probe is rarely needed in pediatric sononeurology.

The probe orientation in neuromuscular ultrasound follows the universal orientation in radiology. The orientation mark is directed toward the sonographer's left side in the axial view (Fig. 13.13) and proximally toward the patient's head in the longitudinal view. Some sonographers use a different orientation in the axial view

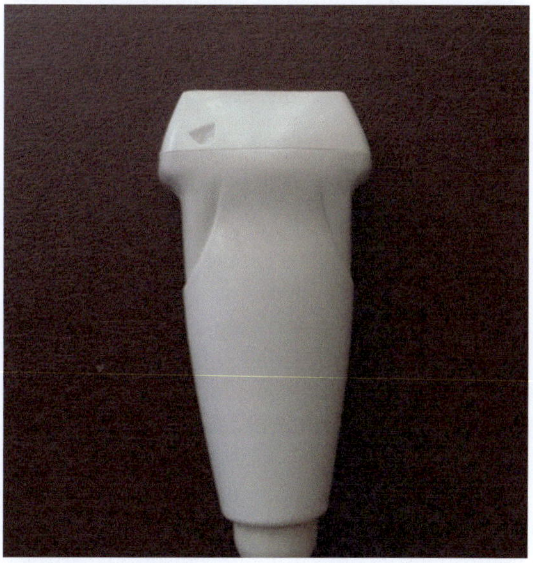

Fig. 13.12 Linear array transducer with medium-sized footprint is suited for pediatric sononeurology

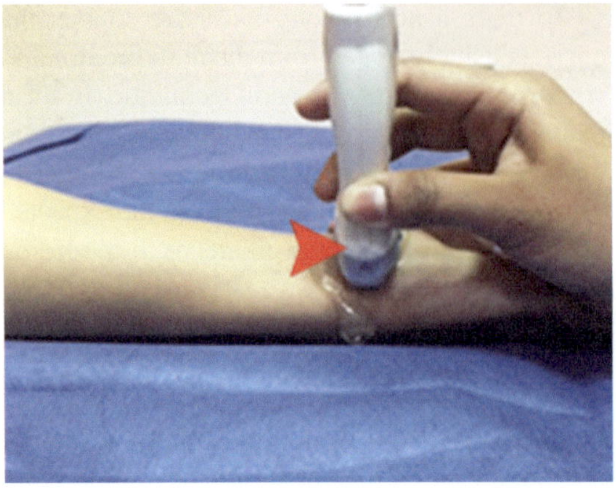

Fig. 13.13 Proper probe handling: the thumb on one side of the probe and the index and middle fingers at the other side with ulnar border in contact with the patient's skin. The orientation mark (arrow) is directed toward the sonographer's left side in the axial view

and direct the mark toward the patient's lateral side whatever the scanning side is. The sonographer is free to adopt either technique as long he/she knows the orientation on the screen and the images are labeled accurately. The probe should be handled between the thumb at one side and the index and middle fingers at the other side with the ulnar border in contact with the patient's skin at all times for easy tracing of the nerves (Fig. 13.13). Continuous adjustment of the frequency, depth, and focus according to the anatomical course of each nerve is mandatory to obtain good quality images at all levels.

The ultrasound gel should be of good consistency and should cover up the proposed tracing path. Large pad of gel is applied over the curvy bony areas to ensure good contact of the probe.

The probe should be kept orthogonal to the target nerve at all times during scanning. This orthogonal orientation is not necessarily achieved by placing the probe perpendicular to the skin. For instance, scanning the brachial plexus at the interscalene level necessitates slight cephalic inclination of the probe to achieve the orthogonal orientation to the brachial plexus. The probe can be inclined on purpose to differentiate between confusing structures using the anisotropic artifact.

The pressure exerted by the probe should be minimal to avoid underestimation of nerve or muscle size. Applying extra pressure by the probe can be used to distinguish collapsible structures like veins or to localize the site of the lesion (ultrasonographic Tinel's sign).

Scanning Planes

Any nerve should be scanned in the axial and longitudinal planes to confirm the pathology in two perpendicular planes. Exception of this rule are the tiny nerves than can only be captured in one view.

Nerve Evaluation

The nerve is evaluated as regards size, shape, echotexture, mobility, and vascularity. The ideal evaluation should also include evaluation of the skeletal muscles that are innervated by the nerve under the study, and evaluation of the surrounding structures includes joints, tendons, and ligaments.

Nerve Size

The most important and sensitive measurement for detection of nerve pathology is the cross-sectional area in the axial view. The cross-sectional area can be calculated by measuring the anteroposterior and the transverse diameters using the distance function of the ultrasound machine or by tracing the nerve using the trace function. The former method is less accurate than the tracing method because the nerves usually have uneven contours. Using the trace function of the machine, the nerve should be traced just inside its hyperechoic rim without the inclusion of its outer border (Fig. 13.14) because in many instances, the outer border of the hyperechoic rim can be hazy. Side-to-side comparison of the cross-sectional area in unilateral lesions is recommended especially when the absolute values are borderline.

Increased cross-sectional area is not pathognomonic to a specific disease but rather is a reaction

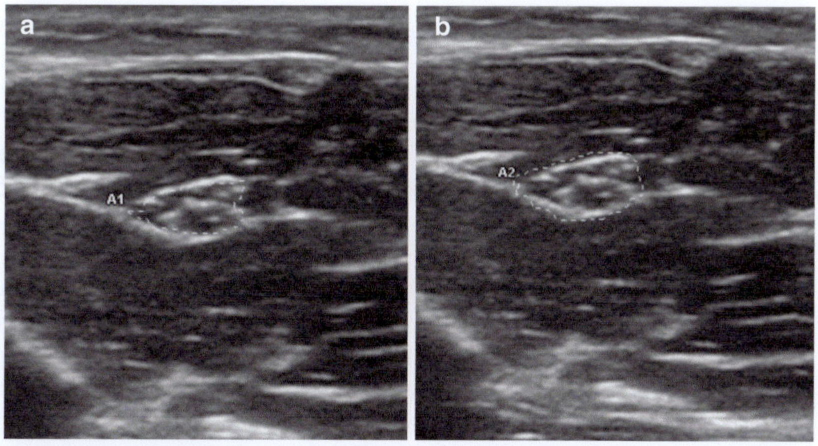

Fig. 13.14 Tracing method for measuring nerve cross-sectional area. (**a**) Correct tracing involves tracing along the inner side of the hyperechoic rim without inclusion of the hyperechoic rim. (**b**) Incorrect tracing involves inclusion of the outer hyperechoic rim

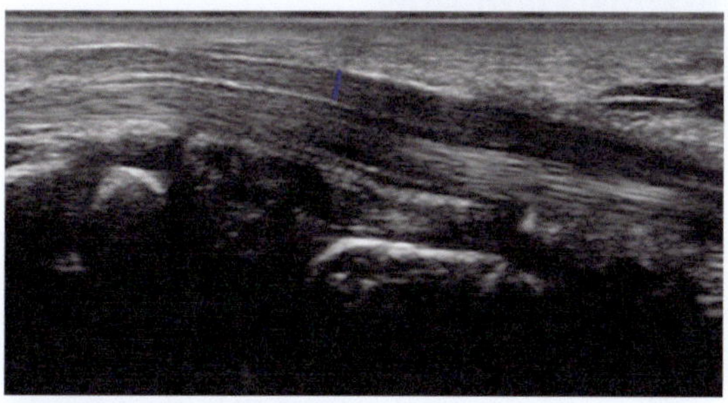

Fig. 13.15 Measurement of nerve diameter in the longitudinal view using the distance function. The distance marks should extend between the inner sides of the outer border

of the nerve to different pathologies. The distribution and the pattern of nerve enlargement are important to reach a diagnosis.

In the longitudinal view, the nerve diameter is measured using the distance function of the machine, and the marks should extend between the inner borders of the hyperechoic rim (Fig. 13.15).

Nerve Shape

Most of the nerves are round or oval. The shape of the nerve may change from one level to another. Therefore, the sonographer should be familiar with the normal shape and the appearance of the nerves at different scanning levels. Change in nerve shape should not be considered pathological unless is associated with change in cross-sectional area and/or echogenicity.

Nerve Echogenicity

The typical echogenic appearance of the nerve is the honeycomb appearance. In neuromuscular disorders, the nerve echogenicity is altered and its pattern differs among different diseases as will be discussed in the next sections.

Nerve Mobility

Although the nerves are less mobile than the tendons, it acquires a gliding movement. The two nerves that are usually assessed for mobility are the median and the ulnar nerves [30]. Median nerve mobility is assessed at the wrist level, and ulnar nerve mobility is assessed at the elbow level. Nerve gliding over a tendon can be evaluated by asking the patient to contract the muscle that underlies the nerve.

The interpretation of an abnormal mobility differs from one nerve to another. The abnormal mobility of the median nerve takes the form of limited mobility on combined flexion of the fingers and the wrist. The limited mobility of the median nerve is observed in entrapment neuropathy or in compression of the nerve by adhesions and scar tissue post-surgery or post-traumatic injuries. In contrast, the abnormal mobility of the ulnar nerve takes the form of excessive medial excursion and denotes nerve subluxation or dislocation. In pediatric neuromuscular ultrasound, assessing nerve mobility is possible only in old children who can follow the sonographer's instructions.

Nerve Vascularity

The nerve vascularity is assessed using color and power Doppler. The normal nerve has no signal on Doppler. Increased vascularity may denote acute inflammation.

Skeletal Muscles

The ideal sonographic workup of a nerve includes assessment of the skeletal muscles that are innervated by the nerve under the study. The denervated muscles have certain sonographic changes that can be helpful in the assessment of the distribution of the lesion and in the follow-up of the patients. The technical details and the principles of muscle scanning will be discussed in the muscle section.

Reference Values of Nerve Cross-Sectional Areas

The reference values of nerve cross-sectional areas in children have not been extensively reported and the available data are scarce [31, 32]. In general, children have smaller nerve cross-sectional area compared to adults, and the cross-sectional area increases from neonatal and infancy stage until adulthood [32]. In children 3 years old or younger, the cross-sectional area of upper limb nerves is about 2/5 to ½ the cross-sectional area in adolescents and adults. At the age 4 to 6, the cross-sectional area is about ¾ the values in adolescents and adults, and by age 11, the ratio between the cross-sectional of children and that of adults may reach 4/5 [32]. For lower limb nerves, the cross-sectional area in children of different age groups from 0 to 11 years is about 1/3 to 2/3 the cross-sectional area in adolescents and adults [32].

The correlation between cross-sectional area and each of height and body mass index is not clear, and the results obtained in the literature are controversial. Whether nerve cross-sectional area in children should be corrected for age, height, weight, and body mass index is an important issue that needs validation and standardization.

Of note, universal use of the published reference values to identify pathologies in children is not recommended, and every EMG lab should set its own reference values.

Neuromuscular Ultrasound in Specific Pediatric Neuropathic Disorders

The neuropathic disorders in children encompass brachial plexus injuries, traumatic peripheral nerve injuries, entrapment mononeuropathy, anterior horn cell diseases (spinal muscle atrophy), and polyneuropathies.

Brachial Plexopathy

Neonatal brachial plexopathy or "obstetric brachial plexus palsy" is the most common brachial plexus lesion in children. The prevalence in different countries ranges from 1.3 to 1.5 per 1000 total births [33]. Although the prevalence is not high, the possible functional and psychological impact when the child reaches the adolescents stage cannot be neglected [34].

Neonatal brachial plexopathy is typically assessed using electrodiagnostic studies to determine the site and the extent of the injury and to predict prognosis which is very important for early surgical interference [35, 36]. MRI and computed tomography myelography provide anatomical and structural assessment [36–38]. Recently, ultrasound attracted the attention as a useful tool in the assessment of brachial plexus injuries in adults and children [39–42] given its well-known advantages of being painless, dynamic, and bedside tool.

Before addressing the utility of ultrasound in the assessment of brachial plexus lesions, a brief anatomical background is presented, and the scanning technique of the brachial plexus in children is described.

Anatomical Background

The brachial plexus is a complex network of uniting and dividing nerves. It extends from the neck to the axilla and consists of five components: roots, trunks, divisions, cords, and terminal branches. The brachial plexus roots are formed by the ventral rami of the C5, C6, C7, and C8 cervical nerves and T1 thoracic nerve. Occasionally, the plexus receives twigs from the C4 root which is known as the prefixed type or receives twigs from the T2 root which is known as the postfixed type. C5 and C6 roots unite to form the superior trunk, C7 root forms the medial (middle) trunk, and C8 and T1 roots unite to form the inferior trunk. Each trunk then divides into anterior and posterior divisions. The anterior divisions of the superior and middle trunks form the lateral cord, the anterior division of the inferior trunk forms the medial cord, and the three posterior divisions of the three trunks unite to form the posterior cord [22, 43, 44].

The roots exit the cervical spine through the intervertebral foramina. The trunks pass between the anterior and middle scalene muscles then pass underneath the clavicle where each trunk divides into anterior and posterior divisions to form the cords. The cords are named according to their relations to the axillary artery: the lateral cord is situated lateral to the artery, the medial cord lies medial to the artery, and the posterior cord lies behind it [43, 44]. The relation of each of the five components of the plexus to the surrounding structures (vertebrae, muscles, and vessels) is of utmost importance because these structures serve as the anatomical landmarks to identify the plexus during ultrasound scanning.

Also, a knowledge of cross-sectional anatomic appearance of the neck is essential for scanning and identification of the brachial plexus. A cross section of the neck at the level of cricoid cartilage shows the trachea lying anteriorly and adjacent to it lies the thyroid gland. Posterolateral to the gland is the carotid sheath. The carotid sheath contains the common carotid artery, the internal jugular vein, and the vagus nerve which lies in the posterolateral wedge between the artery and the vein. The anterior and the middle scalene muscles lie posterolateral to the carotid sheath. The trunks of the brachial plexus are located between the anterior and middle scalene and deep to the sternocleidomastoid muscle. This cross-sectional anatomy of the neck corresponds to the ultrasound image of the interscalene brachial plexus at the level of cricoid cartilage.

Technical Principles of Brachial Plexus Scanning

The basic rules of peripheral nerve scanning apply to brachial plexus scanning as well. A linear array transducer is usually used to scan toddlers and older children. For neonates, a 15–7 MHz small footprint probe (hockey stick probe) may be more appropriate to conform to their short small neck. The optimum frequency ranges from 10 to 18 MHz, but the selection of the frequency depends on the scanning plane, scanning level, the depth of the target structures, and the child's age and body mass index. Scanning obese children with obese neck needs lower frequency transducer. A large pad gel is essential to ensure good contact of the transducer with the skin especially in the supraclavicular scanning plane. The pressure exerted by the probe should be minimal at all times especially before capturing the image and measuring the cross-sectional areas or diameters. At each scanning level, the plexus should be scanned in two views, the axial and the longitudinal views. The longitudinal view can be technically difficult in children at certain levels because of the curved course of the plexus at the neck and the short neck length. In the axial view, the orientation mark of the probe is directed toward the examiner's left side, and in longitudinal view, the mark is directed proximally toward the child's head.

An important point to consider when scanning the plexus is the proper orientation of the probe in relation to the plexus. To obtain the best image, the probe should be inclined 90° to the plexus. To achieve this orthogonal orientation to the plexus, the sonographer needs to incline the probe cranially or caudally according to the scanning level.

Scanning Technique

There are three windows through which the brachial plexus can be visualized. These are the supraclavicular, infraclavicular, and axillary windows. Through the supraclavicular window, the cervical roots and trunks can be visualized at three levels: paravertebral, interscalene, and supraclavicular levels. Scanning the infraclavicular part of the plexus, which is usually challenging in adults, is easier in children. The terminal branches of the plexus are readily visualized at the axillary level and easily traced distally along their entire courses.

In adults, a common approach is to start scanning the plexus at the interscalene level and then tracing it distally to the supraclavicular level and proximally to the paravertebral level. This approach can be followed in infants and older children. In neonates, it is better to start scanning at the supraclavicular level where the plexus can be easily identified and then tracing it proximally to the interscalene and paravertebral levels [45].

In general, the sonographic appearance of the brachial plexus in children is quite similar to that in adults. However, certain differences should be put into consideration. Neonates and infants have brown fat and the nerves have little perineural fibrous tissue. These factors may make it difficult to delineate individual roots/trunks from each other or from the surrounding muscles [45].

The child should be placed in the supine position with the head rotated to the side opposite the side to be scanned. The plexus is scanned first in the axial view by placing the probe transversely above the clavicle and slightly medially. Adjustment of probe rotation and inclination is sometimes needed in this position to obtain the best image. To identify the plexus at this level, the subclavian artery is used as the anatomical landmark. The artery is easily identified by its anechoic appearance, pulsating nature, and Doppler signal. The plexus can then be identified superolateral to the artery and appears as a "bunch of grapes" or "cluster" representing the coalescence of the trunks together (Fig. 13.16). This appearance is quite similar to what is seen in adults. Capturing the plexus in longitudinal view is difficult at this plane because of the clavicle which hinders proper longitudinal orientation. After identification of the supraclavicular plexus, the probe is moved proximally to trace the plexus in the interscalene level. At this level, the trunks are identified as round or oval hypoechoic structures lying between anterior and middle scalenes deep to the sternocleidomastoid muscle (Fig. 13.17). The stacking of the trunks in the interscalene groove in adults which is known as the traffic sign may not be that evident in all children [45]. If the interscalene level is used as the starting scanning point, the probe is positioned at the anterior neck at the level of cricoid cartilage which corresponds to C6 vertebrae level. At this level, the thyroid gland is easily identified by its homogenous and hyperechoic appearance. Moving the probe posterolateral allows visualization of the carotid sheath with its three contents: the common carotid artery, the internal jugular vein, and the vagus nerve. Posterior to the carotid sheath, the trunks appear between anterior and middle scalene

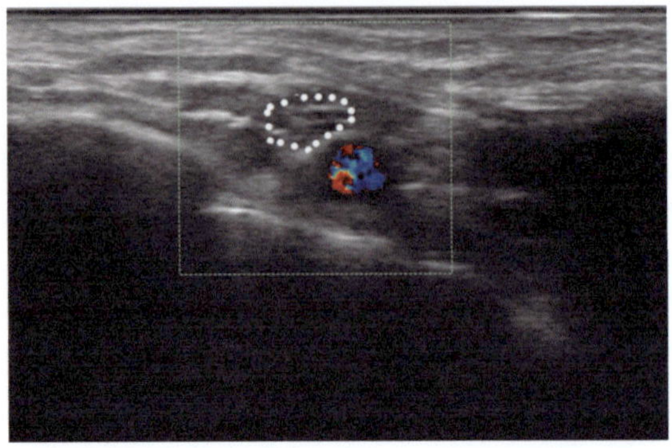

Fig. 13.16 Axial view of the supraclavicular brachial plexus. The plexus (white circled structure) appears as multiple rounded hypoechoic areas coalesced together "punch of grapes" located superolateral to the subclavian artery (color signal)

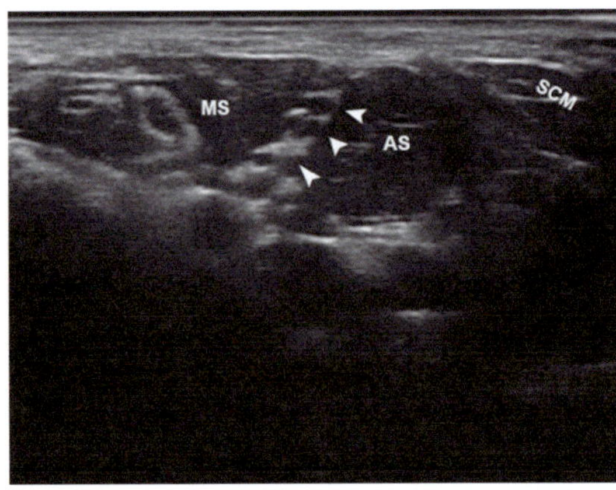

Fig. 13.17 Axial view of the brachial plexus (multiple arrowheads) at the interscalene level between the anterior scalene anteriorly (*AS*) and the middle scalene posteriorly (*MS*), the trunks appear as hypoechoic round/oval structures stacked over each other. SCM Sternocleidomastoid

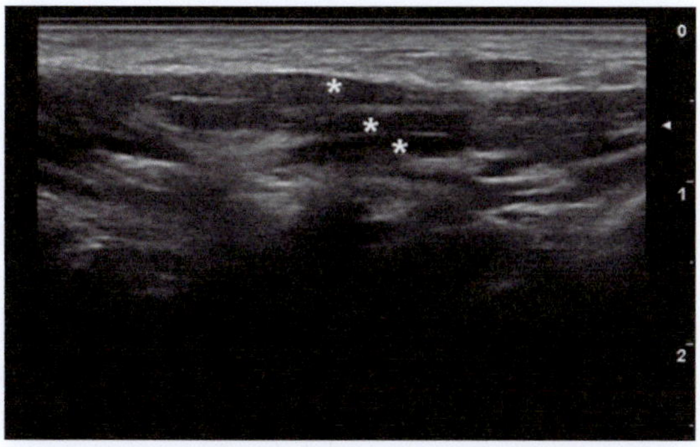

Fig. 13.18 Longitudinal view of the brachial plexus (asterisks) at the interscalene level, the trunks appear as hypoechoic parallel bundles

muscles. From this axial view, the probe can be rotated 90° to assess the trunks in the longitudinal axis where they appear as hypoechoic parallel bundles (Fig. 13.18). Moving the probe cranially, the roots can be visualized and identified through the identification of the tubercles of the transverse processes of the cervical vertebrae [46]. The first transverse process to identify is the C7 process which possesses only a posterior tubercle and lacks anterior tubercle. From C7 root level, the subsequent C6 and C5 roots can be easily identified. At the level of C6 root, the transverse process of the cervical vertebra is characterized by prominent anterior and posterior tubercles. However, the bright hyperechoic appearance of the tubercles which is seen in adults cannot be identified in neonates and infants because the tubercles are still cartilaginous and acquire a hypoechoic appearance. An alternative method to identify the roots is to visually track the trunks from the interscalene level and follow each root. C8 and T1 roots are challenging because of their deep locations [45–47]. The longitudinal view can be obtained by rotating the probe 90° degrees from the axial view.

To scan the infraclavicular part of the plexus, the probe is placed transversely just distal to the mid-clavicle. The axillary artery and vein can be utilized to identify the plexus. It is usually necessary to incline the probe medially to achieve orthogonal orientation of the probe to the axillary vessels and the plexus [48]. The axillary vessels are identified deep to two muscles, the pectoralis major and minor muscles. The lateral cord is the easiest to visualize and is located lateral to the artery. The medial cord lies medial to the artery and the posterior cord lies posterior to the artery.

To scan the plexus at the axillary level, the shoulder is positioned in abduction and external rotation and the probe is placed transversely at the medial axilla. The main terminal branches of the brachial plexus are oriented around the axillary artery in a specific pattern. The median nerve is usually located lateral to the artery. The ulnar nerve is usually medial or caudal to the artery or sometimes, it may be situated between the artery and the vein. The radial nerve lies deep to the artery, and musculocutaneous nerve lies medial to axillary artery in the fascial plane between the biceps and the coracobrachialis. To ensure accurate identification of the different nerves, each nerve is traced distally to the elbow level. The nerves at the axillary plane are multi-fascicular, oval, or rounded in shape with hyperechoic epineurium.

Sonographic Assessment of Brachial plexus

The plexus is typically assessed for size, echotexture, and continuity. The most important measurement is the cross-sectional areas of the plexus or the individual roots. The general rule of measurement applies to the brachial plexus. The cross-sectional area is measured from just inside the hyperechoic rim of the root, the trunk, or the cord using the trace function of the ultrasound machine (Fig. 13.19).

At the supraclavicular level, the cross-sectional area of the whole cluster or the punch of grapes is measured (Fig. 13.19). At the interscalene and paravertebral levels, the cross-sectional area of each trunk/root can be measured separately (Figs. 13.20 and 13.21). An alternative technique at the interscalene level is to measure the cross-sectional area of the three trunks collectively as in Fig. 13.22. This method is useful when the borders of the individual trunks are not clear.

The reference values of the brachial plexus size in children are not sufficiently reported. In neo-

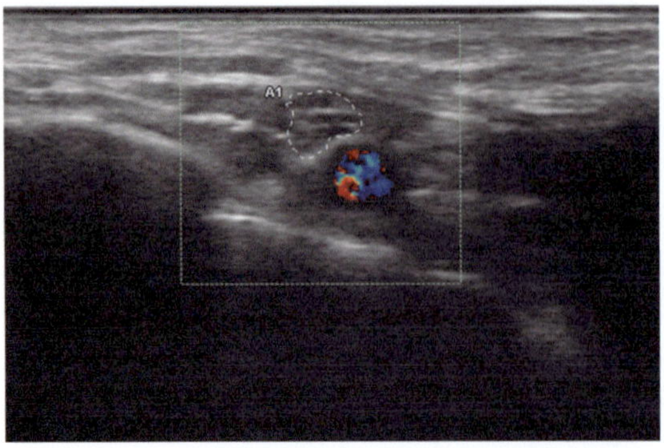

Fig. 13.19 Measurement of the plexus cross-sectional area at the supraclavicular level using the tracing method

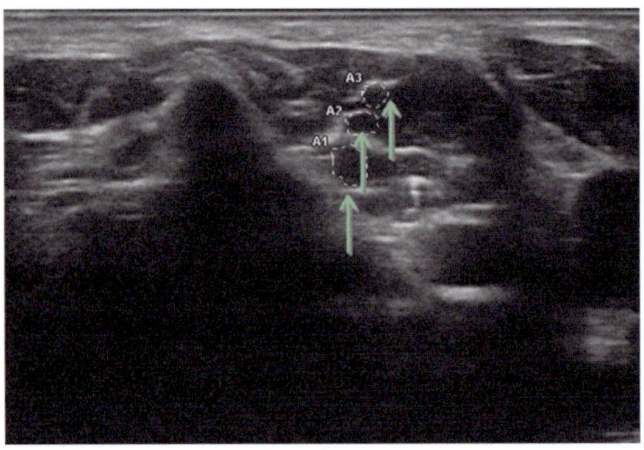

Fig. 13.20 Measurement of the plexus (arrows) cross-sectional area at the interscalene level using the tracing method. Each trunk is measured separately

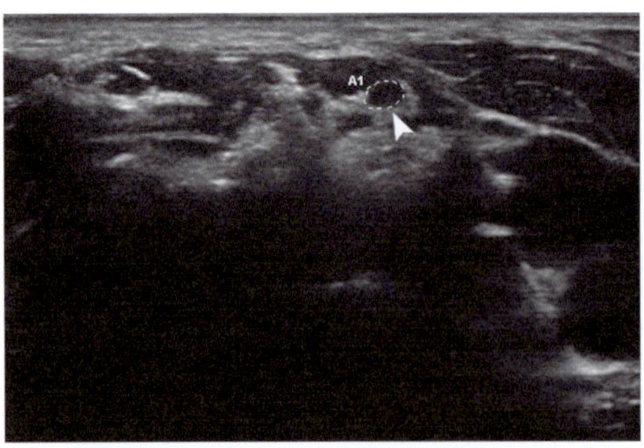

Fig. 13.21 Measurement of the cross-sectional area of C5 root (arrowhead) at the paravertebral level using the tracing method

nates, the median cross-sectional area is 7 mm^2 at the supraclavicular level and 2.1 mm^2 at the paravertebral level, and the median diameter of the nerve roots at the foraminal exit is 1.5 mm [45].

Neuromuscular Ultrasound in Pediatric Brachial Plexopathy

The data available on the value of the ultrasound in pediatric brachial plexopathy is confined to neonatal brachial plexus palsy which is expected since it is the most common brachial plexus injury in pediatric population.

The pathology of neonatal brachial plexus palsy ranges from simple neuropraxia to complete root avulsion. In partial plexus injury (neuropraxia or axonotmesis), the root/trunk may enlarge, and this is reflected in ultrasound by increased cross-sectional area in the axial view (Fig. 13.22) and increased diameter in the longitudinal view. The echogenicity may also change and becomes distorted.

In avulsion injuries and lower trunk lesions, ultrasound is limited and its diagnostic sensitivity is low, whereas in upper and middle trunk lesions, it can accurately detect neuroma [42, 49] making it a useful commentary tool to MRI and electrodiagnostic tests.

Ultrasound can be also used as an indirect method to detect the degree of functional impairment through assessment of thickness and echo intensity of skeletal muscles. The thickness decreases, and the echo intensity increases as the degrees of functional impairment increase [50]. Muscle ultrasound can indirectly determine the distribution and the extent of the plexus injury by screening for atrophy of different muscles supplied by the plexus [41]. Scanning of proximal muscles that are difficult to study or at risk of injury during needle electromyography like serratus anterior, latissimus dorsi, and rhomboids provides an easy painless way to assess these important muscles. Sonographic changes in these muscles in the form of decreased thickness and increased echo intensity in comparison to the healthy side suggest a lesion proximal to the level of trunks. Muscle scanning can also be of value prior to nerve grafting. An atrophic muscle denotes

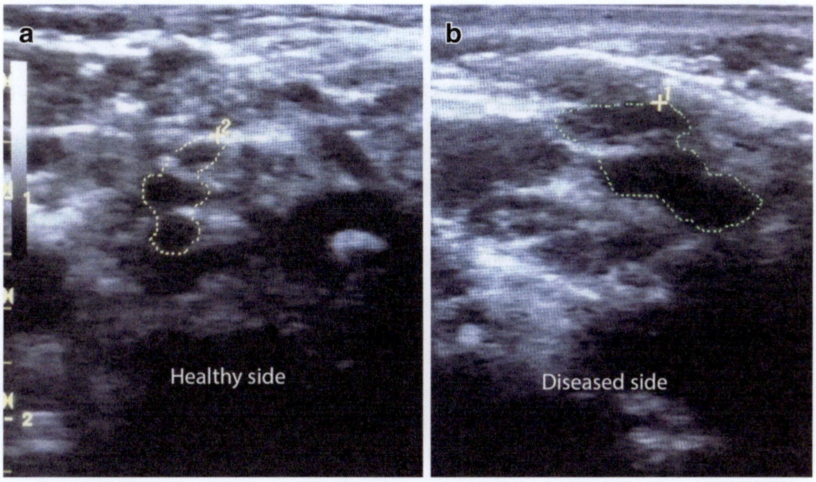

Fig. 13.22 Axial view of the brachial plexus at the interscalene level (arrowheads) in a child with post-traumatic brachial plexus injury showing enlargement of the trunks. (**a**) Healthy side, (**b**) diseased side. Note that the cross-sectional area of the three trunks is measured collectively (not separately) using the trace function

denervation of the nerve innervating the muscle and its unsuitability for nerve grafting [49].

Shoulder joint laxity and dislocation is a well-known complication of neonatal brachial plexus palsy resulting from muscle atrophy and weakness. Identification of such complication is important for optimum management or surgical planning. Reliability of ultrasound in the assessment of humeral position in relation to the glenoid cavity and its ability to detect joint laxity and dislocation add to its value in brachial plexus palsy [51, 52].

In conclusion, the ideal sonographic workup in neonatal brachial plexus palsy includes:

1. Brachial plexus scanning to localize the lesion and detect neuroma and/or scar tissue encasing the plexus
2. Scanning of muscles innervated by different branches of the plexus as an indirect method to determine the extent and distribution of the lesion and to detect the most suitable nerve for grafting if needed
3. Shoulder joint scanning to detect joint laxity or dislocation

Other Traumatic Peripheral Nerve Injuries

Apart from brachial plexus injuries, traumatic nerve injuries of other peripheral nerves are not as common in children as in adults, but the functional impact can be devastating in children. The prevalence of peripheral nerve injuries in children is highest in motorcycle crashes and lowest in bicycle crashes [53].

Electrodiagnostic testing is crucial in the assessment of traumatic nerve injuries. It assesses the functional status of the nerves, localizes the injury, and detects denervation and reinnervation. Nevertheless, the inability of electrodiagnostic tests to differentiate between severe axonotmesis and neurotmesis in the first few weeks of the trauma is a well-known limitation. Moreover, they give no clue about structural factors that may interfere with nerve reinnervation in partial axonal inquires including neuroma and scar tissue that may encase the nerve.

Ultrasound became an attractive tool in the diagnostic workup of traumatic nerve injuries [54–56]. It complements the electrodiagnostic tests and overcomes its shortcomings. Ultrasound assesses nerve continuity and can differentiate between axonotmesis and neurotmesis even in the first few weeks of trauma. It can detect structural compressive causes of nerve injury including nerve entrapment by bone fragment, alteration in the course of a nerve, and post-traumatic nerve swelling [10, 57]. Ultrasound is also reliable in detection of neuroma and nerve encasement by scar tissue [54, 58, 59]. The valuable information obtained via ultrasonography in traumatic nerve injuries makes it an excellent diagnostic and follow-up tool in children. Ultrasound can also be used intraoperatively during nerve repair surgeries for optimum decision making. Intraoperative ultrasound findings have been found to correlate well with histologic cross sections taken during the surgery, accurately identify neuroma, and allow preservation of healthy nerve tissues [60].

Sonographic Workup for Traumatic Peripheral Nerve Injuries

In traumatic peripheral nerve injuries, the anatomy can be significantly altered; so to be able to capture the abnormality, it is recommended to start scanning the nerve in an axial view at a site remote from the site of the trauma and then move the transducer toward the site of the injury. A common approach is to trace the nerve back and forth several times before focusing on the trauma site and observe sudden disappearance of the nerve at any point or any abrupt change in the size or echotexture of the nerve. Nerve transection is suspected if the nerve disappears at a certain point and is replaced by anechoic defect representing nerve gap. To confirm nerve discontinuity, the probe is rotated 90° to obtain the longitudinal view. In the longitudinal view, complete nerve transection appears as anechoic gap with complete loss of the fascicular pattern and the outer nerve sheath [61]. The proximal and distal nerve stumps are usually visualized proximal and distal to the transected segment unless the proximal nerve stump is retracted. Stump neuroma may develop and appears as hypoechoic or anechoic swelling of the proximal and/or the distal nerve ends. The nerve gap between the distal and proximal nerve stumps can be measured using the distance function of the ultrasound machine. The ability of ultrasound to determine the level of transection and to localize the site of distal and proximal nerve stumps via nerve mapping provides valuable information to the surgeon and allows optimum preoperative planning of the surgery. From the surgeon's prospective, knowing the level of nerve stumps allows the surgeon to open directly at the level of stumps and spares the child extensive exploration that may be needed in some patients to find the nerve stumps. In partial transection, the outer epineurium is intact, but the internal nerve fascicles are disrupted. Nerve continuity in partial transection can be confirmed by passive movement of an underlying tendon in infants or by active movement in older children.

If nerve transection is excluded, the nerve should be assessed for the presence/absence of neuroma in continuity, focal nerve swelling, and/or scar tissue compressing or encasing the nerve. In the axial view, neuroma in continuity is suspected if the nerve abruptly enlarges and turns hypoechoic with well-defined borders [59, 62] (Fig. 13.23). In the longitudinal view, neuroma appears as fusiform or spindle-shaped intraneural swelling [62]. Exerting slight pressure on the neuroma by the probe may trigger numbness and tingling in the distribution of the injured nerve "ultrasound Tinel's sign."

Scanning of the muscles innervated by the injured nerve can be a useful adjunct to needle electromyography. A denervated muscle usually shows increased echogenicity and decreased thickness in long-term injuries. Determining which muscles are denervated can indirectly determine which nerve branches are involved.

Lastly, in cases of fractures, the nearby bone profile should be observed for any evidence of callus, bony fragments, or displaced fractures compressing the nerve.

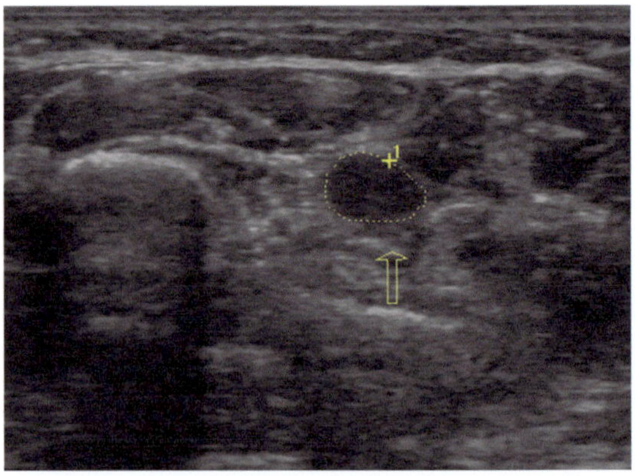

Fig. 13.23 Axial image of the median nerve at the mid-forearm in an 8-year-old child showing post-traumatic neuroma (arrow) appearing as abrupt hypoechoic enlargement of the median nerve

Entrapment Neuropathies

Entrapment neuropathies are considered rare in children, and when it occurs, it commonly develops secondary to metabolic disorders, diabetes, trauma, hereditary polyneuropathy with liability to pressure palsies, juvenile arthritis, and critical illness [63–70].

The most common causes of carpal tunnel syndrome in children are genetic disorders including lysosomal storage diseases, Schwartz-Jampel syndrome, Leri's syndrome, Déjerine-Sottas syndrome, and Weill-Marchesani syndrome [71]. Mucopolysaccharidosis is by far the most common cause of carpal tunnel syndrome, and the prevalence of carpal tunnel syndrome may reach 96% in children with mucopolysaccharidosis type II [72, 73]. The underlying mechanism of carpal tunnel syndrome in mucopolysaccharidosis is related to proteoglycan deposition in the tenosynovium of the flexor tendons [74], thickened flexor retinaculum, and the associated bone dysplasia [75]. Nongenetic causes of carpal tunnel syndrome in children include playing musical instruments, intensive sport training, chronic steroid intake, hemophilia, and scleroderma [76, 77]. Anatomical variations like anomalous palmaris longus and flexor digitorum superficialis inside the carpal tunnel may be risk factors for carpal tunnel syndrome by intruding and compressing on the median nerve during activities of daily living [78]. Idiopathic causes have also been reported [77].

Encountering a child in EMG lab with carpal tunnel syndrome, ulnar neuropathy at the elbow, or other focal neuropathies is uncommon, and when found, the abovementioned causes should be put into consideration and investigated. Electrodiagnosis remains an essential part of the workup of entrapment neuropathy, but in children it is sometimes challenging and thus ultrasound can be a useful complementary tool. The sonographic criterion for focal neuropathy in adults is focal nerve swelling proximal to the site of entrapment. In children, similar finding has been reported. Ultrasound can determine the median nerve alterations in children with mucopolysaccharidosis and thus can be used to screen for carpal tunnel syndrome in those children [79]. The reported sonographic alterations include increased cross-sectional area of the median nerve at the carpal tunnel outlet, increased outlet/forearm cross-sectional area ratio, hypoechogenicity, fascicular enlargement, hypervascularity, and shape alteration [80] (Fig. 13.24). Ultrasound can also identify the structural local causes of carpal tun-

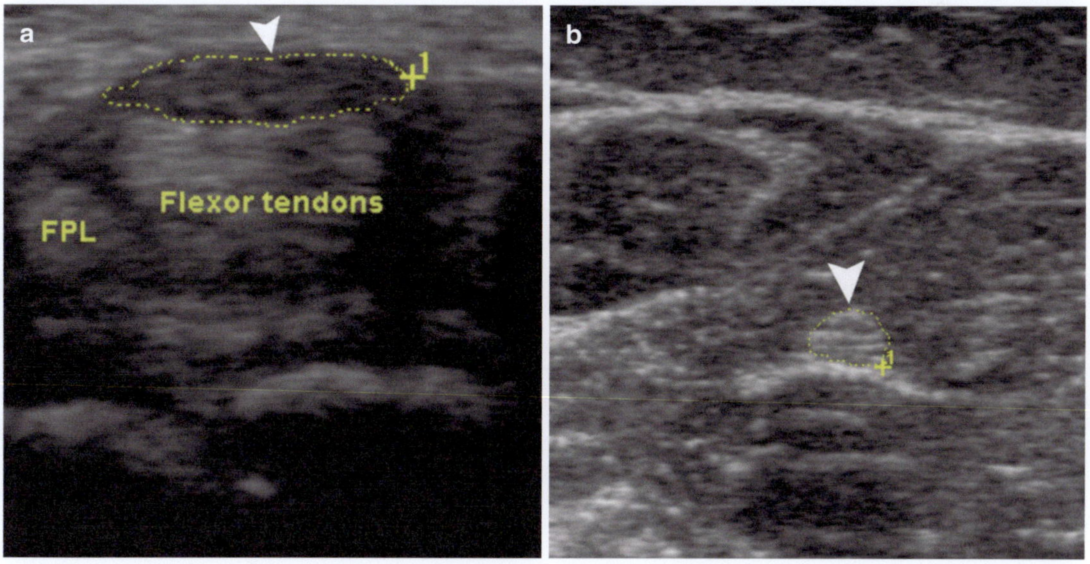

Fig. 13.24 Axial view of the median nerve (arrowhead) at the distal wrist crease (**a**) and mid-forearm (**b**) in a 10-year-old girl with carpal tunnel syndrome. CSA measured 13 mm^2 at the distal wrist crease and 6 mm^2 at the mid-forearm giving a wrist/forearm ratio of 2.1

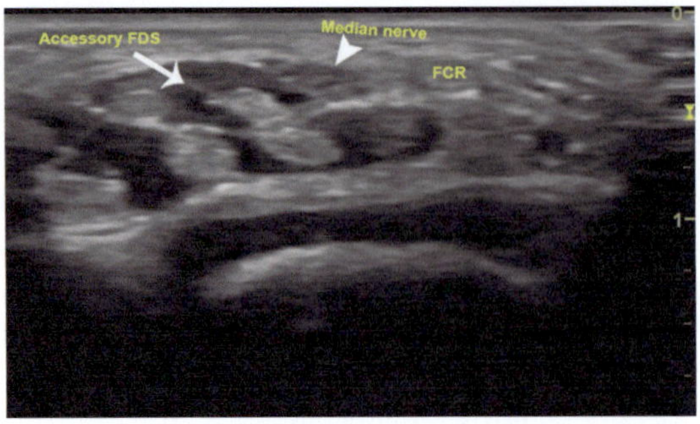

Fig. 13.25 Axial view of the median nerve (arrowhead) inside the carpal tunnel showing accessory flexor digitorum superficialis (long arrow) that appears with finger extension and retracts with finger flexion in a 5-year-old child with carpal tunnel syndrome. The muscle intrudes on the nerve

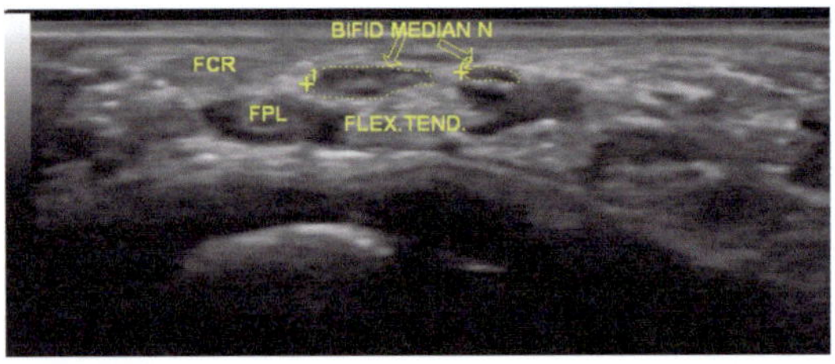

Fig. 13.26 Axial view of the median nerve (arrows) at the wrist showing bifid median nerve in a 5-year-old child

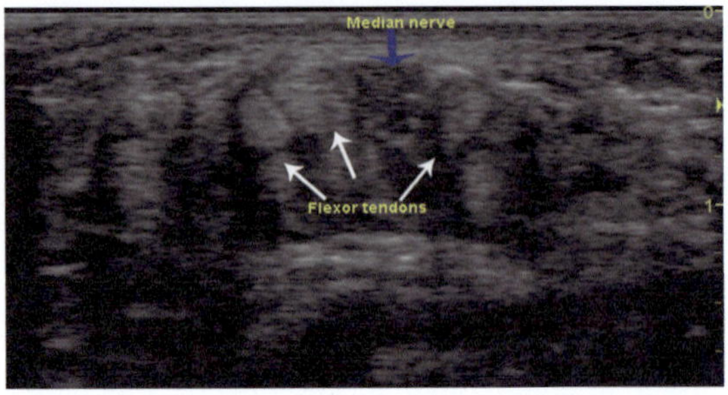

Fig. 13.27 Normal mobility of the median nerve at the wrist (blue arrow) assessed in the axial view in a 10-year-old child. The median nerve dives and becomes surrounded by the flexor tendons on combined finger and wrist flexion

nel syndrome like tenosynovitis of flexor tendons in children with idiopathic juvenile arthritis or secondary to anomalous accessory muscle inside the carpal tunnel that can intrude on the median nerve (Fig. 13.25). Other anatomical variations as bifid median nerve and persistent median artery may be associated with carpal tunnel and can be detected via ultrasound (Fig. 13.26).

Ultrasound can also detect abnormal mobility of the median and ulnar nerves. Normally, the median nerve at the wrist exhibits a degree of excursion at the wrist. With flexion and extension of the index, the median nerve exhibits a transverse sliding movement underneath the flexor retinaculum [81], and on combined finger and wrist flexion, the median nerve dives between the flexor tendons [30] (Fig. 13.27). In carpal tunnel syndrome, this mobility may become reduced [81, 82]. Abnormal ulnar nerve mobility takes the form of anterior displacement. Typically, the ulnar nerve lies behind the medial epicondyle in the ulnar groove and does not displace medially with elbow flexion. The ulnar nerve may subluxate or dislocate. It is considered subluxated if the nerve moves to the tip of the medial epicondyle and is considered dislocated if it moves in front of the medial epicondyle [30]. The prevalence of ulnar nerve displacement in elbows of healthy children has been variably reported ranging from 14–27% for ulnar nerve subluxation to 17–20% for ulnar nerve dislocation [83, 84] with highest incidence in the age group 6–10 years [85]. The incidence in children is less than in adults [83] and may be attributed to smaller space available for ulnar nerve displacement in children [84]. The link between ulnar nerve subluxation/dislocation and ulnar neuropathy is still a matter of debate even in adults. However, detection of a displaced ulnar nerve in children is important prior to surgical management of supracondylar fracture to avoid iatrogenic injury of the ulnar nerve which may occur if the nerve exhibits increased mobility during flexion [86–88].

Sonographic Workup in Focal Neuropathies

Whatever the type of focal neuropathy is, the scanning protocol is almost the same. Scanning should start in the axial view. It is better to scan the nerve under investigation at a site distant from the site of entrapment then tracing it to the expected entrapment site. Median nerve is usually traced from elbow or mid-forearm to the palm, ulnar nerve is traced from the wrist or mid-forearm to the mid-arm level, radial nerve is usually traced from elbow to the proximal arm, and fibular nerve is usually traced from the popliteal fossa to the fibular head/neck levels. During tracing, enlargement of the nerve is observed and the cross-sectional area is measured at the site of maximal enlargement [30]. The cross-sectional area at the site of maximal enlargement is the most reliable parameter in focal neuropathies [89–92]. Recently, it is advisable to not only measure the absolute cross-sectional area but also to measure the cross-sectional area at a healthy segment and calculate diseased/healthy segment cross-sectional area [93, 94] to exclude diffuse nerve enlargements. The upper limit of the cross-sectional area ratio in adults is 1.4 [93, 94]. In children, there are no reports documenting the reference values of cross-sectional area ratio of any nerve. However, the rule logically applies because any nerve gets smaller as it courses distally due to branching and physiological nerve tapering, and thus the ratio between a distal segment and a proximal one is expected to be less than or equal to 1.

The nerve echotexture should be assessed, and any change in the echogenicity of the outer neural sheath or disturbance in the internal fascicular pattern is observed. In entrapment neuropathies, the nerve usually turns hypoechoic, and the typical honeycomb appearance becomes disturbed [95–97]. Nerve vascularity is assessed via color or power Doppler. Hypervascularity denotes acute inflammation and has been found in carpal tunnel syndrome [97, 98]. Assessment of median and ulnar nerve mobility is only possible in toddlers and older children who are cooperative and can actively flex fingers, wrist, and elbow.

The sonographic workup in entrapment neuropathies should also include assessment of the muscles innervated by the nerve under study and assessment of surrounding joints and tendons in addition to observation of any anatomical variations including persistent median artery, bifid median nerve, accessory muscles at the wrist or elbow, and ulnar nerve subluxation/dislocation.

Motor Neuron Diseases

Spinal muscle atrophy is the most common motor neuron disease in children. It is an inherited neuromuscular disorder characterized by motor neuron degeneration leading to progressive muscle atrophy and weakness. Diagnosis depends on genetic testing, nerve conduction, and electromyography studies. The utility of nerve ultrasound in spinal muscle atrophy has not been well investigated and the available literature is scanty. Nerve atrophy has been reported in adults with degenerative motor neuron disorders [13, 14]. However, similar changes in nerve size in spinal muscle atrophy have not been addressed yet.

In contrast, muscle sonographic changes have been reported in spinal muscle atrophy [1, 99–101] and are discussed in this chapter in the muscle section.

Polyneuropathy

Sonographic Workup in Pediatric Polyneuropathy

Nerve scanning in polyneuropathy may take a long time, and although it is a painless, child-friendly tool, the child may get bored, and keeping his/her position and cooperation for a long time can be difficult. To be able to document the pattern of abnormality in polyneuropathy, scanning of multiple nerves of upper and lower limbs at multiple distal and proximal levels may be mandatory. It is recommended to trace at least one nerve from each limb along its entire course and to measure cross-sectional area at different levels including entrapment and non-entrapment sites. Additionally, nerve echogenicity, vascularity, and skeletal muscle assessment should be performed.

The sonographic changes in different types of pediatric polyneuropathies are discussed in the next sections.

Guillain-Barre Syndrome (GBS)

Guillain-Barre syndrome is an autoimmune disorder in which the immune system attacks the peripheral nerves resulting in acute demyelinating sensory and motor polyradiculoneuropathy. The diagnosis depends mainly on the clinical presentation and confirmed by spinal fluid analysis, electrodiagnostic tests, and spinal MRI. The role of ultrasound in the assessment of the generalized peripheral nerve diseases has drawn the attention in the last few years. However, the routine use of ultrasound in the diagnostic workup of generalized polyneuropathy including Guillain-Barre syndrome is not established yet because to date there is no agreement on the diagnostic sonographic criteria for different generalized neuromuscular disorders. Several sonographic alterations in nerve size and echogenicity have been reported in Guillain-Barre syndrome. These changes include focal nerve enlargement of median and ulnar nerves at non-entrapment sites, diffuse enlargement of nerves along their courses, focal enlargement of nerve fascicles even in normally sized nerves, and decreased echogenicity [31, 102]. Other ultrasound measures like intra-nerve cross-sectional variability and side-to-side difference ratio of intra-nerve cross-sectional variability have been found higher in children with post-Guillain-Barre compared to healthy children [103]. It should be emphasized that these sonographic findings are nonspecific and can be seen in different types of peripheral nerve diseases because the observed nerve swelling is just a reaction to different pathologies. Interestingly, temporal changes in nerve size and echotexture have been observed with improvement of the clinical status of patients with GBS; nerve size and echotexture normalize with complete disease resolution [102]. Based on these findings, ultrasound represents an attractive, non-invasive painless follow-up tool in Guillain-Barre syndrome.

Hereditary Polyneuropathies

The most common hereditary neuropathies are Charcot-Marie-Tooth syndrome and hereditary neuropathy with liability to pressure palsies. Charcot-Marie-Tooth is an autosomal dominant sensorimotor polyneuropathy characterized by slowly progressive sensory loss and muscle weakness. Hereditary neuropathy with liability to pressure palsies (HNPP) is an autosomal dominant neuropathy characterized by recurrent episodes of entrapment neuropathies induced by minor trauma or compression of peripheral nerves [104]. This type of neuropathy typically manifests in adolescence, but childhood onset has been reported [105]. Unfortunately, there are no reports on sonographic appearance of nerves in childhood-onset HNPP.

In Charcot-Marie-Tooth syndrome, the nerves enlarge in a diffuse pattern. This is in contrast to acquired demyelinating polyneuropathy in which the nerve may appear normal in size or swells in a regional pattern [106]. Children with Charcot-Marie-Tooth type IA have significantly larger nerve cross-sectional area compared to healthy children. This nerve enlargement correlates with age, weight, height, and disease severity [107]. Based on the available results of the published literature, ultrasound can be used to identify children with Charcot-Marie-Tooth and to differentiate between inherited and acquired polyneuropathy.

Recently, ultrasound scoring system has been developed to differentiate between the different types of polyneuropathy. A modified ultrasound pattern sum score has been useful in differentiation between Charcot-Marie-Tooth and hereditary neuropathy with liability to pressure palsies in adults [108]. However, these scores have not been validated in children.

Other Acquired Pediatric Polyneuropathy

Acute inflammatory demyelinating polyneuropathy is the most common acquired polyneuropathy in children. Although rare in children, chronic inflammatory demyelinating polyneuropathy may also occur under the age of 20 [109–112]. A case of predominately motor autoimmune multifocal polyneuropathy has also been documented in children [113]. The diagnosis of multifocal motor neuropathy can be challenging because it may initially manifest as focal mononeuropathy like cubital tunnel syndrome and focal median nerve mononeuropathy [113]. There are no reports on the value of ultrasound in multifocal motor neuropathy of children, but it definitely can help in the localization of the focal neuropathy and rapid screening of peripheral nerves for multifocal swellings or alterations in the fascicular patterns.

Ultrasound can be helpful in other types of acquired polyneuropathy. In an interesting case of a child with leprosy who developed ulnar neuropathy, ultrasound provided accurate detection of intraneural nerve abscess which was diagnosed clinically as ulnar neuritis [114]. This case report highlights the importance of anatomical structural assessment of neuropathy using neuroimaging.

Skeletal Muscle Ultrasound

Muscle Structure

The primary structural unit of a muscle is the muscle fiber. All skeletal muscles are composed of numerous muscle fibers ranging from 10 to 80 micrometers in diameter. Each muscle fiber contains hundreds and may be thousands of myofibrils which are composed of actin and myosin filaments [115]. Each group of muscle fibers collects to form muscle fascicles. Each muscle fiber is surrounded by a layer of fibrous tissue called the endomysium, and each muscle fascicle is surrounded by perimysium which contains blood vessels and nerves. The whole muscle is surrounded by thick strong epimysium made of fibrous tissue. Of note, ultrasound resolution is about 100 um; thus the smallest structures that can be seen in ultrasound are the muscle fascicles.

The arrangement of the muscle fibers inside the muscle differs. The muscle fibers may orient parallel to the long axis of muscle or oblique to the long axis of a muscle giving a pennate shape. The pennate muscle can take the form of unipennate, bipennate, or multipennate. Muscles can also acquire a fan-shaped or a triangular pattern. These patterns can be well visualized in ultrasound.

Sonographic Appearance of a Normal Muscle

In the axial view, the healthy muscle acquires a speckled or a starry night appearance with the majority of the muscle appearing predominately hypoechoic and interspersed with small hyperechoic foci (Fig. 13.28). The hypoechoic areas represent the muscle fascicles which have the ability to absorb the ultrasound waves. The perimysium reflects the ultrasound waves and thus appears as hyperechoic foci between the muscle fascicles. The outer epimysium appears as bright echogenic border owing to its high reflective property. In the longitudinal view, the muscle appears composed of hypoechoic bundles representing the muscle fascicles with interspersed bright hyperechoic lines representing the perimysium. The fascia and the septa between adjacent muscles appear also as bright hyperechoic lines (Fig. 13.29),

The organizational pattern of muscle fibers (parallel, pennate, or fan-shaped) can be easily identified in the longitudinal view of a muscle by using panoramic mode in the ultrasound machine.

Differentiating a muscle from its tendon is easy. In the axial view, the tendon appears as

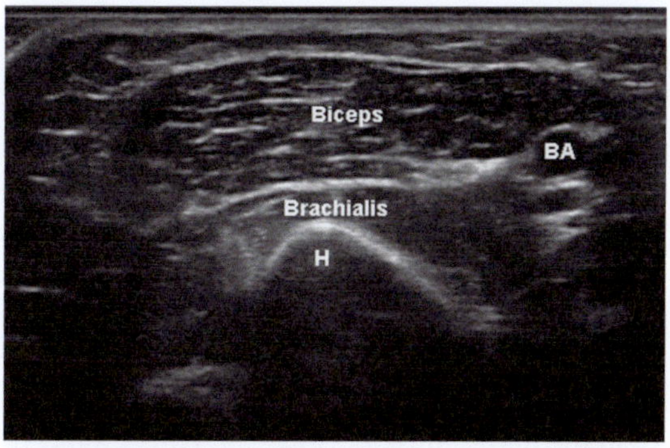

Fig. 13.28 Normal sonographic appearance of the muscle in the axial view

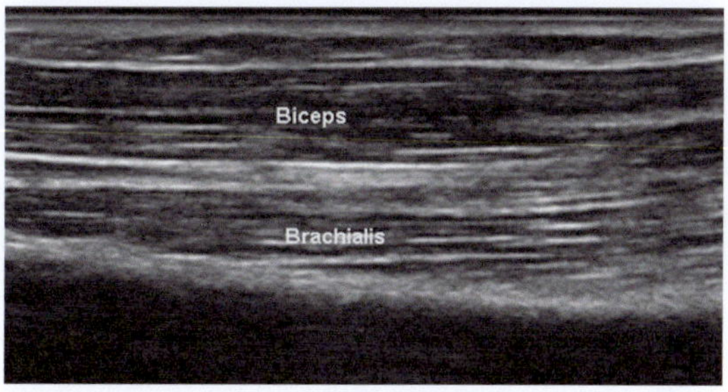

Fig. 13.29 Normal sonographic appearance of the muscle in the longitudinal view

rounded or oval hyperechoic structure. In the longitudinal view, it appears as tightly packed hyperechoic fibrils without hypoechoic interspace Also, the tendon exhibits more anisotropy compared to the healthy muscle.

The sonographic appearance of skeletal muscles in children differs slightly from that in adults. Children have smaller muscle fascicles. Also, the muscles in children exhibit higher echo intensity compared to adults reflecting higher content of connective tissue between muscle fascicles [116].

Scanning Technique of Skeletal Muscles

In infants, a linear array high-frequency transducer is appropriate to scan superficial and deep muscles. A frequency as low as 7.5 MHz can provide enough penetration to scan the muscles in children [117], whereas in adults, a lower frequency as low as 3.5 MHz is needed to reach deep large muscles. A curved array, low-frequency transducer may be needed in older children with high body mass index. The depth is adjusted according to the expected depth of the scanned muscle. Usually a depth of 1–2 cm is chosen for the superficial muscles and a depth of 4–6 cm is suitable for deeper muscles. The focus should be adjusted at the level of scanned muscle. On scanning a nerve, one focal point is recommended to obtain the best resolution. On the other hand, 2–3 focal points may be needed to span the entire muscle. However, care should be taken not to use more than three focal points to avoid decrease in frame rate. Adjusting the correct gain before scanning a muscle is of paramount performance as incorrect gain adjustment may lead to misinterpretation of muscle echogenicity. The correct gain for muscle scanning is the gain at which the muscle appears predominately hypoechoic with clear delineation of fascial planes and intermuscular septa between the muscles. It is better to adjust the gain on a healthy muscle of the child undergoing the study if possible. Having a pre-set program for muscle scanning on the machine is useful to ensure consistency. The bars of the time gain compensation should be kept in the midline in muscle scanning and adjusting time gain compensation is not advisable especially when measuring muscle echogenicity quantitatively. It is very important to keep the machine setting constant when comparing a diseased muscle with a healthy muscle. Equally important is to document the machine settings in the patient's file to be used if follow-up ultrasound studies are needed. If available in the machine, compound imaging and tissue harmonics can substantially improve the quality of the image and provide better delineation of the internal muscle architecture and intermuscular fascia.

The child should lie in a comfortable relaxed position when scanning the muscle as part of the study is to assess the muscles at rest. With active muscle contraction, muscle thickness increases and echogenicity decreases [118, 119], and therefore full child relaxation is important during muscle ultrasound study especially before capturing the image and taking measurements. The probe is held in the same way as in peripheral nerve scanning using the same rules of probe orientation. The muscle should be scanned in two perpendicular planes, axial and longitudinal, and the probe should be kept perpendicular to the muscle at all times. Oblique scanning may overestimate muscle thickness and decrease muscle echogenicity. Clear strong bone profile and delineation of surrounding fascia are signs of proper angle. Also, least pressure should be exerted by the transducer because excessive pressure may dramatically decrease the muscle thickness. Copious amount of gel is preferred for optimal acoustic coupling and to prevent excessive pressure by the probe.

Grayscale Assessment

Grayscale assessment of skeletal muscle includes assessment of muscle thickness, muscle cross-sectional area, muscle echogenicity, and dynamic assessment.

Muscle thickness can be measured in the axial or in the longitudinal views using the distance function of the machine. It is important to

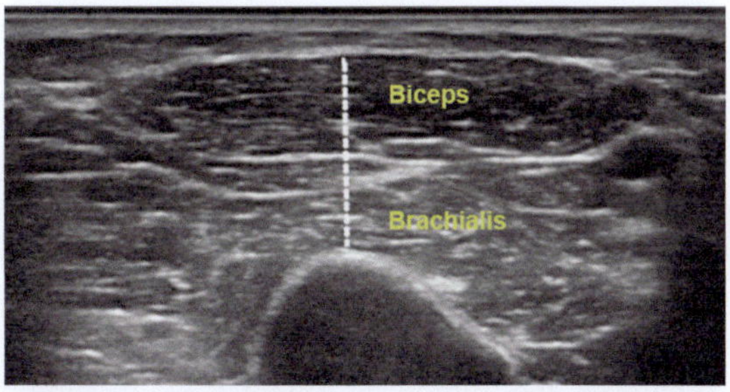

Fig. 13.30 Measurement of muscle thickness of the biceps from a clear bone profile to the superficial edge of the muscle. The disadvantage of this technique is that it includes the underlying brachialis

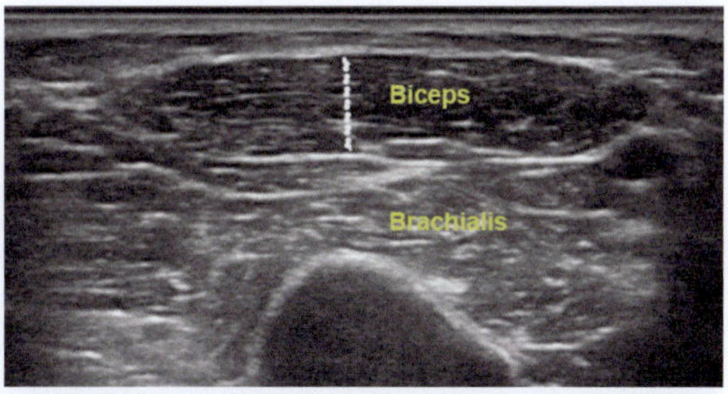

Fig. 13.31 Measurement of biceps thickness by extending the distance caliper from the deep to the superficial aponeurosis

measure the thickness at a specific surface landmark and to use this same surface landmark in side-to-side comparison and in serial follow-up study to ensure objectivity. The anatomical position of the probe should correspond to the main bulk of the muscle. For example, biceps brachii thickness is measured midway between shoulder and elbow (i.e., mid-arm), and quadriceps muscle thickness is measured midway between anterior superior iliac spine and superior patella. Care should be taken to release the pressure by the probe as much as possible prior to measuring muscle thickness. There are two techniques to measure muscle thickness. The first technique is to extend the distance calipers between the superficial border of the muscle and a highly reflective surface usually a bony profile underneath the muscle (Fig. 13.30). The second technique is to measure only the thickness of the muscle of interest by extending the distance caliper between the deep and the superficial aponeurosis of the muscle [120] (Fig. 13.31). The advantage of the first technique is that it uses a fixed landmark (bone profile) and thus is more reliable and reproducible. However, using a bony profile may necessitate measuring the thickness of more than muscle and this in turn may underestimate the thickness of the muscle under the study. The second technique allows assessment of only the muscle in question. However, the surrounding fascia or aponeurosis can be difficult to visualize in neuromuscular disorders especially when there is marked increase in echogenicity.

Abnormal muscle thickness includes muscle atrophy and hypertrophy. Muscle atrophy can be disuse atrophy or pathological atrophy. Pathological atrophy may occur in chronic neuropathic disorders secondary to muscle denervation and may occur in chronic myopathic disorders secondary to muscle weakness. Muscle echogenicity is the factor which differentiates between disuse and myopathic/neuropathic atrophy. Disuse atrophy is associated with normal echogenicity, while pathological atrophy is associated with increased echogenicity. Preserved thickness of the deltoid and calf muscles is observed in children with Duchenne muscular dystrophy [21]. Muscle hypertrophy may occur secondary to extensive exercising in teenagers or caused by intramuscular tumors [16].

Muscle size can also be assessed by measuring the muscle cross-sectional area in the axial view. In adults, it is difficult to capture the whole muscle in one image unless the panoramic view or extended field of view is used [121]. However, in children it is possible to measure the cross-sectional area of a muscle in one image using conventional ultrasonography. The cross-sectional area is measured using the trace function of the machine by following the inner border of the muscle without inclusion of its outer border (Fig. 13.32).

Muscle echogenicity can be assessed qualitatively or quantitatively. Qualitative assessment depends on visual observation of the change in the echotexture of a muscle. The qualitative assessment is subjective and requires familiarity with the normal echotexture of the muscles, and in

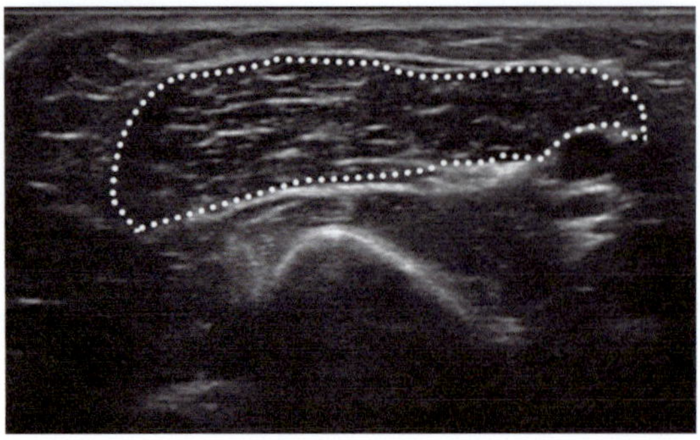

Fig. 13.32 Measurement of muscle cross-sectional area by tracing the inner border of the muscle

many instances it depends on comparison with the contralateral healthy muscle in unilateral disorders. A popular qualitative grading system for muscle echotexture is Heckmatt scale [1]. The scale consists of four grades with grade I representing normal muscle echogenicity and grade IV representing marked increase in echogenicity to the degree that it leads to complete loss of bone echo. The degree of muscle hyper-echogenicity is related to the amount of fat and fibrous tissue within the diseased muscle. The greater the amount of fat and fibrous tissue replacing the muscle fibers, the greater the increased echogenicity [122]. Increased muscle echogenicity is not pathognomonic to a specific disease. It may occur secondary to replacement of muscle fibers by fibrosis or fat in muscle diseases [123], inflammation in myositis or secondary to muscle denervation in axonal lesions. The distribution and the pattern of increased echogenicity may suggest certain disease. Increased echogenicity of the proximal upper and lower limb muscles in a symmetrical fashion may suggest myopathic disorders, while symmetrical bilateral increase in echogenicity of the distal muscles may suggest polyneuropathy. Homogenous hyper-echogenicity within the muscle with preserved muscle thickness was observed in muscle dystrophies, while inhomogeneous hyper-echogenicity with moth-eaten appearance of the muscle was observed in spinal muscle atrophy secondary to degeneration of the anterior horn cell [16, 124]. Pathological decrease in muscle echogenicity was not observed in any disease so far.

Different techniques can be used to quantify muscle echo intensity. The most popular technique is to calculate the mean of gray value of the region of interest (ROI) using the histogram function of offline computer systems like the Adobe Photoshop [125], ImageJ, or similar software. The region of interest can be a whole muscle or a specific region of a muscle [125, 126]. Whatever the region of interest is, it should include muscle tissue without the inclusion of the surrounding fascia [117, 125, 127]. Backscatter analysis is another quantitative technique to measure muscle echo intensity through measuring the amplitudes of the backscattered sound waves [128, 129]. These quantitative tools are highly sensitive and specific compared to the qualitative assessment, and their reliability has been validated in healthy children and in children with neuromuscular disorders [125, 126, 129].

In addition to measuring muscle thickness and echogenicity, other sonographic parameters can be measured. These parameters include pennation angle, fiber angle, and fiber length. Pennation angle is the angle between the deep aponeurosis and the echoes of the interspaces between the fiber bundles and is measured in the longitudinal view [16, 120]. Fiber angle is the angle between the fascicle path and the subcutaneous adipose tissue-muscle interface [116]. The fiber length can be calculated by dividing the muscle thickness by the sin of the pennation angle "fiber length = muscle thickness/sin pennation angle" [130, 131]. The utility of these parameters in routine daily clinical practice is still limited, yet they are useful in the research domain and can provide insights on the relation between muscle architecture and each of joint position, muscle contraction, age, and limb length.

Dynamic Muscle Ultrasound

Dynamic muscle ultrasound refers to the assessment of voluntary and involuntary muscle movements via ultrasonography. Dynamic muscle ultrasound in children may only be possible in older infants and toddlers who can cooperate and respond to instructions to relax or to actively contract a muscle.

To detect involuntary movements, frame rate should be higher than 15/sec to reflect real-time image. The child should lie in a supine relaxed position for this part of assessment, and the probe should be kept steady on the muscle for 10–30 seconds to detect involuntary movement. Involuntary pathological movement should be differentiated from normal arterial pulsations and voluntary muscle activation. Arterial pulsations are rhythmic and localized to one area and display Doppler signal. Voluntary muscle activation results in movement of the whole muscle and alteration of its overall shape.

Ultrasound can detect fasciculation, tremors and cramps, and even fibrillations. Fasciculations appear as spontaneous, random-focal jerky movements which occur irregularly in different parts of the muscle [13, 132]. The sensitivity of ultrasound to detect fasciculations in limb and cranial muscles of adults is higher than needle electromyography [133–139]. The diagnostic sensitivity of electromyography depends on the fasciculation size and the distance of the needle from the fasciculation center [137]. In contrast, ultrasound can noninvasively screen the whole muscle for fasciculations in a rapid and painless way. A scoring system for fasciculations has been used by some researches by counting the number of fasciculations per minute with 0 = absent; 1 = 2–10/min; 2 = 11–49/min; 3 = 50–99/min; and 4 = 100/min [139]. Recently, fasciculation ultrasound score has been developed to diagnose patients with amyotrophic lateral sclerosis and was found to be sensitive and specific [140]. However, such scores have not been developed for children.

In children, fasciculations may occur in spinal muscle atrophy and in chronic polyneuropathy. In a 12-year-old girl with chronic sensorimotor and autonomic peripheral neuropathy, ultrasound identified fasciculations detected simultaneously using surface electromyography [141].

Fibrillations appear as small irregular movements of muscle tissue in all directions without alteration in the overall shape of the muscle. Keeping the muscle warm is recommended when searching for fibrillations because the sensitivity of ultrasound to detect fibrillations decreases with low temperatures [142, 143]. To date, ultrasound sensitivity to detect fibrillations is not as high as its sensitivity to detect fasciculations, and several pitfalls should be put into consideration before interpreting an involuntary movement as fibrillation [143]. However, the diagnostic sensitivity of ultrasound for fibrillations is expected to improve with improvements in the spatial resolution and the processing abilities of ultrasound machines.

Reference Values of Skeletal Muscle Ultrasound Parameters

Reference values of muscle thickness and echo intensity of common muscle groups have been reported [117, 120, 127], but it is important to emphasize that utility of the published reference values in clinical practice requires strict adherence to the technique adopted in the relevant studies including the machine settings, the anatomical measurement site, and the measurement technique.

In general, muscle thickness is smaller in children compared to adults [120]. Reference values of muscle thickness of all muscle groups in children are not available, and the available studies focused on the major muscle groups that are commonly affected in children with neuromuscular disorders like the biceps brachii, forearm muscles, quadriceps, and tibialis anterior [117]. Muscle thickness is dependent on weight up to the age of 16 years [117]. Leg length and muscle force may also influence muscle thickness. Gastrocnemius muscle thickness has been reported to correlate with age and leg length [120], while biceps, forearm muscles, quadriceps, and tibialis anterior thickness have been found to correlate with muscle force [127]. Correction for these factors should be put into consideration when interpreting muscle thickness.

In infants, the muscle appears hypoechoic and the echogenicity increases with age till the age of 5 when the muscle exhibits the same echogenicity as that of adults [144]. On the other hand, echogenicity was found independent on height, weight, or gender [117]. Although quantitative assessment of muscle echogenicity is objective, the published reference values cannot be applied worldwide given the different system settings between ultrasound machine and the different children demographics between different countries.

Muscle Ultrasound in Specific Muscle Disorders

Muscle disorders in children are highly variable and represent a challenge in diagnosis and treatment. Muscle diseases cause pathological and morphological changes in muscle architecture resulting in functional deficits. The pathological changes can be assessed by muscle biopsy, whereas morphological architectural changes can be assessed via neuroimaging including MRI, CT scan, and ultrasonography. Ultrasound has proven itself as an appropriate, reliable tool for the assessment of skeletal muscles with high predictive value to abnormalities in children with neuromuscular disorders [122, 145–147]. Moreover, the majority of muscle diseases in children are progressive, and thus an easy, rapid, noninvasive, painless reliable tool like ultrasound is needed to follow up such patients. Also, ultrasound can be used to guide muscle biopsy or interventions. In the next section, the sonographic appearance of muscles and the value of ultrasound in different muscle diseases are discussed.

Muscular Dystrophy

Muscular dystrophies are a group of inherited progressive muscle disorders. Some of the most common types of muscular dystrophies include Duchenne and Becker muscular dystrophies, limb-girdle muscular dystrophy, and myotonic dystrophy.

Duchenne and Becker muscular dystrophies are genetic progressive disorder characterized by progressive muscle degeneration, wasting, and weakness. The diagnosis depends on clinical examination, electrophysiological studies, laboratory investigations, and muscle biopsy. Neuroimaging adds to the diagnostic workup. The earliest studies of neuromuscular ultrasound were conducted on children with muscular dystrophies [118, 148]. In Duchenne muscular dystrophy, muscle echogenicity increases and bone echo decreases. The increased echo intensity is homogenous and is more evident in proximal muscles (126, 148]. With disease progression, echo intensity of the distal muscles increases, and echo intensity of proximal muscles reaches a plateau [126]. Moreover, increased echo intensity correlates with disease severity and functional and ambulatory status [21, 129].

In muscular dystrophies, ultrasound of skeletal muscles of upper and lower limbs gained most of the interest. However, other muscles are easily accessible via ultrasound in children. Among these muscles are the tongue and submental muscles. In Duchenne muscular dystrophy, tongue thickness increases reflecting hypertrophy, and echo intensity of the mental muscles increases reflecting pathological changes similar to what happens in skeletal muscles [149, 150]. These sonographic changes in tongue and submental muscles gradually progress with increasing age of the patients [149, 150]. The value of muscle ultrasonography in muscular dystrophies lies in its utility as a screening tool prior to muscle biopsy or electromyography and as a noninvasive painless bedside follow-up tool to track disease progression and response to treatment.

Limb-girdle muscular dystrophy is a genetic muscle disease characterized by progressive muscle weakness which predominantly targets the proximal muscles and spares the cranial muscles.

Muscle involvement in limb-girdle muscular dystrophy is selective and focal. Defining this pattern of muscle involvement using neuroimaging can be useful in the diagnosis of limb-girdle muscular dystrophy and differentiating it from other muscle diseases. Selective involvement of vastus muscles and sparing of rectus femoris detected by ultrasonography have been reported in children with limb-girdle muscular dystrophy and correlated with the pathological findings in muscle biopsy [151, 152].

Myotonic dystrophy or dystrophia myotonica (DM) is an autosomal dominant muscle disease.

It encompasses two major types: DM type 1 and DM type 2. Congenital-onset and juvenile-onset myotonic dystrophies are subtypes of DM type 1. The congenital type manifests at birth or shortly after and is characterized by severe muscle weakness and cognitive and developmental impairments. The juvenile type manifests during childhood and is characterized by muscle weakness, cognitive impairments, and myotonia.

Few studies have described the sonographic changes in adults with DM type 1, but none has addressed the congenital and juvenile types. Increased echogenicity has been observed in tibialis anterior, biceps brachii, forearm flexors, and masseter muscles in type 1. In type 2, atrophy of the rectus femoris and masseter muscles was observed in 23% of the patients [153]. The sensitivity of ultrasound to detect myotonia using qualitative visual assessment is low [154]. However, an interesting quantitative sonographic technique to measure muscle relaxation has been found sensitive, specific, and reliable in adult patients with myotonia [154]. This quantitative technique depends on evoking myotonia during ultrasound scanning by percussing the thenar muscle with a reflex hammer and calculating the mean muscle relaxation time from several captured videos. The described percussion technique if furtherly validated can be promising in the future in children in whom the clinical examination of myotonia is difficult as it is a painless, rapid, objective technique and does not require child's cooperation.

Pediatric Inflammatory Myopathies

Pediatric inflammatory myopathies are a group of idiopathic autoimmune inflammatory disorders with predominant affection of the muscle and/or skin. This group of disorders encompasses juvenile dermatomyositis, juvenile myositis, and overlap myositis that associates autoimmune diseases like systemic lupus and systemic sclerosis. The most common type is the juvenile dermatomyositis, and its diagnosis depends on the detection of high serum levels of muscle enzymes, myopathic pattern in electromyography study, and muscle biopsy findings consistent with the disease. The pathological changes include inflammatory infiltrates with perivascular involvement and peri-fascicular muscle atrophy. Detecting muscle inflammation is important for diagnosis and for monitoring treatment. The usual workup includes measurement of serum levels of muscle enzymes, needle electromyography, and muscle biopsy. Both electromyography and muscle biopsy are invasive and cannot be performed serially in children. Ultrasound having many advantages can be a useful alternative.

A peculiar temporal change in the muscle sonographic appearance has been reported in a study conducted on children with juvenile dermatomyositis [155]. The study showed that at the initial stage of the disease, echo intensity of the distal muscles was higher than that of the proximal muscles and reached its highest level after 1–3 months. Additionally, thickness of the proximal muscles was mildly decreased compared to the distal muscles. With the initiation of therapy, muscle echo intensity increased and muscle thickness decreased [155]. This unexpected finding with initiation of the treatment was attributed by the investigators to the anti-edematous effect of steroid and immunosuppressive therapy. With continuation of treatment, muscle thickness and echo intensity normalized within 6–12 months of treatment. In contrary to adult dermatomyositis, juvenile dermatomyositis is associated with perfascial and intramuscular calcifications [156]. Calcifications can be easily visualized by ultrasound and appear as hyperechoic foci with posterior acoustic shadow.

In addition to grayscale assessment which can be used to detect changes in muscle thickness and echogenicity that occur in almost all pediatric muscle diseases, other emerging ultrasound techniques can be of particular importance in myositis. These are power Doppler sonography, contrast-enhanced sonography, and sonoelastography.

Power Doppler can be used to detect intramuscular blood flow. Normally at rest, muscles may exhibit only few scattered Doppler signal [157]. Increased Doppler signal may occur post-exercise [157] or secondary to myositis. Contrast-enhanced ultrasound depends on intravenous administration of contrast agents containing microbubbles which enhances ultrasound backscatter and facilitates assessment of muscle perfusion. Increased muscle perfusion has been reported in myositis using contrast-enhanced ultrasound [158, 159].

Sonoelastography assesses changes in muscle elasticity by measuring degree of tissue displacement in response to applied pressure or force. Muscle stiffness measured using elastography was found increased in adult patients with myositis and correlated with laboratory tests [160]. However, in a study conducted on 18 children with juvenile idiopathic inflammatory myopathy, sonoelastography could not accurately detect active inflammation and the MRI was more superior [161]. The mentioned emerging techniques are still in the initial stage of research, but with further validation, they may add value to the traditional grayscale assessment of skeletal muscles in pediatric neuromuscular disorders.

Muscle Ultrasound in Pediatric Neuropathic Disorders

Muscle ultrasound can be a good noninvasive tool to assess muscle changes secondary to neuropathic disorders and can quickly screen large number of muscles. A denervated muscle shows increased echogenicity due to replacement of muscle tissues by fatty or fibrous tissue. Also, muscle thickness decreases in chronic denervation.

Muscle ultrasound can differentiate between pediatric neuropathic and myopathic disorders based on the pattern and the distribution of muscle abnormalities [162, 163]. Also, predominant affection of distal muscles suggests polyneuropathy rather than myopathy. This distal-proximal sonographic pattern has been found to correlate with clinical and electrophysiological patterns in children with ataxia telangiectasia who develop axonal sensorimotor polyneuropathy [167]. Moreover, muscle ultrasound changes may be evident even before clinical atrophy and weakness [164].

Muscle ultrasound can also help in the localization of the site of the lesion in traumatic nerve injuries and entrapment neuropathies. For example, in anterior interosseus nerve lesion, it is sometimes difficult to localize the lesion using nerve conduction and electromyography. Moreover, the anterior interosseus nerve is too tiny to be directly visualized via ultrasound. Muscle ultrasound can rapidly solve the problem by detecting selective increased echogenicity and decreased thickness of the anterior interosseus nerve-innervated muscles specifically flexor pollicis brevis, lateral half of flexor digitorum profundus, and pronator quadratus [165].

In spinal muscle atrophy, the reported sonographic changes include muscle atrophy, increased echogenicity, and increased subcutaneous tissue thickness [1, 99, 100]. Muscle ultrasound can differentiate between healthy children and children with neuromuscular diseases including those having spinal muscle atrophy. Also, ultrasound can discriminate between myopathy and spinal muscle atrophy based on the pattern of increased echogenicity. In myopathy, muscle hypoechogenicity is homogenous, while in spinal muscle atrophy, muscle hypoechogenicity is heterogeneous [99]. Other quantitative sonographic parameters have been proposed to assess spinal muscle atrophy. These are the muscle/subcutaneous fat luminous ratio and computer-assisted texture analysis [101, 166]. The muscle/subcutaneous fat luminous ratio is the ratio between the muscle luminosity and the overlying subcutaneous fat luminosity measured using the histogram function of computer software. The luminous ratio was found to be high in patients with spinal muscle atrophy compared to controls and correlated with muscle strength in patients [101]. Computer-assisted texture analysis depends on measurement of brightness and micro- and macrostructures of the muscle. Combined use of grayscale analysis and texture was associated with high diagnostic sensitivity in pediatric neuromuscular disorders including spinal muscle atrophy [166]. However, these two mentioned quantitative parameters need further validation before implementing them in clinical practice.

Nowadays, there is a growing interest in investigating the utility of nerve and muscle ultrasound as a marker for diagnosis or disease severity in neuromuscular disorders. The potential of muscle ultrasound to be utilized as a severity marker for polyneuropathy has been studied in adults with Charcot-Marie-Tooth, and the results have shown that quantitative muscle ultrasound of the tibialis anterior and first dorsal interosseus reflects the severity of the polyneuropathy [167]. Whether similar results exist in children with polyneuropathy is as yet unknown.

Other Uses of Muscle Ultrasound

The applications of muscle ultrasound in neuromuscular disorders are not limited to muscle dystrophies and myopathies but extend to other muscle disorders like mitochondrial diseases and upper motor neuron diseases.

Mitochondrial diseases are relatively rare inborn errors of metabolism. It is a multi-organ disease and commonly affects the skeletal muscles. The diagnostic workup includes biochemical analysis, muscle biopsy, and genetic testing. Muscle ultrasound can add to diagnostic workup of mitochondrial disorders given its high predictive value and high specificity [168]. Muscles of children with mitochondrial disorders exhibit increased echo intensity and decreased thickness. However, its sensitivity is proven to be low which limits its utility as a screening test [99, 168].

Ultrasound can be useful in children with cerebral palsy by measuring important muscle parameters that can impact the treatment decision. One of these parameters is muscle volume. Muscle volume is one of the factors that affect the force generating capacity of a muscle [169], and thus measuring muscle volume can be used as an alternative to measuring muscle force in children with disabling neurological disorders. CT and MRI are best suited to measure the muscle volume [170–172], but they are time-consuming and expensive. To measure muscle volume via ultrasound, three-dimensional ultrasonography is the most suitable modality [173]. However, it is not a basic setting in all ultrasound machines. Two-dimensional B-mode ultrasound can be easier than 3-D ultrasonography. Muscle volume can be indirectly calculated using muscle thickness and muscle cross-sectional area measured via 2D ultrasound combined with tibial length measured clinically [174]. Measuring muscle volume via 2D ultrasound has been found to be useful in children with spastic cerebral palsy [174] and thus can be applied in other patients with neurological disorders in whom muscle strength and force cannot be examined properly. Moreover, two-dimensional B-mode ultrasound is reliable in the assessment of changes in muscle architecture including muscle thickness, muscle cross-sectional area, and fascicle angle in children with cerebral palsy and therefore can direct the rehabilitation plan [175].

Elastography in Pediatric Neuromuscular Ultrasound

Elastography is an ultrasound mode that depends on measuring muscle deformation in response to stress or force. In contrast to B-mode ultrasound scanning of a muscle which allows the assessment of muscle architecture and thickness, elastography allows the assessment of the mechanical properties of a muscle, specifically muscle stiffness. The elastography techniques that are commonly used to assess muscle stiffness are strain elastography, acoustic radiation force impulse imaging, and shear wave elastography.

Reliability and feasibility of shear wave elastography in quantification of passive muscle stiffness has been reported in children [176].

Ultrasound is a promising tool in the assessment of muscle spasticity in children. It has been found that shear wave speed was faster in the spastic limb of children with unilateral cerebral palsy compared to the less affected limb reflecting greater muscle stiffness [177]. Also, the shear wave velocity measured by acoustic radiation force impulse and strain ratio was found to be higher in the medial gastrocnemius in children with spastic cerebral palsy compared to healthy children and increases with the severity of spasticity [178, 179]. Post-botulinum toxin injection, ultrasound can detect the decrease in spasticity in response to injection with good reliability [180]. Thus, quantitative elastography can be used in spasticity prior to botulinum toxin injection to select the most appropriate muscle for injection or can be used as an outcome measure post-injection and post-rehabilitation [180–182].

The applications of elastography in children are not limited to spasticity. In Duchenne muscular dystrophy, the mechanical properties of the muscles change, and the muscles become stiffer with disease progression [183, 184] which in turn impact the functional status of the child and rehabilitation. Sonoelastography can detect this increase in muscle stiffness and follow its progression over time [185, 186]. Thus, elastography can be used in combination with grayscale ultrasound in the follow-up of these children.

An interesting application of muscle sonoelastography is its utility in congenital muscular torticollis. The diagnosis of congenital muscle torticollis is usually a clinical one. While B-mode ultrasound can be used to assess the echogenicity and the thickness of sternocleidomastoid and to determine the size of the nodule if present [187] (Fig. 13.33), strain elastography can be used to diagnose torticollis especially when the muscle is isoechoic on B-mode ultrasound [188]. A four-grade scoring system was utilized by a group of researches to grade sternocleidomastoid stiffness in congenital muscle torticollis. The muscle is graded 1 "soft" when the region of interest displays purple or green color and graded 4 "hard" when the region of interest predominately displays red color. This elastography score depends on the size of the sternocleidomastoid mass and the extent of involvement of the muscle, and higher score was observed in children with large mass that involves the entire muscle [189]. Given the advantages of ultrasound being bedside painless imaging tool, it can be used to track the change in size of the nodule or the change in the degree of stiffness in response to treatment through serial follow-up ultrasound scanning.

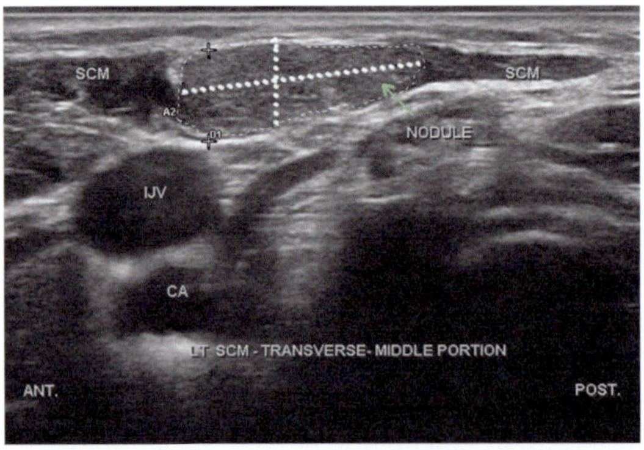

Fig. 13.33 Grayscale assessment of congenital muscular torticollis allows assessment of echogenicity of the sternocleidomastoid nodule (arrow) and measurement of its size (cross-sectional area, anteroposterior and transverse diameters). CA carotid artery, IJV internal jugular vein, SCM sternocleidomastoid

Ultrasound-Guided Procedures in Neuromuscular Ultrasound

Full discussion of interventional neuromuscular ultrasound is beyond the scope of the chapter, but giving a brief review on its applications in pediatrics is worth noting.

Ultrasound-guided procedures can be diagnostic or therapeutic. Diagnostic procedures include ultrasound-guided muscle biopsy, ultrasound-guided nerve biopsy, and ultrasound-guided electromyography. Therapeutic procedures include ultrasound-guided Botox injection, phenol injection, and ultrasound-guided nerve block.

Ultrasound-Guided Diagnostic Procedures

Muscle biopsy is an integral part of the diagnostic workup for pediatric neuromuscular disorders. Muscle sample can be obtained through open surgery under general anesthesia or more commonly percutaneously using needle under local anesthesia. The success of needle muscle biopsy to detect pathological changes depends on the adequacy of the muscle sample. The optimum sample is the sample that is taken from a symptomatic weak but non-atrophic muscle because with severe muscle atrophy, there may be no enough muscle tissue to sample. In traditional unguided muscle biopsy, the choice of muscles for sampling depends on clinical examination and electromyography results. However, the degree of muscle atrophy cannot be accurately determined by clinical examination. Using needle electromyography to choosing the optimum muscle may require inserting the needle in multiple areas of muscle in different limbs and thus can be time-consuming and intolerable to children. Also, unguided muscle biopsy in obese children may lead to the inclusion of large fat mass which decreases the chance to yield pathological findings. Ultrasound can be useful if used prior to or during muscle biopsy. Prior to muscle biopsy, it can determine which muscles exhibit increased echogenicity and can yield histological findings in biopsy. Muscles with moderate increase in echogenicity are the best to sample while muscles with marked increase in echogenicity to the degree that it masks bone profile may be too fibrotic to be sampled. Ultrasound can also determine muscle and subcutaneous layer thickness to avoid sampling severely atrophic muscles and avoid inclusion of large areas of subcutaneous fat. Additionally, performing the biopsy under ultrasound guidance has several advantages compared to the surgical biopsy. It is less time-consuming, more cost-effective, and safe with no associated complications [190, 191]. The technique was also found to be well tolerated by patients including children and was easy to perform [190]. In a study performed on adults, the sonographically obtained samples were diagnostic in 93%, and the surgically obtained samples were diagnostic in 95% of patients with acute neuromuscular disorders [191]. Thus, ultrasound can be used as an alternative to open surgery. On the other hand, when the value of ultrasound scanning was investigated in adult patients undergoing needle muscle biopsy guided by electromyography, ultrasound provided no additional value to electromyography [192]. Whether ultrasound can be used as an alternative to electromyography for muscle selection or not needs further investigation in adults and children to compare their diagnostic success rates.

In contrast to muscle biopsy, nerve biopsy is not a routine procedure in children with neuropathies but it may be needed in certain confusing cases. On reviewing the usefulness of nerve biopsy in 316 children at a tertiary referral center, nerve biopsy confirmed the diagnosis in 29%, modified the diagnosis in 58%, and altered the treatment plan in 25% [193]. The traditional nerve biopsy is performed through an open approach which carries the risk of bleeding and/or infection. Ultrasound can help in reducing these risks and facilitating nerve biopsy procedure. If performed prior to nerve biopsy, ultrasound can guide the site of biopsy based on the sonographic pathological changes and the ultrasound Tinel's sign. Ultrasound Tinel's sign is positive when symptoms are provoked on applying a slight pressure on a diseased nerve or one of its segments. In a patient with mononeuritis multiplex, ultrasound Tinel's sign accurately guided nerve biopsy which revealed vasculitis [194]. However, this sonographic sign is not that applicable in infants and young children who cannot report provocation of symptoms upon probe pressure.

An alternative technique to open nerve biopsy using ultrasound guidance was described by Lolge and colleagues in a case report of adult leprotic neuropathy [195]. They performed core Tru-Cut nerve biopsy of the superficial peroneal nerve using real-time ultrasound which successfully confirmed the diagnosis. This technique is promising and may be of value in children to spare them the open approach.

Ultrasound-Guided Therapeutic Procedures

One of the most common therapeutic procedures performed in children is intramuscular botulinum toxin injection to relieve spasticity in children with cerebral palsy and pediatric dystonia [196–198]. Muscle selection prior to injection depends on clinical examination and electromyography. The injection can be performed blindly depending only on clinical palpation or guided by electrical stimulation and/or electromyography to ensure intramuscular insertion. However, electrical stimulation and electromyography are not best suited for children. Ultrasound can be a good alternative prior to and during the injection. Prior to injection, ultrasound can be used to select the muscles suitable for injection based on the degree of muscle spasticity assessed via sonoelastography. During injection, ultrasound provides real-time imaging and allows accurate identification of the target muscle, needle position and nearby neurovascular structures. Injecting under ultrasound guidance was found to be associated with better clinical and functional improvement of children with cerebral palsy when compared to blinded injection [199].

Recently, ultrasound has been used to guide perineural injection of novel therapeutic agents including vitamin B12 and nerve growth factor in peripheral neuropathy and nerve injury [200, 201]. The current data are obtained from a case report and an experimental study, yet the results are promising and open the door for further validation and trials of other therapeutics agents that may improve or treat neuromuscular disorders.

Ultrasound-guided nerve block in children lies mainly in the scope of anesthesia and is used to improve safety and efficacy of regional anesthesia or to relieve postoperative pain. Nevertheless, it can be used to relieve chronic neuropathic pain [202].

Limitations of Pediatric Neuromuscular Ultrasound

As any diagnostic tool, neuromuscular ultrasound has its own limitations. The limitations in pediatrics include limitations related to the child, limitations related to the ultrasound in general as a diagnostic tool, and limitations related to the pediatric neuromuscular ultrasound field.

The limiting factor related to the child is the need of child's cooperation during muscle ultrasound scanning which may be difficult to achieve in some cases. Although the ultrasound is painless and child-friendly tool, the child may get bored quickly especially if full tracing of multiple nerves or scanning of muscle of the four limbs is needed. In children, the field of view is larger than in adults, but scanning small areas and scanning nerves around curved bones may need probes with small footprint such as the hockey stick probe which may be unavailable in all centers.

The limitations of neuromuscular ultrasound in general include its limited ability to visualize deep lying muscles and nerves due to attenuation. Increasing the depth, decreasing the frequency, adjusting time gain compensation, and using curvilinear probe or trapezoid mode of ultrasound machine partially improve visualization of deep lying nerves and muscles on the expense of high resolution. This limitation is more evident in adults than in children because of difference in body size. Another limitation of ultrasound is its inability to visualize tissues deep to the bone because the bone does not permit transmission of ultrasound beam. This limitation applies on teenagers but not on infants who still have cartilaginous bone that can be easily visualized by ultrasound. Another limitation of nerve ultrasound in general is its low sensitivity to diagnose plexus lesions compared to MRI.

As discussed throughout the chapter, muscle ultrasound can detect muscle atrophy in children with neuromuscular disorders. However, its reliability to detect muscle wasting in critically ill children is low [203].

Pediatric neuromuscular ultrasound is relatively an explored field, and one of the major limitations related to this domain is the lack of reference values for all sonographic measurements of peripheral nerve and skeletal muscles. Setting reference values needs standardization of scanning and measurement techniques among different institutions.

Future Directions

Neuromuscular ultrasound in general is a rapidly evolving specialty, but the applications of nerve and muscle ultrasound in children did not receive the deserved attention till now despite the fact that ultrasound is well suited for children as a bedside, affordable, painless, dynamic, and child-friendly tool. The future directions of pediatric neuromuscular ultrasound from the authors' perspective include setting reference values for nerve and muscle ultrasound, development of diagnostic sonographic criteria to differentiate neuropathic from myopathic disorders and to differentiate between different types of neuropathies and myopathies, development of ultrasound nerve scores, and standardization of quantitative assessment of nerves and muscles.

The utilities of other subdomains of neuromuscular ultrasound in children are expected to gain more attention in the future. Examples of these subdomains are cranial nerve and diaphragm ultrasound. Optic nerve ultrasound is of particular importance in children with increased intracranial tension and is currently used in some centers as a screening test for intracranial hypertension. Diaphragm ultrasound may have the potential to assess or predict respiratory failure in children with myopathies or Guillain-Barre syndrome.

Lastly, emerging ultrasound techniques including three-dimensional and four-dimensional ultrasonography, sonoelastography, contrast-enhanced ultrasonography, and ultrasound-guided interventions are definitely interesting fields for research and clinical practice.

References

1. Heckmatt JZ, Leeman S, Dubowitz V. Ultrasound imaging in the diagnosis of muscle disease. J Pediatr. 1982;101(5):656–60.
2. Buchberger W, Schön G, Strasser K, Jungwirth W. High-resolution ultrasonography of the carpal tunnel. J Ultrasound Med. 1991;10(10):531–7.
3. Chiou HJ, Chou YH, Cheng SP, Hsu CC, Chan RC, Tiu CM, Teng MM, Chang CY. Cubital tunnel syndrome: diagnosis by high-resolution ultrasonography. J Ultrasound Med. 1998;17(10):643–8.
4. Okamoto M, Abe M, Shirai H, Ueda N. Diagnostic ultrasonography of the ulnar nerve in cubital tunnel syndrome. J Hand Surg (Br). 2000;25(5):499–502.
5. Wong SM, Griffith JF, Hui AC, Tang A, Wong KS. Discriminatory sonographic criteria for the diagnosis of carpal tunnel syndrome. Arthritis Rheum. 2002;46(7):1914–21.
6. Park GY, Kim JM, Lee SM. The ultrasonographic and electrodiagnostic findings of ulnar neuropathy at the elbow. Arch Phys Med Rehabil. 2004;85(6):1000–5.
7. Martinoli C, Bianchi S, Pugliese F, Bacigalupo L, Gauglio C, Valle M, Derchi LE. Sonography of entrapment neuropathies in the upper limb (wrist excluded). J Clin Ultrasound. 2004;32(9):438–50.
8. Beekman R, van den Berg LH, Franssen H, Visser LH, van Asseldonk JT, Wokke JH. Ultrasonography shows extensive nerve enlargements in multifocal motor neuropathy. Neurology. 2005;65(2):305–7.
9. Hollister AM, Simoncini A, Sciuk A, Jordan J. High frequency ultrasound evaluation of traumatic peripheral nerve injuries. Neurol Res. 2012;34(1):98–103.
10. Lauretti L, D'Alessandris QG, Granata G, Padua L, Roselli R, Di Bonaventura R, Fernandez E. Ultrasound evaluation in traumatic peripheral nerve lesions: from diagnosis to surgical planning and follow-up. Acta Neurochir. 2015;157(11):1947–51.
11. Grimm A, Heiling B, Schumacher U, Witte OW, Axer H. Ultrasound differentiation of axonal and demyelinating neuropathies. Muscle Nerve. 2014;50(6):976–83.
12. Noto Y, Shiga K, Tsuji Y, Mizuta I, Higuchi Y, Hashiguchi A, Takashima H, Nakagawa M, Mizuno T. Nerve ultrasound depicts peripheral nerve enlargement in patients with genetically distinct Charcot-Marie-Tooth disease. J Neurol Neurosurg Psychiatry. 2015;86(4):378–84.
13. Cartwright MS, Walker FO, Griffin LP, Caress JB. Peripheral nerve and muscle ultrasound in amyotrophic lateral sclerosis. Muscle Nerve. 2011;44(3):346–51.
14. Schreiber S, Abdulla S, Debska-Vielhaber G, Machts J, Dannhardt-Stieger V, Feistner H, Oldag A, Goertler M, Petri S, Kollewe K, Kropf S, Schreiber F, Heinze HJ, Dengler R, Nestor PJ, Vielhaber S. Peripheral nerve ultrasound in amyotrophic lateral sclerosis phenotypes. Muscle Nerve. 2015;51(5):669–75.
15. Adler RS, Garofalo G. Ultrasound in the evaluation of the inflammatory myopathies. Curr Rheumatol Rep. 2009;11(4):302–8.
16. Zaidman CM, van Alfen N. Ultrasound in the assessment of myopathic disorders. J Clin Neurophysiol. 2016;33(2):103–11.
17. Koenig RW, Pedro MT, Heinen CP, Schmidt T, Richter HP, Antoniadis G, Kretschmer T. High-resolution ultrasonography in evaluating peripheral nerve entrapment and trauma. Neurosurg Focus. 2009;26(2):E13.
18. Lee SU, Kim MW, Kim JM. Ultrasound Diagnosis of Double Crush Syndrome of the Ulnar Nerve by the Anconeus Epitrochlearis and a Ganglion. J Korean Neurosurg Soc. 2016;59(1):75–7.
19. Gruber H, Glodny B, Bendix N, Tzankov A, Peer S. High-resolution ultrasound of peripheral neurogenic tumors. Eur Radiol. 2007;17(11):2880–8.
20. Maurits NM, Bollen AE, Windhausen A, De Jager AE, Van Der Hoeven JH. Muscle ultrasound analysis: normal values and differentiation between myopathies and neuropathies. Ultrasound Med Biol. 2003;29(2):215–25.
21. Jansen M, van Alfen N, van der Sanden MW N, van Dijk JP, Pillen S, de Groot IJ. Quantitative muscle ultrasound is a promising longitudinal follow-up tool in Duchenne muscular dystrophy. Neuromuscul Disord. 2012;22(4):306–17.
22. Gray H. Anatomy of the human body. Philadelphia: Lea & Febiger; 1918.
23. Fornage BD. Peripheral nerves of the extremities: imaging with US. Radiology. 1988;167(1):179–82.
24. Silvestri E, Martinoli C, Derchi LE, Bertolotto M, Chiaramondia M, Rosenberg I. Echotexture of peripheral nerves: correlation between US and his-

tologic findings and criteria to differentiate tendons. Radiology. 1995;197(1):291–6.
25. Lee SH, Lee SH, Chan VW, Lee JO, Kim HI. Echotexture and correlated histologic analysis of peripheral nerves important in regional anesthesia. Reg Anesth Pain Med. 2011;36(4):382–6.
26. Matsota PK, Paraskevopoulos TM, Kalimeris KA, Nicolaidou PN, Kostopanagiotou GG. Ultrasound imaging of the musculocutaneous nerve of infants, preschool children, and school children. J Anesth. 2015;29(5):790–3.
27. Erickson SJ. High-resolution imaging of the musculoskeletal system. Radiology. 1997;205(3):593–618.
28. Fornage BD, Rifkin MD. Ultrasound examination of tendons. Radiol Clin N Am. 1988;26(1):87–107.
29. Martinoli C, Derchi LE, Pastorino C, Bertolotto M, Silvestri E. Analysis of echotexture of tendons with US. Radiology. 1993;186(3):839–43.
30. Cartwright MS, Walker FO. Neuromuscular ultrasound in common entrapment neuropathies. Muscle Nerve. 2013;48(5):696–704.
31. Zaidman CM, Al-Lozi M, Pestronk A. Peripheral nerve size in normals and patients with polyneuropathy: an ultrasound study. Muscle Nerve. 2009;40(6):960–6.
32. Cartwright MS, Mayans DR, Gillson NA, Griffin LP, Walker FO. Nerve cross-sectional area in extremes of age. Muscle Nerve. 2013;47(6):890–3.
33. Chauhan SP, Blackwell SB, Ananth CV. Neonatal brachial plexus palsy: incidence, prevalence, and temporal trends. Semin Perinatol. 2014;38(4):210–8.
34. Squitieri L, Larson BP, Chang KW, Yang LJ, Chung KC. Understanding quality of life and patient expectations among adolescents with neonatal brachial plexus palsy: a qualitative and quantitative pilot study. J Hand Surg Am. 2013;38(12):2387–97.e2
35. Van Dijk JG, Pondaag W, Buitenhuis SM, Van Zwet EW, Malessy MJ. Needle electromyography at 1 month predicts paralysis of elbow flexion at 3 months in obstetric brachial plexus lesions. Dev Med Child Neurol. 2012;54(8):753–8.
36. Vanderhave KL, Bovid K, Alpert H, Chang KW, Quint DJ, Leonard JA Jr, Yang LJ. Utility of electrodiagnostic testing and computed tomography myelography in the preoperative evaluation of neonatal brachial plexus palsy. J Neurosurg Pediatr. 2012;9(3):283–9.
37. Yang LJ. Neonatal brachial plexus palsy-management and prognostic factors. Semin Perinatol. 2014;38(4):222–34.
38. Birchansky S, Altman N. Imaging the brachial plexus and peripheral nerves in infants and children. Semin Pediatr Neurol. 2000;7(1):15–25.
39. Graif M, Martinoli C, Rochkind S, Blank A, Trejo L, Weiss J, Kessler A, Derchi LE. Sonographic evaluation of brachial plexus pathology. Eur Radiol. 2004;14(2):193–200.
40. Haber HP, Sinis N, Haerle M, Schaller HE. Sonography of brachial plexus traction injuries. AJR Am J Roentgenol. 2006;186(6):1787–91.
41. Joseph JR, DiPietro MA, Somashekar D, Parmar HA, Yang LJ. Ultrasonography for neonatal brachial plexus palsy. J Neurosurg Pediatr. 2014;14(5):527–31.
42. Smith EC, Xixis KI, Grant GA, Grant SA. Assessment of obstetric brachial plexus injury with preoperative ultrasound. Muscle Nerve. 2016;53(6):946–50.
43. Kattan AE, Borschel GH. Anatomy of the brachial plexus. J Pediatr Rehabil Med. 2011;4(2):107–11.
44. Leinberry CF, Wehbé MA. Brachial plexus anatomy. Hand Clin. 2004;20(1):1–5.
45. Pillen S, Semmekrot B, Meulstee J, Verrips A, Van Alfen N. Ultrasound of the cervical roots and brachial plexus in neonates. Muscle Nerve. 2015;51(1):35–41.
46. Martinoli C, Bianchi S, Santacroce E, Pugliese F, Graif M, Derchi LE. Brachial plexus sonography: a technique for assessing the root level. AJR Am J Roentgenol. 2002;179(3):699–702.
47. Demondion X, Herbinet P, Boutry N, Fontaine C, Francke JP, Cotten A. Sonographic mapping of the normal brachial plexus. AJNR Am J Neuroradiol. 2003;24(7):1303–9.
48. Di Filippo A, Orando S, Luna A, Gianesello L, Boccaccini A, Campolo MC, De Gaudio AR. Ultrasound identification of nerve cords in the infraclavicular fossa: a clinical study. Minerva Anestesiol. 2012;78(4):450–5.
49. Somashekar DK, Di Pietro MA, Joseph JR, Yang LJ, Parmar HA. Utility of ultrasound in noninvasive preoperative workup of neonatal brachial plexus palsy. Pediatr Radiol. 2016;46(5):695–703.
50. Zaidman CM, Holland MR, Noetzel MJ, Park TS, Pestronk A. Newborn brachial plexus palsy: evaluation of severity using quantitative ultrasound of muscle. Muscle Nerve. 2013;47(2):246–54.
51. Bauer AS, Lucas JF, Heyrani N, Anderson RL, Kalish LA, James MA. Ultrasound screening for posterior shoulder dislocation in infants with persistent brachial plexus birth palsy. J Bone Joint Surg Am. 2017;99(9):778–83.
52. Vathana T, Rust S, Mills J, Wilkes D, Browne R, Carter PR, Ezaki M. Intraobserver and interobserver reliability of two ultrasound measures of humeral head position in infants with neonatal brachial plexus palsy. J Bone Joint Surg Am. 2007;89(8):1710–5.
53. Missios S, Bekelis K, Spinner RJ. Traumatic peripheral nerve injuries in children: epidemiology and socioeconomics. J Neurosurg Pediatr. 2014;14(6):688–94.
54. Toros T, Karabay N, Ozaksar K, Sugun TS, Kayalar M, Bal E. Evaluation of peripheral nerves of the upper limb with ultrasonography: a comparison of ultrasonographic examination and the intra-operative findings. J Bone Joint Surg (Br). 2009;91:762–5.
55. Padua L, Di Pasquale A, Liotta G, Granata G, Pazzaglia C, Erra C, Briani C, Coraci D, De Franco P, Antonini G, Martinoli C. Ultrasound as a useful tool in the diagnosis and management of traumatic nerve lesions. Clin Neurophysiol. 2013;124(6):1237–43.

56. Bellavia MA, Cambise C, Coraci D, Maccauro G, Valassina A, Padua L. Ultrasound is a useful tool to evaluate nerve involvement in children with supracondylar humerus fractures. Muscle Nerve. 2017;56(3):E18–20.
57. Ekiz T, Üçpunar F, Yıldız D. Ulnar neuropathy after forearm fracture in a child: the role of peripheral nerve ultrasound in the decision of management. Turk J Phys Med Rehab. 2018;64(x):i–ii.
58. Hobson-Webb LD, Walker FO. Traumatic neuroma diagnosed by ultrasonography. Arch Neurol. 2004;61(8):1322–3.
59. Chen KH, Lee KF, Hsu HC, Huang WC, Hsiao KY, Fang KM. The role of high-resolution ultrasound in the diagnosis of a traumatic neuroma in an injured median nerve. Am J Phys Med Rehabil. 2009;88(9):771–4.
60. Burks SS, Cajigas I, Jose J, Levi AD. Intraoperative imaging in traumatic peripheral nerve lesions: correlating histologic cross-sections with high-resolution ultrasound. Oper Neurosurg (Hagerstown). 2017;13(2):196–203.
61. Cartwright MS, Chloros GD, Walker FO, Wiesler ER, Campbell WW. Diagnostic ultrasound for nerve transection. Muscle Nerve. 2007;35(6):796–9.
62. Peer S, Bodner G. Tumors and tumor-like lesions. In: Peer S, Bodner G, editors. High-resolution sonography of the peripheral nervous system. 2nd ed. New York: Springer; 2010. p. 154–66.
63. Viskochil D, Muenzer J, Guffon N, Garin C, Munoz-Rojas MV, Moy KA, Hutchinson DT. Carpal tunnel syndrome in mucopolysaccharidosis I: a registry-based cohort study. Dev Med Child Neurol. 2017;59(12):1269–75.
64. Trotta D, Verrotti A, Salladini C, Chiarelli F. Diabetic neuropathy in children and adolescents. Pediatr Diabetes. 2004;5(1):44–57.
65. Petratos DV, Stavropoulos NA, Morakis EA, Matsinos GS. Median nerve entrapment and ulnar nerve palsy following elbow dislocation in a child. J Surg Orthop Adv. 2012;21(3):157–61.
66. Dubey V, Saify A, Samant A, Shahane S. Median nerve entrapment after elbow dislocation and the role of ultrasonography – a case report. J Orthop Case Rep. 2017;7(3):21–4.
67. Chrestian N, McMillan H, Poulin C, Campbell C, Vajsar J. Hereditary neuropathy with liability to pressure palsies in childhood: case series and literature update. Neuromuscul Disord. 2015;25(9):693–8.
68. Unal O, Ozçakar L, Cetin A, Kaymak B. Severe bilateral carpal tunnel syndrome in juvenile chronic arthritis. Pediatr Neurol. 2003;29(4):345–8.
69. De Smet L, Wouters C. Severe carpal tunnel syndrome in a patient with juvenile idiopathic arthritis due to proximal migration of hypertrophic lumbrical muscles. Clin Rheumatol. 2004;23(6):552–4.
70. Tan MJ, Kandler R, Baxter PS. Focal neuropathy in children with critical illness. Neuropediatrics. 2003;34(3):149–51.
71. Van Meir N, De Smet L. Carpal tunnel syndrome in children. Acta Orthop Belg. 2003;69(5):387–95.
72. Kwon JY, Ko K, Sohn YB, Kim SJ, Park SW, Kim SH, Cho SY, Jin DK. High prevalence of carpal tunnel syndrome in children with mucopolysaccharidosis type II (hunter syndrome). Am J Med Genet A. 2011;155A(6):1329–35.
73. Yuen A, Dowling G, Johnstone B, Kornberg A, Coombs C. Carpal tunnel syndrome in children with mucopolysaccaridoses. J Child Neurol. 2007;22(3):260–3.
74. Van Heest AE, House J, Krivit W, Walker K. Surgical treatment of carpal tunnel syndrome and trigger digits in children with mucopolysaccharide storage disorders. J Hand Surg. 1998;23(2):236–43.
75. Haddad FS, Hill RA, Jones DH. Triggering in the mucopolysaccharidoses. J Pediatr Orthop. 1998;7(2):138–40.
76. Lamberti PM, Light TR. Carpal tunnel syndrome in children. Hand Clin. 2002;18(2):331–7.
77. Deymeer F, Jones HR Jr. Pediatric median mononeuropathies: a clinical and electromyographic study. Muscle Nerve. 1994;17(7):755–62.
78. Brax P, Destuynder O, Rigaud P, Ridoux PE, Gille P. Carpal tunnel syndrome in children. Apropos of 4 personal cases. Chir Pediatr. 1990;31(6):310–3.
79. Bäumer T, Bühring N, Schelle T, Münchau A, Muschol N. Nerve ultrasound in clinical management of carpal tunnel syndrome in mucopolysaccharidosis. Dev Med Child Neurol. 2016;58(11):1172–9.
80. Bocsa C, Asavoaie C, Bucerzan S, Nascu I, Brumboiu I, Al-Khzouz C. Ultrasonographic evaluation of the median nerve at the level of the carpal tunnel outlet and mid forearm in patients with type II Mucopolysaccharidosis. Med Ultrason. 2016;18(1):36–41.
81. Nakamichi K, Tachibana S. Restricted motion of the median nerve in carpal tunnel syndrome. J Hand Surg (Br). 1995;20(4):460–4.
82. Kuo TT, Lee MR, Liao YY, Chen JP, Hsu YW, Yeh CK. Assessment of median nerve mobility by ultrasound dynamic imaging for diagnosing carpal tunnel syndrome. PLoS One. 2016;11(1):e0147051. https://doi.org/10.1371/journal.pone.0147051.
83. Okamoto M, Abe M, Shirai H, Ueda N. Morphology and dynamics of the ulnar nerve in the cubital tunnel. Observation by ultrasonography. J Hand Surg (Br). 2000;25(1):85–9.
84. Shamsul H, Saw A, John G. Anterior displacement of the ulnar nerve at the elbow in children based on ultrasonography. Malays Orthop J. 2007;1(1):29–33.
85. Erez O, Khalil JG, Legakis JE, Tweedie J, Kaminski E, Reynolds RA. Ultrasound evaluation of ulnar nerve anatomy in the pediatric population. J Pediatr Orthop. 2012;32(6):641–6.
86. Royce RO, Dutkowsky JP, Kasser JR, Rand FR. Neurologic complications after K-wire fixation of supracondylar humerus fractures in children. J Paed Orthop. 1991;11(2):191–4.

87. Brown IC, Zinar DM. Traumatic and iatrogenic neurological complications after supracondylar humerus fractures in children. J Pediatr Orthop. 1995;15(4):440–3.
88. Rasool MN. Ulnar nerve injury after K-wire fixation of supracondylar humerus fractures in children. J Pediatr Orthop. 1998;18(5):686–90.
89. Nakamichi K, Tachibana S. Ultrasonographic measurement of median nerve cross-sectional area in idiopathic carpal tunnel syndrome: diagnostic accuracy. Muscle Nerve. 2002;26(6):798–803.
90. Beekman R, Schoemaker MC, Van Der Plas JP, Van Den Berg LH, Franssen H, Wokke JH, Uitdehaag BM, Visser LH. Diagnostic value of high-resolution sonography in ulnar neuropathy at the elbow. Neurology. 2004;62(5):767–73.
91. Wiesler ER, Chloros GD, Cartwright MS, Shin HW, Walker FO. Ultrasound in the diagnosis of ulnar neuropathy at the cubital tunnel. J Hand Surg Am. 2006;31(7):1088–93.
92. Wiesler ER, Chloros GD, Cartwright MS, Smith BP, Rushing J, Walker FO. The use of diagnostic ultrasound in carpal tunnel syndrome. J Hand Surg Am. 2006;31(5):726–32.
93. Yoon JS, Walker FO, Cartwright MS. Ultrasonographic swelling ratio in the diagnosis of ulnar neuropathy at the elbow. Muscle Nerve. 2008;38(4):1231–5.
94. Hobson-Webb LD, Massey JM, Juel VC, Sanders DB. The ultrasonographic wrist-to-forearm median nerve area ratio in carpal tunnel syndrome. Clin Neurophysiol. 2008;119(6):1353–7.
95. Sernik RA, Abicalaf CA, Pimentel BF, Braga-Baiak A, Braga L, Cerri GG. Ultrasound features of carpal tunnel syndrome: a prospective case-control study. Skelet Radiol. 2008;37(1):49–53.
96. Lee H, Brekelmans GJF, Visser LH. Quantitative assessment of nerve echogenicity as an additional tool for evaluation of common fibular neuropathy. Clin Neurophysiol. 2016;127(1):874–9.
97. Ghasemi-Esfe AR, Khalilzadeh O, Mazloumi M, Vaziri-Bozorg SM, Niri SG, Kahnouji H, Rahmani M. Combination of high-resolution and color Doppler ultrasound in diagnosis of carpal tunnel syndrome. Acta Radiol. 2011;52(2):191–7.
98. Ghanei ME, Karami M, Zarezadeh A, Sarrami AH. Usefulness of combination of grey-scale and color Doppler ultrasound findings in the diagnosis of ulnar nerve entrapment syndrome. J Res Med Sci. 2015;20(4):342–5.
99. Brockmann K, Becker P, Schreiber G, Neubert K, Brunner E, Bönnemann C. Sensitivity and specificity of qualitative muscle ultrasound in assessment of suspected neuromuscular disease in childhood. Neuromuscul Disord. 2007;17(7):517–23.
100. Pillen S, Verrips A, van Alfen N, Arts IM, Sie LT, Zwarts MJ. Quantitative skeletal muscle ultrasound: diagnostic value in childhood neuromuscular disease. Neuromuscul Disord. 2007;17(7):509–16.
101. Wu JS, Darras BT, Rutkove SB. Assessing spinal muscular atrophy with quantitative ultrasound. Neurology. 2010;75(6):526–31.
102. Almeida V, Mariotti P, Veltri S, Erra C, Padua L. Nerve ultrasound follow-up in a child with Guillain-Barré syndrome. Muscle Nerve. 2012;46(2):270–5.
103. Kerasnoudis A, Pitarokoili K, Behrendt V, Gold R, Yoon MS. Correlation of nerve ultrasound, electrophysiological, and clinical findings in post Guillain-Barré syndrome. J Peripher Nerv Syst. 2013;18(3):232–40.
104. Chance PF. Inherited focal, episodic neuropathies: hereditary neuropathy with liability to pressure palsies and hereditary neuralgic amyotrophy. NeuroMolecular Med. 2006;8(1–2):159–74.
105. Antonini G, Luchetti A, Mastrangelo M, Ciambra GL, Di Netta S, Taioli F, Fabrizi GM, Iannetti P. Early-onset hereditary neuropathy with liability to pressure palsy. Neuropediatrics. 2007;38(1):50–4.
106. Zaidman CM, Harms MB, Pestronk A. Ultrasound of inherited vs. acquired demyelinating polyneuropathies. J Neurol. 2013;260(12):3115–21.
107. Yiu EM, Brockley CR, Lee KJ, Carroll K, de Valle K, Kennedy R, Rao P, Delatycki MB, Ryan MM. Peripheral nerve ultrasound in pediatric Charcot-Marie-Tooth disease type 1A. Neurology. 2015;84(6):569–74.
108. Grimm A, Rasenack M, Athanasopoulou IM, Dammeier NM, Lipski C, Wolking S, Vittore D, Décard BF, Axer H. The modified ultrasound pattern sum score mUPSS as additional diagnostic tool for genetically distinct hereditary neuropathies. J Neurol. 2016;263(2):221–30.
109. McLeod JG, Pollard JD, Macaskill P, Mohamed A, Spring P, Khurana V. Prevalence of chronic inflammatory demyelinating polyneuropathy in New South Wales, Australia. Ann Neurol. 1999;46(6):910–3.
110. Iijima M, Koike H, Hattori N, Tamakoshi A, Katsuno M, Tanaka F, Yamamoto M, Arimura K, Sobue G; Refractory Peripheral Neuropathy Study Group of Japan. Prevalence and incidence rates of chronic inflammatory demyelinating polyneuropathy in the Japanese population. J Neurol Neurosurg Psychiatry. 2008;79(9):1040–3.
111. Majumdar A, Hartley L, Manzur AY, King RH, Orrell RW, Muntoni F. A case of severe congenital chronic inflammatory demyelinating polyneuropathy with complete spontaneous remission. Neuromuscul Disord. 2004;14(12):818–21.
112. Pearce J, Pitt M, Martinez A. A neonatal diagnosis of congenital chronic inflammatory demyelinating polyneuropathy. Dev Med Child Neurol. 2005;47(7):489–92.
113. Edelman F, Naddaf E, Waclawik AJ. Upper extremity multifocal neuropathy in a 10-year-old boy associated with NS6S disaccharide antibodies. J Child Neurol. 2015;30(7):945–8.

114. Lugão HB, Frade MA, Mazzer N, Foss NT, Nogueira-Barbosa MH. Leprosy with ulnar nerve abscess: ultrasound findings in a child. Skelet Radiol. 2017;46(1):137–40.
115. Guyton AC, Hall JE. Textbook of medical physiology. Philadelphia: Elsevier; 2006.
116. Debernard L, Robert L, Charleux F, Bensamoun SF. Characterization of muscle architecture in children and adults using magnetic resonance elastography and ultrasound techniques. J Biomech. 2011;44(3):397–401.
117. Scholten RR, Pillen S, Verrips A, Zwarts MJ. Quantitative ultrasonography of skeletal muscles in children: normal values. Muscle Nerve. 2003;27(6):693–8.
118. Heckmatt JZ, Dubowitz V, Leeman S. Detection of pathological change in dystrophic muscle with B-scan ultrasound imaging. Lancet. 1980;1(8183):1389–90.
119. Heckmatt JZ, Pier N, Dubowitz V. Measurement of quadriceps muscle thickness and subcutaneous tissue thickness in normal children by real-time ultrasound imaging. J Clin Ultrasound. 1988;16(3):171–6.
120. Legerlotz K, Smith HK, Hing WA. Variation and reliability of ultrasonographic quantification of the architecture of the medial gastrocnemius muscle in young children. Clin Physiol Funct Imaging. 2010;30(3):198–205.
121. Noorkoiv M, Nosaka K, Blazevich AJ. Assessment of quadriceps muscle cross-sectional area by ultrasound extended-field-of-view imaging. Eur J Appl Physiol. 2010;109(4):631–9.
122. Pillen S, Tak RO, Zwarts MJ, Lammens MM, Verrijp KN, Arts IM, van der Laak JA, Hoogerbrugge PM, van Engelen BG, Verrips A. Skeletal muscle ultrasound: correlation between fibrous tissue and echo intensity. Ultrasound Med Biol. 2009;35(3):443–6.
123. Reimers CD, Schlotter B, Eicke BM, Witt TN. Calf enlargement in neuromuscular diseases: a quantitative ultrasound study in 350 patients and review of the literature. J Neurol Sci. 1996;143(1–2):46–56.
124. van Baalen BA, Stephani U. Muscle fiber type grouping in high resolution ultrasound. Arch Dis Child. 2005;90(11):1189.
125. Pillen S, Scholten RR, Zwarts MJ, Verrips A. Quantitative skeletal muscle ultrasonography in children with suspected neuromuscular disease. Muscle Nerve. 2003;27(6):699–705.
126. Shklyar I, Geisbush TR, Mijialovic AS, Pasternak A, Darras BT, Wu JS, Rutkove SB, Zaidman CM. Quantitative muscle ultrasound in Duchenne muscular dystrophy: a comparison of techniques. Muscle Nerve. 2015;51(2):207–13.
127. Jacobs J, Jansen M, Janssen H, Raijmann W, Van Alfen N, Pillen S. Quantitative muscle ultrasound and muscle force in healthy children: a 4-year follow-up study. Muscle Nerve. 2013;47(6):856–63.
128. Zaidman CM, Holland MR, Anderson CC, Pestronk A. Calibrated quantitative ultrasound imaging of skeletal muscle using backscatter analysis. Muscle Nerve. 2008;38(1):893–8.
129. Zaidman CM, Connolly AM, Malkus EC, Florence JM, Pestronk A. Quantitative ultrasound using backscatter analysis in Duchenne and Becker muscular dystrophy. Neuromuscul Disord. 2010;20(12):805–9.
130. Binzoni T, Bianchi S, Hanquinet S, Kaelin A, Sayegh Y, Dumont M, Jéquier S. Human gastrocnemius medialis pennation angle as a function of age: from newborn to the elderly. J Physiol Anthropol Appl Hum Sci. 2001;20(5):293–8.
131. Shortland AP, Harris CA, Gough M, Robinson RO. Architecture of the medial gastrocnemius in children with spastic diplegia. Dev Med Child Neurol. 2002;44(3):158–63.
132. Walker FO, Donofrio PD, Harpold GJ, Ferrell WG. Sonographic imaging of muscle contraction and fasciculations: a correlation with electromyography. Muscle Nerve. 1990;13(1):33–9.
133. Scheel AK, Toepfer M, Kunkel M, Finkenstaedt M, Reimers CD. Ultrasonographic assessment of the prevalence of fasciculations in lesions of the peripheral nervous system. J Neuroimaging. 1997;7(1):23–7.
134. Reimers CD, Ziemann U, Scheel A, Rieckmann P, Kunkel M, Kurth C. Fasciculations: clinical, electromyographic, and ultrasonographic assessment. J Neurol. 1996;243(8):579–84.
135. Grimm A, Prell T, Decard BF, Schumacher U, Witte OW, Axer H, Grosskreutz J. Muscle ultrasonography as an additional diagnostic tool for the diagnosis of amyotrophic lateral sclerosis. Clin Neurophysiol. 2015;126(4):820–7.
136. Misawa S, Noto Y, Shibuya K, Isose S, Sekiguchi Y, Nasu S, Kuwabara S. Ultrasonographic detection of fasciculations markedly increases diagnostic sensitivity of ALS. Neurology. 2011;77(16):1532–7.
137. Regensburger M, Tenner F, Möbius C, Schramm A. Detection radius of EMG for fasciculations: empiric study combining ultrasonography and electromyography. Clin Neurophysiol. 2017. pii: S1388-2457(17)31145-8.
138. Johansson MT, Ellegaard HR, Tankisi H, Fuglsang-Frederiksen A, Qerama E. Fasciculations in nerve and muscle disorders – a prospective study of muscle ultrasound compared to electromyography. Clin Neurophysiol. 2017;128(11):2250–7.
139. O'gorman CM, Weikamp JG, Baria M, Van Den Engel-Hoek L, Kassardjian C, Van Alfen N, Boon AJ. Detecting fasciculations in cranial nerve innervated muscles with ultrasound in amyotrophic lateral sclerosis. Muscle Nerve. 2017;56(6):1072–6.
140. Tsuji Y, Noto YI, Shiga K, Teramukai S, Nakagawa M, Mizuno T. A muscle ultrasound score in the diagnosis of amyotrophic lateral sclerosis. Clin Neurophysiol. 2017;128(6):1069–74.

141. Oguri M, Saito Y, Okazaki T, Matsumura W, Ohno K, Togawa M, Fukuda C, Saito Y, Nishino I, Maegaki Y. Surface electromyogram and muscle ultrasonography for detection of muscle fasciculations in pediatric peripheral neuropathy. Brain Dev. 2017;39(7):617–20.
142. Pillen S, Nienhuis M, van Dijk JP, Arts IM, van Alfen N, Zwarts MJ. Muscles alive: ultrasound detects fibrillations. Clin Neurophysiol. 2009;120(5):932–6.
143. van Alfen N, Nienhuis M, Zwarts MJ, Pillen S. Detection of fibrillations using muscle ultrasound: diagnostic accuracy and identification of pitfalls. Muscle Nerve. 2011;43(2):178–82.
144. Fischer AQ, Stephens S. Computerized real-time neuromuscular sonography: a new application, techniques and methods. J Child Neurol. 1988;3(1):69–74.
145. Mayans D, Cartwright MS, Walker FO. Neuromuscular ultrasonography: quantifying muscle and nerve measurements. Phys Med Rehabil Clin N Am. 2012;23(1):133–48.
146. Zaidman CM, Wu JS, Wilder S, Darras BT, Rutkove SB. Minimal training is required to reliably perform quantitative ultrasound of muscle. Muscle Nerve. 2014;50(1):124–8.
147. Rahmani N, Mohseni-Bandpei MA, Vameghi R, Salavati M, Abdollahi I. Application of ultrasonography in the assessment of skeletal muscles in children with and without neuromuscular disorders: a systematic review. Ultrasound Med Biol. 2015;41(9):2275–83.
148. Lamminen A, Jääskeläinen J, Rapola J, Suramo I. High-frequency ultrasonography of skeletal muscle in children with neuromuscular disease. J Ultrasound Med. 1988;7(9):505–9.
149. Van Den Engel-Hoek L, Van Alfen N, De Swart BJ, De Groot IJ, Pillen S. Quantitative ultrasound of the tongue and submental muscles in children and young adults. Muscle Nerve. 2012;46(1):31–7.
150. Van den Engel-Hoek L, Erasmus CE, Hendriks JC, Geurts AC, Klein WM, Pillen S, Sie LT, de Swart BJ, de Groot IJ. Oral muscles are progressively affected in Duchenne muscular dystrophy: implications for dysphagia treatment. J Neurol. 2013;260(5):1295–303.
151. Heckmatt JZ, Dubowitz V. Ultrasound imaging and directed needle biopsy in the diagnosis of selective involvement in muscle disease. J Child Neurol. 1987;2(3):205–13.
152. Topaloğlu H, Gücüyener K, Yalaz K, Renda Y, Topçu M, Aysun S, Ozdirim E, Anlar B. Selective involvement of the quadriceps muscle in congenital muscular dystrophies: an ultrasonographic study. Brain Dev. 1992;14(2):84–7.
153. Tieleman AA, Vinke A, van Alfen N, van Dijk JP, Pillen S, van Engelen BG. Skeletal muscle involvement in myotonic dystrophy type 2. A comparative muscle ultrasound study. Neuromuscul Disord. 2012;22(6):492–9.
154. Abraham A, Breiner A, Barnett C, Bril V, Katzberg HD. Quantitative sonographic assessment of myotonia. Muscle Nerve. 2018;57(1):146–9.
155. Habers GE, Van Brussel M, Bhansing KJ, Hoppenreijs EP, Janssen AJ, Van Royen-Kerkhof A, Pillen S. Quantitative muscle ultrasonography in the follow-up of juvenile dermatomyositis. Muscle Nerve. 2015;52(4):540–6.
156. Fleckenstein JL, Reimers CD. Inflammatory myopathies: radiologic evaluation. Radiol Clin N Am. 1996;34(2):427–39.
157. Newman JS, Adler RS, Rubin JM. Power Doppler sonography: use in measuring alterations in muscle blood volume after exercise. AJR Am J Roentgenol. 1997;168(6):1525–30.
158. Weber MA, Krix M, Jappe U, Huttner HB, Hartmann M, Meyding-Lamadé U, Essig M, Fiehn C, Kauczor HU, Delorme S. Pathologic skeletal muscle perfusion in patients with myositis: detection with quantitative contrast-enhanced US – initial results. Radiology. 2006;238(2):640–9.
159. Weber MA, Jappe U, Essig M, Krix M, Ittrich C, Huttner HB, Meyding-Lamadé U, Hartmann M, Kauczor HU, Delorme S. Contrast-enhanced ultrasound in dermatomyositis- and polymyositis. J Neurol. 2006;253(12):1625–32.
160. Botar-Jid C, Damian L, Dudea SM, Vasilescu D, Rednic S, Badea R. The contribution of ultrasonography and sonoelastography in assessment of myositis. Med Ultrason. 2010;12(2):120–6.
161. Berko NS, Hay A, Sterba Y, Wahezi D, Levin TL. Efficacy of ultrasound elastography in detecting active myositis in children: can it replace MRI? Pediatr Radiol. 2015;45(10):1522–8.
162. Heckmatt JZ, Pier N, Dubowitz V. Assessment of quadriceps femoris muscle atrophy and hypertrophy in neuromuscular disease in children. J Clin Ultrasound. 1988;16(3):177–81.
163. Schmidt R, Voit T. Ultrasound measurement of quadriceps muscle in the first year of life. Neuropediatrics. 1992;24(1):36–42.
164. Verhagen MM, van Alfen N, Pillen S, Weemaes CM, Yntema JL, Hiel JA, Ter Laak H, van Deuren M, Broeks A, Willemsen MA. Neuromuscular abnormalities in ataxia telangiectasia: a clinical, electrophysiological and muscle ultrasound study. Neuropediatrics. 2007;38(3):117–21.
165. Hide IG, Grainger AJ, Naisby GP, Campbell RS. Sonographic findings in the anterior interosseous nerve syndrome. J Clin Ultrasound. 1999;27(8):459–64.
166. Pohle R, Fischer D, von Rohden L. Computer-supported tissue characterization in musculoskeletal ultrasonography. Ultraschall Med. 2000;21(6):245–52.
167. Shahrizaila N, Noto Y, Simon NG, Huynh W, Shibuya K, Matamala JM, Dharmadasa T, Devenney E, Kennerson ML, Nicholson GA, Kiernan MC. Quantitative muscle ultrasound as a bio-

marker in Charcot-Marie-Tooth neuropathy. Clin Neurophysiol. 2017;128(1):227–32.
168. Pillen S, Morava E, Van Keimpema M, Ter Laak HJ, De Vries MC, Rodenburg RJ, Zwarts MJ. Skeletal muscle ultrasonography in children with a dysfunction in the oxidative phosphorylation system. Neuropediatrics. 2006;37(3):142–7.
169. Fukunaga T, Miyatani M, Tachi M, Kouzaki M, Kawakami Y, Kanehisa H. Muscle volume is a major determinant of joint torque in humans. Acta Physiol Scand. 2001;172(4):249–55.
170. Akagi R, Takai Y, Ohta M, Kanehisa H, Kawakami Y, Fukunaga T. Muscle volume compared to cross-sectional area is more appropriate for evaluating muscle strength in young and elderly individuals. Age Ageing. 2009;38(5):564–9.
171. Pitcher CA, Elliott CM, Williams SA, Licari MK, Kuenzel A, Shipman PJ, Valentine JP, Reid SL. Childhood muscle morphology and strength: alterations over six months of growth. Muscle Nerve. 2012;46(3):360–6.
172. Rice CL, Cunningham DA, Paterson DH, Lefcoe MS. A comparison of anthropometry with computed tomography in limbs of young and aged men. J Gerontol. 1990;45(5):M175–9.
173. Barber L, Barrett R, Lichtwark G. Validation of a freehand 3D ultrasound system for morphological measures of the medial gastrocnemius muscle. J Biomech. 2009;42(9):1313–9.
174. Park ES, Sim E, Rha DW, Jung S. Estimation of gastrocnemius muscle volume using ultrasonography in children with spastic cerebral palsy. Yonsei Med J. 2014;55(4):1115–22.
175. Moreau NG, Teefey SA, Damiano DL. In vivo muscle architecture and size of the rectus femoris and vastus lateralis in children and adolescents with cerebral palsy. Dev Med Child Neurol. 2009;51(10):800–6.
176. Brandenburg JE, Eby SF, Song P, Zhao H, Landry BW, Kingsley-Berg S, Bamlet WR, Chen S, Sieck GC, An KN. Feasibility and reliability of quantifying passive muscle stiffness in young children by using shear wave ultrasound elastography. J Ultrasound Med. 2015;34(4):663–70.
177. Lee SS, Gaebler-Spira D, Zhang LQ, Rymer WZ, Steele KM. Use of shear wave ultrasound elastography to quantify muscle properties in cerebral palsy. Clin Biomech (Bristol, Avon). 2016;31:20–8.
178. Bilgici MC, Bekci T, Ulus Y, Ozyurek H, Aydin OF, Tomak L, Selcuk MB. Quantitative assessment of muscular stiffness in children with cerebral palsy using acoustic radiation force impulse (ARFI) ultrasound elastography. J Med Ultrason (2001). 2017. https://doi.org/10.1007/s10396-017-0824-3. [Epub ahead of print].
179. Kwon DR, Park GY, Lee SU, Chung I. Spastic cerebral palsy in children: dynamic sonoelastographic findings of medial gastrocnemius. Radiology. 2012;263(3):794–801.
180. Ceyhan Bilgici M, Bekci T, Ulus Y, Bilgici A, Tomak L, Selcuk MB. Quantitative assessment of muscle stiffness with acoustic radiation force impulse elastography after botulinum toxin A injection in children with cerebral palsy. J Med Ultrason (2001). 2018;45(1):137–41.
181. Park GY, Kwon DR. Sonoelastographic evaluation of medial gastrocnemius muscles intrinsic stiffness after rehabilitation therapy with botulinum toxin a injection in spastic cerebral palsy. Arch Phys Med Rehabil. 2012;93(11):2085–9.
182. Picelli A, La Marchina E, Gajofatto F, Pontillo A, Vangelista A, Filippini R, Baricich A, Cisari C, Smania N. Sonographic and clinical effects of botulinum toxin Type A combined with extracorporeal shock wave therapy on spastic muscles of children with cerebral palsy. Dev Neurorehabil. 2017;20(3):160–4.
183. Cornu C, Goubel F, Fardeau M. Stiffness of knee extensors in Duchenne muscular dystrophy. Muscle Nerve. 1998;21(2):1772–4.
184. Cornu C, Goubel F, Fardeau M. Muscle and joint elastic properties during elbow flexion in Duchenne muscular dystrophy. J Physiol. 2001;533(Pt 2):605–16.
185. Lacourpaille L, Hug F, Guével A, Péréon Y, Magot A, Hogrel JY, Nordez A. Non-invasive assessment of muscle stiffness in patients with Duchenne muscular dystrophy. Muscle Nerve. 2015;51(2):284–6.
186. Lacourpaille L, Gross R, Hug F, Guével A, Péréon Y, Magot A, Hogrel JY, Nordez A. Effects of Duchenne muscular dystrophy on muscle stiffness and response to electrically-induced muscle contraction: a 12-month follow-up. Neuromuscul Disord. 2017;27(3):214–20.
187. Cheng JC, Metreweli C, Chen TM, Tang S. Correlation of ultrasonographic imaging of congenital muscular torticollis with clinical assessment in infants. Ultrasound Med Biol. 2000;26(8):1237–41.
188. Lee SY, Park HJ, Choi YJ, Choi SH, Kook SH, Rho MH, Chung EC. Value of adding sonoelastography to conventional ultrasound in patients with congenital muscular torticollis. Pediatr Radiol. 2013;43(12):1566–72.
189. Kwon DR, Park GY. Diagnostic value of real-time sonoelastography in congenital muscular torticollis. J Ultrasound Med. 2012;31(5):721–7.
190. Lindequist S, Larsen C, Schrøder HD. Ultrasound guided needle biopsy of skeletal muscle in neuromuscular disease. Acta Radiol. 1990;31(4):411–3.
191. O'Sullivan PJ, Gorman GM, Hardiman OM, Farrell MJ, Logan PM. Sonographically guided percutaneous muscle biopsy in diagnosis of neuromuscular disease: a useful alternative to open surgical biopsy. J Ultrasound Med. 2006;25(1):1–6.
192. Billakota S, Dejesus-Acosta C, Gable K, Massey EW, Hobson-Webb LD. Ultrasound in EMG-guided

biopsies: a prospective, randomized pilot trial. Muscle Nerve. 2016;54(4):786–8.
193. Ida CM, Dyck PJ, Dyck PJ, Engelstad JK, Wang W, Selcen D, Bodensteiner JB, Mauermann ML, Klein CJ. Pediatric nerve biopsy diagnostic and treatment utility in tertiary care referral. Pediatr Neurol. 2016;58:3–11.
194. Chipman JN, Mott RT, Stanton CA, Cartwright MS. Ultrasonographic tinel sign. Muscle Nerve. 2009;40(6):1033–5.
195. Lolge SJ, Morani AC, Chaubal NG, Khopkar US. Sonographically guided nerve biopsy. J Ultrasound Med. 2005;24(10):1427–30.
196. Houltram J, Noble I, Boyd RN, Corry I, Flett P, Graham HK. Botulinum toxin Type A in the management of equinus in children with cerebral palsy: an evidence-based economic evaluation. Eur J Neurol. 2001;(Suppl 5):194–202.
197. Chang HJ, Hong BY, Lee SJ, Lee S, Park JH, Kwon JY. Efficacy and Safety of Letibotulinum Toxin A for the Treatment of Dynamic Equinus Foot Deformity in Children with Cerebral Palsy: A Randomized Controlled Trial. Toxins (Basel). 2017;18(9;8):pii. E252
198. Roubertie A, Mariani LL, Fernandez-Alvarez E, Doummar D, Roze E. Treatment for dystonia in childhood. Eur J Neurol. 2012;19(10):1292–9.
199. Py AG, Zein Addeen G, Perrier Y, Carlier RY, Picard A. Evaluation of the effectiveness of botulinum toxin injections in the lower limb muscles of children with cerebral palsy. Preliminary prospective study of the advantages of ultrasound guidance. Ann Phys Rehabil Med. 2009;52(3):215–23.
200. Chen CH, Huang YK, Jaw FS. Ultrasound-guided perineural vitamin B12 injection for peripheral neuropathy. J Med Ultrasound. 2015;23(2):104–6.
201. Li HF, Wang YR, Huo HP, Wang YX, Tang J. Neuroprotective effects of ultrasound-guided nerve growth factor injections after sciatic nerve injury. Neural Regen Res. 2015;10(11):1846–55.
202. Shah RD, Suresh S. Applications of regional anaesthesia in paediatrics. Br J Anaesth. 2013;111(Suppl 1):i114–24.
203. Fivez T, Hendrickx A, Van Herpe T, Vlasselaers D, Desmet L, Van den Berghe G, Mesotten D. An analysis of reliability and accuracy of muscle thickness ultrasonography in critically ill children and adults. JPEN J Parenter Enteral Nutr. 2016;40(7):944–9.

Part III

US in Juvenile Inflammatory Musculoskeletal Conditions

14 Juvenile Inflammatory Arthritis

Johannes Roth

Rationale for Using Ultrasonography in Juvenile Arthritis: The "Why"

Juvenile idiopathic arthritis (JIA) is a potentially debilitating, chronic disease which affects children and adolescents of all ages but has an overall peak incidence around 2 years of age [1]. It is divided into several subgroups with some subgroups (oligoarticular JIA) affecting predominantly large joints, specifically the knee as the most commonly affected one followed by the ankle and wrist, whereas in polyarticular JIA the small joints are also affected in a higher percentage [2]. Dactylitis as a specific type of involvement of the fingers can be found in oligoarticular JIA as well as the subgroup of psoriatic arthritis. Finally, the enthesitis-related arthritis subgroup of JIA is characterized by involvement of peripheral entheses in addition to synovitis. The involvement of the axial skeleton is much less frequent in children and tends to occur more often in adolescents presenting with the disease.

J. Roth (✉)
University of Ottawa, Ottawa, ON, Canada

Division of Pediatric Dermatology and Rheumatology, Children's Hospital of Eastern Ontario, Ottawa, ON, Canada
e-mail: jroth@cheo.on.ca

Treatment options have evolved dramatically over the past two decades [2] and it has become clear that appropriate guidance of these treatments is necessary in order to apply them optimally and improve outcomes. An extensive body of data in adults with RA but also other rheumatic diseases has shown that a targeted treatment approach (treat to target or T2T) in rheumatoid arthritis (RA) patients ensuring low disease activity (LDA) leads to improved outcomes. In such a strategy, frequent adjustments of therapy according to quantitative indices, irrespective of therapy, are being made. It has been shown that the strategy of tight control, aiming for remission, is more important than the individual medications [3].

There are few studies in the context of JIA, but early data show that standardized disease activity assessments and a regular target review combined with clinical decision support tools and the inclusion of the patient/parents improve outcomes as measured by JADAS scores significantly [4].

The pillars of a T2T strategy are:

- A defined target
- A measurement tool for the target
- Treatment options to achieve the target

Traditionally the target has been defined clinically as remission or low disease activity corresponding to the absence of inflammatory disease activity, including extra-articular manifestations [5].

Y. El Miedany (ed.), *Pediatric Musculoskeletal Ultrasonography*,
https://doi.org/10.1007/978-3-030-17824-6_14

In the context of JIA, the clinical assessment might not be sufficient though. For example, the time spent in inactive disease before MTX withdrawal is relevant with regard to the flare risk in patients with JIA, and clinical predictors for a lower likelihood of flare like shorter disease duration, older age at diagnosis, and shorter time to clinically inactive disease have been identified. These statistical parameters nevertheless still amount to guessing when it comes to taking treatment decisions in individual patients [6, 7].

A look at a specialty working closely with rheumatologists in the care of patients with uveitis, ophthalmologists, demonstrates that visualization of inflammation through slit lamp examinations and other assessments may have significant advantages over a clinical assessment only to monitor inflammation objectively before damage has actually occurred.

It is not surprising therefore to see an increased interest in the addition of imaging methods in the management of JIA and among the available methods musculoskeletal ultrasonography (MSUS) and MRI are favorites given the lack of radiation and the ability to provide a complete assessment including structural parameters as well as measures of inflammation [8].

MSUS may have unique advantages given the ability to assess several joints without sedation even in young children at the point of care and at a much lower cost than MRI [8].

Specific techniques used are B-mode ultrasonography and Doppler ultrasonography [8], the latter without any preference for Power-Doppler or Color-Doppler. More specialized techniques like the determination of the resistance index are not part of the routine clinical care yet and have not been evaluated in pediatric patients.

MSUS and Subclinical Disease Activity

Several studies in JIA have shown that MSUS is more sensitive than the clinical examination in the assessment of joint inflammation [9–13]. These studies would typically find discrepancies in the number of active joints between the clinical exam and ultrasonography with overall 30% of joints assessed as normal on physical exam showing signs of synovitis on MSUS. They do have limitations including the lack of information on normal ultrasound anatomy in children which affects the ability to determine what should be considered pathologic. Until recently there was also an absence of commonly agreed definitions for pathology on ultrasound and several of the published studies use scoring and grading systems that have not been validated for children.

Finally, it may be difficult to draw firm conclusions from a single cross-sectional assessment as is the case in most of these studies. In an interesting prospective trial using precise definitions of pathology [14], MSUS showed a strong sensitivity to change with a standardized response mean of 2.44 in B-mode and 1.23 in power Doppler ultrasound. 13/20 (65.0%) joints with US abnormalities were in clinical remission, and 6/21 (28.6%) patients in the ACRp90 responders group showed persistence of synovial abnormalities on MSUS. It has been shown that these imaging abnormalities correspond to histologic findings of inflammation [15].

A lack of clear definitions of synovitis and misinterpretation of low-grade, likely physiologic Doppler signals might also explain why some of the existing literature has yielded conflicting results including the inability of the presence of ultrasound findings to predict disease flares [16, 17]. In contrast, in a recent study on 88 patients in clinical remission in whom 44 joints were assessed clinically and with MSUS, the latter was abnormal in 20/88 (22.7%) patients at baseline [18]. At the 4 years follow-up, 41/88 (46.6%) patients experienced a flare with 38.2% MSUS-negative and 75% MSUS-positive at baseline. MSUS abnormalities resulted in an OR of flare of R = 3.8, 95% (CI 1.2 to 11.5), and the combination of B-mode and power Doppler had a higher predictive value of relapse (65%, 13/20) than B-mode alone (33%, 6/18).

Synovitis in Children on MSUS: How to Discriminate from Physiologic Findings

Through various international consensus efforts, definitions for the components of the normal pediatric joint have been issued [8, 19]. These include a clear description of the epiphyseal bone with the interruption of the bone contour at the growth plate, the variable amount of cartilage as described above, and the presence of hyperechoic signals within the cartilage that represent vascular channels as well as physiologic blood flow detectable as Doppler signals that can be demonstrated in any part of the joint (Fig. 14.1).

The intraarticular fat and physiologic blood flow within the joint have also been described [19]. In addition, the reliable imaging of ossification [20] and the reliable detection of Doppler signals (mean 1.5) in the cartilage, physis, and fat pad have been demonstrated [20]. Finally, normative data [21, 22] for most joints have been published providing further orientation for differentiating pathologic from physiologic findings.

Given the significant physiologic blood flow found in all areas of the joints of children, it is important to identify the joint capsule in order to determine the intraarticular space but at the same time differentiate this intraarticular space from the intrasynovial area as Doppler signals found outside the intrasynovial area might be intraarticular (inside the joint capsule) but if extrasynovial will not qualify to be a sign of synovitis [8, 19, 20]. In some joints like the hip joint, the synovial membrane is directly lining the joint capsule on its insides, but in the majority of joints like the elbow joint or ankle joint, there is intracapsular fat which is extrasynovial, i.e., going from superficial to deep the joint capsule comes first followed by intracapsular fat and connective tissue followed by the synovial membrane defining the intrasynovial space. In the presence of a joint effusion, this intracapsular fat/connective tissue might be displaced and even appear thinned out. In children (but also adults) the joint capsule itself can often be shown very nicely as a fibrillar structure (Fig. 14.2).

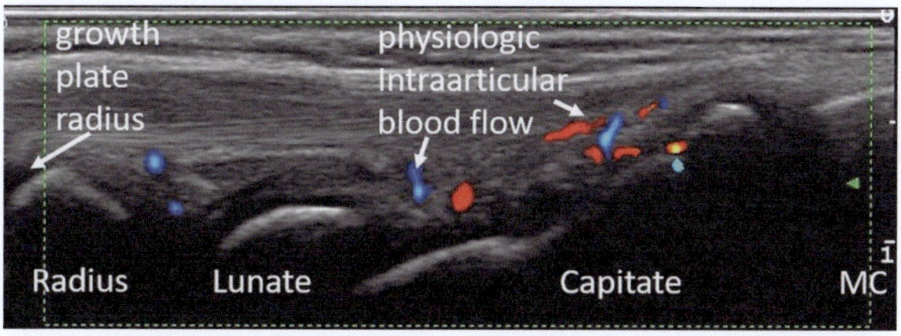

Fig. 14.1 Normal wrist joint showing features of pediatric anatomy. On the proximal end (left) an interruption of the bone (radius) can be seen which represents the growth plate. Blood flow can be seen in the intraarticular but extrasynovial area.

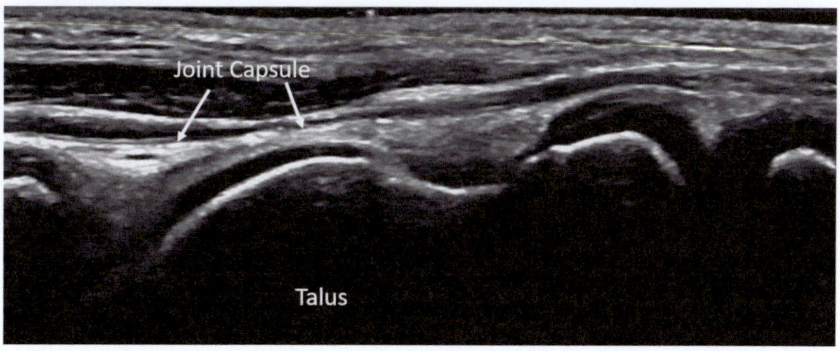

Fig. 14.2 Joint capsule in the tibiotalar joint. A longitudinal view of the tibiotalar and talonavicular joint is shown with the incompletely ossified cartilage in the talonavicular joint and the clear depiction of the joint capsule as a fibrillar structure in the tibiotalar joint

Synovitis

As in adults, the assessment of synovitis by US requires the use of both B-mode and Doppler mode, and an international consensus on the definition of synovitis in children has been published (Fig. 14.3 and [23]).

Given the complex anatomy of many joints, it is nevertheless extremely important to clearly identify the synovial recess on B-mode and differentiate this recess from other connective tissues, which might be intraarticular but extra-synovial [23] and can mimic the presence of an abnormal synovial thickening/effusion. Only Doppler signals within an area of synovial hypertrophy will clearly be suggestive of increased blood flow as part of the inflammatory process. This clear emphasis on the precise intrasynovial and not just intraarticular location of the Doppler signals represents an evolution of and differentiation from the existing definition in adults [23]. It is especially important in the pediatric context with the significant presence of intraarticular but physiologic blood flow that can be depicted with Doppler ultrasonography. However, the technical limitations affecting the sensitivity of Doppler especially for large joints where the joint recess is located relatively deep [23] should be taken into account. Therefore, the Omeract definition of an US-detected synovitis in children reflects the different anatomy of the joints by allowing the diagnosis of synovitis based on B-mode only (i.e., presence of synovial thickening and/or effusion, without Doppler signal). It also emphasizes the need to define the use of this technology in a more detailed way with variations of its use according to the different joints. A "one-size-fits-all" approach is therefore not possible, and the limitations of the technique need to be discussed clearly in order to ensure its appropriate use, and to take into account the different quality of the Doppler mode according to the type of the US equipment [24]. The possibility of the presence of physiologic Doppler signal in any area of the joint including the synovial recess [23] requires the sonographer to recognize and distinguish them from truly pathologic findings. For instance, feeding vessels can traverse the synovial recess but can be easily recognized by their direct trajectory into the bone/cartilage. Interesting aspects that need to be clarified in future longitudinal studies are the hyperemia and therefore increased visibility of feeding vessels in states of inflammation as well as peri-synovial and even periarticular hyperemia that might be an important sign of inflammatory activity but has not been studied systematically yet. An example of synovitis is shown in Fig. 14.4.

There is no preference with regard to the two main Doppler techniques that are being used in US at this point: power Doppler and color Doppler [24]. Whereas the sensitivity of power Doppler was considered superior in the detection of low velocity blood flow as seen in the inflamed synovium in the past, this is no longer universally true. Instead the question of which technique should be used to obtain maximum sensitivity very much depends on the ultrasound machine and the optimization of settings [24].

Fig. 14.3 Definition of synovitis in children on MSUS according to [23]

Synovitis detection by US in children includes the assessment of B-mode and Doppler mode (color or power Doppler) findings.

Synovitis can be detected on the basis of B-mode findings alone. Synovitis cannot be detected based on color/power Doppler findings alone.

B mode findings include synovial effusion and synovial hypertrophy.

A synovial effusion is defined as an abnormal, intraarticular, anechoic or hypoechoic material that is displaceable.

Synovial hypertrophy is defined as an abnormal, intraarticular, hypoechoic material that is non-displaceable. Color/power Doppler signals must be detected within synovial hypertrophy to be considered as a sign of synovitis.

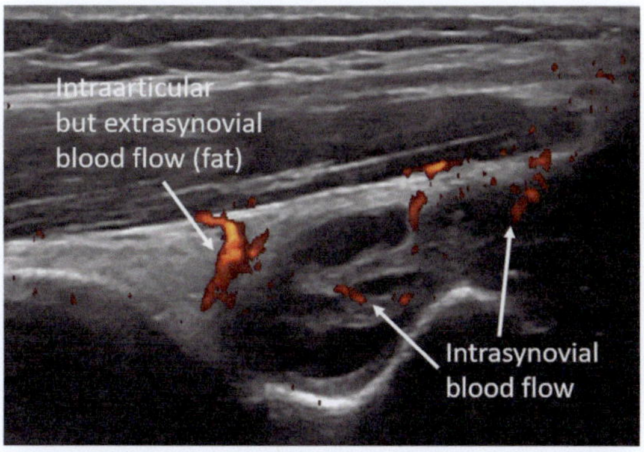

Fig. 14.4 Synovitis. Posterior longitudinal view of the elbow joint with intraarticular hyperechoic fat (bright) and synovial proliferation and fluid (hypo- to anechoic). Doppler signals can be seen in an intraarticular but extrasynovial location and also in a true intrasynovial location

Assessing Damage

Cartilage Thickness

As one of the cardinal features of damage in inflammatory arthritis is cartilage loss, US might play an important role in the monitoring of patients with chronic arthritis. In order to be able to interpret cartilage thickness in children with diseases like JIA, solid reference data studying cartilage thickness in healthy children and adolescents will be necessary. Unfortunately, only limited data are available thus far. Several publications have studied cartilage thickness in the knee joint, wrist and fingers [25, 26]. The data are provided according to age but not according to pubertal stage, which will limit the applicability. In addition, fairly high variability among observers has been documented for some of the joints, which is probably not surprising given the irregular shape of the secondary ossification centers in the epiphyses. The measurement of cartilage thickness might therefore prove challenging in pediatric rheumatology, and special care should be taken when applying normative data scales to assess a given patient's results. Another option for the assessment of cartilage is to assess the integrity of the cartilage surface. The first sign of cartilage damage is in fact the loss of the clear depiction of the cartilage surface and the cartilage surface interface sign even before cartilage thickness is compromised.

Erosions

Ultrasound has been shown to be more sensitive than radiographs and—depending on the location and the age—equally sensitive than MRI for the demonstration of erosions in adults and children. Whereas bone erosions might overall be less common in JIA than RA they still occur and are an important sign of joint damage. Not many publications have studied the appearance of bone erosions in JIA with ultrasound. It does seem however that the location can be more epiphyseal than commonly in adults where the location might be more meta-epiphyseal [27]. This is likely due to the fact that the epiphyseal cartilage especially in younger children is vascularized and allows inflammatory cells and lytic factors to invade more easily and cause destruction. A recent publication has demonstrated excellent interobserver reliability in demonstrating bone erosions in children with JIA [28].

Assessing Damage Beyond Cartilage/Bone Lesions

The radiographic assessment of joints in JIA is very much limited to the assessment of structural damage related to cartilage and bone lesions. From a functional point of view, damage to soft tissue structures may be even more important, and this would include tendon tears or partial tears, ligament lesions, and lesions to other structures supporting the normal function of the musculoskeletal system. One example would be the damage to pulleys keeping the flexor tendons of the fingers in place which may become compro-

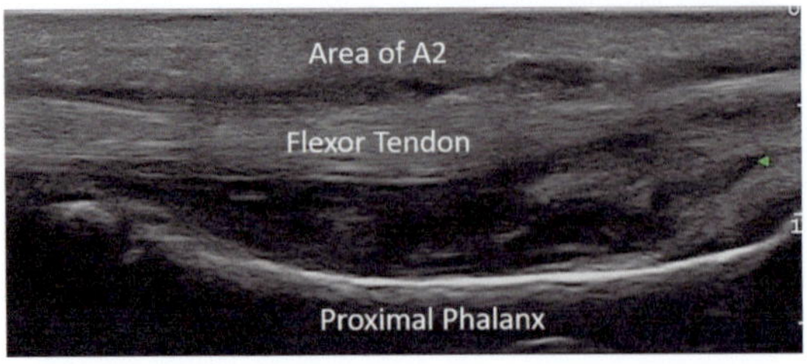

Fig. 14.5 Damage to the A2 pulley. Damage to the A2 pulley leads to "bow-stringing" of the flexor tendon along the proximal phalanx of the finger. Also note the tenosynovitis

mised secondary to chronic inflammation with a lack of proper guidance of the tendon as a result. In the more significant cases, it will lead to the so-called bow-stringing of the flexor tendon (Fig. 14.5).

Scoring Synovitis

The objective analysis or quantification of ultrasound findings is important for the serial clinical assessment and also the comparability among providers but is also needed for the use of MSUS as an outcome measure in research.

Whereas in a clinical context a descriptive approach, for example, "effusion in the tibiotalar joint with increased Doppler," potentially adding measurements, may be sufficient, a graduation of findings is important when trying to assess change over time. This can be done with qualitative terms, for example, mild, moderate, and severe, but the clear definition and reliability of such terms may be a challenge. At this point semiquantitative scoring systems are most widely used especially in adults. For children several scoring systems have been suggested, but the scoring definitions do not clearly apply to referenced illustrations [29] nor do general descriptions adequately apply to all joints and all views [30]. The development of dedicated scoring systems for individual joints may be superior to general scores for all joints. The knee joint is currently the only joint for which dedicated scoring systems are available [31–33], but only one of these systems includes the suprapatellar as well as the parapatellar recesses [34].

Challenges in obtaining objective findings remain related to the variability in equipment, but these can be mitigated by ensuring the optimization of settings, especially frequency and PRF (see section on technical aspects of ultrasonography), and avoiding the use of standardized settings given the variable anatomy and physical dimensions in children.

MSUS as a Tool to Monitor JIA

When trying to use MSUS as a tool to monitor JIA, one essential question is how many joints should be assessed at which time-points. For none of the two questions, the literature will give very clear answers at this point, but it might be reasonable to assume that MSUS can be a useful adjunct to the clinical assessment at any major clinical decision point, including diagnosis, remission, flare, change of treatment, and the planning of a joint injection.

Especially when trying to determine subclinical disease activity in clinical remission, the number of joints that should be assessed is also important.

In one study a 44 joint count was compared with a 10 joint count including the bilateral knee, tibiotalar, wrist, elbow, and 2MCP joints, and this selection was able to identify 100% of patients that did show B-mode and power Doppler findings in the more extensive 44 joint count suggesting that such a more limited joint count with an emphasis on large joints may be sufficient in JIA [29].

MSUS of JIA Versus RA

The body of evidence for the use of MSUS in rheumatoid arthritis (RA) is even larger than in JIA. MSUS contributes significantly in early diagnosis of both RF/ACPA-positive and RF/ACPA-negative patients and has an important role in the detection of subclinical arthritis. MSUS detects 50% more synovitic joints than clinical exam (fingers and toes). In another study 66% of patients had subclinical disease detectable by US and in many reclassification occurred to polyarticular disease course. MSUS is predictive of response and structural progression, and especially power Doppler predicts flare [35–38].

Other Roles of MSUS in a T2T Approach of JIA

Similar to the situation in RA, MSUS may significantly contribute to the management of JIA by supporting early diagnosis (an essential step to even implement T2T) and by capturing the full picture and guiding specific therapy by demonstrating pathology in many areas of the joint, enthesis, and tendon. Many joints are complex and do require the assessment of multiple synovial recesses, tendon sheaths, the paratenon, and entheses.

MSUS is important in the precise planning of joint injections and will increase the options for joint injections as part of T2T even in difficult locations.

Finally, it allows the inclusion of patient and parents in the decision-making process through the visual illustration of abstract concepts like inflammation and can help when there is discordance between the patient symptoms and the physician clinical assessment.

In summary MSUS is an important measurement tool in the care for children with JIA and a T2T approach. It helps to determine relevant subclinical disease activity, is applicable for most joints, has to be embedded in the overall clinical assessment of course, but is well-tolerated and benefits on many levels including patient interaction.

References

1. Minden K, Niewerth M, Listing J, Biedermann T, Bollow M, Schöntube M, Zink A. Long-term outcome in patients with juvenile idiopathic arthritis. Arthritis Rheum. 2002;46(9):2392–401.
2. Ravelli A, Martini A. Juvenile idiopathic arthritis. Lancet. 2007;369(9563):767–78.
3. Smolen JS, Aletaha D, Bijlsma JW, Breedveld FC, Boumpas D, Burmester G, Combe B, Cutolo M, de Wit M, Dougados M, Emery P, Gibofsky A, Gomez-Reino JJ, Haraoui B, Kalden J, Keystone EC, Kvien TK, McInnes I, Martin-Mola E, Montecucco C, Schoels M, van der Heijde D, T2T Expert Committee. Treating rheumatoid arthritis to target: recommendations of an international task force. Ann Rheum Dis. 2010;69(4):631–7.
4. Buckley L, Ware E, Kreher G, Wiater L, Mehta J, Burnham J. Improving outcomes using a treat to target approach and clinical decision support in polyarticular juvenile idiopathic arthritis [abstract]. Arthritis Rheumatol. 2017;69(suppl 10)
5. Wallace CA, Ruperto N, Giannini E, Childhood Arthritis and Rheumatology Research Alliance, Pediatric Rheumatology International Trials Organization, Pediatric Rheumatology Collaborative Study Group. Preliminary criteria for clinical remission for select categories of juvenile idiopathic arthritis. J Rheumatol. 2004;31(11):2290–4.
6. Klotsche J, Minden K, Niewerth M, Horneff G. Time spent in inactive disease before MTX withdrawal is relevant with regard to the flare risk in patients with JIA. Ann Rheum Dis. 2018;77(7):996–1002.
7. Lovell DJ, Johnson AL, Huang B, Gottlieb BS, Morris PW, Kimura Y, Onel K, Li SC, Grom AA, Taylor J, Brunner HI, Huggins JL, Nocton JJ, Haines KA, Edelheit BS, Shishov M, Jung LK, Williams CB, Tesher MS, Costanzo DM, Zemel LS, Dare JA, Passo MH, Ede KC, Olson JC, Cassidy EA, Griffin TA, Wagner-Weiner L, Weiss JE, Vogler LB, Rouster-Stevens KA, Beukelman T, Cron RQ, Kietz D, Schikler K, Schmidt KM, Mehta J, Wahezi DM, Ting TV, Verbsky JW, Eberhard BA, Spalding S, Chen C, Giannini EH. Risk, timing, and predictors of disease flare after discontinuation of anti-tumor necrosis factor therapy in children with polyarticular forms of juvenile idiopathic arthritis with clinically inactive disease. Arthritis Rheumatol. 2018;70(9):1508–18.
8. Roth J, Jousse-Joulin S, Magni-Manzoni S, Rodríguez A, Tzaribachev N, Iagnocco A, Naredo E, D'Agostino MA, Collado P, Outcome Measures in Rheumatology Ultrasound Group. Definitions for the sonographic features of joints in healthy children. Arthritis Care Res. 2015;67:136–42.
9. Haslam K, McCann L, Wyat S, et al. The detection of subclinical synovitis by ultrasound in oligoarticular juvenile idiopathic arthritis: a pilot study. Rheumatology. 2010;49:123–7.
10. Magni-Manzoni S, Epis O, Ravelli A, et al. Comparison of clinical versus ultrasound-determined synovitis in juvenile idio- pathic arthritis. Arthritis Rheum. 2009;61:1497–504.
11. Breton S, Jousse-Joulin S, Cangemi C, et al. Comparison of clinical and ultrasonographic evaluations for peripheral synovitis in juvenile idiopathic arthritis. Semin Arthritis Rheum. 2011;41:272–8.
12. Filippou G, Cantarini L, Bertoli I, Picerno V, Frediani B, Galeazzi M. Ultrasonography vs. clinical examination in children with suspected arthritis. Does it make

sense to use polyarticular ultraso- nographic screening? Clin Exp Rheumatol. 2011;29:345–50.
13. Rebollo-Plo M, Koujok K, Weisser C, Jurencak BA, Roth J. Ultrasound findings in patients with juvenile idiopathic arthritis in clinical remission. Arthritis Care Res. 2011;63:1013–9.
14. Lanni S, van Dijkhuizen EHP, Vanoni F, Viola S, Magnaguagno F, Magnano GM, Gandolfo C, Ravelli A, Malattia C. Ultrasound changes in synovial abnormalities induced by treatment in juvenile idiopathic arthritis. Clin Exp Rheumatol. 2018;36(2):329–34.
15. Anandarajah A, Thiele R, Giampoli E, Monu J, Seo GS, Feng C, Ritchlin CT. Patients with rheumatoid arthritis in clinical remission manifest persistent joint inflammation on histologic and imaging studies. J Rheumatol. 2014;41:2153–60.
16. Magni-Manzoni S, Scirè CA, Ravelli A, Klersy C, Rossi S, Muratore V, Visconti C, Lanni S, Merli P, Montecucco C. Ultrasound-detected synovial abnormalities are frequent in clinically inactive juvenile idiopathic arthritis, but do not predict a flare of synovitis. Ann Rheum Dis. 2013;72(2):223–8.
17. Zhao Y, Rascoff NE, Iyer RS, Thapa M, Reichley L, Oron AP, Wallace CA. Flares of disease in children with clinically inactive juvenile idiopathic arthritis were not correlated with ultrasound findings. J Rheumatol. 2018;45(6):851–7.
18. De Lucia O, Ravagnani V, Pregnolato F, Hila A, Pontikaki I, Gattinara M, Romano M, Gerloni V, Pieropan S, Murgo A, Rossini M, Cimaz R, Meroni PL. Baseline ultrasound examination as possible predictor of relapse in patients affected by juvenile idiopathic arthritis (JIA). Ann Rheum Dis. 2018;77(10):1426–31.
19. Collado P, Windschall D, Vojinovic J, Magni-Manzoni S, Balint P, Bruyn GAW, Hernandez-Diaz C, Nieto JC, Ravagnani V, Tzaribachev N, Iagnocco A, D'Agostino MA, Naredo E, OMERACT ultrasound subtask force on pediatric. Amendment of the OMERACT ultrasound definitions of joints' features in healthy children when using the DOPPLER technique. Pediatr Rheumatol Online J. 2018;16(1):23.
20. Windschall D, Collado P, Vojinovic J, Magni-Manzoni S, Balint P, Bruyn GAW, Hernandez-Diaz C, Nieto JC, Ravagnani V, Tzaribachev N, Iagnocco A, D'Agostino MA, Naredo E, OMERACT paediatric ultrasound subtask force. Age-related vascularization and ossification of joints in children: an international pilot study to test multi-observer ultrasound reliability. Arthritis Care Res (Hoboken). 2017; https://doi.org/10.1002/acr.23335.
21. Trauzeddel R, Windschall D, Trauzeddel RF, Nirschl C, Ganser G, Palm-Beden K, Berendes R, Haller M, Krumrey-Langkammerer M, Nimtz-Talaska A, Schoof P, Lehmann H. Arthrosonographic reference values of the shoulder joint in healthy children and adolescents: a cross-sectional multicentre ultrasound study. Klin Padiatr. 2017;229(5):293–301.
22. Trauzeddel RF, Lehmann H, Windschall D, Ganser G, Berendes R, Haller M, Krumrey-Langkammerer M, Palm-Beden K, Nimtz-Talaska A, Nirschl C, Schoof P, Trauzeddel R. Age-dependent arthrosonographic reference values of the hip joint in healthy children and adolescents – a cross-sectional multicenter ultrasound study. Pediatr Radiol. 2017;47(10):1329–36.
23. Roth J, Ravagnani V, Backhaus M, Balint P, Bruns A, Bruyn GA, Collado P, De la Cruz L, Guillaume-Czitrom S, Herlin T, Hernandez C, Iagnocco A, Jousse-Joulin S, Lanni S, Lilleby V, Malattia C, Magni-Manzoni S, Modesto C, Rodriguez A, Nieto JC, Ohrndorf S, Rossi-Semerano L, Selvaag AM, Swen N, Ting TV, Tzaribachev N, Vega-Fernandez P, Vojinovic J, Windschall D, D'Agostino MA, Naredo E, OMERACT Ultrasound Group. Preliminary definitions for the sonographic features of synovitis in children. Arthritis Care Res (Hoboken). 2017;69(8):1217–23.
24. Torp-Pedersen S, Christensen R, Szkudlarek M, Ellegaard K, D'Agostino MA, Iagnocco A, et al. Power and color Doppler ultrasound settings for inflammatory flow: impact on scoring of disease activity in patients with rheumatoid arthritis. Arthritis Rheumatol. 2015;67(2):386–95.
25. Spannow AH, Pfeiffer-Jensen M, Andersen NT, Herlin T, Stenbøg E. Ultrasonographic measurements of joint cartilage thickness in healthy children: age- and sex-related standard reference values. J Rheumatol. 2010;37(12):2595–601.
26. Pradsgaard DØ, Fiirgaard B, Spannow AH, Heuck C, Herlin T. Cartilage thickness of the knee joint in juvenile idiopathic arthritis: comparative assessment by ultrasonography and magnetic resonance imaging. J Rheumatol. 2015;42(3):534–40.
27. Karmazyn B, Bowyer SL, Schmidt KM, et al. US findings of metacarpophalangeal joints in children with idiopathic juvenile arthritis. Pediatr Radiol. 2007;37:475–82.
28. Ventura-Ríos L, Faugier E, Barzola L, De la Cruz-Becerra LB, Sánchez-Bringas G, García AR, Maldonado R, Roth J, Hernández-Díaz C. Reliability of ultrasonography to detect inflammatory lesions and structural damage in juvenile idiopathic arthritis. Pediatr Rheumatol Online J. 2018;16(1):58.
29. Collado P, Naredo E, Calvo C, Gamir ML, Calvo I, Garcia ML, et al. Reduced joint assessment vs comprehensive assessment for ultrasound detection of synovitis in juvenile idiopathic arthritis. Rheumatology (Oxford). 2013;52(8):1477–84.
30. Vojinovic J, Magni-Manzoni S, Collado P, Windschall D, Ravagnani V, Hernandez-Diaz C, Nieto Gonzales JC, Malattia C, Tzaribachev N, Susic G, Damjanov N, Guillaume Czitrom S, Herlin T, Lanni S, Bruyn G, Iagnocco A, Terslev A, D'Agostino MA, Naredo E. SAT0636 ultrasonography definitions for synovitis grading in children: the OMERACT pediatric ultrasound task force. Ann Rheum Dis. 2017;76:1015.
31. Algergawy S, Haliem T, Al-Shaer O. Clinical, laboratory, and ultrasound assessment of the knee in juvenile rheumatoid arthritis. Clin Med Insights Arthritis Musculoskelet Disord. 2011;4:21–7.

32. Hirsch G, O'Neill T, Kitas G, Klocke R. Distribution of effusion in knee arthritis as measured by high-resolution ultrasound. Clin Rheumatol. 2012;31(8):1243–6.
33. Beitinger N, Ehrenstein B, Schreiner B, Fleck M, Grifka J, Luring C, et al. The value of colour Doppler sonography of the knee joint: a useful tool to discriminate inflammatory from non-inflammatory disease? Rheumatology (Oxford). 2013;52(8):1425–8.
34. Ting TV, Vega-Fernandez P, Oberle EJ, De Ranieri D, Bukulmez H, Lin C, Moser D, Barrowman NJ, Zhao Y, Benham HM, Tasan L, Thatayatikom A, Roth J, CARRA JIA Ultrasound Workgroup. A novel ultrasound image acquisition protocol and scoring system for the pediatric knee. Arthritis Care Res (Hoboken). 2018; https://doi.org/10.1002/acr.23746.
35. Saleem B, Brown AK, Quinn M, Karim Z, Hensor EM, Conaghan P, Peterfy C, Wakefield RJ, Emery P. Can flare be predicted in DMARD treated RA patients in remission, and is it important? A cohort study. Ann Rheum Dis. 2012;71(8):1316–21.
36. Saleem B, Brown AK, Keen H, Nizam S, Freeston J, Karim Z, Quinn M, Wakefield R, Hensor E, Conaghan PG, Emery P. Disease remission state in patients treated with the combination of tumor necrosis factor blockade and methotrexate or with disease-modifying antirheumatic drugs: a clinical and imaging comparative study. Arthritis Rheum. 2009;60(7):1915–22.
37. Brown AK, Conaghan PG, Karim Z, Quinn MA, Ikeda K, Peterfy CG, Hensor E, Wakefield RJ, O'Connor PJ, Emery P. An explanation for the apparent dissociation between clinical remission and continued structural deterioration in rheumatoid arthritis. Arthritis Rheum. 2008;58(10):2958–67.
38. Brown AK, Quinn MA, Karim Z, Conaghan PG, Peterfy CG, Hensor E, Wakefield RJ, O'Connor PJ, Emery P. Presence of significant synovitis in rheumatoid arthritis patients with disease-modifying antirheumatic drug-induced clinical remission: evidence from an imaging study may explain structural progression. Arthritis Rheum. 2006;54(12):3761–73.

Juvenile Spondyloarthropathies

15

Goumy Laurence and Jousse-Joulin Sandrine

Juvenile idiopathic arthritis (JIA) is the most common rheumatic condition of childhood, affecting 3 to 4 per 1000 children [1]. The International League of Associations for Rheumatology (ILAR) criteria defines seven categories of arthritis [2]. The category called enthesitis-related arthritis represents 20% of JIA. Enthesitis is defined as the association of one type of arthritis and one enthesitis or one arthritis and at least two other elements: sacroiliac pain, inflammatory spine, HLAB27 positivity, anterior uveitis, spondyloarthropathy, or inflammatory enterocolopathy. It can also be associated with extra-articular manifestations, such as eye, heart, cutaneous, or digestive conditions. Even if the axial involvement can be possible in children, enthesitis is more involved and common than the adult form of spondyloarthropathy [3–5]. Detection of enthesitis in children remains a subjective examination because it is depending only on clinical examination, and 30% of healthy children may complain pain at enthesis level, if evaluated with a dolorimeter [6]. On the other hand, imaging studies in JIA reported examples of subclinical enthesitis that may be related to a persistent chronic activity of the disease [7, 8].

G. Laurence
Pediatric Department, CHU, Angers, France

J.-J. Sandrine (✉)
Rheumatology Department, Cavale Blanche Hospital and Brest Occidentale University, Brest, France
e-mail: sandrine.jousse-joulin@chu-brest.fr

Enthesitis is typically defined as an inflammation of the insertion of tendons, ligaments, aponeurosis, and capsules into the bone, and it is considered a pathological, clinical, and imaging hallmark of the spondyloarthritis (SpA) group in adults. For the time being, the diagnosis of enthesitis in children is pivotal, being important criteria for enthesitis-related arthritis (ERA) subtype of juvenile idiopathic arthritis (JIA). ERA is associated with HLA–B27. Among patients with JIA, 11–16% have ERA [9].

Imaging technique has being developed to assess entheses in children. Over the last few years, MSKUS coupled with power Doppler (US-PD) has been proven accurate for assessing tendon and joint disease in adults. In several studies, US-PD was used to detect asymptomatic peripheral enthesitis in adults with SPA [10, 11]. Musculoskeletal ultrasonography combined with power Doppler (MSKUS-PD) has been used in few studies to detect enthesitis in children, in whom cartilage growth and vascularization patterns differ from those in adults.

Indeed, MSKUS is an ideal technique to evaluate the pediatric population for children aged less than 5 years, because it uses no radiation, nor anesthesia-like traditional plain radiography and magnetic resonance image (MRI) [12].

Definition Enthesis as an organ concept has been developed [13], but its applicability in children

Y. El Miedany (ed.), *Pediatric Musculoskeletal Ultrasonography*,
https://doi.org/10.1007/978-3-030-17824-6_15

remains a problem because of the peculiar characteristics of the normal immature entheses, so different from adult enthesis, particularly in term of tendon/bone interface and vascularization [14–16]. The use of MSKUS in children is challenging because of the growing skeleton (i.e., increase ratio of cartilage, vascularization of cartilage, ossification centers) compared to adults. It took time to develop normal definitions of joints in healthy children [17] and after in a context of JIA [18]. Normal definitions of entheses have been recently described [15] in different groups of age and showed the difficulty to assess the development of entheses in lower limb at different ages and also the vascularization of the different entheses in B mode. However, with the normal definitions published, pathological findings could be identified.

The entheses is a real entity and is defined as an enthesis organ concept by McGonagle [19]. This concept is based on the environment of the structures which are attached between tendon and bone. The entheses most commonly involved in children are the plantar aponeurosis, calcaneal enthesitis, and distal and proximal patellar ligament insertions [20].

We describe in this chapter the interest to use MSKUS in the normal development of entheses in lower limbs with some pathological findings as the most common apophysitis (i.e., Osgood-Schlatter disease and Sever's disease).

Normal Development of Lower Limb Enthesis

The enthesis is a complex structure including several components: the insertion of the tendon in fibro cartilage, the bursae, the fat, the ligament, the capsule, and the nail matrix. All these components are often in contiguity.

MRI is an excellent imaging modality to see all these components, but because of its accessibility, costs, and the need of sedation for very young child, it is easier to use ultrasonography (US) for the diagnosis. US has many advantages in the assessment of the different enthesis. It is a real time process and we can assess all enthesis in the same time without radiation, without sedation, and also with the presence of parents.

Achilles Tendon

Achilles enthuses is considered as the archetypal enthesis organ and is described as the "premiere enthuse." However, with growth, the development of enthesis changes and it is very important to have knowledge concerning the different steps of the normal development of enthesis to recognize enthesis pathology. It is been clearly described by Fornage and Grechenig as follows: (1) from 2 months to 3 years, no ossification of the secondary center of calcaneus is visible; (2) from 4 to 6 years, early signs of the secondary ossification center appear; (3) from 7 to 11 years, the posterior bony contour of the primary ossification center of the calcaneus has got a wavy appearance; and (4) from 12 to 18 years, the secondary ossification center then appears and full ossification of the apophyseal cartilage occurs. Figures 15.1, 15.2, 15.3, and 15.4 represent the development of the Achilles tendon at the different age groups.

Vascularization of Enthesis As described in the recent literature [15], cartilage is vascularized

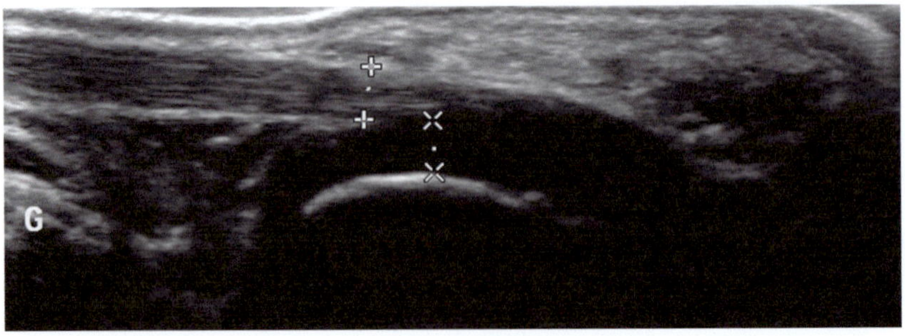

Fig. 15.1 Calcaneal tendon with its insertion on calcaneus. 3 years old

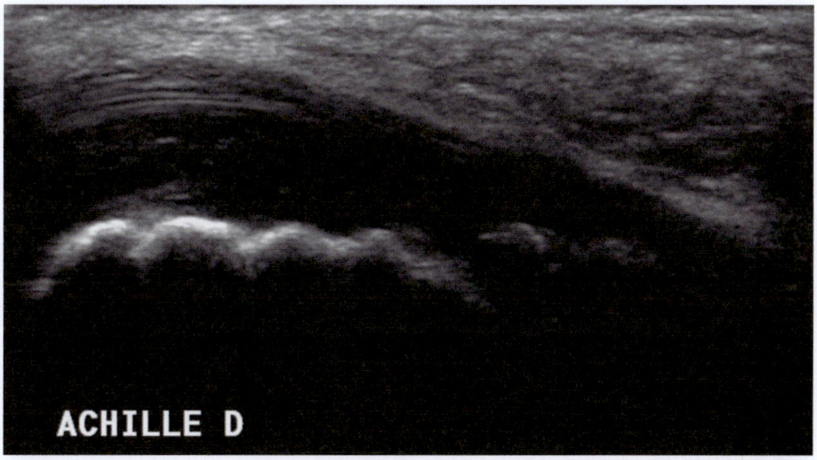

Fig. 15.2 Calcaneal tendon with its insertion on calcaneus and the developpement of the secondary ossification center. 4 years old

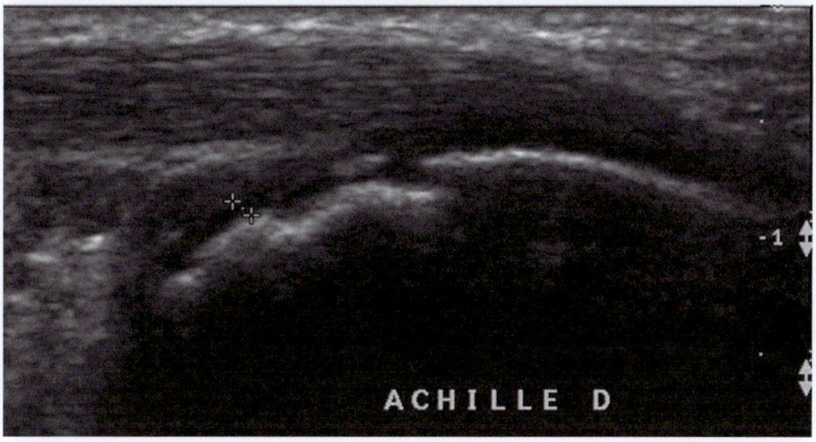

Fig. 15.3 Calcaneal tendon and its insertion on calcaneus. The secondary ossification center is presnt and easily visible as a hyperechoic line. 13 years old

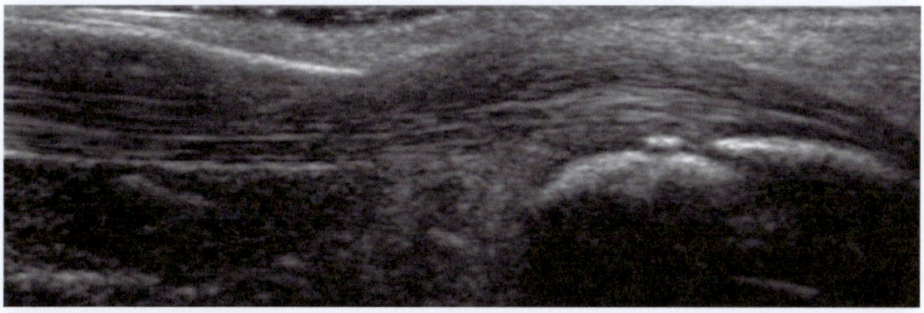

Fig. 15.4 Calcaneal tendon and its insertion on calcaneus. The secondary ossification center is almost fused with the calcaneus bone. 15 years old

in children but disappears in the same time of the decrease of cartilage.

Grechenig and associates [14] used color Doppler to show vascularization at the apophyseal cartilage in the first group (2 months to 3 years) in 76% of cases. This appearance of vascularization has been found in one case in adolescents (12–18 years). Recently, Jousse-Joulin S et al. also showed apophyseal cartilage vascularization in different age group as follows: presence of apophyseal cartilage vascularization in 2–4 years old age group in 1/14 (7%), 5–7 years old age group in 4/22 (18%), and 8–12 years old age group in 2/24 (8%) and no vascularization in 13–16 years old age group.

Quadricipital Enthesis

The development of the quadricipital enthesis is associated with the development of the patella. But, the description of the normal development of the patella is very scarce in the literature and we found only one paper [21].

The apparition of the ossification center and its vascularization have been recently described [15] and it seem to appear after 4 years old. However according to the different age groups, we can see ossification center as follows:

Ossification center is present in 2–4 years old age group in 11/17 (65%), 5–7 years old age group in 22/22 (100%), 8–12 in years old age group in 24/24 (100%), and 13–16 years old age group in 17/17 (100%). The vascularization of the patella is also present when cartilage is present in 2–4 years old age group in 6/13 (46%) and 5–7 years old age group in 7/22 (32%) and not present after 7 years.

Patellar Ligament

Insertion at the Lower Patellar Pole The development of the patellar ligament enthesis is important to know because of the pathology at this area. It is the location of Jumper's knee disease and Sinding-Larsen-Johansson disease [22–26] at the lower pole of the patella and the Osgood-Schlatter disease at the tibial tuberosity insertion. However, before knowing these conditions, we need to know the normal evolution of these two enthesis sites.

The proximal patellar ligament is attached to the patella with is completely cartilaginous under 4 years and with growth, the ossification center of the patella appears and some cartilage remains until 7–8 years. This persistent cartilage during the growth is vascularized (Figs. 15.5 and 15.6).

Insertion at the Tibial Tuberosity Ehrenborg and Engfeldt [27] described development of the tibial tuberosity in four phases:

1. Cartilage phase: development of a separate growth plate associated with the tibial tuberosity (Fig. 15.7)
2. Apophyseal phase: development of a secondary ossification center in the distal portion of the tuberosity (see Fig. 15.8)
3. Epiphyseal phase: coalescence of the ossification centers of the tuberosity and the proximal tibial epiphysis (see Fig. 15.9)
4. Bone phase: closure of the contiguous growth plates of the proximal tibia and tuberosity (see Fig. 15.10)

We now know that the vascularization for this entheseal site is very important and remains present until adolescence [15]. Apophyseal distal patellar ligament enthesis cartilage vascularization is present in 1/9 (11%) of the 2–4 years old age group, 11/22 (50%) of the 5–7 years old age group, 17/24 (71%) of the 8–12 in years old age group, and 5/17 (29%) of the 13–16 years old age group.

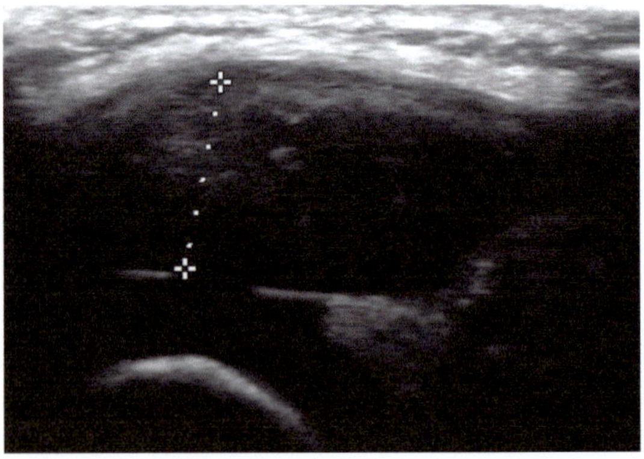

Fig. 15.5 Hypoechoic cartilage of the patella which is not yet ossified. 3 years old

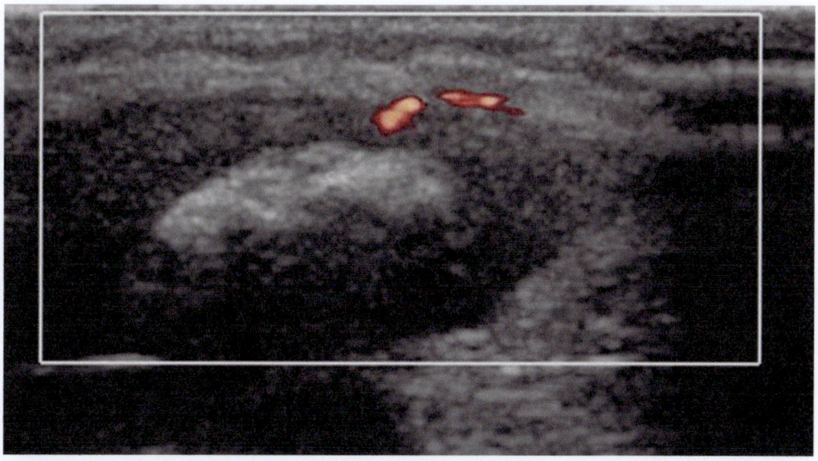

Fig. 15.6 Normal cartilage vascularisation of the patella. 7 years old

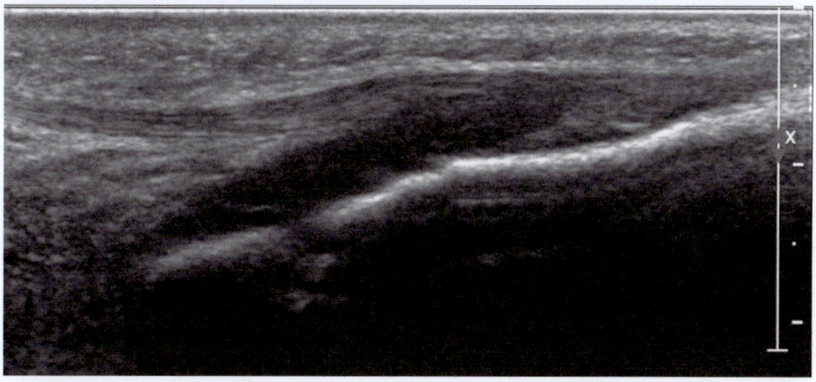

Fig. 15.7 Cartilage phase of the tibial tuvberosity. The secondary ossification is not yet present. 6 years old

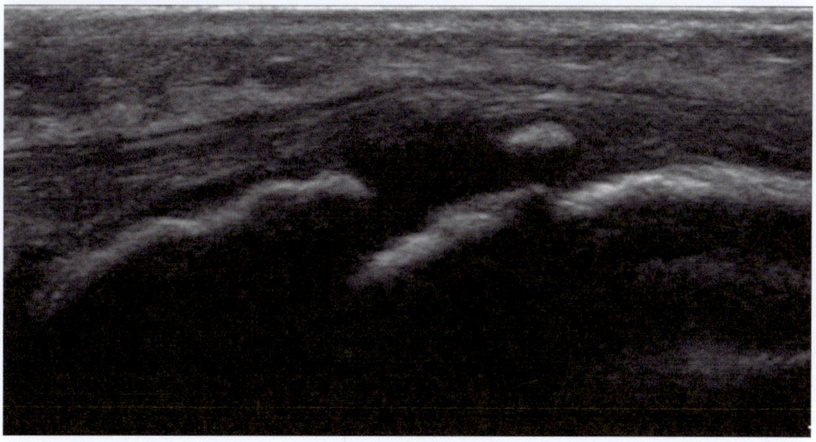

Fig. 15.8 Apparition of the secondary ossification center of the tibial tuberosity. 8 years old

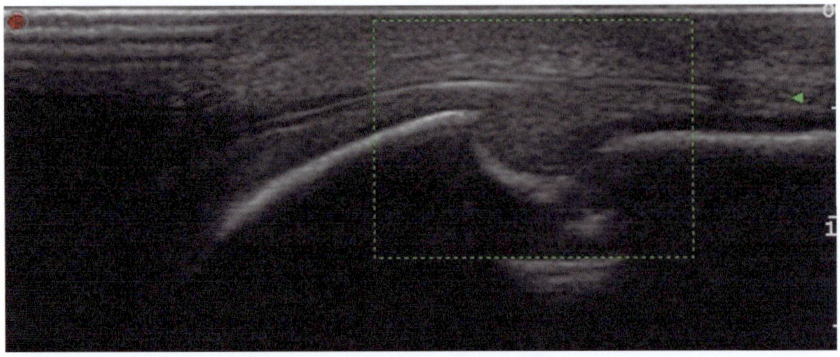

Fig. 15.9 Bone fusion between the tibial tuberosity and the secondary ossification center. 12 years old

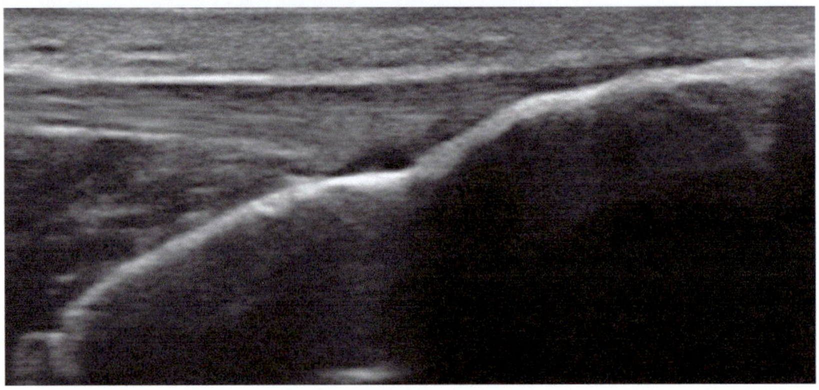

Fig. 15.10 Complete fusion between the tibial tuberosity and the secondary ossification center. Normal aspect as in adult of the tibial tuberosity. 15 years old

Apophysitis

It is a very frequent mechanical pathology encountered in young children. It corresponds to an insertional tendinopathy at an apophyseal site and could lead to an avulsion of osteochondral fragments [28].

The most common examples described are Osgood-Schlatter disease at the tibial tuberosity entheseal site and Sever's disease at the Achilles apophyseal site. This condition is frequent in children during growth and corresponds either with a simple tendinopathy or traction of the ossification center, which can be seen by clinical examination in adult period or using US (Fig. 15.16). The differential diagnosis between apophysitis and enthesitis, as a manifestation of juvenile spondyloarthropathy, can be achieved through patient history and clinical exam as the imaging features. The tendinopathies symptomatology increases with sport activities, whereas in ERA the morning stiffness and the improvement with effort is present. Indeed, tendinopathy involves one site, whereas ERA involves multiple entheseal sites with synovitis. Concerning US imaging, ERA shows inflammation in the entheseal insertion with some bone irregularities (Figs. 15.11, 15.12, 15.13, and 15.14), and Osgood-Schlatter disease or Sever's disease shows thickened tendon and osteochondral traction (Fig. 15.15).

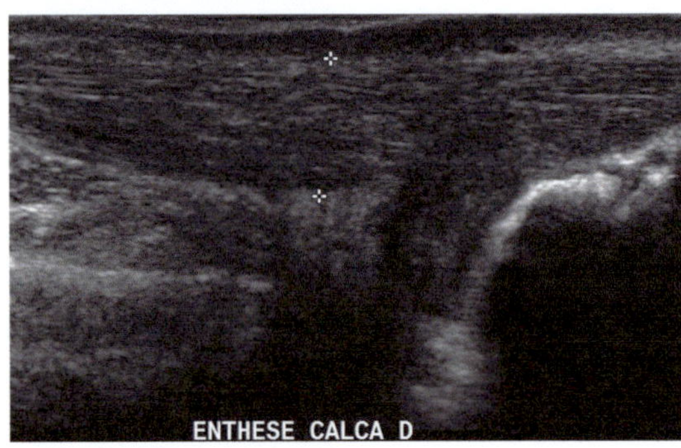

Fig. 15.11 Abnormal fusiform aspect of the calcaneal tendon with its bony irregular insertion on calcaneus

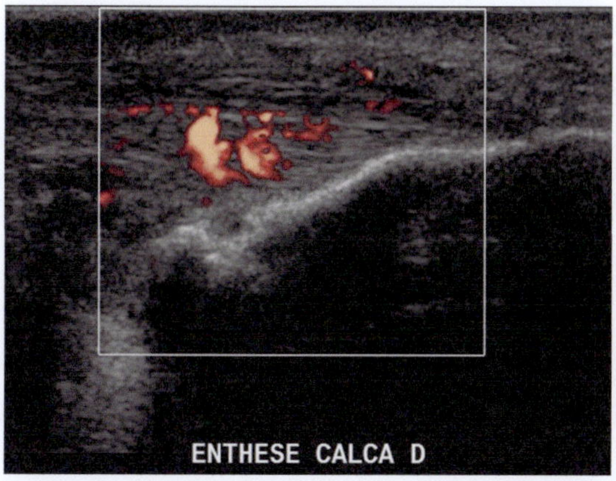

Fig. 15.12 Longitudinal scan of calcaneal tendon with its insertion on calcaneus. Doppler mode shows inflammation at the level of this enthesitis

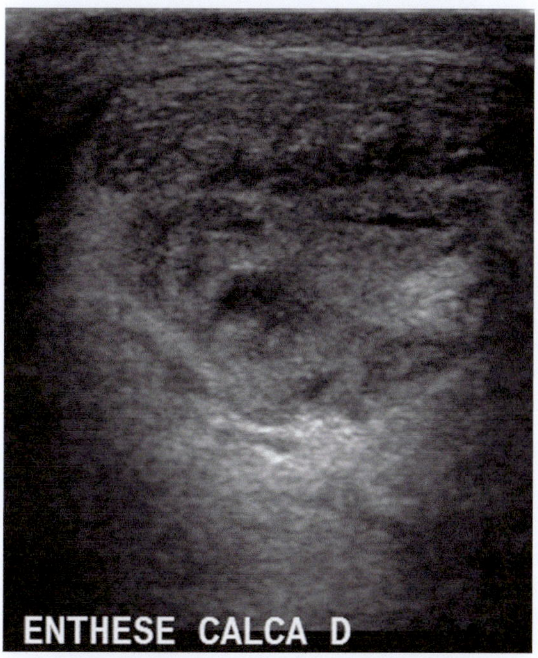

Fig. 15.13 Transversal scan of the calcaneal tendon showing irregular contour and round aspect. Abnormal B mode calcaneal image suspected of enthesitis or tendinitis

Arthritis

Enthesitis-related arthritis children concerns enthesitis but also arthritis [2] and as well as JIA especially at the onset. These arthritides are assumed to be no different than those of the other forms of JIA in a US point of view and have the same definitions.

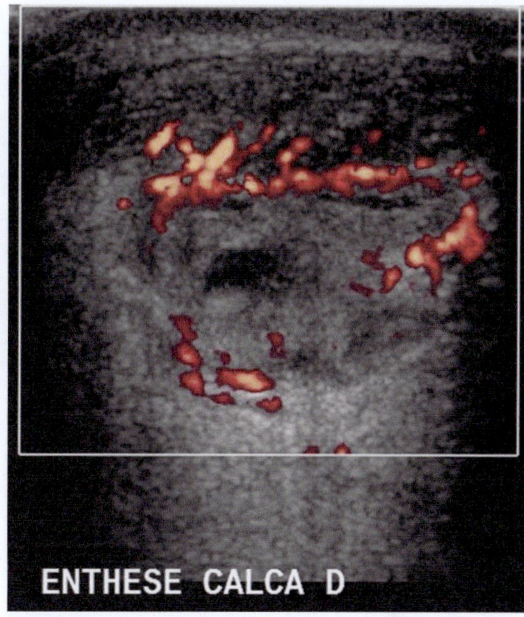

Fig. 15.14 Transvesal scan of the calcaneal tendon using Doppler mode and showing abnormal inflammation inside the tendon

Normal sonographic features of joints in healthy children have been described by Roth et al. [18] giving a reference for synovitis diagnosis in children. Spannow et al. [29] as well as Pradsgaard et al. [30] gave normal measurements of joint cartilage thickness with age- and sex-related standard reference values.

A recent review has been done by Basra et al. [31] with a description of what should be examined by US in children with recommendations for the peculiarities of the joint ultrasound in children (Fig. 15.16). Ultrasound definitions of arthritis in adults were agreed upon in 2005 by the OMERACT group [32] and widely used in children with EULAR-PREs recommendations in 2015 [33]. More recently, OMERACT preliminary definitions for EULAR recommendations for imaging in spondyloarthritis exist but only for the adults [34].

Nonetheless, one must keep in mind the overlap of US imaging between inflammatory synovitis and joint infection (Nguyen [35]).

One of the important contribution of US in JIA is to see exactly which joints are involved with consequences for classification of the child in the right subtype. Indeed many studies have shown the superiority of US to detect synovitis in chil-

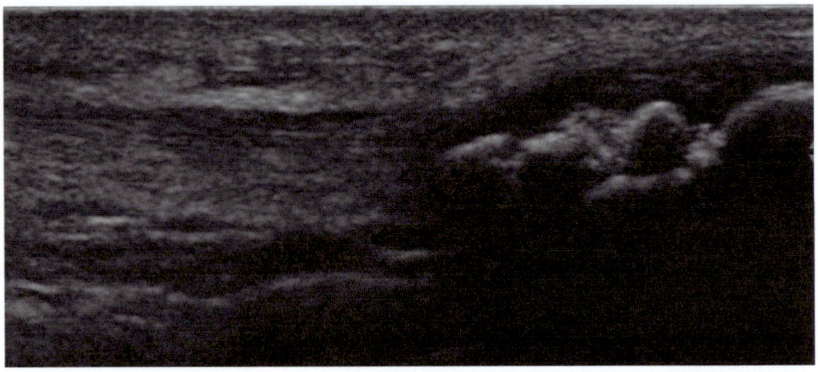

Fig. 15.15 Longitudinal scan of the tibial tuberosity. The secondary ossification center is not fused with the tibial tuberosity. This image is typical of Ogood -Schlatter disease in a 7 years old boy

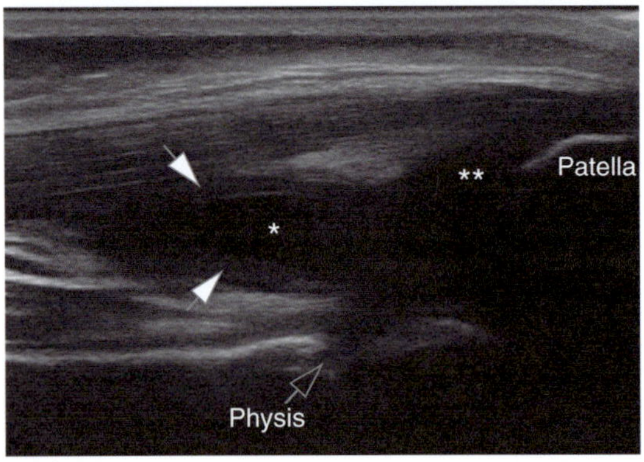

Fig. 15.16 Five years old girl with enthesitis-related arthritis. Knee longitudinal view supra patellar recessus synovitis (plain arrow) effusion (∗) and normal patellar cartilage (∗∗)

dren [36–38] but also its high value for the hip frequently involved in jSPA (Fig. 15.17) and difficult to assess clinically [39]. In our experience, US is also very useful to explore midfoot and toes (Figs. 15.18 and 15.19), but unfortunately, there is no studies addressing these subjects.

Moreover, US can help to distinguish between joint synovitis and tenosynovitis especially in ankles (Rooney) [40] which are often implicated in jSPA. US is also able to detect active disease in juvenile idiopathic arthritis [41] with a good sensitivity and reliability, and it has been shown by Shahin et al. [42] a good correlation between Power Doppler sonography and levels of circulating inflammatory cytokines. However, the significance of subclinical US synovitis in JIA remains undetermined [43, 44], but recent works showed that Power Doppler signal should be a good predictor of clinical flare [45, 46].

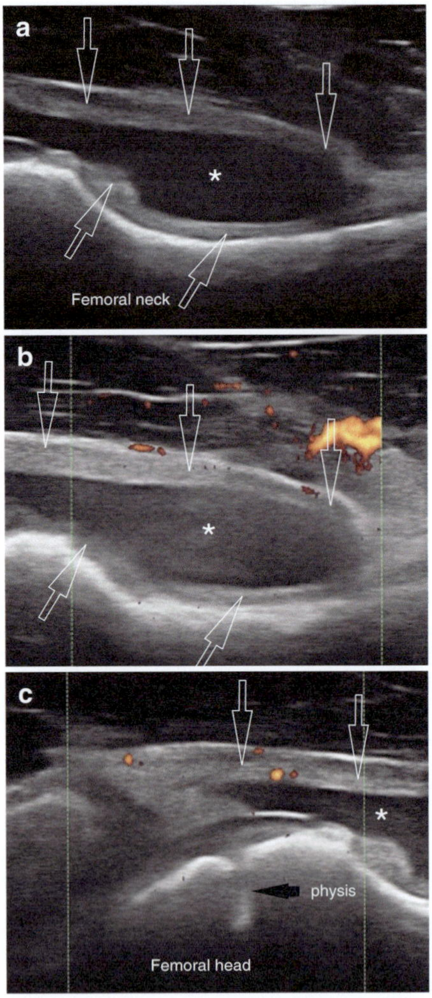

Fig. 15.17 Eight years old boy with juvenile spondyloarthritis. Hip synovitis (arrows) and effusion (∗). (**a**) Longitudinal view on femoral neck mode B. (**b**) Longitudinal view on femoral neck mode Doppler puissance. (**c**) Longitudinal view on femoral head and cotyle mode Doppler puissance

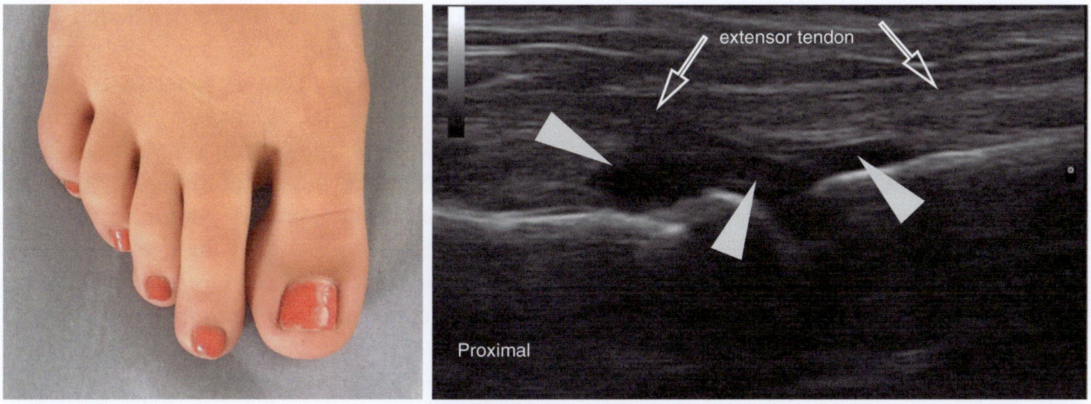

Fig. 15.18 Fifteen years old girl with psoriatic arthritis: 2nd métatarsophalangeal joint, longitudinal view synovitis (arrows)

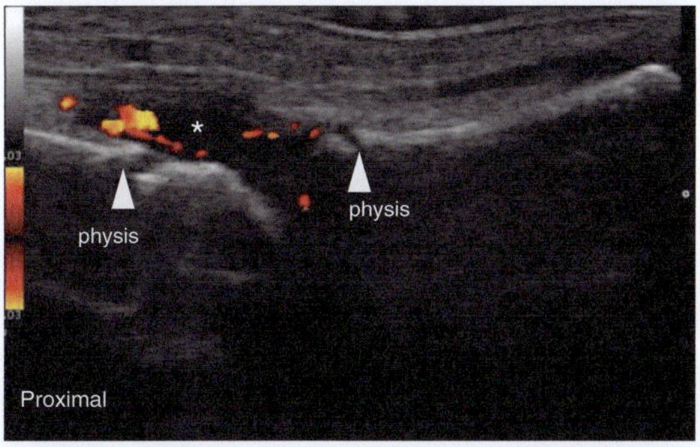

Fig. 15.19 Nine years old boy with psoriatic rheumatism: 2nd métatarsophangeal joint, longitudinal view active synovitis with positivity of power Doppler and effusion (∗)

Another point needs to be taken into consideration concerning the usefulness of US in pediatric MSK is its utility as in adults to guide and follow up steroid injection in joints with two studies on the ankle [47] and the wrist [48] and in a more recent retrospective study for tendon sheath injections [49]. Follow up of systemic medication may also be very useful [50, 51].

Today, many questions remain unknown and we are lacking specific studies addressing US synovitis and enthesitis follow-up in jSPA.

MR Imaging Modality

Until now, MRI is well known to be an important imaging modality for diagnosing and monitoring axial disease in JIA.

In a child referred for joint pain or effusion, dactylitis, or chronic back pain, the diagnosis of spondyloarthritis often remains challenging, especially in the axial form. Burgos Vargas et al. [52] and Goirand et al. [53] showed a low rate of symptomatic axial disease at onset but with a marked increase (60% of axial involvement after 5 years in 114 patients seen in a tertiary center), and some studies showed a worse prognosis in children with spondyloarthritis compared with adults [54]. Moreover, Bou Antoun et al. [55] showed a high rate of MRI sacroiliitis in children with ERA diagnosis as well as Stoll et al. in 2010 [56], even in the absence of suggestive symptoms or physical examination findings. Recent advances in management of SpA have made diagnostic ascertainment crucial, since biological agents have become available and proven major efficacy in axial SpA, especially, at the beginning of the disease.

In the same time, progress in imaging modalities with MRI has made possible an earlier diagnosis and a better prognosis for these patients. This and limitations of radiographic evaluation for sacroiliac joint, especially, in children have made MRI the first imaging technique for sacroiliac assessment in children (Weiss) [57].

Sacroiliac joint anatomy is complex and needs to be known for a correct MRI interpretation [58]. The joint is composed of two compartments: inferior and anterior cartilage-covered compartment correspond to a symphysis and superior; and posterior ligamentous portion compartment correspond to syndesmosis and contain strong interosseous ligament. Between both there is a transition zone of fibrocartilage [59, 60].

Evaluation of sacroiliac imaging remains difficult in the adults because of variation in joint anatomy [61] and influence of physical activity especially for the runners and in postpartum [62] and even more in children for the same reasons and due to growth cartilage presence depending on the age of the patient.

In 1997, Bollow et al. [63] described normal MRI sacroiliac joints findings in 102 children. The major differences with adults were cartilaginous connections between sacroiliac joints and the sacral foramina at the level of the intervertebral disks of the sacrum late in the adolescence. This ossification is completed earlier in girls than boys and this is the same for lateral apophysis of the sacral wings which is completed in all girls of 17 years old and sometimes only partially in boys at that age. As in adults, they underlined some pitfalls in children sacroiliac joints assessment as transitional vertebrae, accessory joint, and pelvic asymmetry (more frequent in females).

Twenty years later, in 2017, Zejden et al. [64] described normal anatomy of sacroiliac joints in children. They showed an important variation of normal osseous structure in children's sacroiliac joints with a progressive ossification between the sacral vertebrae. Ossified nuclei anterolateral at S1 and/or in the joint space were observed until the age of 18 years and occurred in 77% of individuals ≥13 years with intraarticular localization in 64% of girls and 60% of boys. More important, joint facet defects >3 mm occurred in 17% located to both the iliac and sacral joint facets.

The ASAS group (Assessment of Spondyloarthritis International Society) has recently revised the criteria of MRI lesion definitions for sacroiliitis in adults [58, 65–67]:

As before, sacroiliitis elementarylesions are divided in active lesions (Figs. 15.20 a–c, 15.21 and 15.22 a–c) and structural lesions (Figs. 15.20 a–c, 15.21 and 15.22 a–c).

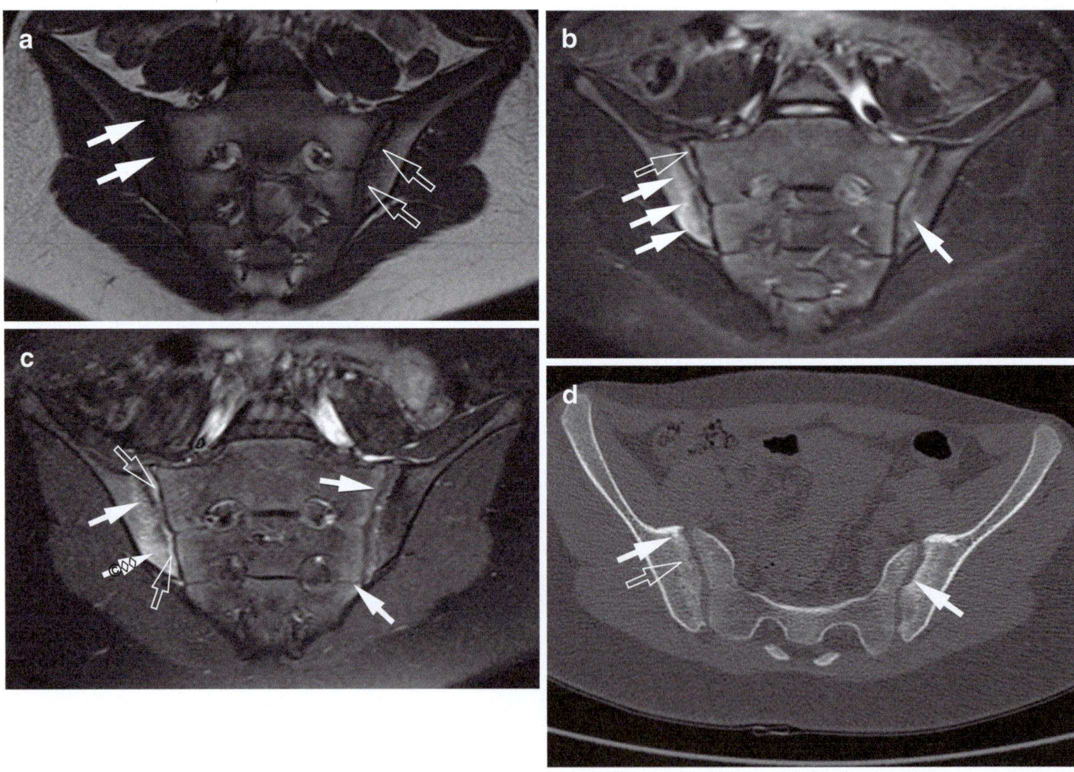

Fig. 15.20 Fourteen years old girl: (**a**) Coronal T1 sequence. Bone marrow edema (plain arrows) and erosions (empty arrows). (**b**) Coronal STIR sequence. Bone marrow edema (plain arrows) and synovitis (empty arrows). (**c**) Coronal FAT SAT contrast sequence. Bone marrow edema (plain arrows) and synovitis (empty arrows). (**d**) Tomodensitometry axial showing bone condensation (plain arrows) and erosion (empty arrow)

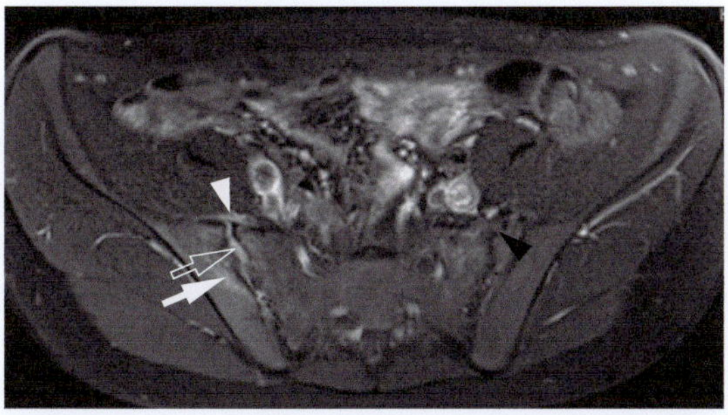

Fig. 15.21 Fourteen years old boy: axial FAT SAT contrast enhanced sequence. Bone marrow edema (plain arrow), synovitis (empty arrow) and enthesitis (short arrow). On the opposite side, there are older lesions with a fusion onset in the anterior portion of the sacroiliac joint (black arrow)

Active lesions are defined as subchondral bone edema, enthesitis, and joint space enhancement (which means increased signal in contrast-enhanced images in the joints space of the cartilaginous portion of the sacroiliac joint and replaces the term synovitis and capsulitis). Bone marrow edema is defined as increased signal intensity in the bone marrow on short tau inversion recovery (STIR) or T2-weighted fat-saturated (T2FS) sequence. It must be present in typical anatomical areas for spondyloarthritis inflammation, i.e., in the joint subchondral areas. But as ever seen, bone marrow edema may occurs in healthy persons and in patients with other diseases, including mechanical diseases such as degenerative changes, osteitis condensans ilii, insufficiency fractures, as well as tumor of infection [67]. Enthesitis is an increased signal in bone marrow and/or soft issue on STIR or T1FS post-contrast sequences at ligaments and tendons attach sites. It's frequent in spondyloarthritis and rare in other diagnosis or healthy persons. It can be found in the three parts of the joint and also on other sites of the pelvis (e.g., pelvic symphysis, big and small trochanter, iliac crest). Capsulitis is defined by an increase signal on STIR and/or T1FS post-gadolinium images where synovium is present in the anterior and inferior portion of the joint. However, it is not possible to distinguish between capsule and synovium with MRI and therefore capsulitis is globally evaluated with synovitis. Synovitis is well visualized with gadolinium contrast enhancement with an increased volume of synovium. It needs contrast to be separated from joint effusion, and the added value of contrast for synovitis visualization is yet unexplored. All these reasons have made the concept of joint space enhancement emerged in the last work of the ASAS group [65].

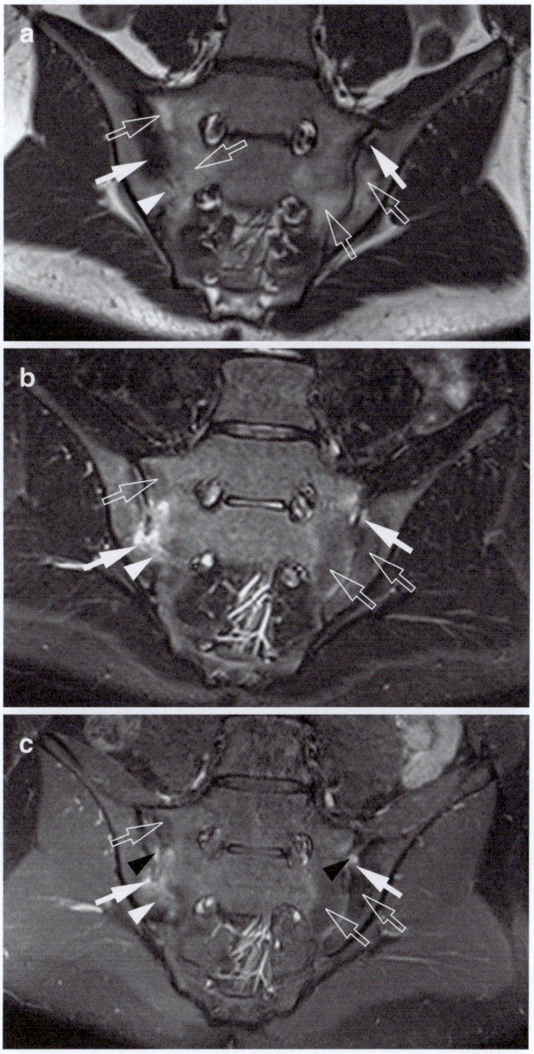

Fig. 15.22 Sixteen years old boy with inflammatory back pain for 7 years. (**a**) Coronal T1 sequence. Bone marrow edema (plain arrows), fat metaplasia (empty arrows) and joint fusion (short arrow). (**b**) Coronal T2 STIR sequence. Bone marrow edema (plain arrows), fat metaplasia (empty arrows) and joint fusion (short arrow). (**c**) Coronal FAT SAT contrast enhanced sequence. Bone marrow edema (plain arrows), fat metaplasia (empty arrows), joint fusion (short arrow) and synovitis (short black arrow)

Structural lesions appear later (i.e., erosions, fat metaplasia, backfill, ankylosis, and sclerosis). Erosions are both a cortical defect (loss of the dark signal of the subchondral bone plate) and bone marrow matrix defect. They are very specific for the diagnosis of SpA. Erosions may be difficult to assess on T1-weighted sequences and better visualized on high-resolution thin-slice MRI sequences. Fat metaplasia is the reason for a subchondral increased signal intensity in the bone marrow on T1 and decreased signal on STIR or T2FS sequences. It indicates previous inflammation and may reflect a reparative process associated with an increased propensity toward ankylosis, but it may also be seen in normal elderly individuals and in case of degenerative disease. Backfill is the presence of high T1 signal intensity within an erosion or erosive cavitation at the joint surface. It may represent a synovial metaplasia or ongoing new born formation and is very specific for sacroiliitis in SpA with 96% specificity. Moreover, backfill has a high prevalence in patients with sacroiliitis and a sensitivity of 38% [68].

Finally, ankylosis is a continuity of bright marrow signal in T1 sequences across the joint space connecting the ileum and sacrum. It is very specific for SpA but occurs at the end stage of the disease and is not suitable for early diagnosis. It can also be seen in septic sacroiliitis, trauma, and diffuse idiopathic skeletal hyperostosis. Sclerosis is an area with very low signal intensity on all sequences located in the subchondral bone with a depth of at least 5 mm. It has a moderate specificity of 70% [58] and is frequent in mechanical diseases. Moreover for these authors, the association of bone marrow edema and sclerosis decreases the specificity for a diagnosis of SpA compared with the presence of bone marrow edema alone.

One must be careful to assess the diagnosis of sacroiliitis and if bone marrow edema remains the most important and common MRI features and its specificity is low. A global appreciation of all features with several lesions is mandatory avoiding false positive or negative MRI reports [69].

Inflammatory changes in the sacroiliac joints are frequent in juvenile spondyloarthritis [70] and in ERA diagnosed patients [55] sometimes before any clinical manifestation [55–57], but the classification or diagnostic criteria used in adults seems to be not applicable in juvenile patients.

Bollow in 1998 [71] studied prospectively 100 children with suspected juvenile spondyloarthritis and 30 controls found 42.9% of active inflammatory changes in sacroiliac joints while radiographs remains normal. Even chronic lesions were detected more frequently on MRI (14.3%) than on radiographs (6.7%). Patients with MRI active lesions had higher levels of CRP and longer history of illness.

More recently Jaremko in 2014 [72], in a retrospective study on 26 patients and 35 controls, showed a high diagnostic utility for diagnostic for MRI (likelihood ratios LR = 9.4) without any false positive. They emphasize the presence of bone marrow edema in 20% of patients and 9% of controls. Fat infiltration was less frequent in patients but even more in controls with LR = 4.5 for fat infiltration and 3.1 for bone marrow edema. Sclerosis was also seen in controls and had a poor utility. Erosions had a good utility for diagnosis (LR = 6.7) even if it can be present in controls. Importantly, most patients have multiple erosions and that can help in case of doubt for a particular image interpretation.

Herregod et al. [69] conducted, in 2017, a retrospective study on all MRI for suspected juvenile spondyloarthropathy in 109 patients. They evaluated each examination results with either a global assessment or with the ASAS adult definition. Those patients clinically having a juvenile spondyloarthritis were considered positive with the expert global assessment and only half (12/23) had fulfilled the ASAS criteria. In the 62 patients clinically not having spondyloarthritis, 7 were found MRI positive with the global assessment and among them only 2 were ASAS MRI positive. Importantly none of the ASAS MRI negative were found positive with the global assessment and conversely all ASAS MRI positive were also positive with the global assessment had the same specificity and a slightly lower sensitivity (49%) as in adults, but ASAS definition had a much lower sensitivity (26% versus 67–79%) and a better specificity. The most important differences between these two evaluations were in the global assessment that bone marrow edema was present only on one slice or location, or presence of synovitis capsulitis enthesitis, or structural lesions without bone marrow edema. Including bone marrow edema only on one slice in the definition, the authors found the sensitivity rose from 26% to 36% with a lowering of specificity only from 97% to 95%. One of the explanations for somewhat different sacroiliac joints changes in children and adolescents compared with adults is the persistence of growth-related edematous changes, sometimes the smaller size of the joint and lack of a clear delineation of minor osseous structures by MRI because of the slice thickness; suggested a pediatric-specific definition of MRI positive sacroiliitis including BME lesions visible only on one slice, synovitis, and capsulitis.

The authors suggested inclusion of bone marrow edema on only one slice, synovitis, and capsulitis in the definition of ASAS MRI criteria for children.

MRI is very useful for sacroiliac exploration but can also explore pelvic entheses. Herregods et al. in 2015 [73] showed a high association (74%) between presence of sacroiliitis and pelvic enthesitis in children on the MRI (without contrast enhancement as in ASAS guidelines) [74]. Moreover, pelvic enthesitis was found in 15% with clinically evident enthesitis but also in 17% of children without any clinical pelvic enthesitis. Given that the existence of pelvic enthesitis may be helpful for spondyloarthropathy diagnosis in children, pediatric rheumatologists and radiologist have to keep in mind these data and look at the different pelvic entheses sites with attention. Yilmaz et al. [75] had the same results in a smaller study.

MRI may also have a role in monitoring patients. Lin et al. [76] conducted a study in 2014 and confirmed the valuable role or MRI in the initial evaluation and showed the important role of MRI evaluation for treatment monitoring of children with spondyloarthropathy. Moreover, synovial enhancement was significantly reduced after treatment, but unlike adults, synovial enhancement may be detected without accompanying bone marrow edema, which suggests gadolinium contrast may be an important component in the assessment of children with spondyloarthropathy. Another goal of this work was to study association between clinical manifestation and MRI. One must emphasize the high association between hip arthritis and sacroiliitis. Indeed, hip arthritis was found in 79% of children with hip pain and associated with sacroiliitis in 90% of subjects. The same results were found by Stoll et al. [56]. Later Herregods et al. [73] found an association between pelvic enthesitis and sacroiliitis in 31% of children. Pelvis enthesitis was always associated with either sacroiliitis or hip arthritis. During outcome, they emphasize the absence of correlation between the bone marrow edema presence and the clinical outcome because of possible secondary osteoarthritis and mechanical change. All must keep in mind that bone marrow edema does not always reflect active inflammation.

MRI is very useful to explore sacroiliac joints but can also explore lumbar spine. Vendhan et al. in 2014 [77] conducted a retrospective study in 79 children diagnosed as enthesitis-related arthritis and having low back pain and 21 controls. They showed that the majority (67%) of ERA cases with sacroiliitis had abnormalities of the lumbar spine and particularly apophyseal joints synovitis and interspinous ligaments inflammatory changes. Interestingly, 71% of patients with normal sacroiliac imaging had abnormalities of the lumbar spine. Even if a small number of children are concerned (7 in this study) it can be helpful for the diagnosis in case of normal sacroiliac findings and inflammatory low back pain.

All these studies used different MRI sequences with contrast use. But the necessity of contrast enhancement is still not clear.

Herregods et al. in 2015 [78] conducted a prospective study on 80 children suspected for sacroiliitis and found a similar sensitivity and specificity for sacroiliitis for STIR and T1/Gado sequences as well as for bone marrow edema, capsulitis, and enthesitis. Weiss et al. [79] in the same time showed the same results in 51 patients with the presence of bone marrow edema but also of synovitis and capsulitis. Nevertheless, contrast administration may help to confirm the presence of synovitis in cases with a high STIR signal in the joint alone [68].

Another technique has been described by Vendhan et al. [80] for quantifying sacroiliac inflammation in children with enthesitis-related arthritis using a diffusion-based quantification technique. They showed in a retrospective study on 10 patients and 10 controls a very good correlation with STIR sequence with a good reproducibility, and this technique could be useful to quantify inflammation and efficacy of therapy. However it needs further refinement and validation.

Recently the contrast enhancement safety has been questioned both in adults and children with possible nephrogenic systemic fibrosis in patients with a poor renal function and also gadolinium deposition in the brain of the patients with normal renal function. Macrocyclic formulation is recommended for their best stability. Therefore the necessity of using gadolinium-based contrast agent in children have to be considered carefully for each examination [81, 82].

Finally even if MRI criteria for sacroiliitis are still missing in children, and despite the fact that classification of juvenile idiopathic arthritis remains unclear for juvenile spondyloarthritis diagnosis, it is a key feature for diagnosis of sacroiliitis in children. The risk for having sacroiliitis in case of suspicion of juvenile spondyloarthritis is the presence of B27 HLA, high CRP levels [79], and presence of hip arthritis [78]. Pelvic MRI should be proposed in each of these situations and maybe in undifferentiated arthritis because of the presence of sacroiliitis at the beginning of the disease in about 10% of children without any back pain of sacroiliac tenderness [55–57].

References

1. Petty RE, Laxer RM, Lindsley CB, Wedderburn LR. Textbook of pediatric rheumatology. 7th ed. Philadelphia: Elsevier; 2016.
2. Petty RE, Southwood TR, Manners P, Baum J, Glass DN, Goldenberg J, et al. International league of associations for rheumatology classification of juvenile idiopathic arthritis: second revision, Edmonton, 2001. J Rheumatol. 2004;31(2):390–2.
3. Azouz EM, Duffy CM. Juvenile spondyloarthropathies: clinical manifestations and medical imaging. Skelet Radiol. 1995;24:399–408.
4. Burgos-Vargas R, Clark P. Axial involvement in the seronegative enthesopathy and arthropathy syndrome and its progression to ankylosing spondylitis. J Rheumatol. 1989;16:192–7.
5. Hofer M. Spondylarthropathies in children—are they different from those in adults? Best Pract Res Clin Rheumatol. 2006;20:315–28.
6. Weiss PF, Chauvin NA, Klink AJ, Localio R, Feudtner C, Jaramillo D, Colbert RA, Sherry DD, Keren R. Detection of enthesitis in children with enthesitis-related arthritis: dolorimetry compared to ultrasonography. Arthritis Rheumatol. 2014 Jan;66(1):218–27.
7. Jousse-Joulin S, Breton S, Cangemi C, Fenoll B, Bressolette L, de Parscau L, Saraux A, Devauchelle-Pensec V. Ultrasonography for detecting enthesitis in juvenile idiopathic arthritis. Arthritis Care Res (Hoboken). 2011 Jun;63(6):849–55.
8. Shenoy S, Aggarwal A. Sonologic enthesitis in children with enthesitis-related arthritis. Clin Exp Rheumatol. 2016 Jan–Feb;34(1):143–7.
9. Burgos-Vargas R, Vazquez-Mellado J. The early clinical recognition of juvenile-onset ankylosing spondylitis and its differentiation from juvenile rheumatoid arthritis. Arthritis Rheum. 1995;38:835–44.
10. Balint PV, Kane D, Wilson H, McInnes IB, Sturrock RD. Ultrasonography of entheseal insertions in the lower limb in spondyloarthropathy. Ann Rheum Dis. 2002;61:905–10.
11. McGonagle D, Marzo-Ortega H, Benjamin M, Emery P. Report on the second international enthesitis workshop. Arthritis Rheum. 2003;48:896–905.
12. Magni-Manzoni S. Ultrasound in juvenile idiopathic arthritis. Pediatr Rheumatol Online J. 2016 May 27;14(1):33.
13. Shaw HM, Vázquez OT, McGonagle D, Bydder G, Santer RM, Benjamin M. Development of the human Achilles tendon enthesis organ. J Anat. 2008 Dec;213(6):718–24.
14. Grechenig W, Mayr JM, Peicha G, Hammerl R, Schatz B, Grechenig S. Sonoanatomy of the Achilles tendon insertion in children. J Clin Ultrasound. 2004;32(7):338–43.
15. Jousse-Joulin S, Cangemi C, Gerard S, Gestin S, Bressollette L, de Parscau L, Devauchelle-Pensec V, Saraux A. Normal sonoanatomy of the paediatric entheses including echostructure and vascularisation changes during growth. Eur Radiol. 2015 Jul;25(7):2143–52.
16. Chauvin NA, Ho-Fung V, Jaramillo D, Edgar JC, Weiss PF. Ultrasound of the joints and entheses in healthy children. Pediatr Radiol. 2015 Aug;45(9):1344–54.
17. Roth J, Ravagnani V, Backhaus M, Balint P, Bruns A, Bruyn GA, Collado P, De la Cruz L, Guillaume-Czitrom S, Herlin T, Hernandez C, Iagnocco A, Jousse-Joulin S, Lanni S, Lilleby V, Malattia C, Magni-Manzoni S, Modesto C, Rodriguez A, Nieto JC, Ohrndorf S, Rossi-Semerano L, Selvaag AM, Swen N, Ting TV, Tzaribachev N, Vega-Fernandez P, Vojinovic J, Windschall D, D'Agostino MA, Naredo E, OMERACT ultrasound group. Preliminary definitions for the sonographic features of synovitis in children. Arthritis Care Res (Hoboken). 2017 Aug;69(8):1217–23.

18. Roth J, Jousse-Joulin S, Magni-Manzoni S, Rodriguez A, Tzaribachev N, Iagnocco A, Naredo E, D'Agostino MA, Collado P, Outcome Measures in Rheumatology Ultrasound Group. Definitions for the sonographic features of joints in healthy children. Arthritis Care Res (Hoboken). 2015 Jan;67(1):136–42.
19. Benjamin M, Moriggl B, Brenner E, et al. The "enthesis organ" concept: why enthesopathies may not present as focal insertional disorders. Arthritis Rheum. 2004;50:3306–13.
20. Petty R, Cassidy JT. Juvenile ankylosing spondylitis. In: Textbook of pediatric rheumatology. 4th ed. Philadelphia: WB Saunders; 2001. p. 323–44.
21. Walker J, Rang M, Daneman A. Ultrasonography of the unossified patella in young children. J Pediatr Orthop. 1991;11:100–92.
22. Blazina M, Kerlan RK, Jobe F, et al. Jumper's knee. Orthop Clin North Am. 1973;4:665–78.
23. Gisslen K, Alfredson H. Neovascularisation and pain in jumper's knee: a prospective clinical and sonographic study in elite junior volleyball players. Br J Sports Med. 2005;39:423–8.
24. Terslev L, Qvistgaard E, Torp-Pedersen S, et al. Ultrasound and power Doppler findings in jumper's knee. Preliminary observations. Eur J Ultrasound. 2001;13:183–9.
25. Davies S, Baudonin CJ, King JB, Perry JD. Ultrasound, computed tomography and magnetic resonance imaging in patellar tendonitis. Clin Radiol. 1991;43:52.
26. McLoughlin R, Raber EL, Vellet AD, et al. Patellar tendinitis: MR imaging features, with suggested pathogenesis and proposed classification. Radiology. 1995;197:843–8.
27. Ehrenborg G, Engfeldt B. The insertion of the ligamentum patellae on the tibial tuberosity. Some views in connection with the Osgood-Schlatter lesion. Acta Chir Scand. 1961;121(Jun–Jul):491–9.
28. Ogden JA, Southwick WO. Osgood-Schlatter's disease and tibial tuberosity development. Clin Orthop Relat Res. 1976;116:180–9.
29. Spannow AH, Pfeiffer-Jensen M, Andersen NT, et al. Ultrasonographic measurements of joint cartilage thickness in healthy children: age- and sex-related standard reference values. J Rheumatol. 2010;37:2595–601.
30. Pradsgaard D, Spannow AH, Heuck CW, et al. Joint cartilage thickness measured by ultrasound in juvenile idiopathic arthritis. Pediatr Rheumatol. 2012;10(Suppl 1):A35.
31. Basra HAS, Humphries PD. Juvenile idiopathic arthritis: what is the utility of ultrasound? Br J Radiol. 2017;90:20160920.
32. Wakefield RJ, Balint PV, Szkudlarek M, et al. Musculoskeletal ultrasound including definitions for ultrasonographic pathology. J Rheumatol. 2005;32:2485–7.
33. Colebatch-Bourn AN, Edwards CJ, Collado P, et al. EULAR-PRes points to consider for the use of imaging in the diagnosis and management of juvenile idiopathic arthritis in clinical practice. Ann Rheum Dis. 2015;74:1946–57.
34. Uson J, Loza E, Möller, et al. Recommendations for the use of ultrasound and magnetic resonance in patients with spondyloarthritis, including psoriatic arthritis, and patients with juvenile idiopathic arthritis. Reumatol Clin. 2018;14(1):27–35.
35. Nguyen JC, Lee KS, Thapa, et al. US evaluation of juvenile idiopathic arthritis and osteoarticular infection. Radiographics. 2017;37(4):1181–201.
36. Erik Nielsen H, Strandberg C, Andersen S, et al. Ultrasonographic examination in juvenile idiopathic arthritis is better than clinical examination for identification of intraarticular disease. Dan Med J. 2013;60:3.
37. Magni-Manzoni S, Epis O, Ravelli A, et al. Comparison of clinical versus ultrasound-determined synovitis in juvenile idiopathic arthritis. Arthritis Care Res. 2009;61:1497–504.
38. Haslam KE, McCann LJ, Wyatt S, et al. The detection of subclinical synovitis by ultrasound in oligoarticular juvenile idiopathic arthritis: a pilot study. Rheumatology (Oxford). 2010;49:123.
39. Shelmerdine SC, Di Paolo PL, Tanturri de Horatio L, et al. Imaging of the hip in juvenile idiopathic arthritis. Pediatr Radiol. 2018;48(6):811–7.
40. Rooney ME, McAllister C, Burns JF. Ankle disease in juvenile idiopathic arthritis: ultrasound findings in clinically swollen ankles. J Rheumatol. 2009;36:1725–9.
41. Janow GL, Panghaal V, Trinh A, et al. Detection of active disease in juvenile idiopathic arthritis: sensitivity and specificity of the physical examination vs ultrasound. J Rheumatol. 2011;38:2671–4.
42. Shahin AA, Shaker OG, Kamal N, et al. Circulating interleukin-6, soluble interleukin-2 receptors, tumor necrosis factor alpha, and interleukin-10 levels in juvenile chronic arthritis: correlations with soft tissue vascularity assessed by power Doppler sonography. Rheumatol Int. 2002;22:84–8.
43. Magni-Manzoni S, Scire CA, Ravelli A, et al. Ultrasound-detected synovial abnormalities are frequent in clinically inactive juvenile idiopathic arthritis, but do not predict a flare of synovitis. Ann Rheum Dis. 2013;72:223–8.
44. Zhao Y, Rascoff NE, Iyer RS, et al. Flares of disease in children with clinically inactive juvenile idiopathic arthritis were not correlated with ultrasound findings. J Rheumatol. 2018;45(6):851–7.
45. Miotto E, Silva VB, Mitraud SAV, Furtado, et al. Patients with juvenile idiopathic arthritis in clinical remission with positive power Doppler signal in joint ultrasonography have an increased rate of clinical flare: a prospective study. Pediatr Rheumatol Online J. 2017;15(1):80.
46. De Lucia O, Ravagnani V, Pregnolato, et al. Baseline ultrasound examination as possible predictor of relapse in patients affected by juvenile idiopathic arthritis (JIA). Ann Rheum Dis. 2018;77:1426–31.

47. Court-Payen M, Nielsen S, Zak M, et al. Ultrasonography and color Doppler in juvenile idiopathic arthritis: diagnosis and follow-up of ultrasound-guided steroid injection in the ankle region. A descriptive interventional study. Pediatr Rheumatol Online J. 2011;9:4.
48. Laurell L, Court-Payen M, Nielsen S, et al. Ultrasonography and color Doppler in juvenile idiopathic arthritis: diagnosis and follow-up of ultrasound-guided steroid injection in the wrist region. A descriptive interventional study. Pediatr Rheumatol Online J. 2012;10:11.
49. Peters SE, Laxer RM, Connolly BL, Parra DA. Ultrasound-guided steroid tendon sheath injections in juvenile idiopathic arthritis: a 10-year single-center retrospective study. Pediatr Rheumatol Online J. 2017;15(1):22.
50. Lovell DJ, Giannini EH, Reiff A, et al. Etanercept in children with polyarticular juvenile rheumatoid arthritis. N Engl J Med. 2000;342:763–9.
51. Lanni S, van Dijkhuizen EHP, Vanoni F, et al. Ultrasound changes in synovial abnormalities induced by treatment in juvenile idiopathic arthritis. Clin Exp Rheumatol. 2018;36(2):329–34.
52. Burgos-Vargas R, et al. Pediatr Rheumatol. 2012;10:14.
53. Goirand M, Breton S, Chevallier F, et al. Clinical features of children with enthesitis-related juvenile idiopathic arthritis/juvenile spondyloarthritis followed in a French tertiary care pediatric rheumatology centre. Pediatr Rheumatol. 2018;16:21.
54. Stone M, Warren RW, Bruckel J, et al. Juvenile-onset ankylosing spondylitis is associated with worse functional outcomes than adult-onset ankylosing spondylitis. Arthritis Rheum. 2005;53(3):445–51.
55. Bou Antoun M, Adamsbaum C, Semerano L, et al. Clinical predictors of magnetic resonance imaging-detected sacroiliitis in children with enthesitis related arthritis. Joint Bone Spine. 2017;84:699–702.
56. Stoll ML, Bhore R, Dempsey-Robertson M, Punaro M. Spondyloarthritis in a pediatric population: risk factors for sacroiliitis. J Rheumatol. 2010;37(11):2042–8.
57. Weiss PF, Xiao R, Biko DM, Chauvin NA. Assessment of Sacroiliitis at diagnosis of juvenile spondyloarthritis by radiography, magnetic resonance imaging, and clinical examination. Arthritis Care Res (Hoboken). 2016;68:187–94.
58. Jans L, Egund N, Eshed I, et al. Sacroiliitis in axial spondyloarthritis: assessing morphology and activity. Semin Musculoskelet Radiol. 2018;22(2):180–8.
59. Egund N, Juik AG. Anatomy and histology of the sacroiliac joints. Semin Musculoskelet Radiol. 2014;18(03):332–9.
60. Puhakka KB, Melsen F, Jurik AG, et al. MR imaging of the normal sacroiliac joint with correlation to histology. Skelet Radiol. 2004;33(01):15–28.
61. El Rafei M, Badr S, Lefebvre G, et al. Sacroiliac joints: anatomical variations on MR images. Eur Radiol. 2018 Jun 6; https://doi.org/10.1007/s00330-018-5540-x.
62. De Winter J, de Hooge M, van de Sande M, et al. Magnetic resonance imaging of the sacroiliac joints indicating sacroiliitis according to the assessment of spondyloarthritis international society definition in healthy individuals, runners, and women with postpartum back pain. Arthritis Rheumatol. 2018 Mar 7; https://doi.org/10.1002/art.40475.
63. Bollow M, Braun J, Kannenberg J, et al. Normal morphology of sacroiliac joints in children: magnetic resonance studies related to age and sex. Skelet Radiol. 1997;26:697–704.
64. Zejden A, Jurik AG. Anatomy of the sacroiliac joints in children and adolescents by computed tomography. Pediatr Rheumatol. 2017;15:82.
65. Maksymowych WP, Lambert RG, Østergaard M, et al. MRI lesion definitions in axial spondyloarthritis: a consensus reappraisal from the assessments in spondyloarthritis international society (ASAS). Ann Rheum Dis. 2018;77:356–7.
66. Lambert GW, Bakker PA, Van der Heijde D, Weber U, Rudwaleit M, et al. Defining active sacroiliitis on MRI for classification of axial spondyloarthritis: update by the ASAS MRI working group. Ann Rheum Dis. 2016;75:1958–63.
67. Rudweileit M, Jurik AG, Hermann KG, et al. Defining active sacroiliitis on magnetic resonance imaging (MRI) for classification of axial spondyloarthritis: a consensual approach by the ASAS/OMERACT MRI group. Ann Rheum Dis. 2009;68(10):1520–7.
68. Laloo F, Herregods N, Varkas G, et al. MR signals in the sacroiliac joint space in spondyloarthritis: a new sign. Eur Radiol. 2017;27(05):2024–30.
69. Herregods N, Dehoorne J, Van den Bosch F, et al. ASAS definition for sacroiliitis on MRI in SpA: applicable to children? Pediatr Rheumatol. 2017;15:24.
70. Strom H, Lindvall N, Hellstrom B, Rosenthal L. Clinical, HLA, and roentgenological follow up study of patients with juvenile arthritis: comparison between the long term outcome of transient and persistent arthritis in children. Ann Rheum Dis. 1989;48:918–23.
71. Bollow M, Braun J, Biedermann T, et al. Use of contrast-enhanced MR imaging to detect sacroiliitis in children. Skelet Radiol. 1998;27:606–16.
72. Jaremko JL, Liu L, Winn NJ, et al. Diagnostic utility of magnetic resonance imaging and radiography in juvenile spondyloarthritis: evaluation of the sacroiliac joints in controls and affected subjects. J Rheumatol. 2014;41(5):963–70.
73. Herregods N, Dehoorne J, Pattyn E, et al. Diagnositic value of pelvic enthesitis on MRI of the sacroiliac joints in enthesitis related arthritis. Pediatr Rheumatol. 2015;13:46.
74. Sieper J, Rudwaleit M, Baraliakos X, et al. The assessment of spondyloarthritis international society (ASAS) handbook: a guide to assess spondyloarthritis. Ann Rheum Dis. 2009;68:ii1–44E.
75. Yilmaz MH, Ozbayrak M, Kasapcopur O, et al. Pelvic MRI findings of juvenile-onset ankylosing spondylitis. Clin Rheumatol. 2010;29(9):1007–13.

76. Lin C, MacKenzie JD, Courtier JL, et al. Magnetic resonance imaging findings in juvenile spondyloarthropathy and effects of treatment observed on subsequent imaging. Pediatr Rheumatol. 2014;12:25.
77. Vendhan K, Sen D, Fisher C, et al. Inflammatory changes of the lumbar spine in children and adolescents with enthesitis-related arthritis: magnetic resonance imaging findings. Arthritis Care Res. 2014;66(1):40–6.
78. Herregods N, Jaremko JL, Baraliakos X, et al. Limited role of gadolinium to detect active sacroiliitis on MRI in juvenile spondyloarthritis. Skelet Radiol. 2015;44(11):1637–46.
79. Weiss PF, Xiao R, Biko DM, et al. Detection of inflammatory sacroiliitis in children with magnetic resonance imaging: is gadolinium contrast enhancement necessary? Arthritis Rheumatol. 2015;67(8):2250–6.
80. Vendhan K, Bray TJ, Atkinson D, et al. A diffusion-based quantification technique for assessment of sacroiliitis in adolescents with enthesitis-related arthritis. Br J Radiol. 2016;89(1059):20150775.
81. Pasquini L, Napolitano A, Visconti E, et al. Gadolinium-based contrast agent-related toxicities. CNS Drugs. 2018;32(3):229–40.
82. Soares BP, Lequin MH, Huisman TAGM. Safety of contrast material use in children. Magn Reson Imaging Clin N Am. 2017;25(4):779–85.

Part IV

Musculoskeletal US in Standard Pediatric Practice

Pediatric Musculoskeletal Ultrasonography: A Clinician's Tool

16

Alice Leahy

The usefulness of ultrasound (U/S) in paediatric rheumatology has been well established and is extensively covered elsewhere in this book. The emphasis in this chapter is therefore to look more specifically at what ultrasound in the hands of the clinician, rather than the radiologist, can bring to the management of children in paediatric rheumatology clinics. The use of U/S for guiding joint injections is also dealt with elsewhere, so this chapter will focus on diagnostic use.

The following areas will be covered:

- Uses of U/S in clinical settings
- Advantages of clinician scanning vs radiology scanning
- The specific challenges for the paediatric rheumatologist scanning children: how their images differ from those of adult joints
- Subclinical inflammation, prediction of flares/remission: update of the evidence
- Future directions

In the adult rheumatology world the use of ultrasound by rheumatologists is established, and increasing numbers of consultants are now routinely scanning patients in clinic. In the UK now a majority of adult rheumatology trainees are opting to train in ultrasonography. Training courses and materials are abundant, and U/S training is a part of the curriculum for specialist certification (albeit still an optional module). Scanning patients' joints in clinic is an integral part of many services, and is one of the ways in which early arthritis is picked up, remission is diagnosed, and response to treatment is assessed.

Paediatric rheumatologists have been slower to take up ultrasound scanning, and some of the reasons for this will be discussed. Ultrasound scans of children's joints are usually performed by radiologists, usually in a separate department, and often require another visit to the hospital sometime after the paediatric rheumatology clinic appointment. A recent survey looked at attitudes of paediatric rheumatologists in Europe and North America to MSK U/S [1]. There was only a 36% response rate to the survey, but of those who responded only 34% were doing ultrasound themselves (41% of Europeans, 28% of North Americans). Reasons cited for not doing it included a fear of excessive workload, and satisfaction with the service they received from their radiology departments. Both of these obstacles to change will be addressed in this chapter.

A. Leahy (✉)
Paediatric Rheumatology, University Hospital Southampton, Southampton, UK
e-mail: Alice.Leahy@uhs.nhs.uk

Y. El Miedany (ed.), *Pediatric Musculoskeletal Ultrasonography*,
https://doi.org/10.1007/978-3-030-17824-6_16

How Can Ultrasound Serve Us in the Context of a Clinical Consultation?

- *Reassurance for the 'worried well'*:

A significant proportion of the children that we see in paediatric rheumatology clinics have non-inflammatory or 'mechanical' joint symptoms and seek reassurance that they do not have arthritis.

In most cases this reassurance can be given as a verbal explanation based on careful history taking and joint examination. However, we sometimes find that patients or their parents remain worried and convinced that their child has a rheumatological disease underlying their symptoms.

Performing an ultrasound scan, showing the child and parents the normal looking joint and pointing out the absence of pathology (effusion, positive Doppler, etc.) can be an extremely useful adjunct in this situation, by enhancing the patient's understanding of normal and abnormal joints and showing what seems like objective 'proof' of joint health, reinforcing the opinion of the examining physician.

Many people seem to find the scan images more persuasive than verbal reassurances based on examination, and leave the consultation more satisfied and able to proceed with physiotherapy exercises. We know that ultrasound has a high negative predictive value [2], allowing us to confidently rule out inflammatory activity in the face of a normal scan combined with normal clinical examination.

- *Enhancing the clinical encounter and improving compliance*:

When patients with Juvenile idiopathic arthritis (JIA) are found to have active synovitis, the paediatric rheumatologist responds by initiating or escalating treatment.

There are some patients and families who, for a variety of reasons, are resistant to starting immune suppression, resulting in sometimes difficult discussions trying to 'persuade' them into compliance.

In some cases it may be that the reluctance is caused by, or compounded by, an inability to see or understand the meaning of active synovitis and its potential to cause long-term joint damage.

Undertaking an ultrasound scan of the joint can contribute in a positive way to this interaction. Showing the child and their parents the abnormal joint, pointing out the effusion, the thickened synovium, and the positive Doppler (the 'fire' in the joint) can make it much easier to conceptualise the pathology, especially when compared with another normal joint.

Many people are visual learners, and do not fully grasp things until they see them, often finding it hard to believe there is a potentially serious problem in a joint which may not be causing much pain or functional difficulty to the child (Figs. 16.1 and 16.2).

In this situation the ultrasound scan, as an integral part of the clinical interaction, clearly needs to be performed by the clinician leading the discussion, rather than postponed and done in a radiology department by someone with no knowledge of the family. This is another example of how, in order to be optimally effective, ultrasound needs to be integrated into the conversation between the patient and their treating physician.

- *As a therapeutic intervention*:

As well as demonstrating absence of pathology to the 'worried well', ultrasound in the clinic room can be extremely helpful as a way of reassuring children who have had arthritis and who have gone into remission on treatment, or stayed in remission off treatment.

- *Providing us with an additional clinical tool when signs are not obvious*:

Our clinical examination can often yield equivocal findings, for example when there is only very subtle (or no) swelling, when the patient is obese, when we are querying active synovitis in a treated joint with persistent swelling/stiffness but no heat, or in patients with learning difficulty who may sometimes not complain

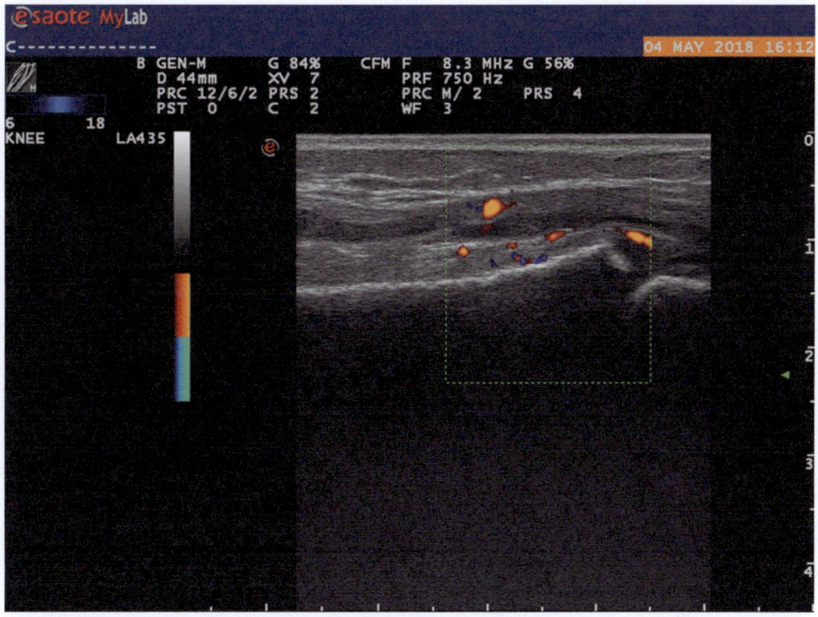

Fig. 16.1 Effusion, synovial hypertrophy, and positive PD signal in the knee of a child whose parents did not believe the diagnosis of JIA, because of the child's lack of pain and disability. After demonstrating the ultrasound findings and comparing them with the normal appearances on the contralateral knee, the family was happy to move on and accept the diagnosis and treatment without further delay

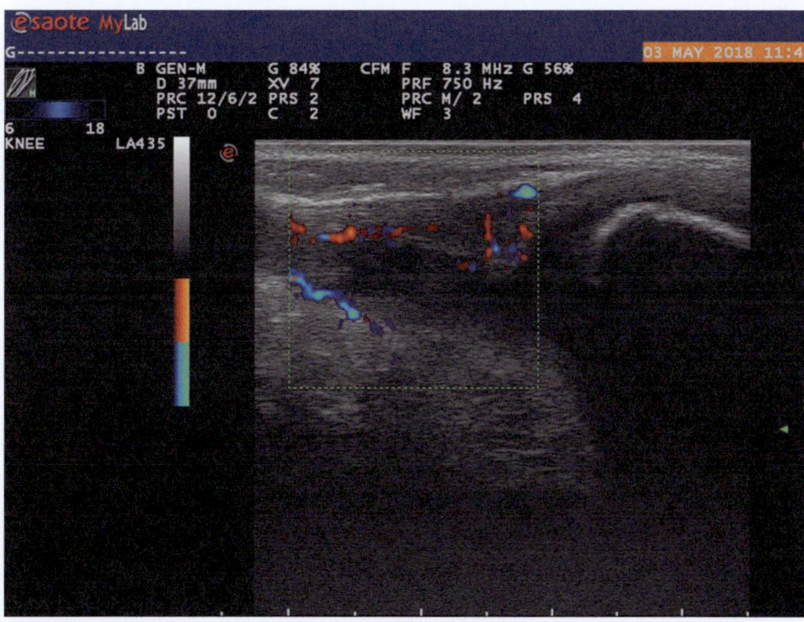

Fig. 16.2 Effusion, synovial thickening, and positive PD signal in a child who had come off treatment for his JIA 1 year previously, and could not accept that he had relapsed and needed treatment again. The swelling in the knee was subtle and he had little in the way of symptoms. Demonstration of the ultrasound abnormalities played a significant role in the conversation, and the family eventually allowed a joint injection

of pain or tenderness, and who may also be significantly hypermobile (Fig. 16.3).

- *Improving anatomical accuracy:*

Children may present with generalised swelling in a joint (particularly a wrist or an ankle) so that it is sometimes difficult to determine clinically which structures are affected (Fig. 16.4).

U/S has been shown to be superior to clinical examination at distinguishing between synovitis and tenosynovitis [3]. This allows for the correct structures to be targeted, e.g. by tendon sheath rather than intra-articular steroid injection.

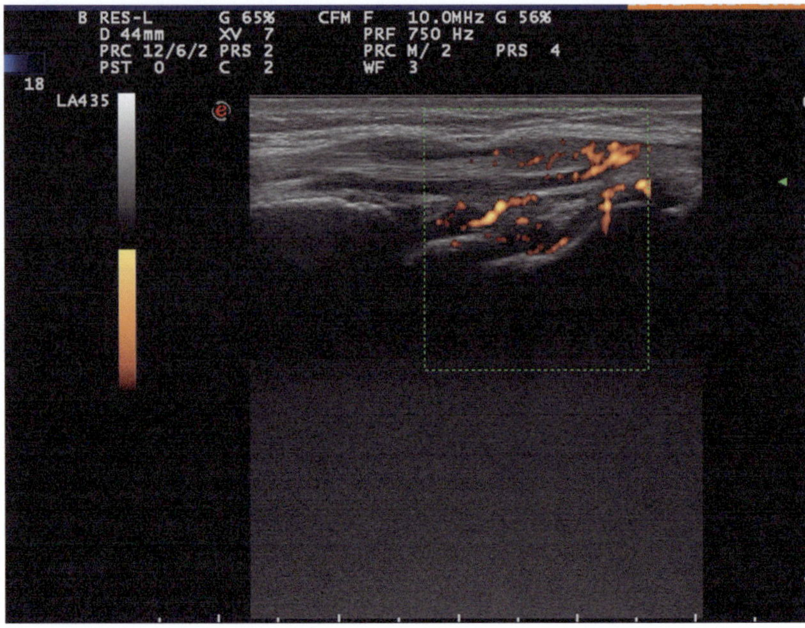

Fig. 16.3 Wrist scan from a girl with Trisomy 21 presenting with subtle loss of range in finger and toe joints. Asymptomatic wrists, clinically very little to find. U/S shows active synovitis and tenosynovitis

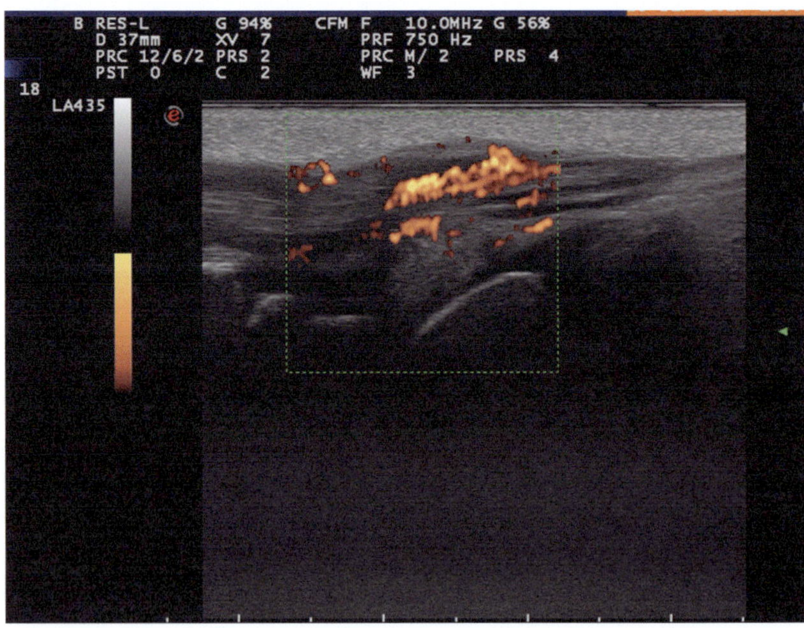

Fig. 16.4 Wrist scan of a child with boggy swollen tender wrist, listed for joint injection. U/S shows predominantly tenosynovitis

- *Detection of subclinical synovitis:*

We know that ultrasound is better at detecting synovitis than clinical examination [4]. We also know that U/S correlates well with MRI [5, 6], which is held to be the gold standard for detection of inflammatory joint disease (and itself correlates well with histological findings).

We do not yet however have the evidence to understand the clinical significance of ultrasound-detected synovitis in the context of negative clinical findings, or 'subclinical' synovitis [7].

Part of the reason why it has not yet been possible to demonstrate the ability of subclinical synovitis on U/S to predict disease flare is likely due to the lack of data showing ultrasound findings in normal joints up until recently.

It is easy to over-diagnose effusions in young children because of the presence of hypo-echoic hyaline cartilage, and to over-interpret positive power Doppler signals around the growth plates.

These limitations will be dealt with in depth later on in this chapter.

- *Monitoring treatment response:*

After initiating or escalating treatment for JIA, we need readily available and accurate means to determine response to treatment, thus allowing us to 'treat to target' effectively.

Comparing U/S images from before and after treatments during follow-up clinic appointments allows us to know in a timely fashion whether the treatment is having an effect, without the need to wait for confirmation from the radiology department.

- *Guided injections:*

The role of ultrasound in guiding intra-articular steroid injections has been established, especially in adults. This aspect of its clinical use will be covered in a separate chapter in this book.

The Advantages of Clinician Scanning over Radiology Scanning

One of the frequently heard objections to the development of clinician scanning from the paediatric rheumatology community is that the service many departments receive from their radiology colleagues is extremely good.

With a responsive radiology team, able to do ultrasound scans without significant delay or inconvenience for the patient, what is the advantage to the paediatric rheumatologist of going to great lengths and expense to deliver the same service themselves?

It is only once you have started scanning in clinic yourself that you come to realise that however excellent and prompt the radiologist-delivered service is, it can never be anywhere near as useful and flexible as that provided by the clinician with his or her scanner in the clinic room for every consultation. Some of the reasons for this include:

- The clinician can scan as many joints as they need at any given time.
- Scans will be undertaken during the clinic visit, thus obviating the need for a separate radiology department appointment. Not only does this improve the experience for patients and families, but it also reduces delays in diagnosis and treatment by giving the clinician an immediate answer to their clinical question.
- The clinician will scan joints on a background of intimate knowledge of the child's symptoms, signs, and history, thus giving a much better understanding of the clinical context of the imaging.
- The child will usually know and trust the clinician which may improve compliance with the procedure, especially in younger children.
- The scan will take place in a familiar environment which again may improve compliance and enhance the patient experience.
- If a clinician can scan, and has access to a portable scanner, they are then at liberty to scan wherever the procedure is needed, for example on inpatients on the ward, in theatres, and in outreach clinics in other hospitals.
- As well as being able to scan anywhere, the clinician with a scanner is also able to scan at any time without having to depend on the availability of a suitable radiologist. This includes out of hours or at weekends, before and after clinic hours.

This kind of flexibility and responsiveness can never be reproduced even in the most resource-rich and compliant radiology department. Just as cardiologists will never now relinquish their mastery of echocardiography having taken it out of radiologists' hands, for the paediatric rheumatologist skilled in the use of ultrasound in children's joints there is no turning back.

The Challenges of Clinician Scanning

1. Ultrasound scanners are expensive and many clinicians have struggled to persuade hospital managers to fund what is perceived to be non-essential kit.

In the author's case the money for both scanners (one main-frame machine used in clinic and one portable one for use around the hospital and in outreach clinics) was raised by parents quite quickly. Parents and patients understood the potential advantage to them of having in-clinic scanning, and were thus highly motivated to fundraise.

Since then, having been persuaded of the benefits to the service, and to the over-subscribed radiology department, the author's hospital management have been willing to pay for upkeep and repairs.

Companies are often able to offer cheaper ex-demonstration machines, and will waive VAT when payment is coming from charitable funds.

2. It is not easy to learn to scan children's joints. There are very few skilled clinician-sonographers around to teach and train others, and in the author's experience most radiologists do not have the time or inclination to train rheumatologists how to scan either.

There are MSK ultrasound courses in Europe and North America, but these are almost exclusively adult oriented. Paediatric courses are infrequent and geographically sparse. Whilst attending adult U/S courses is useful initially, to gain familiarity with the principles and techniques of scanning, and to get used to navigating the controls, the focus on these courses is towards adult type pathologies.

3. Similarly there is a paucity of teaching resources for those wishing to learn to scan children's joints. There are online courses and image atlases for adult rheumatologists but very few similar materials for paediatricians.

Up until recently the main obstacle to developing teaching materials for budding clinician-ultrasonographers in paediatric rheumatology has been the lack of data on normal values in children. The sonographic appearances of children's joints change with growth and development, making distinction between normal and pathology much more challenging for the learner. Atlases of normal appearances from infancy to full skeletal development are still in relatively early stages of development [8].

4. Evidence for the usefulness of ultrasound by clinicians is lacking. Much of the focus on the use of ultrasound in rheumatology is around the detection of 'subclinical' synovitis.

Thus far, for reasons explained later in this chapter, the evidence to support this function in paediatric rheumatology has been mixed [7, 9, 10] unlike in the adult world, where evidence to support the ability of ultrasound to pick up clinically significant synovitis missed by clinical examiners is robust [11].

Whilst there are many other important uses of ultrasound in clinic, as outlined above, the uncertainty of its reliability in this area may put some clinicians off committing to it, and potentially weaken business cases put to managers.

5. Not all joints are amenable to ultrasound. Ultrasound is not useful in the detection of spinal or temporomandibular arthritis.

Some joints are more challenging to scan than others; this author has found glenohumeral and subtalar joints difficult to master although that is by no means a universal experience.

Hip joints are easy to scan in slim children but can it be very difficult to get useful images in obese subjects.

6. Another very common concern raised by sceptical clinicians is that there simply is not

enough time in a busy clinic to include ultrasound as a routine adjunct to clinical examination.

Up until now this author has not had to reduce clinic numbers or lengthen clinic times to absorb scanning time. In most situations the scan takes a matter of minutes and can actually reduce the amount of time needed for explanation or 'persuasion'.

However, we do not currently scan every child every time they come to clinic. Nor do we scan a significant number of clinically normal joints routinely. If robust evidence emerges (as we suspect it will) to show the usefulness of ultrasound in detecting 'subclinical' synovitis in children, then the imperative to scan more joints, in more children, on more occasions may change the shape of our clinics and necessitate longer appointments.

Scanning a sample of joints which are clinically normal, either to confirm/refute a diagnosis of remission, or to produce an accurate joint count and thus determine ILAR classification status, in all children with JIA, could increase clinic time from 15 to 20 or 25 minutes per patient depending on the chosen joint sample size [12–14].

The Particular Challenges of Scanning Children's Joints

One of the reasons why ultrasound has not been taken up by paediatric rheumatologists with the enthusiasm of their adult counterparts is the difficulty interpreting children's images in the light of the changing appearances according to age and skeletal development, and the lack of easily accessible normal data for all age groups across childhood.

The key sources of difficulty in interpreting U/S images, especially for people who are used to scanning adults:

1. The growing edges of ossification centres are often uneven or ragged and can thus be confused with erosions by a sonographer unfamiliar with scanning healthy children's joints (Fig. 16.5).
2. In children there can be prominent vascularisation of the epiphysis, and anastomosis of metaphyseal and epiphyseal vessels through the growth plate (feeding vessels). This normal physiological vascularity can be detected on ultrasound and potentially mistaken for pathological PD signal, as can reverberation

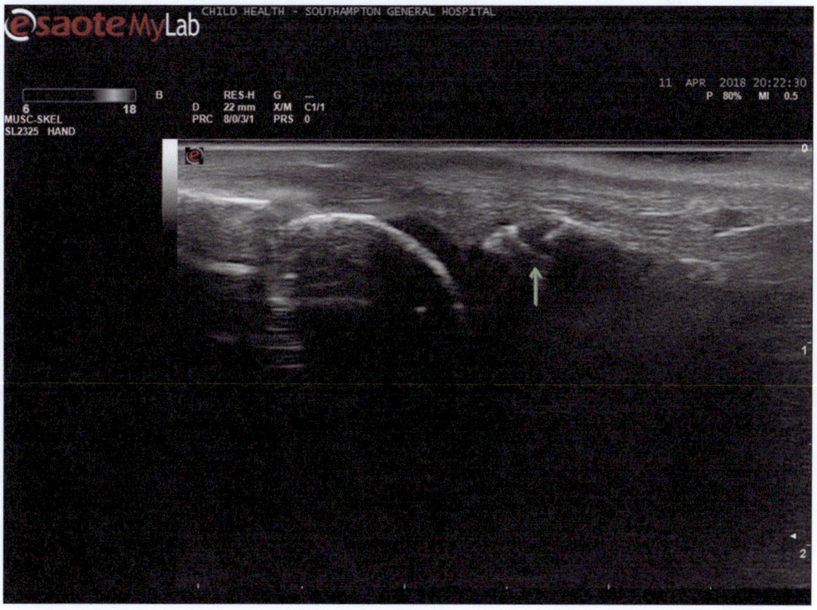

Fig. 16.5 Irregular appearance of growth plate in finger of healthy child

from nearby large vessels (Figs. 16.6, 16.7, 16.8, 16.9, 16.10, and 16.11).

3. At birth a large percentage of infant bone consists of unossified cartilage. Ossification centres in the epiphyses gradually enlarge with growth until the child reaches full skeletal maturation in late puberty. There is therefore wide age-related variation in the thickness of articular cartilage. To a sonographer used to scanning adults' joints, the wide anechoic cartilaginous space can easily be mistaken for effusion (Figs. 16.7, 16.12, and 16.13).

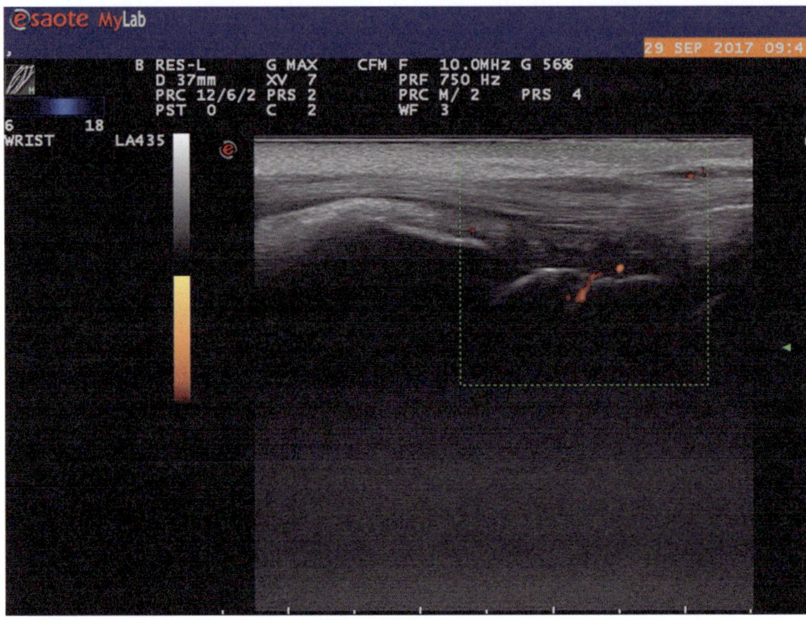

Fig. 16.6 An example of a feeder vessel in the wrist of a healthy child

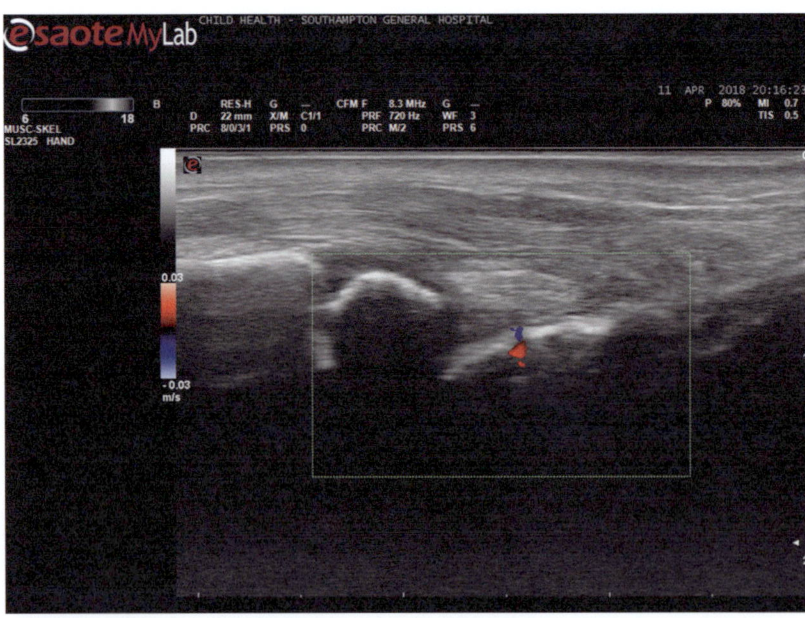

Fig. 16.7 Doppler signal in wrist of healthy child. Note the colour box in this image is not correctly placed at the top of the picture, but the findings were unchanged when it was correctly positioned

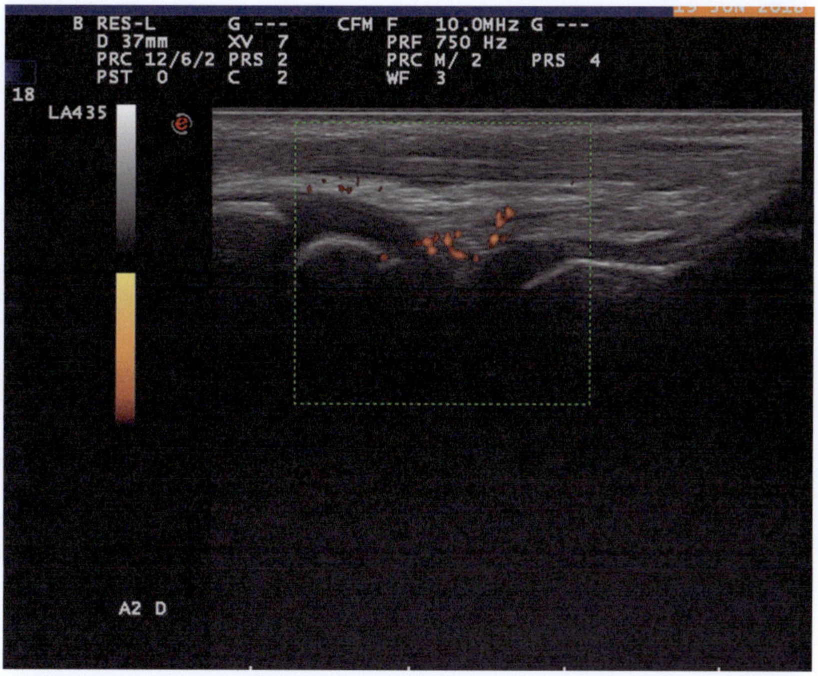

Fig. 16.8 Greyscale image of the same child showing growth plate in carpal bone corresponding to Doppler signal in previous image

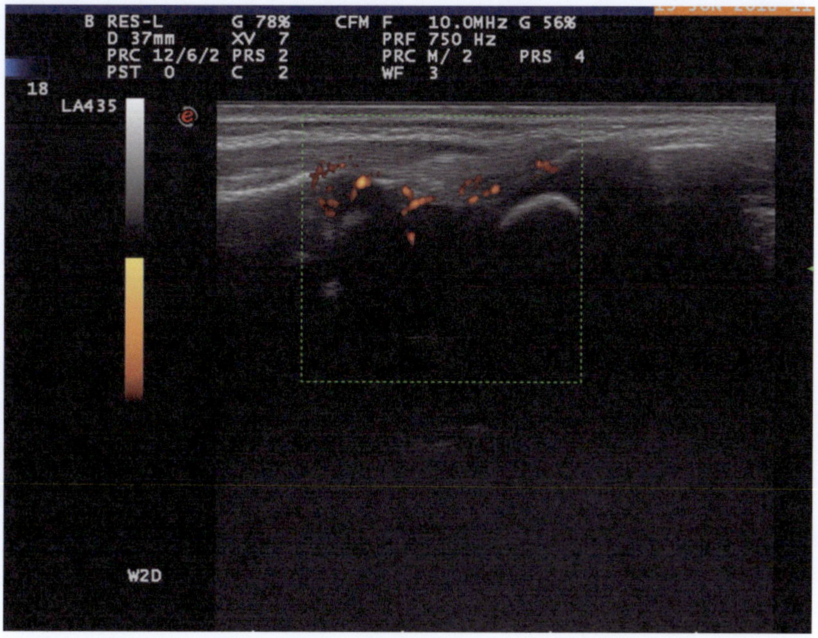

Fig. 16.9 Longitudinal images of tibiotalar joint in healthy children (aged 7, 5, and 3 clockwise from top right) showing wide anechoic articular cartilage

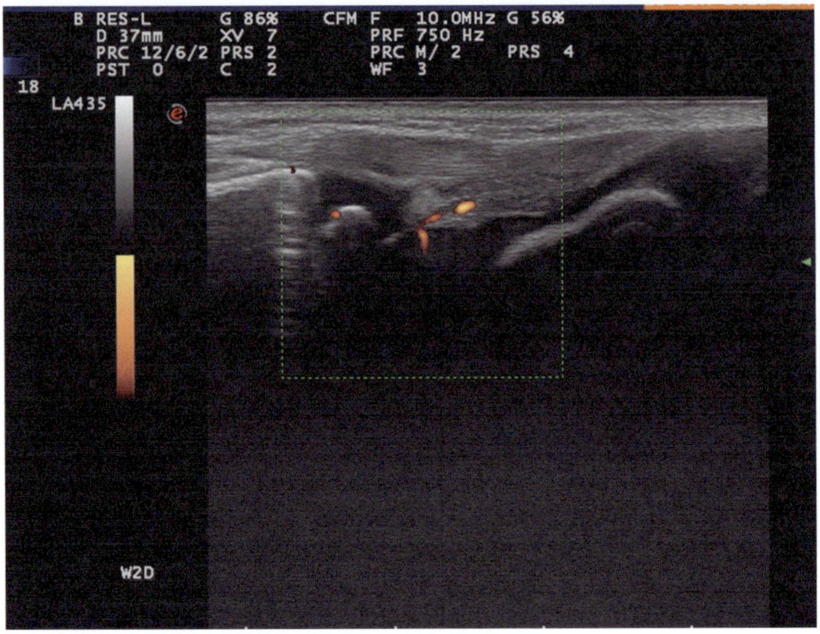

Fig. 16.10 Doppler signal in ankle of healthy child without JIA

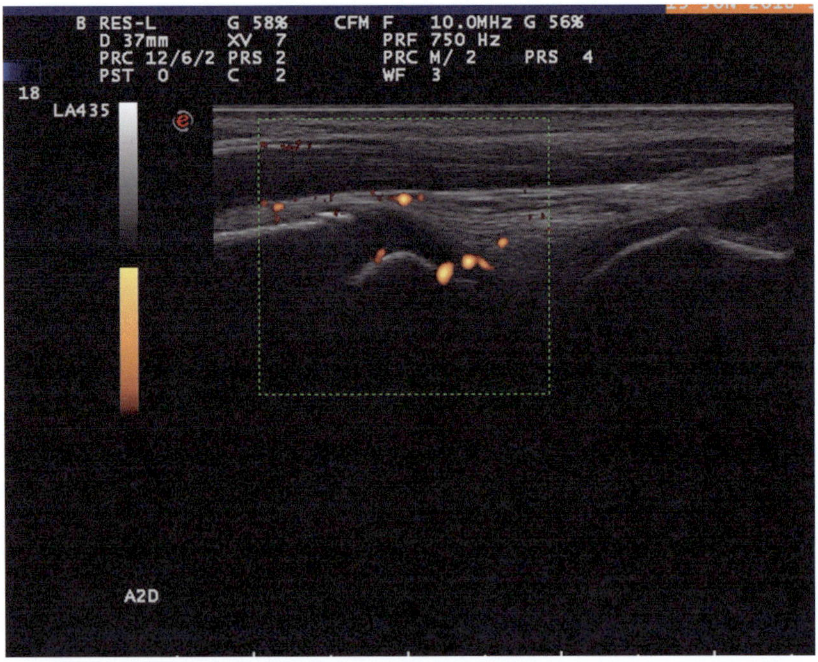

Fig. 16.11 Doppler signal in wrist of healthy child without JIA. Note significant reverberation from unseen (in this view) overlying blood vessel. When seen in transverse view, the relationship to the vessel is clear, and it cannot thus be mistaken for synovitis

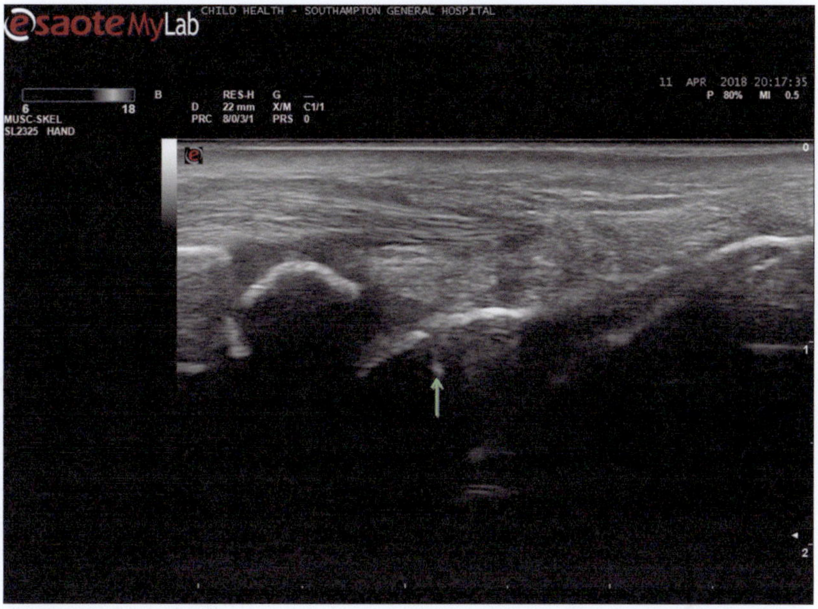

Fig. 16.12 Doppler signal in wrist of healthy child without JIA

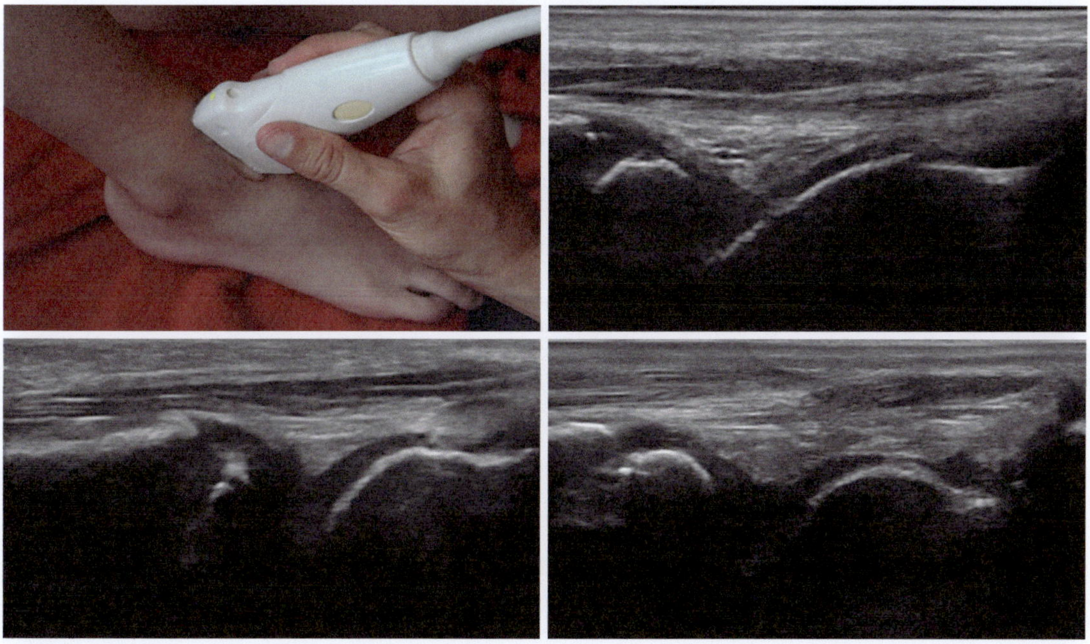

Fig. 16.13 Doppler signal in ankle of healthy child without JIA, showing feeder vessel as well as reverberation from overlying vessel

The Role of Ultrasound in Detecting Subclinical Synovitis

We know that ultrasound has better sensitivity than clinical examination in terms of picking up synovitis. Ultrasound correlates well with MRI, which in turn correlates well with histological findings [15, 16].

Some patients thought to be in remission based on clinical findings show abnormalities on ultrasound suggestive of persistent synovitis [17].

The question that remains un-answered relates to the significance of these abnormal ultrasound findings in the context of clinical remission. Are they a true reflection of ongoing disease activity? Can subclinical synovitis found on ultrasound be used to guide treatment decisions or to form the basis for a joint count which will place the child into an ILAR subtype?

In adults there is now a growing body of evidence to show the usefulness of subclinical synovitis as a predictor of disease flare in patients in clinical remission [11, 18, 19, 26].

However the evidence in children remains inconclusive. Janow et al. in 2011 [10] did demonstrate progression to clinically detected active synovitis in children with abnormal baseline U/S of clinically inactive joints. But Magni-Manzoni et al. [7] in 2013 showed that ultrasound-detected subclinical synovitis did not predict disease flare. However, the study authors conceded that part of the reason for that might have been the lack of standardised definitions of the appearances of healthy joints. We know that the presence of synovial thickening may persist after acute inflammation has been controlled, and that small effusions may be found in healthy joints. The poor predictive value of power Doppler however was unexpected. However, as discussed above, the presence of Doppler signal may have been wrongly attributed to inflammation, instead of the physiological finding described in healthy growing joints. The study used a semi-quantitative scoring system to describe PD signals [20–23] which has not been validated in children, and does not take into account these normal variants in growing joints. All but two joints described as having positive Doppler signal were given the lowest possible score; the youngest children tended to have greater prevalence of Doppler signal and most of these stayed in remission despite this finding. In the light of subsequent work, it now seems likely that low-grade Doppler activity is a physiological finding, especially in younger children.

A more recent study [9] with similar numbers of subjects did show a correlation between positive PD on ultrasound and subsequent disease flare in children who were in clinical remission on treatment.

The work needed to describe and define the ultrasound appearances in normal joints is already underway [8, 24, 25]. Up till now however these have been conducted in relatively small numbers of healthy children.

With the scarcity of data on the appearance of healthy joints on ultrasound it has not yet been possible to draw up definitions of pathological appearances. It will take much larger studies of healthy joints to be able to define the thresholds between normal and pathological signs, and only then will it be possible to look at whether or not sonographic synovitis is a helpful marker of active disease in the context of clinical remission.

Future Directions

Until we have established the usefulness of detecting subclinical synovitis, it seems unlikely that there will be a big increase in the uptake of in-clinic scanning amongst paediatric rheumatologists. Whilst there are many benefits to clinician scanning, as described above, the cost and effort involved in developing this skill may be prohibitive without the extra more 'scientific' justification. Definitions of pathology, founded on robust data on normal appearances at different stages of growth and development, will hopefully enable ultrasound to become an established part of clinical practice in paediatric rheumatology. Once we have accumulated the necessary evidence we will then be in a position to:

- Use U/S as one of a panel of predictive biomarkers
- Develop training courses and materials
- Develop a module for trainees to be incorporated into curriculum
- Bring about full integration of U/S into clinical practice

Conclusions

Some of the benefits of using ultrasound in clinic are hard to quantify, and will need qualitative research to explore, but will also be very familiar to rheumatologists who use it routinely in clinical practice. These benefits derive from ultrasound's role in communication between patients and clinicians. The rheumatologist comes to rely upon the ability of the timely scan to reassure, to reinforce, to enhance, to convince, and sometimes to help to persuade. Ultrasound used in this way can sometimes fulfil a therapeutic as well as diagnostic role.

To be an effective tool it is best used contemporaneously, so as to be an integral part of the physician/patient/parent interaction. By sending the patient away to be scanned by a new person, in a different place at a different time we lose the impact and immediacy of a scan performed by a trusted and familiar person with an understanding and knowledge of the patient's particular story and needs.

At a rather more 'scientific' level ultrasound is known to be able to detect synovitis in clinically normal joints. We are still in the early stages of understanding the significance of these 'subclinical' findings, but there is growing evidence in paediatrics, and robust evidence in adult practice, that ultrasound will be part of a panel of biomarkers used to predict or confirm remission, response to treatment, and relapse on or off treatment. Current evidence suggests that whilst synovial hypertrophy may persist in inactive joints, and small effusions may be present in healthy joints, the presence of moderate- or high-grade (yet to be defined) Doppler signal, coinciding with greyscale changes, is very likely to prove significant in this context.

Once we have the evidence to support this hypothesis we will then be able to use ultrasound to produce accurate joint counts for the purposes of attributing ILAR classification status to our patients, and to help inform decisions about starting or stopping medications as well as improving the accuracy of joint counts for research purposes.

However, confirmation that subclinical synovitis carries important diagnostic and prognostic significance will also mean that it becomes imperative to scan a large number of joints (numbers yet to be defined) in all JIA children at every appointment. Clearly this cannot be accommodated by even the most amenable radiology department, so there will be a need for a huge increase in the number of paediatric rheumatologists competent in scanning children's joints, which in turn will have very significant implications for training in this specialty, just as there was when cardiologists began to take over echocardiography from radiologists.

Hence the importance of continued efforts to produce robust data on the normal appearances of all joints at all ages, to define pathology based on those, to develop learning materials using banks of images, and with these to build training modules into paediatric rheumatology curriculums.

References

1. Magni-Manzoni S, Collado P, Jousse-Joulin S, Naredo E, D'Agostino M-A, Muratore V, Merli P, Roth J on Behalf of the Paediatric Ultrasound Group of the OMERACT Ultrasound Task Force. Current state of musculoskeletal ultrasound in paediatric rheumatology: results of an international survey. Rheumatology. 2014;53:491–96. https://doi.org/10.1093/rheumatology/ket368.
2. Cellerini M, Salti S, Trapani S, D'Elia G, Falcini F, Villari N. Correlation between clinical and ultrasound assessment of the knee in children with monoarticular or pauci-articular juvenile rheumatoid arthritis. Pediatr Radiol. 1999;29:117–23.
3. Rooney ME, McAllister C, Burns JF. Ankle disease in juvenile idiopathic arthritis: ultrasound findings in clinically swollen ankles. J Rheumatol. 2009;36:1725–9.
4. Pascoli L, Wright S, McAllister C, Rooney M. Prospective evaluation of clinical and ultrasound findings in ankle disease in juvenile idiopathic arthri-

tis: importance of ankle ultrasound. J Rheumatol. 2010;37(11):2409–14. https://doi.org/10.3899/jrheum.091262. Epub 2010 Sep 15.
5. El-Miedany YM, Housny IH, Mansour HM, Mourad HG, Mehanna AM, Megeed MA. Ultrasound versus MRI in the evaluation of juvenile idiopathic arthritis of the knee. Joint Bone Spine. 2001;68:222–30.
6. Magni-Manzoni S, Epis O, Ravelli A, Klersy C, Veisconti C, Lanni S, et al. Comparison of clinical versus ultrasound determined synovitis in juvenile idiopathic arthritis. Arthritis Rheum. 2009;61:1497–504.
7. Magni-Manzoni S, Scirè C, Ravelli A, Klersy C, Rossi S, Muratore V, Visconti C, Lanni S, Merli P, Montecucco C. Ultrasound-detected synovial abnormalities are frequent in clinically inactive juvenile idiopathic arthritis, but do not predict a flare of synovitis. Ann Rheum Dis. 2013;72(2):223–8. https://doi.org/10.1136/annrheumdis-2011-201264.
8. Collado P, Vojinovic P, Nieto J, Windschall D, Magni-Manzoni S, Bruyn G, Iagnocco A, D'Agostino M, Naredo E on Behalf of the OMERACT Ultrasound Paediatric Group. Toward standardized musculoskeletal ultrasound in pediatric rheumatology: normal age-related ultrasound findings. Arthritis Care Res. 2016;68(3):348–56. https://doi.org/10.1002/acr.22670.
9. Miotto e Silva V, Mitraud S, Furtado R, Natour J, Len C, Terreri M. Patients with juvenile idiopathic arthritis in clinical remission with positive power Doppler signal in joint ultrasonography have an increased rate of clinical flare: a prospective study. Pediatr Rheumatol. 2017;15:80. https://doi.org/10.1186/s12969-017-0208-7.
10. Janow GL, Panghaal V, Trinh A, Badger D, Levin TL, Ilowite NT. Detection of active disease in juvenile idiopathic arthritis: sensitivity and specificity of the physical examination vs ultrasound. J Rheumatol. 2011;38(12):2671–4. https://doi.org/10.3899/jrheum.110360.
11. Scirè C, Montecucco C, Codullo V, Epis O, Todoerti M, Caporali R. Ultrasonographic evaluation of joint involvement in early rheumatoid arthritis in clinical remission: power Doppler signal predicts short-term relapse. Rheumatology. 2009;48:1092–7. https://doi.org/10.1093/rheumatology/kep171.
12. Naredo E, Gamero F, Bonilla G, Uson J, Carmona L, Laffon A. Ultrasonographic assessment of inflammatory activity in rheumatoid arthritis: comparison of extended versus reduced joint evaluation. Clin Exp Rheumatol. 2005;23:881–4.
13. Backhaus M, Ohrndorf S, Kellner H, et al. Evaluation of a novel 7-joint ultrasound score in daily rheumatologic practice: a pilot project. Arthritis Rheum. 2009;61:1194–201.
14. Collado P, Naredo E, Calvo C, ECO-JIA Study Group, et al. Reduced joint assessment vs comprehensive assessment for ultrasound detection of synovitis in juvenile idiopathic arthritis. Rheumatology. 2013;52:1477–84.
15. Collado P, Jousse-Joulin S, Alcalde M, Naredo E, D'Agostino M. Is ultrasound a validated imaging tool for the diagnosis and management of synovitis in juvenile idiopathic arthritis? A systematic literature review. Arthritis Care Res. 2012;64(7):1011–9. https://doi.org/10.1002/acr.21644.
16. Gaffney K, Cookson J, Blake D, Coumbe A, Blades S. Quantification of rheumatoid synovitis by magnetic resonance imaging. Arthritis Rheum. 1995;38:1610–7.
17. Rebollo-Polo M, Koujok K, Weisser C, Jurencak R, Bruns A, Roth J. Ultrasound findings on patients with juvenile idiopathic arthritis in clinical remission. Arthritis Care Res. 2011;63(7):1013–9. https://doi.org/10.1002/acr.20478.
18. Bruyn GA, Naredo E, Iagnocco A, Balint PV, Backhaus M, Gandjbakhch F, et al. The OMERACT ultrasound working group 10 years on: update at OMERACT 12. J Rheumatol. 2015;42(11):2172–6. https://doi.org/10.3899/jrheum.141462.
19. Naredo E, Wakefield RJ, Iagnocco A, Terslev L, Filippucci E, Gandjbakhch F, et al. The OMERACT ultrasound task force—status and perspectives. J Rheumatol. 2011;38(9):2063–7. https://doi.org/10.3899/jrheum.110425.
20. Backhaus M, Burmester GR, Gerber T, et al. Guidelines for musculoskeletal ultrasound in rheumatology. Ann Rheum Dis. 2001;60:641–9.
21. Wakefield RJ, Balint PV, Szkudlarek M, et al. Musculoskeletal ultrasound including definitions for ultrasonographic pathology. J Rheumatol. 2005;32:2485–7.
22. Naredo E, Collado P, Cruz A, et al. Longitudinal power Doppler ultrasonographic assessment of joint inflammatory activity in early rheumatoid arthritis: predictive value in disease activity and radiologic progression. Arthritis Rheum. 2007;57:116–24.
23. Naredo E, Rodríguez M, Campos C, et al. Validity, reproducibility, and responsiveness of a twelve-joint simplified power doppler ultrasonographic assessment of joint inflammation in rheumatoid arthritis. Arthritis Rheum. 2008;59:515–22.
24. Roth J, Jousse-Joulin S, Magni-Manzoni S, Rodriguez A, Tzaribachev N, Iagnocco A, Naredo E, D'Agostino M, Collado P. Definitions for the sonographic features of joints in healthy children. Arthritis Care Res. 2015;67(1):136–42. https://doi.org/10.1002/acr.22410.
25. Collado P, Windschall D, Vojinovic J, Magni-Manzoni S, Balint P, Bruyn G, Hernandez-Diaz C, Nieto J, Ravagnani V, Tzaribachev N, Iagnocco A, D'Agostino M, Naredo E. Amendment of the OMERACT ultrasound definitions of joints features in healthy children when using the DOPPLER technique. Pediatr Rheumatol. 2018;16:23. https://doi.org/10.1186/s12969-018-0240-2.
26. Brown AK, Conaghan PG, Karim Z, Quinn MA, Ikeda K, Peterfy CG, et al. An explanation for the apparent dissociation between clinical remission and continued structural deterioration in rheumatoid arthritis. Arthritis Rheum. 2008;58:2958–67.

Reporting Ultrasound Diagnosis and Findings

17

Anna Ciechomska

Introduction

Musculoskeletal ultrasound is becoming a popular technique supplementing physical examination in the *outpatient* clinic. Lack of radiation makes it a preferable imaging modality in paediatrics. When performed in the clinic, the formal reporting is frequently missing as the scan is considered a part of clinical assessment. The images are rarely stored to the picture archiving and communication system (PACS) which is usually not available outside radiology departments.

Meanwhile, the ultrasound report is a legal document and forms part of medical documentation. The responsibility for its accuracy lies with the person performing or verifying the scan. The report should therefore include specific information according to standards of best practice published by Royal College of Radiologists [1–3].

The purpose of this chapter is to familiarise readers with these standards for safe and effective performance.

Writing the Report

The official report should contain:

1. Patient's name and ID.
2. Name of patient's healthcare provider.
3. Location of ultrasound facility and contact information.
4. Date of the referral, scan, and report.
5. Clinical information provided in the referral letter including clinical problem and reason for the referral.
6. Region of the examination performed.
7. Name and position of the person performing the scan.
8. Description including normal sonoanatomy (structures assessed) and pathological findings:
   (a) Location
   (b) Size, accompanied by measurements (each pathological finding should be assessed and documented in two perpendicular planes)
   (c) Internal characteristics including sound attenuation (echogenicity and echo structure).
   (d) Blood flow characteristics (with grading if relevant)
   (e) Response to compression (compressible, movable, painful)
   (f) Borders/outline
   (g) Comparison with collateral side if relevant
   (h) Dynamic examination if relevant
9. Limitations and recommendations for additional studies.

A. Ciechomska (✉)
University Hospital Wishaw, Wishaw, UK

Y. El Miedany (ed.), *Pediatric Musculoskeletal Ultrasonography*,
https://doi.org/10.1007/978-3-030-17824-6_17

10. Impression or conclusion – this part should be an answer to main clinical question, include specific diagnosis where certain or a list of differential diagnoses. Further investigations or a specialist referral should be suggested if required.
11. Action taken – as joint aspiration, guided steroid injection, specialist referral.

The style of the report varies depending on the local practice. It should be concise and easy to understand, without ambiguity. Only the common abbreviation can be used with less common terms given in full. The irrelevant findings can be omitted and technical terms used only when the diagnosis is unclear and second opinion is sought (Table 17.1). The significance of measurements and appearances should be explained. Template for specific type or region of ultrasound examination can be used and the completely normal report can be abbreviated.

The report should be completed and transmitted to the referrer in a timely fashion in accor-

Table 17.1 Description of normal and common abnormal findings in musculoskeletal ultrasound using technical terms and its interpretation

	Normal	Abnormal	Interpretation
Bone	Smooth outline, hyperechoic contour with acoustic shadowing. Cortical break *can be seen* at location of growth plate in children	Irregular outline, cortical lesion seen in two planes	Erosion
		Bone overgrowth on the edges of the joint line	Osteophytes
		Bone overgrowth at the insertion of joint capsule, ligaments, tendons	Enthesophytes
Hyaline cartilage	Thickness depends on patient's age, anechoic, echoic dots (vessels), blood flow occasionally seen in young children. Ossification centres vary in appearance depending on patient's age	Thinning of cartilage, increased echogenicity, irregular subchondral bone	Chondromalacia
		Irregularity/fragmentation of ossification centres	Associated with injury or inflammation
Synovial tissue	Not seen	Thickening of synovial tissue	Synovial hypertrophy
		Increased vascularity	Synovitis
		Grade 1 Grade 2 Grade 3	Mild Moderate Marked
Synovial fluid	Not seen or modest	Moderate to marked increase in anechoic joint content	Effusion
Ligament	Fibrillar structure, anisotropy, no evidence of blood flow	Thickening of the ligament, decreased echogenicity, blurred echo structure, increased vascularity of ligament enthesis	Enthesitis
		Thickening, decreased echogenicity, blurred echo structure, +/−increased vascularity; Disrupted continuity Associated joint instability	Injury Partial or complete tear
		Hyperechoic lesions with acoustic shadowing	Calcifications
		Iso- or hyperechoic lesions with various acoustic shadowing	Urate deposits
		Thickening, decreased echogenicity, lack of anisotropy, blurred echo structure, increased vascularity	Tendinopathy

Table 17.1 (continued)

	Normal	Abnormal	Interpretation
Tendons	Fibrillar structure, anisotropy, no evidence of blood flow	Thickening of the tendon, decreased echogenicity, blurred echo structure, increased vascularity of tendon enthesis	Enthesitis
		Hypoechoic lesions, reduced thickness, disrupted continuity	Partial, longitudinal, complete tears
		Hyperechoic lesions with acoustic shadowing	Calcifications
		Iso- or hyperechoic slurred lesions with various acoustic shadowing	Urate deposits
		Solitary lesion within the tendon	Nodule (rheumatoid, tophi, other)
Tendon sheaths	Not seen	Hypoechoic tissue with or without increased vascularity surrounding tendon	Tenosynovitis
		Anechoic fluid surrounding tendon	Effusion
		Restricted tendon gliding on dynamic examination	Adhesions, tendon nodules, stenosing tenosynovitis
Retinaculum	Thin, fibrillar structure surrounding tendons in specific locations	Thickening of retinaculum, decreased echogenicity, increased vascularity, irregular bone at insertion	Enthesitis
		Thickening of the retinaculum with restriction in tendon passing on dynamic examination with or without increased vascularity	Stenosing tenosynovitis (when related to A1 pulley) De Quervain's tenosynovitis (when related to first compartment extensors)
Nerves	Hypoechoic fascicles surrounded by thin, hyperechoic epineurium	Thickening of the nerve, decreased echogenicity, blurred echostructure, thickening of epineurium; flattening of the nerve at the site of compression	Entrapment

dance *with* national guidelines. *In case of critical and urgent findings, reporter is obliged to inform the referrer using local alert mechanisms.*

When the ultrasound scan supplements the physical examination during patient visit in clinic and is performed and reported by clinician for their own use, then only the region of examination, interpretation, and diagnosis are included in the report which becomes a part of clinic letter.

Person performing ultrasound examination should work only within scope of their practice and competence. Systematic audit of practice, learning feedback, and attendance on multidisciplinary team meetings should be applied to maintain high-quality practice.

Image Capture

Ultrasound images constitute an important medical documentation. The abnormal finding (including measurements and vascularity) should be *captured* as clearly as possible and in two perpendicular planes. Common bone landmarks, site markers, and labelling on image are used for better orientation.

Images should be captured and labelled with minimum dataset which includes name, ID (e.g., CHI number), date of birth, gender, and postcode. Entering of data is time-consuming exercise and therefore often omitted when scan is performed in a busy outpatient clinic. When the ultrasound scanner is connected to PACS, patient demographics are easily accessible using DICOM modality work-list (DMWL). In such situation, the images are acquired, stored and are accessible to review in the DICOM format.

When the departmental scanner is not connected to PACS, the images are archived locally. The internal memory drive of the scanner allows storing of large number of images and clips which can be useful for monitoring of treatment.

For the safety of patients' data, the images should not be transferred on the external memory drives unless the encrypted systems are used. This however can pose a problem when transferring images from the local memory drive of scanner. The cooperation between the ultrasound manufacturer representative and hospital IT might be required to allow for transferring data for teaching purposes. Some scanners are equipped with a software which allow blinding of patients' data for image transfer.

Conclusions

- Ultrasound report is a legal document and should be composed according to standards of best clinical practice.
- The report can be included in clinical letter when examination is performed by the person responsible for patient's care.
- The ultrasound images are important part of medical documentation.
- The images labelled with patients' personal data should be transferred using encrypted systems.

References

1. Royal College of Radiologists: Standards for the communication of radiological reports and fail-safe alert notification. Clin Radiol. 2016;BFCR(16)4. https://www.rcr.ac.uk/publication/standards-communication-radiological-reports-and-fail-safe-alert-notification. Accessed 1 Jun 2016.
2. Royal College of Radiologists: Standards for the provision of an ultrasound service. Clin Radiol. 2014;BFCR(14)17. https://www.rcr.ac.uk/publication/standards-provision-ultrasound-service. Accessed 5 Dec 2014.
3. Royal College of Radiologists: Standards for interpretation and reporting of imaging investigations. 2nd ed. Clin Radiol. 2018;BFCR(18)1. https://www.rcr.ac.uk/publication/standards-interpretation-and-reporting-imaging-investigations-second-edition. Mar 2018.

18 US Guided Interventional Procedures in Paediatrics

Daniel Windschall and Johannes Roth

Introduction

In oligoarticular JIA, in particular, injections of corticosteroids into joints play an important and established role in anti-inflammatory treatment [1–5]. The knee is the most commonly affected and injected joint in JIA, but all peripheral joints can be safely and effectively injected with CS via ultrasound guidance. Ultrasound guidance improves the precise identification of the target as well as the accuracy of the needle placement within the joint space, tendon sheath, or around the enthesis [6–8]. It can be challenging to inject very small joint regions in younger children without any imaging guidance, and incorrectly placed CS injections can potentially damage the cartilage and soft tissue structures in these younger patients. Ultrasound techniques have undergone marked development over the last two decades, so that all joint and tendon structures are clearly shown by the newer high-resolution ultrasound devices. High-frequency ultrasound probes with frequencies of up to 20 MHz help to safely guide the needle into the targeted structure. Studies have shown that ultrasound guidance increases the safety and efficacy of intraarticular injections in rheumatic patients [9–13]. Ultrasound guidance of the needle has no negative side effects in pediatric patients and does not increase the time required for the injection procedure.

D. Windschall (✉)
Pediatric Clinic, Asklepios Hospital Weissenfels, Weissenfels, Germany

University of Halle-Wittenberg, Halle, Germany
e-mail: d.windschall@asklepios.com

J. Roth (✉)
University of Ottawa, Ottawa, ON, Canada

Division of Pediatric Dermatology and Rheumatology, Children's Hospital of Eastern Ontario, Ottawa, ON, Canada
e-mail: jroth@cheo.on.ca

Indications

While the most important and established role of ultrasound consists of guiding injections of CS in pediatric rheumatology, there are various other indications in the management of patients with joint or tendon complaints.

First, ultrasound guidance may help to identify the underlying diagnosis in a child with arthritis or tenosynovitis by precisely guiding the needle into the targeted structure (e.g., intraarticular fluid) for aspiration [14]. In the initial round of differential diagnosis of joint inflammation, it may be very important to differentiate between septic arthritis, infection-related arthritis like Lyme arthritis, chronic rheumatic diseases, and traumatic lesions.

Second, ultrasound guidance helps to avoid side effects related to the inadvertent perforation and injury of vessels, tendons, nerves, cartilage, or bone structures.

Y. El Miedany (ed.), *Pediatric Musculoskeletal Ultrasonography*,
https://doi.org/10.1007/978-3-030-17824-6_18

Third, the correct delivery of CS at the site of inflammation in joints or tendons may substantially increase the chance for a successful outcome. This may especially be true in younger children with a higher percentage of cartilage of the immature bone.

Ultrasound-guided corticosteroid injections are mostly established in the management of oligo-JIA to resolve synovitis but may also support the treatment of a polyarticular disease course by addressing treatment-resistant joints or providing temporary treatment until other systemic treatment modalities may come into effect. This includes joints that would be difficult to inject with imaging (e.g., hip joints, very small joints) and may be especially important for joints that will lead to significant impairment when damaged due to ongoing disease activity or improperly placed injections (e.g., hip joints) [1, 2].

Ultrasound guidance may also help to inject CS into tendon sheaths, around entheses or inflamed bursae.

Efficacy and Safety

Several studies have reported impressive response rates to joint injections in JIA especially when using triamcinolone hexacetonide (TCH), which has become the gold standard for joint injections in JIA [3–6]. Other substances, such as triamcinolone acetonide, are reportedly not as effective as TCH [15]. However, TCH joint injections have potential side effects, most of which are related to incorrect placement of the injectate. A very common adverse effect seen after intraarticular injections with CS is subcutaneous atrophy or hypopigmentation above the injected joint region. One strategy to avoid such adverse effects is to use a more soluble steroid preparation like betamethasone or methylprednisolone when injecting the smaller joints of children, such as the finger joints, midfoot joints, or toes. However, most of the more soluble preparations result in a shorter duration of efficacy of the joint injection. Another strategy to avoid such adverse effects is to improve the accuracy of needle positioning using ultrasound guidance.

A more frequent potential consequence of intraarticular injections is periarticular or intraarticular calcification. Other rare adverse events include transient suppression of endogenous cortisol production, avascular necrosis of the femoral head, local inflammatory reactions, local bleeding, or infection. Ultrasound guidance not only increases the safety of intraarticular steroid injection by reducing the likelihood of adverse events but also improves the efficacy via the correct placement of the CS within the targeted structure [9–12].

Technical Aspects of Ultrasound-Guided Injections

Before starting the procedure of an ultrasound-guided injection, you have to clearly identify your target by ultrasound. Especially in children it is fundamental to have an advanced knowledge of the sonographic presentation of the pediatric immature skeleton including secondary ossification zones with the growth plate and a higher percentage of cartilage related to age [16–18]. The vascularization of pediatric joints detected by color or power Doppler ultrasound appears different with a higher amount of physiological feeding vessels [19–21].

After the target has been identified, the required length and caliber of the needle need to be chosen and adapted to the depth and size of the target.

After the selection of an injectate, e.g., TCH, a decision has to be taken between guiding the needle in-plane and out-of-plane (illustration). The advantage of a direct ultrasound-guided injection is a real-time visualization of the needle tip allowing for the exact adjustment of depth and the target. The needle is best visualized when it is parallel to the probe in the long axis. Reverberation and metal artifacts may help to clearly identify the needle (Fig. 18.1a and b).

If the insertion site is in close proximity to the probe a sterile probe cover and gel have to be used to avoid any contamination. Only when a non-touch technique will be guaranteed at all times non-sterile gloves may be sufficient.

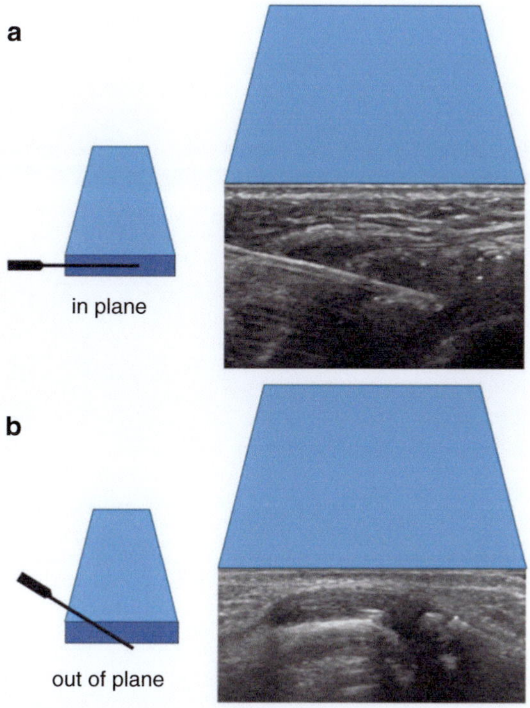

Fig. 18.1 (**a**) In-plane direction of the needle parallel to the probe (injection of a subtalar joint). (**b**) Out-of-plane direction of the needle crossing the probe (injection of a small finger joint)

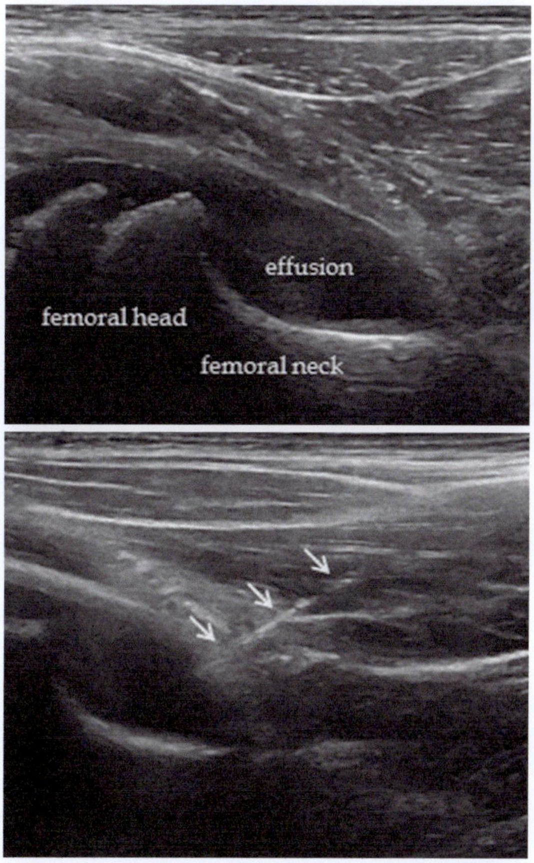

Fig. 18.2 In-plane injection of the ventral hip recess (arrows marking the needle) in a 6-year-old male SJIA patient

Prior to the insertion of the needle, it is important to ensure that the patient as well as the person performing the injection has a comfortable position also in relation to the equipment. The need for sedation has to be decided according to the age of the patient and the number of joints to be injected. An informed consent from the parents and/or the patient has to be obtained before the procedure.

Examples for Ultrasound-Guided Injections in Juvenile Idiopathic Arthritis

Coxitis

In some patients, the hip joint is only accessed to aspirate synovial fluid for the diagnosis of septic arthritis or transient hip arthritis. However, ultrasound-guided CS injections are a very well-established treatment modality in patients with JIA with coxitis, which occurs more commonly in those with RF-negative or RF-positive polyarthritis, enthesitis-associated arthritis, or systemic arthritis.

The patient lies in the supine position. Younger children should be sedated for the injection procedure. The strictly aseptic technique includes the use of a sterile probe cover filled with sterile ultrasound transmission gel. The ultrasound probe is placed along the longitudinal axis of the femoral neck to reveal the joint effusion in the anterior recess. The anterior recess should be accessed by a long needle, e.g., a spinal needle, to safely reach the recess. The needle is guided longitudinally through the joint capsule into the anterior recess (Fig. 18.2). After successful aspiration of the effusion, a small amount of sodium chloride should be injected and checked by ultrasound. After the correct needle placement is confirmed, the CS can be injected. Some sodium chloride should be injected through the needle while it is being withdrawn to avoid subcutaneous atrophy.

Knee Arthritis

The knee is the most commonly affected joint in JIA. In particular, young patients with oligo-JIA often experience knee involvement. Such patients will often receive CS injections to achieve fast improvement and short-term relief of symptoms. Some patients require only treatment with CS injections, without any systemic antirheumatic drugs. Ultrasound guidance is not always necessary for knee injections but may help in specific conditions, such as in very young and small children, in cases where the effusion is already partly organized, a large amount of synovial hypertrophy is present or with smaller amounts of effusion, and to improve the efficacy and safety of the steroid injection. In the case of a persistent suprapatellar plica, it may be necessary to inject both compartments.

The patient lies in the supine position. The knee may be flexed by 30°. The ultrasound probe is placed along the transverse suprapatellar axis of the knee to reveal the joint effusion in the suprapatellar recess. The suprapatellar recess should be accessed from the lateral side to safely reach the effusion within the recess (Fig. 18.3). Before introducing the needle, the superior and lateral margins of the patella should be identified as anatomic landmarks. The needle is guided with mild anterior-posterior angulation of the probe. After successful aspiration of the effusion, a small amount of sodium chloride should be injected and checked by ultrasound. After the correct needle placement is confirmed, the CS can be injected. Some sodium chloride should be injected through the needle while it is being withdrawn to avoid subcutaneous atrophy.

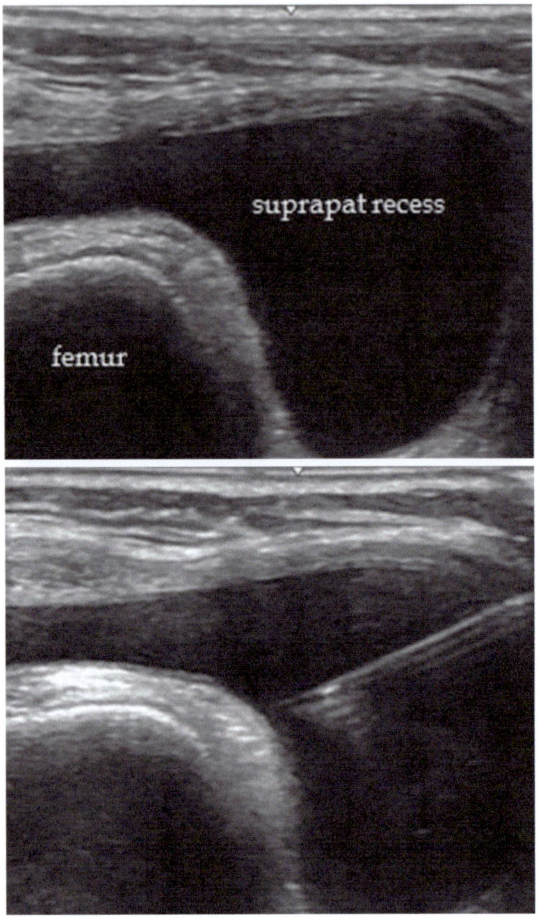

Fig. 18.3 In-plane injection from lateral of the suprapatellar recess in a 6-year-old female JIA patient

Tibiotalar Joint and Subtalar Joint

The ankle joints are very commonly affected in JIA. Particularly, in those with oligoarticular arthritis, local CS injection into the tibiotalar or subtalar joints may substantially improve the course of JIA.

The patient lies in the supine position. For the injection of the upper ankle joint (tibiotalar joint), the foot may be positioned flat on the ground. The ultrasound probe is placed along the longitudinal axis of the tibiotalar joint, revealing the joint effusion between the distal tibial epiphysis and the talus. In many patients, the effusion extends along the entire body of the talus and into the area of the head of the talus. For the tibiotalar joint, the needle should be

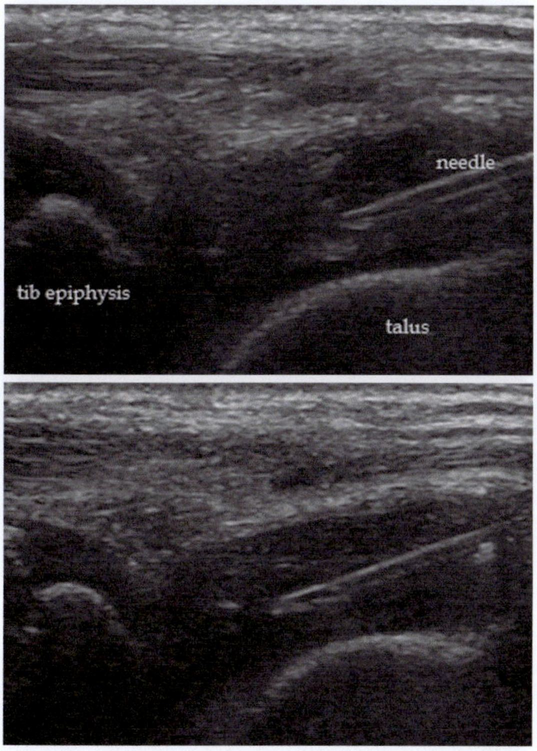

Fig. 18.4 Dorsally in-plane injection of the tibiotalar joint in a 3-year-old female JIA patient

inserted from the anterior aspect distally to the probe (Fig. 18.4). The needle is guided longitudinally, with an anterior-posterior angulation of the probe of about 40–60°. After successful aspiration of the effusion (if desired), a small amount of sodium chloride can be injected and checked by ultrasound. After confirming the correct needle placement, the steroid can be injected. Some sodium chloride should be injected through the needle while it is being withdrawn to avoid subcutaneous atrophy. An alternative approach of injection of the tibiotalar joint would be in transverse view if the effusion can be clearly identified. This has the advantage that the needle will be more parallel to the probe with better visibility and the needle trajectory may be shorter.

The subtalar joint is visualized on a lateral transverse scan of the talocalcaneal aspect of the joint. It may be located in the posterior aspect of the joint but the synovial recess may also extend into the area of the sinus tarsi, which does not contain synovial tissue in the healthy joint. The needle can be inserted from the lateral side, optimally guided by a small hockey stick applicator. To identify the effusion and joint space, the foot should be moved to the supine position under ultrasound imaging. In case the distension of the synovial recess is better visible on the medial aspect, the subtalar joint can also be accessed medially.

Midfoot

It can be challenging to inject CS into the small talotarsal or intertarsal joints in younger children, as the joint spaces are very narrow. Ultrasound may help to detect a small amount of effusion or synovial hypertrophy, which can be injected under ultrasound guidance. Most midfoot joints can be injected with CS under ultrasound guidance (Fig. 18.5). One significant advantage is the fact that the injectate only needs to be injected into the distended synovial recess and the needle does not need to be placed in between the bones of the midfoot.

The patient lies in the supine position. The ultrasound probe is usually placed along the longitudinal axis of the small midfoot joints to reveal the targeted structure. The needle is guided with anterior-posterior angulation.

Wrist

The pediatric wrist is always a challenging joint to inject if one wants to aim to the precise area of inflammation as it is divided into four synovial compartments, and inflammation may also be present in tendon sheaths running along the wrist. Depending on the region of effusion or synovial hypertrophy (e.g., radiocarpal or midcarpal recess), the wrist can be injected in different places. The wrist is usually injected distally to the probe, which is placed in the longitudinal axis of the targeted structure. The needle is guided safely to the recess with an anterior-posterior angulation. In younger children, it is very important to distinguish between hypo- or anechoic cartilage and anechoic effusion. A dynamic examination before the injection that

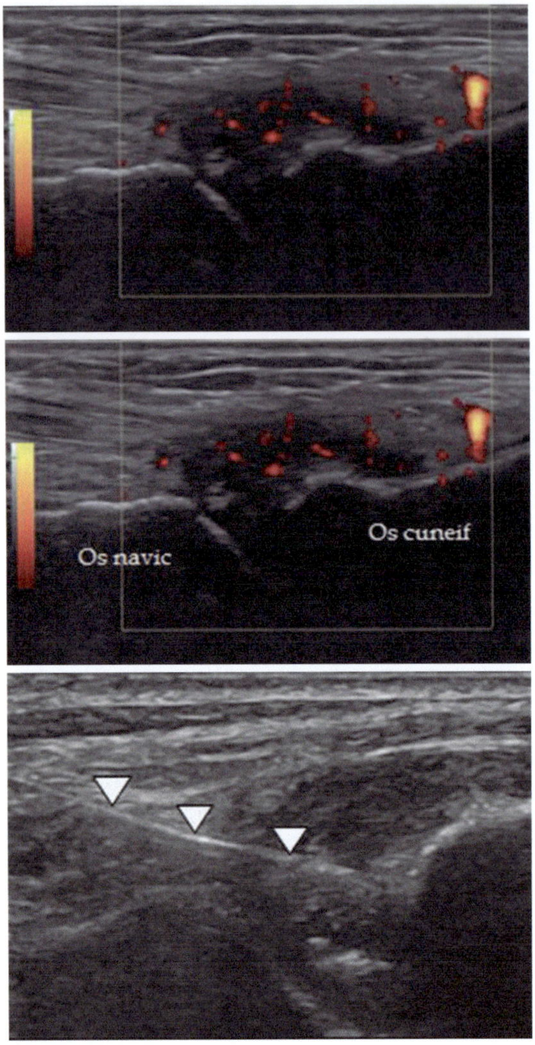

Fig. 18.5 In-plane injection (arrows showing the needle) of the talonavicular joint in the dorsal midfoot region of a 7-year-old JIA patient

enables the visualization of the hyperechoic boundary line between cartilage and effusion helps to better discriminate both structures.

Finger Joints

Incorrect placement of the needle in the small finger joints of children easily leads to soft tissue damage, with potential tendon contracture. Therefore, it is very important that the steroid injection reaches the targeted structure precisely. Ultrasound guidance with small hockey stick probes optimizes the safety and efficacy of CS injection into the finger joints of children. The small finger joints may be injected with the transducer placed in the longitudinal axis of the joint or in transverse.

Tenosynovitis

Paratenonitis and tenosynovitis are common in JIA. The involvement of the extensor tendons of the wrist or the tibialis posterior tendon of the foot is very often detected by ultrasound in patients with JIA. Tenosynovitis is characterized by distension of the tendon sheath with anechoic or hypoechoic fluid, which is sometimes combined with synovial hypertrophy within the tendon sheath and thickening of the tendons. The tendons appear hyperechoic within the anechoic fluid, and may demonstrate hypervascularization. A very gentle way to inject the tendon sheaths is with the probe placed transversely to the tendon sheaths (Fig. 18.6). It is possible to inject more than one tendon sheath during each injection procedure. Before the injection of the steroid, an injection of a few ml of sodium chloride may help confirm the correct placement of the needle and expands the space available for the steroid injection. Sodium chloride should be injected through the needle while it is being withdrawn to avoid soft tissue atrophy [22, 23]. In the case of long stretches of tendon sheaths being inflamed, it may be advantageous to inject in the long axis to ensure placement of the CS along the entire region of pathology and if necessary move the needle further during the injection.

Bursitis

Bursitis is very common in JIA and is sometimes asymptomatic and only detected by ultrasound. However, some patients with JIA

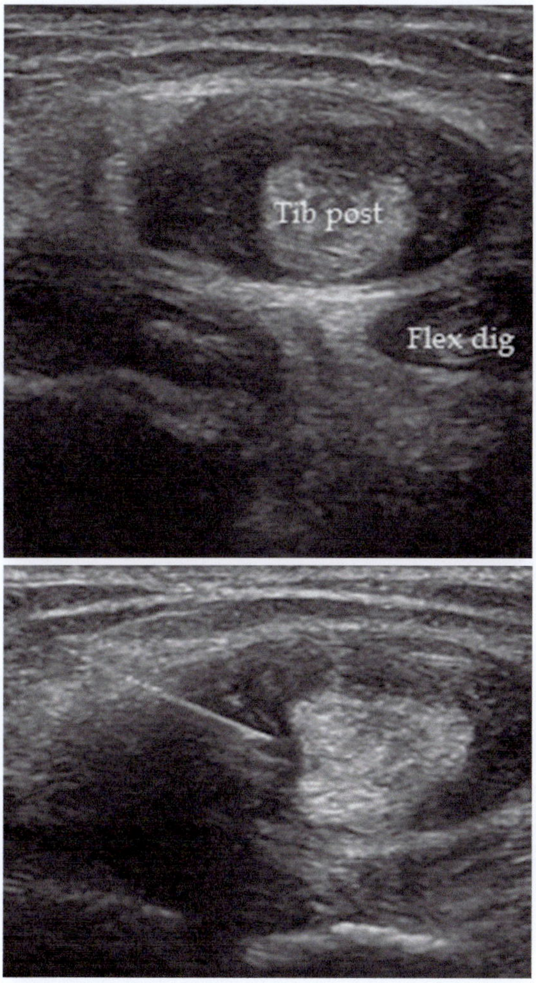

Fig. 18.6 In-plane injection (corticosteroid) of the tibialis posterior tendon sheath in a 13-year-old female patient with JIA

bursitis are symptomatic and experience pain, swelling, and loss of function, e.g., active bursitis infrapatellaris profunda. Steroid injection of the affected bursa can be a very effective therapeutic approach to achieve short- and long-term relief of symptoms and improve function. As one example, the bursa infrapatellaris profunda can be injected from the lateral or medial aspects, while the transducer is placed in short axis relative to the bursa. The needle is guided under the probe to the enlarged bursa with a mild anterior-posterior angulation (Fig. 18.7).

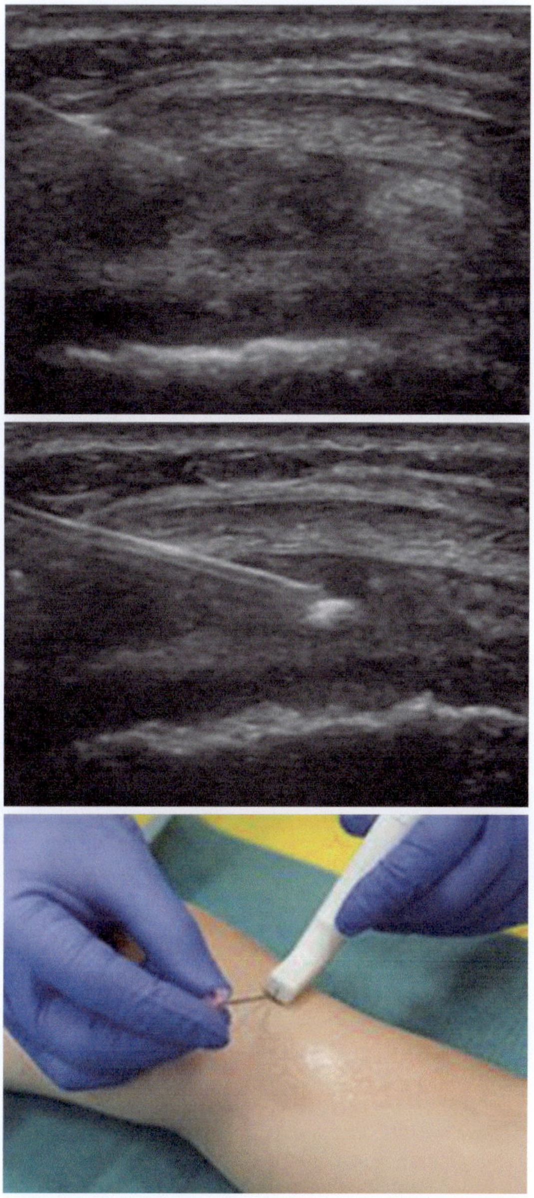

Fig. 18.7 In-plane injection (corticosteroid) of the Bursa infrapatellaris profunda in a 10-year-old JIA patient

References

1. Scott C, et al. A reappraisal of intra-articular corticosteroid therapy in juvenile idiopathic arthritis. Clin Exp Rheumatol. 2010;28(5):774–81.
2. Dent PB, Walker N. Intra-articular corticosteroids in the treatment of juvenile rheumatoid arthritis. Curr Opin Rheumatol. 1998;10:475–80.

3. Beukelmann et al. Usage of intra-articular corticosteroid injections for the treatment of juvenile idiopathic arthritis: a survey of pediatric rheumatologists in the United States and Canada. Clin Exp Rheumatol. 2008;26:700–3.
4. Breit W, et al. A subgroup-specific evaluation of the efficacy of intraarticular triamcinolone hexacetonide in juvenile chronic arthritis. J Rheumatol. 2000;27:2696–702.
5. Gotte AC. Intra-articular corticosteroids in the treatment of juvenile idiopathic arthritis: safety, efficacy, and features affecting outcome. Open Access Rheumatol Res Rev. 2009;1:37–49.
6. Young CM, et al. Ultrasound-guided corticosteroid injection therapy for juvenile idiopathic arthritis: 12-year care experience. Pediatr Radiol. 2012;42:1481–9.
7. Bruyn G, Schmidt W. How to perform ultrasound guided injections. Best Pract Res Clin Rheumatol. 2009;23:269–79.
8. Parra D. Technical tips to perform safe and effective Ultrasound Guided steroid joint injections in children. Pediatr Rheumatol. 2015;13:2.
9. Koski JM. Ultrasound guided injections in rheumatology. J Rheumatol. 2000;27:2131.
10. d'Agostino MA, Ayral X, Baron G, et al. Impact of ultrasound imaging on local corticosteroid injections of symptomatic ankle, hind-, and mid-foot in chronic inflammatory diseases. Arthritis Rheum. 2005;53:284.
11. Balint PV, Kane D, Hunter J, et al. Ultrasound guided versus conventional joint and soft tissue fluid aspiration in rheumatology practice: a pilot study. J Rheumatol. 2002;29:2209.
12. Naredo E, Cabero F, Beneyto P, et al. A randomized comparative study of short term response to blind injection versus sonographic-guided injection of local corticosteroids in patients with painful shoulder. J Rheumatol. 2004;31:308.
13. Sibbitt WL Jr, Peisajovich A, Michael AA, et al. Does sonographic needle guidance affect the clinical outcome of intraarticular injections? J Rheumatol. 2009;36:1892.
14. Weitoft T, Uddenfeldt P. Importance of synovial fluid aspiration when injecting intra-articular corticosteroids. Ann Rheum Dis. 2000;59:233–5.
15. Zulian F, et al. Comparison of intra-articular triamcinolone hexacetonide and triamcinolone acetonide in oligoarticular juvenile idiopathic arthritis. Rheumatology. 2003;42:1254–9.
16. Roth J, Jousse-Joulin S, Magni-Manzoni S, Rodriguez A, Tzaribachev N, Iagnocco A, et al. Outcome measures in Rheumatology Ultrasound Group. Definitions for the sonographic features of joints in healthy children. Arthritis Care Res. 2015;67:136–42.
17. Collado P, Vojinovic J, Nieto JC, Windschall D, Magni Manzoni S, Bruyn GAW, on behalf of the OMERACT Ultrasound Group, et al. Toward standardized musculoskeletal ultrasound in paediatric rheumatology: normal age-related ultrasound findings. Arthritis Care Res. 2016;68:348–56.
18. Collado P, Windschall D, Vojinovic J, et al. Amendment of the OMERACT ultrasound definitions of joints' features in healthy children when using the DOPPLER technique. Pediatr Rheumatol Online J. 2018;16:23.
19. Windschall D, Collado P, Vojinovic J, et al. Age-related vascularization and ossification of joints in children: an international pilot study to test multiobserver ultrasound reliability. Arthritis Care Res. 2017. https://doi.org/10.1002/acr.23335.
20. Roth J, Ravagnani V, Backhaus M, et al. Preliminary definitions for the sonographic features of synovitis in children. Arthritis Care Res. 2017;69:1217–23.
21. Breton S, Jousse-Joulin S, Cangemi C, de Parscau L, Colin D, Bressolette L, et al. Comparison of clinical and ultrasonographic evaluations for peripheral synovitis in juvenile idiopathic arthritis. Semin Arthritis Rheum. 2011;41:272–8.
22. Gutierrez M, et al. Short-term efficacy to conventional blind injection versus ultrasound-guided injection of local corticosteroids in tenosynovitis in patients with inflammatory chronic arthritis: a randomized comparative study. Joint Bone Spine. 2016;83:161–6.
23. Peters, et al. Ultrasound-guided steroid tendon sheath injections in juvenile idiopathic arthritis: a 10-year single-center retrospective study. Pediatr Rheumatol. 2017;15:22.

Part V

Sports Medicine

US in Children with Sports Injuries

19

Jeimylo C. de Castro

Introduction

Injuries of the musculoskeletal system among children during sports activities represent about 3–11% per year with boys twice as affected as girls with injuries more severe among the boys [1]. Schmidt and Hollwarth noted the frequency of sports injuries to be more common in the upper extremity (43.8%) as compared to the lower extremity (34.5%) and 16% involving the head and has a peak age of 12 years old [2]. Auringer and colleagues, however, noted a higher frequency in the lower extremities in pediatric sports injuries [3].

The growing musculoskeletal system of a child is unique as ligaments and tendons are relatively stronger than its attachment, namely, the epiphyseal plate. Thus, in a severe sports trauma, the epiphyseal plate being the weaker segment gives way [1, 4, 5] subsequently damaging the growth plate [4, 5]. With these injuries, the disturbance can result in limb length discrepancy, angular deformity, and long-term disability [6]. Other details consequent to these pathologies will not be covered in this discussion.

J. C. de Castro (✉)
Physical Medicine and Rehabilitation Department, The Medical City-South Luzon, Santa Rosa, Laguna, Philippines

SMARTMD Center for Non-Surgical Pain Interventions, Makati City, Philippines

Immature bones during the adolescent stage behave differently as physiologic loading may be beneficial to bone, while excessive strains can injure the joints. Sudden overload, however, may render the bones to bow due to increasing bone stiffness and diminishing resistance to impact [7]. Low-intensity training can stimulate bone growth, while the reverse is true for high-intensity training [8] (Fig. 19.1).

With an increasing frequency and the peculiar features of pediatric sports injury, there is a need for imaging specific areas in the musculoskeletal system using ultrasound. Radiographs are still used as a screening modality for the evaluation of bone defects. Magnetic resonance imaging remains to be the imaging modality of choice for joint and soft tissue injuries [9]. The advantage of using ultrasound in pediatric sports injuries is due to its portability, accessibility, high resolution, and its ability to scan dynamically. Its main disadvantage includes operator dependence and steep learning curve [10].

Lower Extremities

Osgood-Schlatter Disease

This condition was first described in 1903 by Robert Osgood and Carl Schlatter [11, 12]. This is a repetitive traction injury of the apophysis involving the anterior tibia by the quadriceps

Y. El Miedany (ed.), *Pediatric Musculoskeletal Ultrasonography*,
https://doi.org/10.1007/978-3-030-17824-6_19

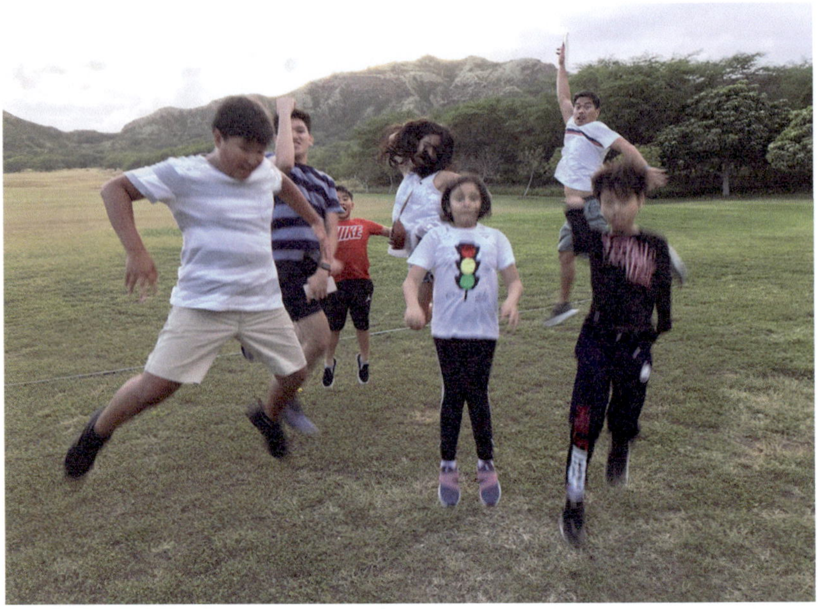

Fig. 19.1 The dynamic activities of children imposing upon their young and immature musculoskeletal system the forces and loads in their varied activities

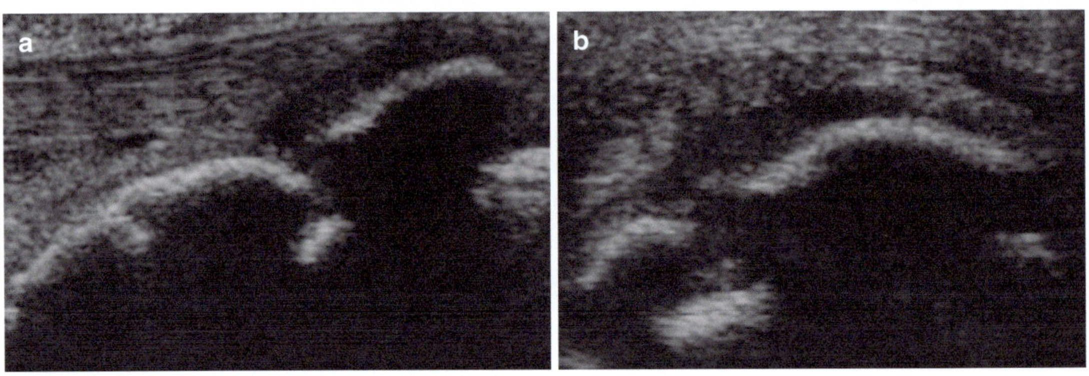

Fig. 19.2 Normal ultrasound images of a child in longitudinal (**a**) and short axis (**b**) view at the distal knee where the patellar tendon is inserted. No hypoechoic swelling is seen in these views

muscle. This typically affects boys at the age of 10–14 years old especially those playing soccer, basketball, and volleyball [13] and other jumping sports [9] (Fig. 19.2). The symptoms include pain, swelling, and tenderness at the proximal anterior tibial tuberosity [14]. It is bilateral in 20–30% of cases [9].

Ultrasound findings showed cartilage swelling, fragmentation of the secondary ossification center of the tibial tuberosity, inflammation of the tendons with thickening of the patellar tendon and increased signal on power Doppler, and bursitis [13, 15, 16] (Fig. 19.3).

The amount of power Doppler signal correlates with the intensity of pain [14]. Three types of Osgood-Schlatter based on ultrasound findings were observed by Czyrny [12]: type 1, delamination of the internal ossification center; type 2, delamination tear or fracture of the epiphyseal part of the tibial tuberosity; and type 3, delamination tear of the ossification center producing in irregular deformation of the tuberosity [12].

Sinding-Larsen-Johansson Disease

This is a rarer condition described as an osteochondrosis of the patella. Patients affected are usually younger than Osgood-Schlatter disease. It is likewise caused by repetitive microtrauma and

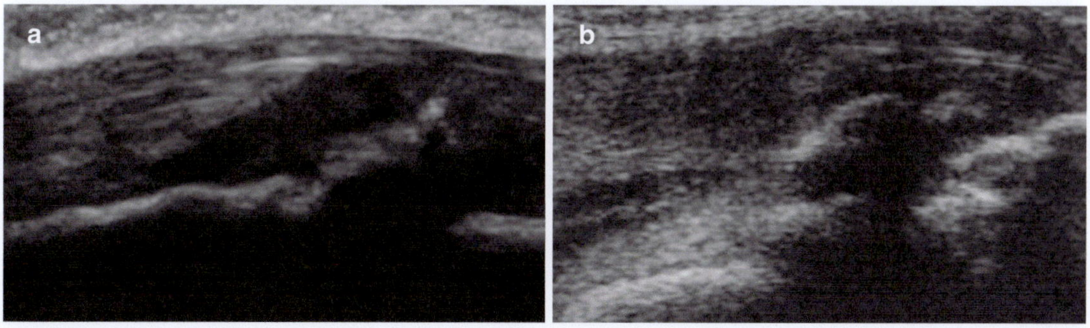

Fig. 19.3 These are longitudinal views of a child showing cartilage swelling (**a**) and irregular fragmentation (**b**) of the tibial tuberosity with relative thickening of the patellar tendon

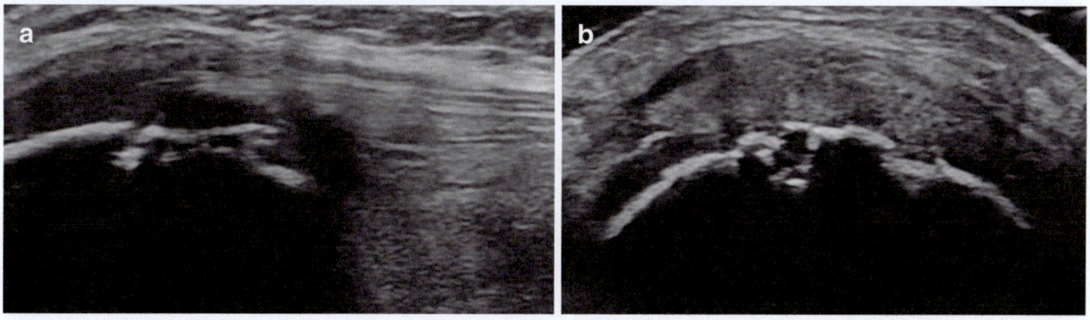

Fig. 19.4 (**a**) Longitudinal axis view of the knee showing the bony contour irregularities with hypoechoic tendon thickening and echogenic Hoffa's fat pad. (**b**) Short axis view of the same child showing bony cortical irregularity of the inferior pole of the patella and hypoechoic swelling of the proximal patellar tendon. (With permission from Dr. Taco Geertsma)

excessive prolong stress. Pain over the anterior knee is marked during extreme knee flexion. In this condition, ultrasound shows the lower pole of the patella to be fragmented and hypoechoic with swelling of the cartilage at the insertion site of the patellar tendon [14, 16] (Fig. 19.4).

Osteochondritis Dissecans of the Knee

This is a repetitive, nontraumatic, and localized process wherein a focus of subchondral bone and adjacent articular cartilage separates from the surrounding bone most commonly affecting the skeletally immature male athletes [9, 17, 18]. According to Research in Osteochondritis Dissecans of the Knee Group, it is defined as a focal, idiopathic alteration of subchondral bone with risk for stability and disruption of adjacent articular cartilage that may result in premature osteoarthritis [19]. This is commonly affecting the knee joint and is considered one of the severest injuries affecting athlete due to the intensity of fragmentation and with poor reparative capability of the cartilage [14]. Although etiology is not certain, mechanical and traumatic factors form part of the etiology. There is noted "failure of the process of the endochondral ossification of the articular complex" [19]. This commonly occurs at the lateral aspect of the medial femoral condyle [19] and less frequently at the lateral femoral condyle. The sonographic features depend upon the stage of the lesion. The early stage is characterized by a localized subchondral bony flattening with a normal articular surface. In more advanced stage, however, it shows non-displaced to slightly displaced fragments with double hyperechoic areas [20]. Gregerson and Rasmussen in their preliminary study of the osteochondritis dissecans showed a hypoechoic material found in most of the defects which is due to the resorption of bone with replacement of granulation tissue or fibrocartilage. The echogenic spots with posterior acoustic shadowing represent the separated subchondral bone and degenerative calcifications in the articular cartilage or were part of the repair process [21].

Sever's Disease

This is an overuse injury of the posterior ankle affecting the apophysis of the calcaneus frequently seen in physically active children usually those involved in running and jumping sports between the ages of 8 and 10 for girls and 10 and 12 for boys. The Achilles tendon inserts in the calcaneus apophysis (Fig. 19.5). The apophysis of the os calcis is an epiphyseal plate that develops along the posterior border of the bone [22]. Ultrasound findings showed the presence of Achilles tendinitis and/or retrocalcaneal bursitis. There is also a fragmentation of secondary nucleus of ossification of calcaneus [22].

Apophyseal Avulsion Fractures

This is one of the most common acute injuries in pediatric sports injuries. It usually involved the apophysis of the pelvis although it can involve other sites in the lower extremities. And in the pelvis, the most commonly involved area is the ischial tuberosity [23]. In this type of injury, there is a strong tendency to avulse completely from the bone unlike that seen in epiphysis [9] (Fig. 19.6).

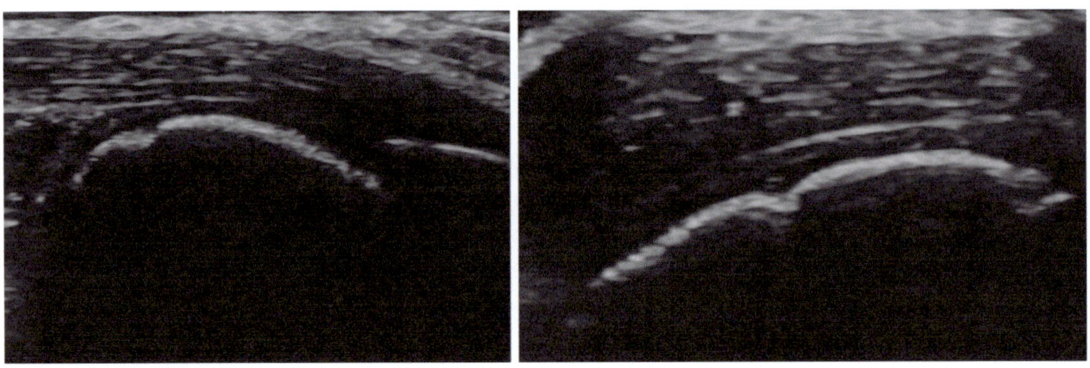

Fig. 19.5 These are the normal longitudinal and short axis views of the posterior ankle of a 9-year-old male child showing the apophysis of the calcaneus which are the usual site to evaluate in a patient with posterior ankle pain as in the case of a Sever's disease

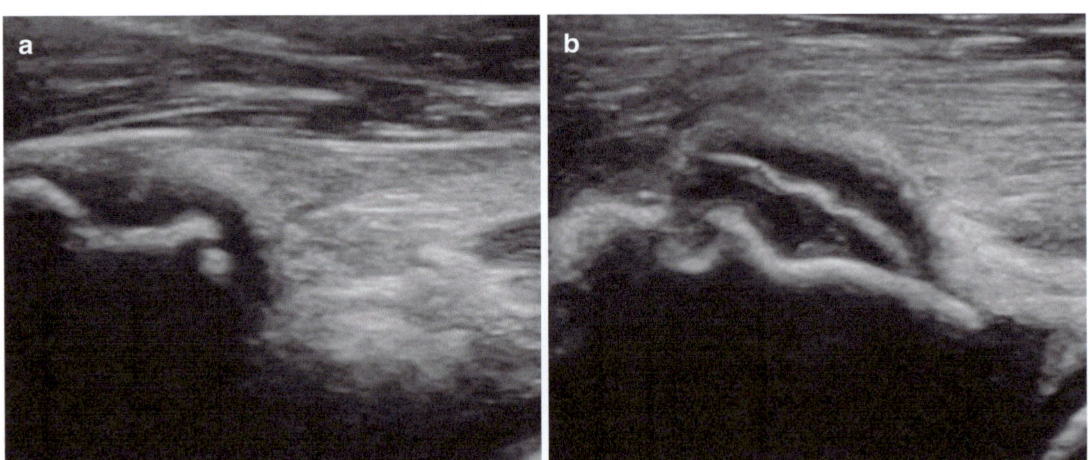

Fig. 19.6 (**a**) Normal ultrasound images of the rectus femoris as it inserts at the anterior superior iliac spine. (**b**) Post-traumatic changes in the apophysis of the rectus femoris insertion in a 9-year-old girl. (With permission from Dr. Taco Geertsma)

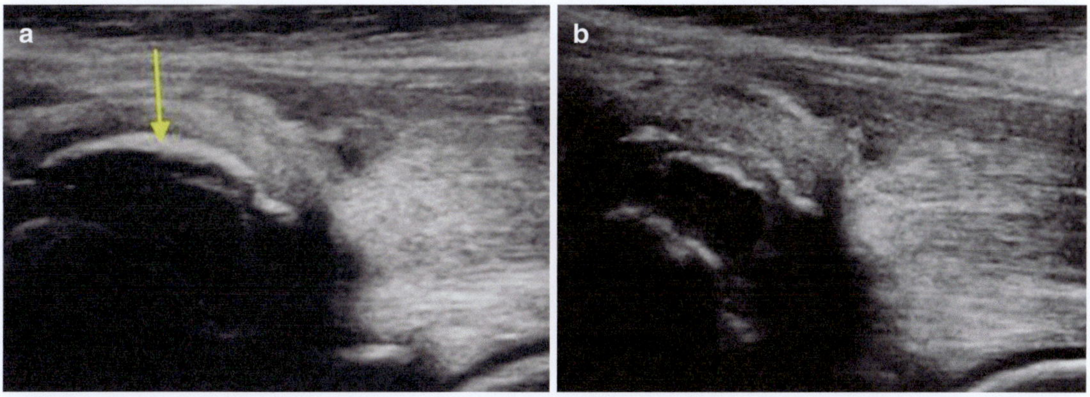

Fig. 19.7 (**a**) Normal ultrasound image of the anterior superior iliac spine. (**b**) An ultrasound image showing the avulsion of the apophysis of the anterior superior iliac spine. (With permission from Dr. Taco Geertsma)

Sonographic criteria for diagnosis include four criteria: a hypoechogenic zone, an increased distance to the apophysis, dislocation of the apophysis, and mobility of the apophysis on dynamic examination. These criteria are correlated with edema, lysis, avulsion, and unstable avulsion of the apophysis [24]. Power Doppler though is not helpful for chronic injuries [25] (Fig. 19.7).

Upper Extremity

Osteochondritis Dissecans (OCD) of the Capitellum

It is a repetitive overhead or upper extremity weight-bearing activity where a segment of articular cartilage separates from the subchondral bone involving 11–23-year-old adolescents with boys more affected than girls [26]. The prevalence of OCD of the humeral capitellum is about 3–4% among baseball players [27]. Although common as sports injuries among children, it can also occur in nonsporting children. It affects the dominant arm especially in little league baseball pitchers and gymnasts, due to the loading of the lateral elbow on valgus motion. Patient will usually complain of lateral elbow pain with inability to fully extend the elbow. There is usually tenderness over the lateral elbow [1]. Elbow OCD must be distinguished with Panner's disease or osteochondrosis of the capitellum which is seen in younger children between 4 and 12 years old. This condition is characterized by ischemia and necrosis of the capitellar epiphysis with consequent regeneration and recalcification but is usually self-limiting and resolves with rest [26]. Sonography of the elbow is done at the anterolateral aspect of the capitellum as this is the most commonly affected. It shows non-displaced (stable) or slightly displaced (unstable) fragments as double-high echogenic areas in the capitellar subchondral bone. Once the fragment is completely displaced, the osteochondral defect was usually observed in the capitellum. This defect is often repaired with fibrocartilaginous tissue and thus appears in ultrasound as a hypoechoic structure at the surface of the defect. The outline of the cartilaginous tissue is irregular in unstable lesions and is intact in stable lesions. The free bone fragment in unstable lesions may be sometimes difficult to detect by ultrasound. The free bone usually appears as a highly echoic fragment overlying the intact subchondral bone [28]. These sonographic findings are consistent with surgical and MR assessment in about 89% [28].

Shoulder Instability

Shoulder instability is one of the common injuries affecting adolescents. Anterior shoulder instability secondary to trauma is one such condition involving the glenohumeral joint. Glenohumeral instability is defined as the inability to maintain the humeral head inside the center of the glenoid fossa [29]. Patients can either be injured in traumatic or atraumatic causes.

Patients with traumatic etiology which comprise 90% of patients usually have unidirectional anterior instability with labral detachment (Bankart lesion) but with atraumatic instability are usually multidirectional, and patient presents with bilateral hyperlaxity but no labral pathology. The recurrence of the former responds better with surgery but the latter is better stabilized with physical rehabilitation [29]. A study by Owens identified patients with an increased glenoid height-to-width ratio as measured on sagittal-oblique MRI having an increased risk for anterior shoulder instability [30]. Male athletes between 14 and 16 years old have a greater tendency to developed recurrent shoulder dislocation within 1 year of shoulder dislocation [31]. Surgically treated patients have better results in terms of sports performance as compared with other conservative measures like physical therapy and immobilization in external rotation [32] because of its high recurrence rates [33, 34]. Details of different surgical interventions will not be discussed here.

Traumatic posterior shoulder instability is observed in about 2–10% of cases [35, 36]. Nonsurgical treatment is successful in about 65–80% of patients [32]. Increased glenoid retroversion was associated with this kind of shoulder instability [36].

Atraumatic posterior shoulder instability in pediatric patients does not have clear-cut causes although it may be associated with swimming, throwing, hitting, or overhead serving. This is associated with multidirectional instability of the shoulder and is characterized by recurrent dislocation but in the absence of pain and spontaneous reduction [29, 37].

Although MRI remains to be the most common and reliable diagnostic tool for diagnosis, ultrasound is an emerging imaging tool for its diagnosis. Hammar and colleagues proposed the following ultrasound criteria for shoulder instability which includes a labral tear with the presence of hypoechoic zone larger than 2 mm at the base of the labrum, a degenerated labrum, the absence of labrum and/or degenerated labrum, and a vacuum phenomenon (gas) between the glenoid and the labrum and movement of the labrum during dynamic imaging [38]. The criterion for a degenerated labrum was a small anterior labrum, with an altered configuration, that was smaller than the ipsilateral posterior labrum and smaller than the anterior labrum on the normal side [38]. For anterior ligamental-capsular rupture, the criteria include a discontinuity or irregular texture of the anterior capsular complex with an irregular movement during dynamic imaging [12].

Clavicular Fractures and Other Fractures

One of the most common sports injuries among children and adolescents is clavicular fracture with torus fracture being the most common type [39–41]. Standardized assessment and treatment was established by FACTS (Function after Adolescent Clavicle Trauma and Surgery) using the commonly used radiographic parameters of shortening, angulation, and displacement [39].

Fractures in children can be viewed differently in ultrasound than its radiographic images. Eksioglu and colleagues in their study of 39 pediatric patients with fracture aged 1 to 14 have observed unique characteristics by ultrasound [40]. Whether the fracture is complete or incomplete, the most valuable finding is subperiosteal hematoma (Fig. 19.8).

Other findings include cortical disruption, bending sign, and reverberating echo. Subperiosteal hematoma is defined as a periosteal elevation. There is also periosteal thickening, hyperemia, and soft tissue edema [42]. Due to the thicker and stronger periosteum seen among children than in adults, the periosteum tends to readily elevate from the diaphyseal and metaphyseal region of the bones. Thus, the periosteum is easily injured among children. Reverberation appears in ultrasound as a reflection of ultrasound waves from the medullary bone instead of the cortical bone which is especially seen in complete greenstick fractures. It is rarely seen in torus fractures. Bending sign is usually seen in incomplete fractures such that any deformation of the cortex even without gapping can be seen in ultrasound. Cortical disruption on the other hand is defined as gapping in

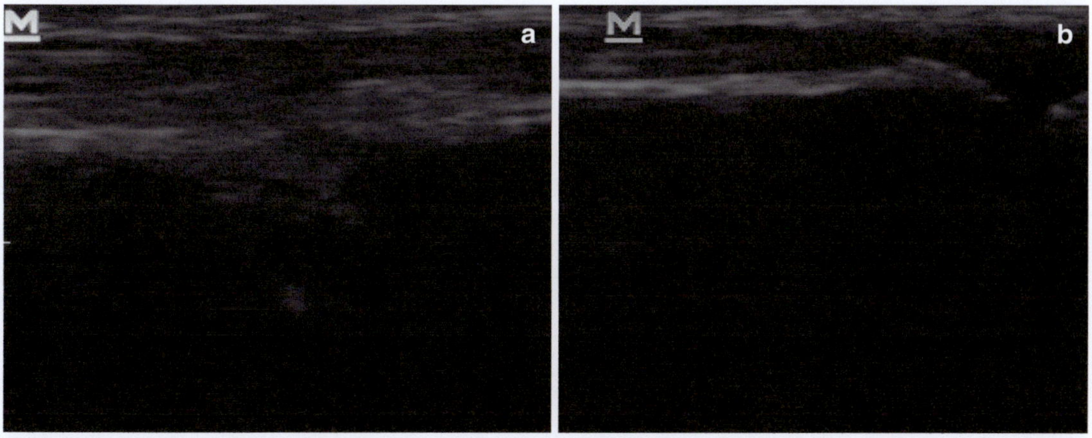

Fig. 19.8 An ultrasound image of the longitudinal view of the non-displaced fracture (**a**, **b**) of the distal radius of a 9-year-old girl who sustained a fall. Notice the subperiosteal edema on the first image

cortical continuity and can be due to microfractures. It can be seen in complete, torus, and greenstick fractures [40]. With an added portability and tolerability of pediatric patients, ultrasound was found to be better than radiograph in detecting and confirming fractures among children [41, 43–45]. It was less dependable however for fractures adjacent to joints, lesions of the small bones of hand and foot, non-displaced epiphyseal fracture (Salter-Harris type 1), or those with fracture line less than 1 mm [43]. The number of negative radiographic results can be a good reason why ultrasound can be an effective modality in detecting fractures in children especially when this group of patients appears irritable and resistant to questioning and does not cooperate during physical examination [43].

Sonographic findings of non-displaced physeal injury include thickening of the perichondral ring with edema and hyperemia, physeal widening, cortical interruption, and bony fragments at the physis [42]. In case of doubt, the presence of abnormality can be confirmed by checking the contralateral side.

Medial Elbow Injuries

Medial elbow pain and injuries among children constitute a spectrum of other disorders that include medial epicondylar apophysitis, medial epicondyle avulsions, ulnar collateral ligament tears or sprains, common wrist flexors strains, and pronator strains (Fig. 19.9).

All of these come about as repetitive or overuse injuries in sports especially during the early acceleration or late cocking phase of throwing such as that of "Little Leaguer's Elbow" and in this case may injure the ulnar collateral ligament (UCL) [46, 47] (Fig. 19.10). More severe injuries however especially among young children may lead to frank avulsions of the medial epicondyle. With this type of injury, the physis is the most susceptible in younger patient due to their immature skeleton rather than the ulnar collateral ligament [46]. In patients with ulnar collateral ligament injury, it is important to assess the overlying common flexor-pronator mass as it is usually concomitantly injured [47].

Ultrasound images of pathology are shown as focal hypoechoic heterogeneity and ligamentous thickening for partial tear of the UCL and disruption of the UCL with widening of the ulnotrochlear joint for full-thickness tear. Dynamic imaging may be required to determine between the incomplete and complete tears with valgus stress maneuvers indicating an instability [47]. The hypoechoic thickening of the UCL alone with no history of trauma however should be interpreted with caution as these changes can occur especially for those asymptomatic young baseball players over time as they age as noted by studies made by Atanda and colleagues [48].

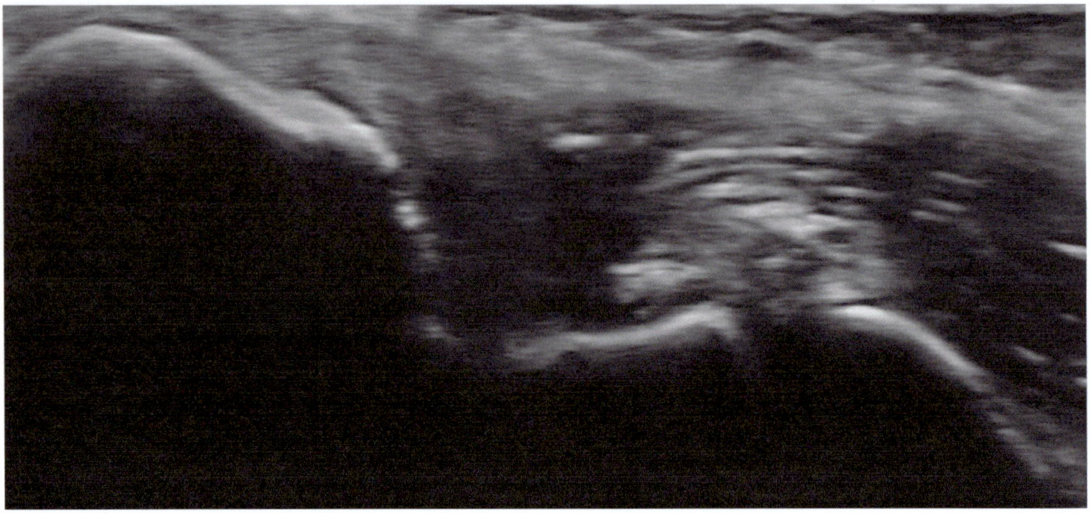

Fig. 19.9 A longitudinal axis view of the normal medial elbow showing the insertion of the common flexor tendons at the medial epicondyle of the distal humerus

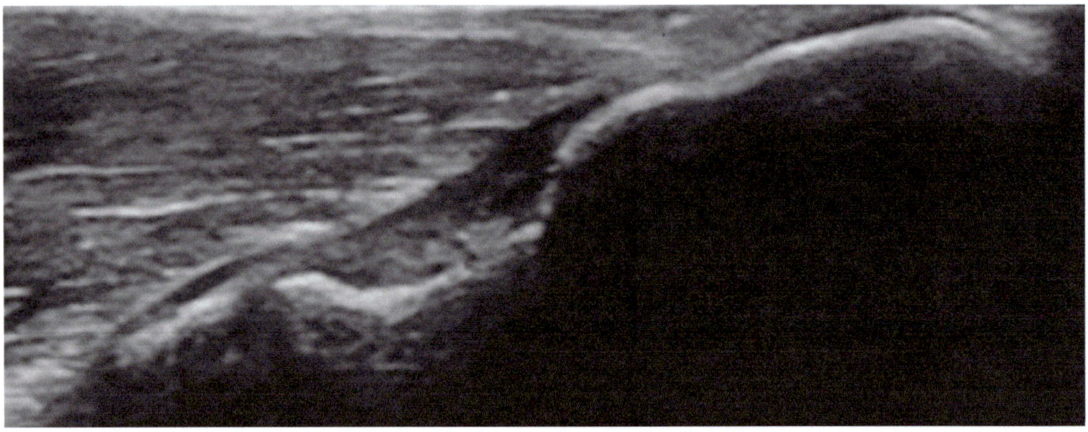

Fig. 19.10 Normal ultrasound of the longitudinal axis view of the ulnar collateral ligament where it originates from the anterior and inferior surfaces of the medial epicondyle and inserts into the coronoid process of the ulna

Medial epicondyle fractures are commonly seen among overhead and upper extremity weight-bearing athletes. Accurate measurements of medial epicondyle fracture displacements are necessary since displacement is important in decision-making for surgical intervention [36]. Except for fracture dislocation, which has significant limitations in flexion-extension motions as compared to isolated fractures only, most patients, however, had minimal clinical or functional disabilities [49]. Radiography would still be the best screening imaging modality for this type of conditions. The most common findings are displacement and fragmentation of the medial epicondyle apophysis [50, 51]. MRI may prove useful when radiographs are normal and when patients are suspected of having possible medial epicondylar apophysitis and other sports-related injuries [52]. Ultrasound may show a discontinuity of the medial epicondyle [53] with medial epicondyle irregularity and fragmentation [54].

Children with sports injuries present with a dynamic and peculiar musculoskeletal characteristic due to its developing nature. Although there are existing imaging modalities which we can utilize to make a diagnosis, such as radiographs, CT, and MRI scans, the portability of ultrasound and its usage for dynamic imaging prove to be a useful addition for making a quick and early diagnosis. This also means that with an early detection, it will provide a safe and quicker intervention especially in the field coverage of sports activities. The use of ultrasound however should be seen as a complementary means of coming up to a diagnosis rather than adversarial [55]. Although operator-dependent and with a long learning curve, musculoskeletal sonography in sports medicine has proven itself to be invaluable in the diagnosis of sports-related musculoskeletal abnormalities [10] and may guide clinicians as to what other modality is needed in the diagnosis in the pediatric population [56].

References

1. Shanmugam C, Maffulli N. Sports injuries in children. Br Med Bull. 2008;86(1):33–57.
2. Schmidt B, Hollwarth ME. Sports accidents in children and adolescents. Z Kinderchir. 1989;44:357–62.
3. Auringer ST, Anthony EY. Common pediatric sports injuries. Semin Musculoskelet Radiol. 1999;3(3):247–56.
4. Bright RW, Burstein AH, Elmore SM. Epiphyseal-plate cartilage: a biomechanical and histological analysis of failure modes. J Bone Joint Surg Am. 1974;56:688–703.
5. Flachsman R, Broom ND, Hardy AE, et al. Why is the adolescent joint particularly susceptible to osteochondral shear fracture? Clin Orthop Relat Res. 2000;381:212–21.
6. Caine D, DiFiori J, Maffuli N. Physeal injuries in children's and youth sports: reasons for concern. Br J Sports Med. 2006;40:749–60.
7. Maffulli N, Baxter-Jones AD. Common skeletal injuries in young athletes. Sports Med. 1995;19:137–49.
8. Booth FW, Goiuld EW. Effects of training and disuse on connective tissue. Exerc Sport Sci Rev. 1975;3:83–112.
9. O'Dell MC, Jaramillo D, Bancroft L, Varich L, Logsdon G, Servaes S. Imaging of sports-related injuries of the lower extremity in pediatric patients. Radiographics. 2016;36(6):1807.
10. Jacobson JA. Ultrasound in sports medicine. Radiol Clin N Am. 2002;40(2):363–86.
11. Osgood RB. Lesions of the tibial tubercle occurring during adolescence. Clin Orthop Relat Res. 1993;6:1903.
12. Czyrny Z. Osgood-Schlatter disease in ultrasound diagnostics – a pictorial essay. Med Ultrason. 2010;12(4):323–35.
13. Draghi F, Danesino GM, Coscia D, Precerutti M, Pagani C. Overload syndromes of the knee in adolescents: sonographic findings. J Ultrasound. 2008;11(4):151–7.
14. Suzue N, Matsuura T, Iwame T, Higashino K, Sakai T, Hamada D, et al. State of the art ultrasonographic findings in lower extremity sports injuries. The J of Med Investigation. 2015;62:109–13.
15. Ogden JA, Southwick WO. Osgood-Schlatter's disease and tibial tuberosity development. Clin Orthop Relat Res. 1976;(116):180–9.
16. De Flaviis L, Nessi R, Scaglione P, Balconi G, Albisetti W, Derchi LE. Ultrasonic diagnosis of Osgood-Schlatter and Sinding-Larsen-Johansson disease of the knee. Skelet Radiol. 1989;18(3):193–7.
17. Crawford DC, Safran MR. Osteochondritis dissecans of the knee. J Am Acad Orthop Surg. 2006;14(2):90–100.
18. Eismann EA, Pettit RJ, Wall EJ, Myer GD. Management strategies for osteochondritis dissecans of the knee in the skeletally immature athlete. J Orthop Sports Phys Ther. 2014;44(9):665–79.
19. Grimm NL, Weiss JM, Kessler JI, Aoki SK. Oseochondritis dissecans of the: pathoanatomy, epidemiology, and diagnosis. Clin Sports Med. 2014;33(2):181–8.
20. Berna-Serna JD, Martinez F, Reus M, Berna-Mestre JD. Osteochondritis dessicans of the knee: sonographically guided percutaneous drilling. J Ultrasound Med. 2008;27:255–9.
21. Gregersen HE, Rasmussen OS. Ultrasonography of osteochondritis dissecans of the knee: a preliminary report. Acta Ragiologica. 1989;30(5):552–4.
22. Hosgoren B, Koktener A, Dilmen G. Ultrasonography of the calcaneus in Sever's disease. Indian Pediatr. 2005;42:801–3.
23. Ferlic PW, Sadoghi P, Singer G, Kraus T, Eberl R. Treatment for ischial tuberosity avulsion fractures in adolescent athletes. Knee Surg Sports Traumatol Arthrosc. 2014;22(4):893–7.
24. Lazovic D, Wegner U, Peters G, Gosse F. Ultrasound for diagnosis of apophyseal injuries. Knee Surg Sports Traumatol Arthrosc. 1996;3(4):234–7.
25. Pisacano RM, Miller TT. Comparing sonography with MR imaging of apophyseal injuries of the pelvis in four boys. Am J Roentgenol. 2003;181:223–30.
26. Bergen CJA, van den Ende KIM, Brinke BT, Eygendaal D. Osteochondritis dissecans of the capitellum in adolescents. World J Orthop. 2016;7(2):102–8.
27. Kida Y, Morihara T, Kotoura Y, Hojo T, Tachiiri H, Sukenari T, Iwata Y, Furukawa R, Oda R, Arai Y, et al. Prevalence and clinical characteristics of osteochondritis dissecans of the humeral capitellum among adolescent baseball players. Am J Sports Med. 2014;42:1963–71.
28. Takahara M, Ogino T, Tsuchida H, Takagi M, Kashiwa H, Nambu T. Sonographic assessment of

osteochondritis dissecans of the humeral capitellum. Am J Roentgenol. 2000;174(2):411–5.
29. Cil A, Kocher M. Treatment of pediatric shoulder instability. J Pediatr Orthop. 2010;30:S3–6.
30. Owens BD, Campbell SE, Cameroon KL. Risk factors for anterior glenohumeral instability. Am J Sports Med. 2014;42:2591–6.
31. Leroux T, Ogilve-Harris D, Veillete C, et al. The epidemiology of primary anterior shoulder dislocation in patients aged 10 to 16 years. Am J Sports Med. 2015;43:2111–7.
32. Lawton R, Choudhury S, Mansat P, Cofield R, Stans A. Pediatric shoulder instability: presentation, findings, treatment and outcomes. J Pediatr Orthop. 2002;22(1):52–61.
33. Gigis I, Heikenfeld R, Kapinas A, et al. Arthroscopic versus conservative treatment of first anterior dislocation of the shoulder in adolescents. J Pediatr Orthop. 2014;34:421–5.
34. Longo UG, van der Linde JA, Loppini M, et al. Surgical versus nonoperative treatment in patients up to 18 years old with traumatic shoulder instability: a systematic review and quantitative synthesis of the literature. Arthroscopy. 2016;32:944–52.
35. Arciero RA, Mazzocca AD. Traumatic posterior shoulder subluxation with labral injury: suture anchor technique. Tech Should Elbow Surg. 2004;5:13–24.
36. Beck JJ, Richmond CJ, Tompkins MA, Heyer A, Shea KG, Cruz AI. What's new in pediatric upper extremity sports injuries? J Pediatr Orthop. 2018;38(2):e73–7.
37. Good CR, MacGillivray JD. Traumatic shoulder dislocation in the adolescent athlete: advances in surgical treatment. Curr Opin Pediatr. 2005;17:25–9.
38. Hammar MV, Wintzell GB, Astrom GO, Larsson S, Elvin A. Role of US in the preoperative evaluation of patients with anterior shoulder instability. Radiology. 2001;219(1):29.
39. Li Y, Donohue KS, Robbins CB, et al. Reliability of radiographic assessments of adolescent midshaft clavicle fractures by the FACTS multicenter study group. J Orthop Trauma. 2017;31:479–84.
40. Eksioglu F, Altinok D, Uslu MM, Gudemez E. Ultrasonographic findings in pediatric fractures. The Turkish J of Pediatr. 2003;45:136–40.
41. Cross KP, Warkentine FH, Kim IK, Gracely E, Paul RI. Bedside ultrasound diagnosis of clavicle fractures in the pediatric emergency department. Acad Emerg Med. 2010;17(7):687–93.
42. Hoffman DF, Adams E, Bianchi S. Ultrasonography of fractures in sports medicine. Br J Sports Med. 2015;49:152–60.
43. Hubner U, Schlicht W, Outzen S, Barthel M, Halsband H. Ultrasound in the diagnosis of fractures in children. J Bone Joint Surg Br. 2000;82(8):1170–3.
44. Lazar RD, Waters PM, Jaramillo D. The use of ultrasonography in the diagnosis of occult fracture of the radial neck. J Bone Joint Surg. 1998;80-A:1361–3.
45. Wang CC, Linden KL, Otero HJ. Sonographic evaluation of fractures in children. J Diag Med Sonography. 2017;33(3):200–7.
46. Crowther M. Elbow pain in pediatrics. Curr Rev Musculoskelet Med. 2009;2(2):83–7.
47. Konin GP, Nazarian LN, Walz DM. Ultrasound of the elbow: indications, technique, normal anatomy and pathologic conditions. Radiographics. 2013;33:4.
48. Atanda A Jr, Averill LW, Wallace M, et al. Factors related to increased ulnar collateral ligament thickness on stress sonography of the elbow in asymptomatic youth and adolescent baseball players. Am J Sports Med. 2017;44:3179–87.
49. Knapik DM, Fausett CL, Gilmore A, et al. Outcomes of non-operative pediatric medial humeral epicondyle fractures with and without associated elbow dislocation. J Pediatr Orthop. 2017;37:e224–8.
50. Hang DW, Chao CM, Hang YS. A clinical and roentgenographic study of little league elbow. Am J Sports Med. 2004;32:79–84.
51. Gore RM, Rogers LF, Bowerman J, et al. Osseous manifestations of elbow stress associated with sports activities. A J Roentgen. 1980;134:971–7.
52. Iyer RS, Thapa MM, Khanna PC, Chew FS. Pediatric bone imaging: imaging elbow trauma in children—a review of acute and chronic injuries. A J Roentgen. 2012;198(5):1053–68.
53. Lin CW, Chen YH, Chen WS. Application of ultrasound and ultrasound-guided intervention for evaluating elbow joint pathologies. J Med Ultrasound. 2012;20(2):87–95.
54. Harada M, Takahara M, Sasaki J, Mura N, Ito T, Ogino T. Using sonography for the early detection of elbow injuries among young baseball players. Am J Roentgenol. 2006;187(6):1436–41.
55. Lento PH, Primack S. Advances and utility of diagnostic ultrasound in musculoskeletal medicine. Curr Rev Musculoskelet Med. 2008;1(1):24–31.
56. Hryhorczuk AL, Restrepo R, Lee EY. Pediatric musculoskeletal ultrasound: practical imaging approach. Am J Roentgenol. 2016;206(5):W62–72.

Part VI

Recent Developments in Pediatric Ultrasonography

Advances in Pediatric Musculoskeletal Ultrasonography

20

Alessandra Bruns

Introduction

In relatively recent years, ultrasound (US) imaging has progressed rapidly improving the diagnostic accuracy in several rheumatic conditions, and it is currently considered a first-line research tool for several musculoskeletal diseases. Better transducer technology is now available increasing B-mode image quality as well as information from Doppler imaging. Additionally, new US technologies such as three-dimensional (3D) US, elastography (ES), and fusion imaging (FI) are able to increase the traditional role of US. The purpose of this chapter is to bring this new technology closer to pediatric rheumatologist and to summarize some of its possible clinical applications.

A. Bruns (✉)
Division of Rheumatology, Sherbrooke University, Sherbrooke, QC, Canada

MSK Ultrasound Courses, Sherbrooke University, Sherbrooke, QC, Canada

Pediatric Rheumatology & Musculoskeletal Ultrasound, McGill University, Montreal, QC, Canada

EULAR Working Group Anatomy for the Image, Zürich, Switzerland

OMERACT Ultrasound Pediatric Group, Zürich, Switzerland
e-mail: alessandra.bruns@usherbrooke.ca

Content

Three-Dimensional Ultrasound (3D US)

In the clinical setting, this technology has been mostly used in obstetrics [1–3], urology [4], and cardiology [5]. In recent years, it has also demonstrated its potential role in some adult rheumatologic conditions such as rheumatoid arthritis (RA) [6], spondyloarthritis (SPA) [7], and rotator cuff pathology [8]. There are several 3D US image acquisition techniques [9].In rheumatological practice, a volumetric probe (a large footprint probe that covers a relatively wide anatomical area) (Fig. 20.1) is used in order to obtain a 3D US image in an automatic manner and in a few seconds. The image acquisition, in both grayscale and power Doppler (PD) modes, is performed by an automatic sweeping scan movement of the piezoelectric crystals located inside the probe. This technique offers virtual operator independence due to transducer automated sweeping. In order to generate the US images, the operator places the volumetric probe with a steady hand on the chosen anatomical area which is covered by a generous layer of acoustic gel and then presses the acquisition button. After 4 s, the ultrasound images are ready to be examined on longitudinal, transverse, and coronal planes and on 3D reconstruction as well. The stored US images are also available to be examined at any time and without the presence of the patient. It is important to stress

Y. El Miedany (ed.), *Pediatric Musculoskeletal Ultrasonography*,
https://doi.org/10.1007/978-3-030-17824-6_20

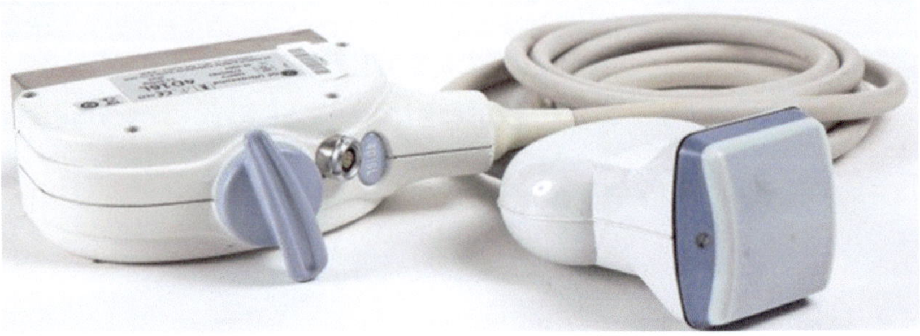

Fig. 20.1 Volumetric probe

that even though 3D US seems to be not operator dependent, the diagnostic quality of the US volumetric images is influenced by the ultrasonographer knowledge of anatomic landmarks, the correct placement of the probe, the use of an appropriate amount of acoustic gel, and finally the avoidance of probe movement. A very recent study where 31 RA patients underwent examination of seven joints (491 anatomic sites) by 2D and 3D US for synovitis and tenosynovitis in B and PD modes and erosions in B-mode revealed that 15% of the 3D scans could not be properly evaluated due to technical issues with the image acquisition (nonachievement of minimum standard of image quality) [10]. Although image acquisition time is shorter than with 2D US, image reconstruction and interpretation can be time-consuming, and its accurate evaluation still depends on previous training. The 3D PDUS is considered a reliable imaging technique due to its capability to assess synovial vascularity in inflamed wrists of RA patients when compared with clinical symptoms and the gold standard contrast-enhanced magnetic resonance imaging (MRI) [11]. 3D PDUS allows the spatial demonstration of synovial blood vessels in the peri- and intra-articular region of inflamed joints in patients with RA [12]. Furthermore, several studies have confirmed good-to-excellent agreement in both qualitative and semiquantitative assessments of joint inflammation and bone erosions between 3D US and conventional 2D US when examining RA hand and wrist joints [10, 13–15]. Acebes et al. [10] found that a higher level of agreement was attained for patient global scores than for individual joints. Naredo et al. [15] reported that 3D US may even improve the reliability for inflammatory changes of the hand and wrist in patients with RA, but they did not show a significant inter-modality agreement for bone erosions. A recent study [16] that investigated the performance of 3D US in the detection of bone erosions in hand and wrist joints of radiographically nonerosive RA patients compared to computed tomography (CT) as the reference method revealed that 3D US exhibited a sensitivity of 90% and a specificity of 55% in identifying erosive patients, suggesting that the majority of erosive patients identified by 3D US were correctly classified. However, more than 50% of the cortical breaks detected with 3D US were not considerate CT true erosions showing that at a single erosion level, misclassification can occur on 3D US. Contrary to Naredo et al. [15], Lai et al. [17] did not find any relevant advantage of a 3D transducer with respect to the 2D US assessment in wrist inflammation in RA patients. Due to the possible observation of synovial blood vessels and angiogenesis in patients with synovitis by 3D PDUS imaging, this method can play a key role in monitoring anti-inflammatory and biological therapy in RA as shown by some studies [18–21]. Another important advantage for therapy monitoring which has a major impact on follow-up examinations of synovitis is the fact that due to the sweep over the entire joint, the 3D imaging provides a true 3D perspective of the whole anatomical region which can be processed immediately for objective quantification (Fig. 20.2). In the case of conventional 2D US, only the directly accessible part of the inflamed joint region can be imaged. Four-dimensional US (real-time 3D US)-guided biopsy is feasible and can improve visualization of biopsy procedures by using multiplanar views as shown by [22]. Although the accuracy is comparable to that of conventional 2D biopsy, this technique may be helpful for biopsy of lesions

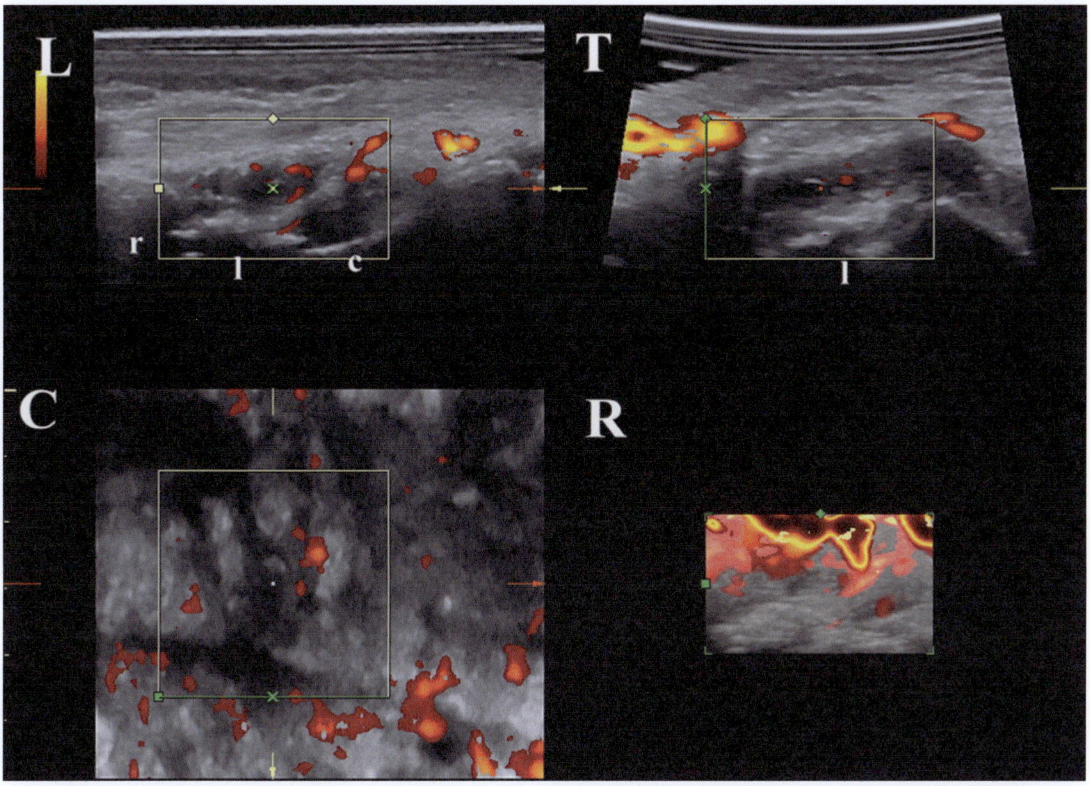

Fig. 20.2 Volumetric PD US image of the dorsal aspect of the radiocarpal and midcarpal joints in an RA patient (21).Wrist was globally scored moderately on both B-mode and PD-mode. r radius, l lunate, c capitate, L longitudinal, T transverse, C coronal, R reconstruction volume. (Courtesy of I. Möller, MD)

with close relation to relevant anatomical structures. It's relevant to stress that a potential use of this technique imaging may be in guiding synovial and tenosynovial biopsies. In spondyloarthritis (SPA), similar findings comparing conventional 2D and 3D US have been shown for Achilles tendon involvement [7] as well as for the presence and change of calcaneal bone erosions [23]. Further studies are needed to validate this technique in psoriatic arthritis. Regarding the pediatric population and the musculoskeletal (MSK) system, there are a number of studies on the potential applications of this method mainly in infant hip dysplasia [24–27]. 3D US can display the full acetabular shape, improving the assessment accuracy of developmental dysplasia of the hip. To date, there is no data in the medical literature about this innovative technique and its use in the diagnosis and/or follow-up of inflammatory arthritis in children. One important limitation of the application of this imaging tool is the size and shape of the 3D transducer which can decrease its ability to study the MSK system of this age range. Another disadvantage is the fact that the image acquisition process does not allow for movement, thus preventing the possibility of obtaining a dynamic image which is an essential part of the examination of tendons in children and adults. Even though its image resolution is inferior to conventional 2D US, 3D US can be used for training and education, as it is an ideal tool to demonstrate complex anatomy and vasculature (Fig. 20.3) and the 3D volume can be virtually rescanned without the patient's presence. The improvement of transducer technology with higher resolution and smaller size may allow pediatric MSK 3D US to become a promising imaging tool for assisting the diagnosis and follow-up of some of the pediatric rheumatologic diseases (Fig. 20.4).

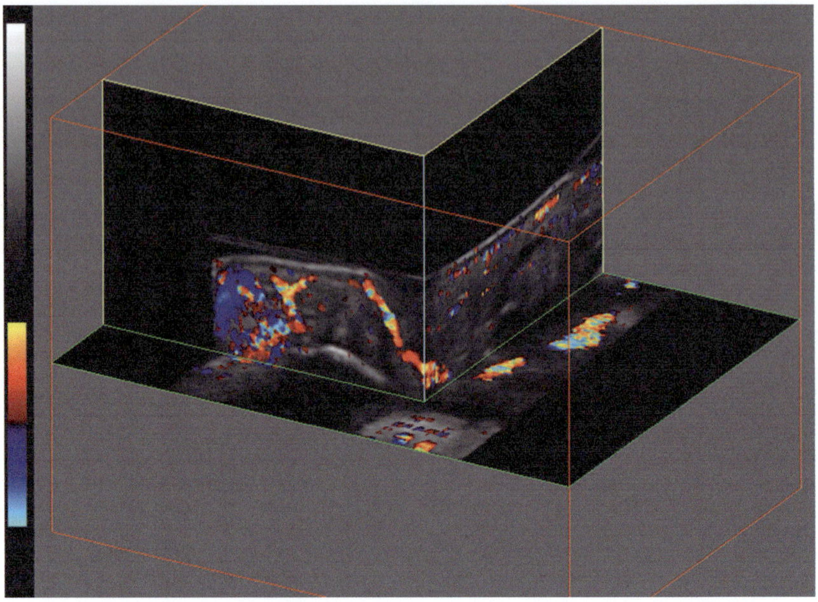

Fig. 20.3 Normal vessel branch of a finger in 3D block. (Courtesy of M. Ammitzbøll-Danielsen, MD)

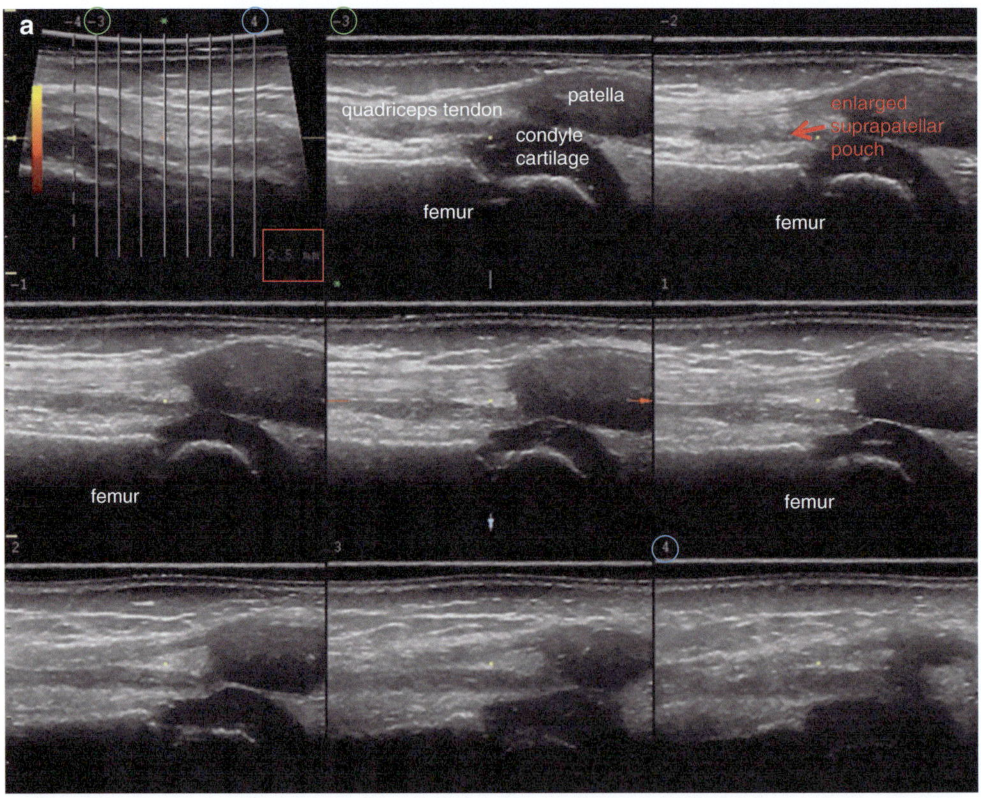

Fig. 20.4 3D data of synovitis of the right knee of a 3-year-old girl with juvenile idiopathic arthritis. Each image is a mosaic of nine ultrasound images showing mild suprapatellar pouch enlargement due to synovitis. (**a**) One transverse view of the one in the upper left corner and eight longitudinal views parallel to each other and distance of 2.5 mm between each other; (**b**) one longitudinal view of the one in the upper left corner and eight transverse views parallel to each other and distance of 2.5 mm between each other;(**c**) one longitudinal view of the one in the upper left corner and eight coronal views parallel to each other and distance of 2.5 mm between each other. (Courtesy of E. Filippucci, MD)

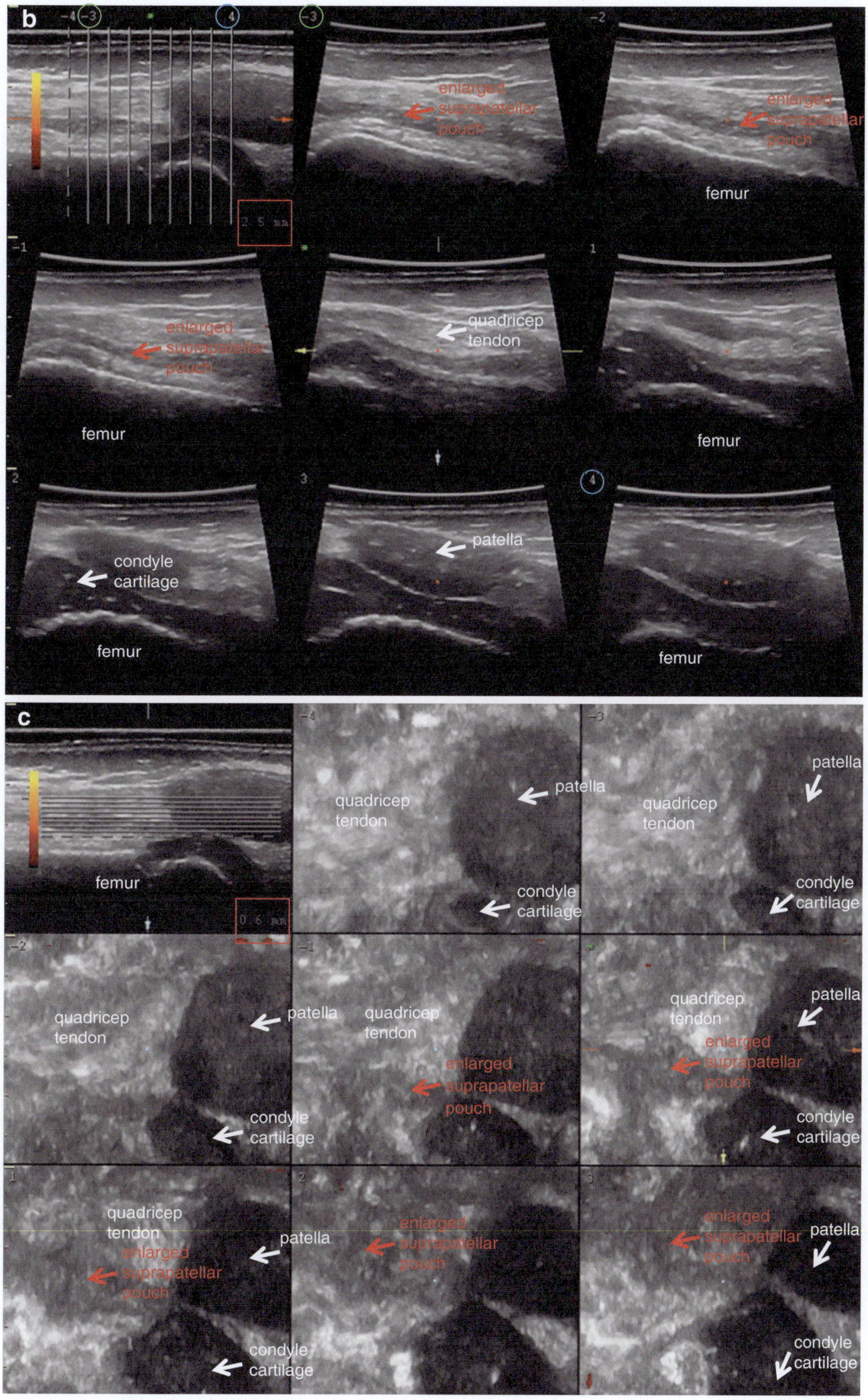

Fig. 20.4 (continued)

Ultrasound Elastography (Sonoelastography)

Ultrasound is an essential tool in medical imaging. New recent applications as elastography (ES) can contribute to the assessment of rheumatic diseases. In addition to the information obtained from B-mode and Doppler ultrasonography, ES can provide a different form of tissue evaluation as it may show pathologic changes before its detection on B-mode imaging. Besides that, since the pathological and the surrounding healthy tissue may often present the same echogenicity on conventional US, it is sometimes difficult to distinguish between them [28].

Tissue elasticity assessment by ES is based on the principle that tissue compression produces strain (displacement) which is lower in harder and less compressible tissues and higher in softer and more compressible ones [29].

There are currently two main methods used to perform ES in the clinical setting: strain or compression ES (the most common one) and shear-wave ES. Essentially, strain ES measures the elasticity of the tissue through the collection of US echo data before and after a slight compression applied from the transducer by repetitive manual pressure and, thus, a qualitative, color-coded *strain map* termed elastogram is obtained. Different grades of elasticity are frequently super-imposed on the related B-mode image in order to show anatomical localization using diverse coloring (yellow to red in soft tissues and green and blue representing hard ones). A potential disadvantage of this image modality is the variability in the pressure applied to the tissue, which might affect reproducibility. Tissue shifting due to unilateral compression is another relevant issue; the use of a gel standoff pad can help to reduce this problem. It is recommended to apply at least three cycles of compression and decompression for an ideal assessment [30]; however, it is important to stress that repeated compressions may cause excessive preload of the tissues modifying tissue elasticity. To address this problem, there is a visual indicator scale on the machine that monitors the relationship between pressure exerted and tissue strain. If the pressure decreases or increases below a certain level, the pattern of the elasticity image changes considerably.

Unlike strain elastography, shear-wave elastography allows the determination of the actual tissue elasticity since it applies a vibration to tissues through a focused US pulse generated by a linear transducer, which by itself provides a local stress generating tissue displacement without the need for manual compression. The vibration within the tissues creates shear waves (transverse waves) which are perpendicular to the US pulse and propagate faster in stiffer tissues. A quantitative color-coded elastogram on the US screen displays shear-wave velocities in meters per second or tissue elasticity in kilopascals [31]. Shear-wave ES is thus likely to be more objective and reproducible than strain ES due to direct assessment of tissue elasticity, with the possibility to obtain quantitative measurements. A major limitation of this imaging tool is the fact that very deep (>9 cm from the skin) or very superficial structures cannot be assessed [32]. Shallow depths may be compensated by using a gel standoff pad.

Additionally, shear-wave ES is sensitive to transducer pressure and angle similar to strain ES [33]. Shear-wave measurements are potentially affected by the way the anatomical structure is evaluated (long vs short axis) due to anisotropy as well as the size and shape of the region of interest. The heating generated by the repetitive use of the shear-wave ES may modify the measurements and cause tissue damage. This is compensated by a cooling delay. Finally, cystic structures are not well analyzed owing to the fact that shear waves are not generated within fluids [34]. Tissue elasticity changes caused by tumors have already been evaluated in breast [35–38], thyroid [39, 40], and prostate cancers [41, 42]. Despite the recent advances in tumor diagnosis with ES, biopsy still remains the gold standard. However, it is now considered the standard imaging tool in the assessment of liver fibrosis, even, replacing biopsy in many cases [43].

Recently, ES has been proven useful in the evaluation of rheumatic disorders such as tendinosis [44] (Achilles tendon [45, 46], supraspinatus tendon [47], common extensor tendon of the elbow

[48], SPA (Achilles tendon abnormalities) [49]), polymyalgia rheumatica (subacromial-subdeltoid bursitis) [50], carpal tunnel syndrome [51], Sjögren's syndrome (salivary tissue assessment) [52], gout (gouty arthritis) [53], adhesive capsulitis of the shoulder (coracohumeral ligament) [54], and inflammatory myopathies [55, 56]. Regarding systemic sclerosis (SSc), a very recent systematic review about US assessment of the skin in SSc which included three studies on strain ES and three studies on shear-wave ES showed significantly higher shear-wave velocities in SSc patients than in controls [57]. To date, there is little information regarding the elastographic appearance of the synovium in rheumatoid arthritis. Recently, a cross-sectional study presented as a poster (*FRI0525—Sammel AM* et al. *2016*) evaluated nine patients with low to moderate activity of RA and five controls with shear-wave elastography of the MCP joints. The authors found significantly lower maximum shear-wave velocity in RA patients than in controls (6.38 m/s vs 6.99 m/s $p = 0.042$). In MSK disorders in children, ES has been mostly used to evaluate muscle elasticity in healthy subjects (at rest and after exercise) [58] and in patients with congenital muscle torticollis [59, 60], cerebral palsy [61], myositis [56], and in Bethlem myopathy, a congenital muscle dystrophy [62].Regarding cerebral palsy, ES was equally used to guide botulinum toxin injections into contracted muscle fibers, identified as hard (blue) on the elastogram [63]. A recent study [56] that evaluated inflammatory myopathies (dermatomyositis (41,2%), polymyositis (29,4%), systemic lupus erythematosus overlap (11.8%), juvenile dermatomyositis (5.9%), mixed connective tissue disease (5.9%), and RA overlap (5.9%)) by physical examination, imaging (MRI and strain ES), and histopathology showed alteration in the normal muscle elastogram, with predominance of stiff appearance of pathological muscles. Besides that, the authors also found a correlation between sonographic stiffness and the inflammatory changes on muscle biopsy suggesting that strain ES could be an important tool in identifying and measuring the degree of muscular inflammation. In contrast, Berko N et al. [64] who evaluated the performance of strain ES in the diagnosis of juvenile idiopathic inflammatory myopathy compared to MRI showed no association between abnormal muscle appearance on the elastogram and muscle edema detected on MRI ($P > 0.999$). Muscle elasticity was assessed based on a comparison with previously published findings of muscle elasticity in a cohort of normal children of similar age and gender [58]. The areas of signal abnormality seen on MRI in patients with active inflammatory myopathy correspond to areas of muscle edema. A possible explanation for the absence of correlation between ES and MRI is the fact that sonoelastography might not be able to detect small changes in fluid related to muscle inflammation seen on MRI as well as the smaller area of the muscle able to be evaluated with ES. Patients with JDM often have heterogeneous areas of affected muscle, and therefore it is possible that the area of muscle analyzed on the ES studies was not an area of active disease.

Other potential limitations of strain ES in assessing skeletal muscles are related to reproducibility, and it is possible that other ES tools, such as shear-wave ES and magnetic resonance elastography [65], may be useful in the assessment of muscular diseases. However, it is important to note that understanding and interpreting color elastograms and shear-wave velocities requires knowledge of the basic ultrasound physics of shear-wave ES. More research is needed to establish the role of ES in assessing myositis and other muscle disorders. To date, this image modality is unlikely to replace muscle biopsy for the diagnosis of muscular pathologies.

Fusion Imaging

Another interesting approach is the fusion imaging (FI) which software may be integrated into high-end US machines. This imaging modality overlaps information from previously performed computed tomography (CT) or MRI on to real-time image acquisition by US scanning with better illustrations of bony and certain soft-tissue lesions. This is particularly promising for intra-articular guided infiltrations, improving injection accuracy, especially into the sacroiliac joints. Bony landmarks are provided by the CT scan and the needle placement is guided by real-time US [66]. With respect to rheumatic diseases, the FI applications have already been evaluated in the hand and wrist joints of patients with RA and osteoarthritis [67] and in shoulder pathology [68].

Regarding the pediatric population, the major limitations to the use of this technology are the difficulty that children have to tolerate MRI exam without sedation and the well-established risk for developing a radiation-related cancer when exposed to CT scan. However, young patients with chronic sacroiliitis who require several infiltrations of the sacroiliac joints already have the necessary information from previously performed CT scan reducing repeated radiation exposure [66].

Conclusion

New developments in US imaging such as 3D US and ES have potential applications in pediatric rheumatic diseases. An interdisciplinary approach between pediatric rheumatologists and radiologists is essential to spread information on the advantages of using such imaging tools. This cooperation might certainly result in optimal patient management. Besides that, despite all advances in imaging diagnosis, much remains to be done regarding pediatric rheumatology.

References

1. Tonni G, Araujo Junior E. Three-dimensional ultrasound in obstetrics practice: myth or reality? Rev Bras Ginecol Obstet. 2014;36(4):143–5.
2. Goncalves LF, Lee W, Espinoza J, Romero R. Three- and 4-dimensional ultrasound in obstetric practice: does it help? J Ultrasound Med. 2005;24(12):1599–624.
3. Kurjak A, Miskovic B, Andonotopo W, Stanojevic M, Azumendi G, Vrcic H. How useful is 3D and 4D ultrasound in perinatal medicine? J Perinat Med. 2007;35(1):10–27.
4. Cool DW, Connolly MJ, Sherebrin S, Eagleson R, Izawa JI, Amann J, et al. Repeat prostate biopsy accuracy: simulator-based comparison of two- and three-dimensional transrectal US modalities. Radiology. 2010;254(2):587–94.
5. Surkova E, Muraru D, Aruta P, Romeo G, Bidviene J, Cherata D, et al. Current clinical applications of three-dimensional echocardiography: when the technique makes the difference. Curr Cardiol Rep. 2016;18(11):109.
6. Filippucci E, Meenagh G, Epis O, Iagnocco A, Riente L, Delle Sedie A, et al. Ultrasound imaging for the rheumatologist. XIII. New trends. Three-dimensional ultrasonography. Clin Exp Rheumatol. 2008;26(1):1–4.
7. Iagnocco A, Riente L, Delle Sedie A, Filippucci E, Salaffi F, Meenagh G, et al. Ultrasound imaging for the rheumatologist. XXII. Achilles tendon involvement in spondyloarthritis. A multi-Centre study using high frequency volumetric probe. Clin Exp Rheumatol. 2009;27(4):547–51.
8. Wallny TA, Schild RL, Schulze Bertelsbeck D, Hansmann ME, Kraft CN. Three-dimensional ultrasonography in the diagnosis of rotator cuff lesions. Ultrasound Med Biol. 2001;27(6):745–9.
9. Downey DB, Fenster A, Williams JC. Clinical utility of three-dimensional US. Radiographics. 2000;20(2):559–71.
10. Acebes C, McKay N, Ciechomska A, Alcorn N, Harvie JP, Robson B, et al. Level of agreement between three-dimensional volumetric ultrasound and real-time conventional ultrasound in the assessment of synovitis, tenosynovitis and erosions in rheumatoid arthritis patients. Rheumatol Int. 2017;37(2):197–205.
11. Strunk J, Klingenberger P, Strube K, Bachmann G, Muller-Ladner U, Kluge A. Three-dimensional Doppler sonographic vascular imaging in regions with increased MR enhancement in inflamed wrists of patients with rheumatoid arthritis. Joint Bone Spine. 2006;73(5):518–22.
12. Strunk J, Lange U. Three-dimensional power Doppler sonographic visualization of synovial angiogenesis in rheumatoid arthritis. J Rheumatol. 2004;31(5):1004–6.
13. Filippucci E, Meenagh G, De Agustin JJ, De Miguel E, Iagnocco A, Mayordomo L, et al. Level of agreement between rheumatologists on US image acquisition using a 3D volumetric probe. Clin Exp Rheumatol. 2007;25(1):116.
14. Filippucci E, Meenagh G, Delle Sedie A, Salaffi F, Riente L, Iagnocco A, et al. Ultrasound imaging for the rheumatologist. XX. Sonographic assessment of hand and wrist joint involvement in rheumatoid arthritis: comparison between two- and three-dimensional ultrasonography. Clin Exp Rheumatol. 2009;27(2):197–200.
15. Naredo E, Moller I, Acebes C, Batlle-Gualda E, Brito E, de Agustin JJ, et al. Three-dimensional volumetric ultrasonography. Does it improve reliabililty of musculoskeletal ultrasound? Clin Exp Rheumatol. 2010;28(1):79–82.
16. Peluso G, Bosello SL, Gremese E, Mirone L, Di Gregorio F, Di Molfetta V, et al. Detection of bone erosions in early rheumatoid arthritis: 3D ultrasonography versus computed tomography. Clin Rheumatol. 2015;34(7):1181–6.
17. Lai KL, Chen DY, Chen YH, Huang WN, Hsieh TY, Hsieh CW, et al. Assessment of wrist joint

inflammation in patients with rheumatoid arthritis by quantitative two- and three-dimensional power Doppler ultrasonography. Clin Exp Rheumatol. 2014;32(5):674–9.
18. Meenagh G, Filippucci E, Abbattista T, Busilacchi P, Grassi W. Three-dimensional power Doppler sonography in short-term therapy monitoring of rheumatoid synovitis. Rheumatology (Oxford). 2007;46(11):1736.
19. Strunk J, Strube K, Muller-Ladner U, Lange U. Three dimensional power Doppler ultrasonography confirms early reduction of synovial perfusion after intra-articular steroid injection. Ann Rheum Dis. 2006;65(3):411–2.
20. Strunk J, Strube K, Rumbaur C, Lange U, Muller-Ladner U. Interobserver agreement in two- and three-dimensional power Doppler sonographic assessment of synovial vascularity during anti-inflammatory treatment in patients with rheumatoid arthritis. Ultraschall Med. 2007;28(4):409–15.
21. Naredo E, Acebes C, Brito E, de Agustin JJ, de Miguel E, Mayordomo L, et al. Three-dimensional volumetric ultrasound: a valid method for blinded assessment of response to therapy in rheumatoid arthritis. J Rheumatol. 2013;40(3):253–60.
22. Albrecht H, Stroszczynski C, Felix R, Hunerbein M. Real time 3D (4D) ultrasound-guided percutaneous biopsy of solid tumours. Ultraschall Med. 2006;27(4):324–8.
23. de Miguel E, Falcao S, Castillo C, Plasencia C, Garcia M, Branco JC, et al. Enthesis erosion in spondyloarthritis is not a persistent structural lesion. Ann Rheum Dis. 2011;70(11):2008–10.
24. Diederichs C, Heath A, Hareendranathan AR, Zonoobi D, Kuntze G, Dulai S, et al. Cross-modality validation of acetabular surface models using 3-d ultrasound versus magnetic resonance imaging in normal and dysplastic infant hips. Ultrasound Med Biol. 2016;42(9):2308–14.
25. Mabee MG, Hareendranathan AR, Thompson RB, Dulai S, Jaremko JL. An index for diagnosing infant hip dysplasia using 3-D ultrasound: the acetabular contact angle. Pediatr Radiol. 2016;46(7):1023–31.
26. Jaremko JL, Mabee M, Swami VG, Jamieson L, Chow K, Thompson RB. Potential for change in US diagnosis of hip dysplasia solely caused by changes in probe orientation: patterns of alpha-angle variation revealed by using three-dimensional US. Radiology. 2014;273(3):870–8.
27. Hareendranathan AR, Zonoobi D, Mabee M, Diederichs C, Punithakumar K, Noga M, et al. Semiautomatic classification of acetabular shape from three-dimensional ultrasound for diagnosis of infant hip dysplasia using geometric features. Int J Comput Assist Radiol Surg. 2017;12(3):439–47.
28. Frey H. Realtime elastography. A new ultrasound procedure for the reconstruction of tissue elasticity. Radiologe. 2003;43(10):850–5.
29. Garra BS. Imaging and estimation of tissue elasticity by ultrasound. Ultrasound Q. 2007;23(4):255–68.
30. Klauser AS, Faschingbauer R, Jaschke WR. Is sonoelastography of value in assessing tendons? Semin Musculoskelet Radiol. 2010;14(3):323–33.
31. Taljanovic MS, Gimber LH, Becker GW, Latt LD, Klauser AS, Melville DM, et al. Shear-wave elastography: basic physics and musculoskeletal applications. Radiographics. 2017;37(3):855–70.
32. Winn N, Lalam R, Cassar-Pullicino V. Sonoelastography in the musculoskeletal system: current role and future directions. World J Radiol. 2016;8(11):868–79.
33. Kot BC, Zhang ZJ, Lee AW, Leung VY, Fu SN. Elastic modulus of muscle and tendon with shear wave ultrasound elastography: variations with different technical settings. PLoS One. 2012;7(8):e44348.
34. Elkateb Hachemi M, Calle S, Remenieras JP. Transient displacement induced in shear wave elastography: comparison between analytical results and ultrasound measurements. Ultrasonics. 2006;44(Suppl 1):e221–5.
35. Itoh A, Ueno E, Tohno E, Kamma H, Takahashi H, Shiina T, et al. Breast disease: clinical application of US elastography for diagnosis. Radiology. 2006;239(2):341–50.
36. Evans A, Whelehan P, Thomson K, McLean D, Brauer K, Purdie C, et al. Invasive breast cancer: relationship between shear-wave elastographic findings and histologic prognostic factors. Radiology. 2012;263(3):673–7.
37. Tozaki M, Isobe S, Sakamoto M. Combination of elastography and tissue quantification using the acoustic radiation force impulse (ARFI) technology for differential diagnosis of breast masses. Jpn J Radiol. 2012;30(8):659–70.
38. Carlsen J, Ewertsen C, Sletting S, Vejborg I, Schafer FK, Cosgrove D, et al. Ultrasound elastography in breast cancer diagnosis. Ultraschall Med. 2015;36(6):550–62; quiz 63-5.
39. Bojunga J, Dauth N, Berner C, Meyer G, Holzer K, Voelkl L, et al. Acoustic radiation force impulse imaging for differentiation of thyroid nodules. PLoS One. 2012;7(8):e42735.
40. Azizi G, Keller JM, Mayo ML, Piper K, Puett D, Earp KM, et al. Thyroid nodules and shear wave elastography: a new tool in thyroid cancer detection. Ultrasound Med Biol. 2015;41(11):2855–65.
41. Correas JM, Tissier AM, Khairoune A, Vassiliu V, Mejean A, Helenon O, et al. Prostate cancer: diagnostic performance of real-time shear-wave elastography. Radiology. 2015;275(1):280–9.
42. Woo S, Suh CH, Kim SY, Cho JY, Kim SH. Shear-wave elastography for detection of prostate cancer: a systematic review and diagnostic meta-analysis. AJR Am J Roentgenol. 2017;209(4):806–14.
43. Barr RG, Ferraioli G, Palmeri ML, Goodman ZD, Garcia-Tsao G, Rubin J, et al. Elastography assessment of liver fibrosis: society of radiologists in ultrasound consensus conference statement. Ultrasound Q. 2016;32(2):94–107.
44. Fusini F, Langella F, Busilacchi A, Tudisco C, Gigante A, Masse A, et al. Real-time sonoelastography: prin-

ciples and clinical applications in tendon disorders. A systematic review. Muscles Ligaments Tendons J. 2017;7(3):467–77.
45. De Zordo T, Chhem R, Smekal V, Feuchtner G, Reindl M, Fink C, et al. Real-time sonoelastography: findings in patients with symptomatic achilles tendons and comparison to healthy volunteers. Ultraschall Med. 2010;31(4):394–400.
46. Tan S, Kudas S, Ozcan AS, Ipek A, Karaoglanoglu M, Arslan H, et al. Real-time sonoelastography of the Achilles tendon: pattern description in healthy subjects and patients with surgically repaired complete ruptures. Skelet Radiol. 2012;41(9):1067–72.
47. Lee SU, Joo SY, Kim SK, Lee SH, Park SR, Jeong C. Real-time sonoelastography in the diagnosis of rotator cuff tendinopathy. J Shoulder Elb Surg. 2016;25(5):723–9.
48. Klauser AS, Pamminger M, Halpern EJ, Abd Ellah MMH, Moriggl B, Taljanovic MS, et al. Extensor tendinopathy of the elbow assessed with sonoelastography: histologic correlation. Eur Radiol. 2017;27(8):3460–6.
49. Turan A, Tufan A, Mercan R, Teber MA, Tezcan ME, Bitik B, et al. Real-time sonoelastography of Achilles tendon in patients with ankylosing spondylitis. Skelet Radiol. 2013;42(8):1113–8.
50. Silvestri E, Garlaschi G, Bartolini B, Minetti G, Schettini D, D'Auria MC, et al. Sonoelastography can help in the localization of soft tissue damage in polymyalgia rheumatica (PMR). Clin Exp Rheumatol. 2007;25(5):796.
51. Orman G, Ozben S, Huseyinoglu N, Duymus M, Orman KG. Ultrasound elastographic evaluation in the diagnosis of carpal tunnel syndrome: initial findings. Ultrasound Med Biol. 2013;39(7):1184–9.
52. Hofauer B, Mansour N, Heiser C, Gahleitner C, Thuermel K, Bas M, et al. Sonoelastographic modalities in the evaluation of salivary gland characteristics in Sjogren's syndrome. Ultrasound Med Biol. 2016;42(9):2130–9.
53. Tang Y, Yan F, Yang Y, Xiang X, Wang L, Zhang L, et al. Value of shear wave Elastography in the diagnosis of gouty and non-gouty arthritis. Ultrasound Med Biol. 2017;43(5):884–92.
54. Wu CH, Chen WS, Wang TG. Elasticity of the Coracohumeral ligament in patients with adhesive capsulitis of the shoulder. Radiology. 2016;278(2):458–64.
55. Botar-Jid C, Damian L, Dudea SM, Vasilescu D, Rednic S, Badea R. The contribution of ultrasonography and sonoelastography in assessment of myositis. Med Ultrason. 2010;12(2):120–6.
56. Song Y, Lee S, Yoo DH, Jang KS, Bae J. Strain sonoelastography of inflammatory myopathies: comparison with clinical examination, magnetic resonance imaging and pathologic findings. Br J Radiol. 2016;89(1065):20160283.
57. Santiago T, Santiago M, Ruaro B, Salvador MJ, Cutolo M, da Silva JAP. Ultrasonography for the assessment of skin in systemic sclerosis: a systematic review. Arthritis Care Res (Hoboken). 2018;
58. Berko NS, Fitzgerald EF, Amaral TD, Payares M, Levin TL. Ultrasound elastography in children: establishing the normal range of muscle elasticity. Pediatr Radiol. 2014;44(2):158–63.
59. Lee SY, Park HJ, Choi YJ, Choi SH, Kook SH, Rho MH, et al. Value of adding sonoelastography to conventional ultrasound in patients with congenital muscular torticollis. Pediatr Radiol. 2013;43(12):1566–72.
60. Park GY, Kwon DR, Kwon DG. Shear wave sonoelastography in infants with congenital muscular torticollis. Medicine (Baltimore). 2018;97(6):e9818.
61. Kwon DR, Park GY, Lee SU, Chung I. Spastic cerebral palsy in children: dynamic sonoelastographic findings of medial gastrocnemius. Radiology. 2012;263(3):794–801.
62. Drakonaki EE, Allen GM. Magnetic resonance imaging, ultrasound and real-time ultrasound elastography of the thigh muscles in congenital muscle dystrophy. Skelet Radiol. 2010;39(4):391–6.
63. Vasilescu D, Vasilescu D, Dudea S, Botar-Jid C, Sfrangeu S, Cosma D. Sonoelastography contribution in cerebral palsy spasticity treatment assessment, preliminary report: a systematic review of the literature apropos of seven patients. Med Ultrason. 2010;12(4):306–10.
64. Berko NS, Hay A, Sterba Y, Wahezi D, Levin TL. Efficacy of ultrasound elastography in detecting active myositis in children: can it replace MRI? Pediatr Radiol. 2015;45(10):1522–8.
65. McCullough MB, Domire ZJ, Reed AM, Amin S, Ytterberg SR, Chen Q, et al. Evaluation of muscles affected by myositis using magnetic resonance elastography. Muscle Nerve. 2011;43(4):585–90.
66. Klauser AS, De Zordo T, Feuchtner GM, Djedovic G, Weiler RB, Faschingbauer R, et al. Fusion of real-time US with CT images to guide sacroiliac joint injection in vitro and in vivo. Radiology. 2010;256(2):547–53.
67. Iagnocco A, Perella C, D'Agostino MA, Sabatini E, Valesini G, Conaghan PG. Magnetic resonance and ultrasonography real-time fusion imaging of the hand and wrist in osteoarthritis and rheumatoid arthritis. Rheumatology (Oxford). 2011;50(8):1409–13.
68. Liu J, Zhan W, Zhou M, Zhang X, Hu Y, Zhu Y. The feasibility study of US-MRI virtual navigation in the shoulder. Clin Imaging. 2012;36(6):803–9.

Index

Y. El Miedany (ed.), *Pediatric Musculoskeletal Ultrasonography*,
https://doi.org/10.1007/978-3-030-17824-6

T

W